ENDOTHELIAL DYSFUNCTION - OLD CONCEPTS AND NEW CHALLENGES

Edited by **Helena Lenasi**

Endothelial Dysfunction - Old Concepts and New Challenges
http://dx.doi.org/10.5772/intechopen.68656
Edited by Helena Lenasi

Contributors

Cristina Sena, Fernanda Carrilho, Raquel Seiça, Vera Nevzorova, Tatyana Brodskaya, Natalia Zakharchuk, Carmen Diniz, Joana Beatriz Sousa, Francesca Caccuri, Pietro Mazzuca, Arnaldo Caruso, Katarzyna Korybalska, Marina Ziganshina, Ekaterina L. Yarotskaya, Gennady T. Sukhikh, Nicolai Bovin, Ezequiel Álvarez, Mercedes González-Peteiro, Beatriz Paradela-Dobarro, José R. González-Juanatey, Julia Carracedo, Rafael Ramirez-Carracedo, Matilde Alique, Rafael Ramirez-Chamond, Yu Wang, Joyce Gonzales, An Aerts, Bjorn Baselet, Raghda Ramadan, Abderrafi Mohammed Benotmane, Sarah Baatout, Pierre Sonveaux, Domokos Gero, Luiza Rusu, Richard Minshall, Claudio Aguayo, Felipe Zuñiga, Estefania Nova-Lamperti, Valeska Ormazabal, Carlos Escudero, Andres Rodriguez, Meriem Rezgaoui, Kurt Herlitz, Ines Drenjančević, Ivana Jukić, Ana Stupin, Anita Ćosić, Martina Mihalj, Marko Stupin, Kristina Selthofer-Relatic, Helena Lenasi

First published in London, United Kingdom, 2018 by IntechOpen
IntechOpen is the global imprint of INTECHOPEN LIMITED, registered in England and Wales, registration number: 11086078, The Shard, 25th floor, 32 London Bridge Street
London, SE19SG – United Kingdom
Printed in Croatia

British Library Cataloguing-in-Publication Data
A catalogue record for this book is available from the British Library

Additional hard copies can be obtained from orders@intechopen.com

Endothelial Dysfunction - Old Concepts and New Challenges, Edited by Helena Lenasi
p. cm.
Print ISBN 978-1-78984-253-1
Online ISBN 978-1-78984-254-8

For EU product safety concerns:
IN TECH d.o.o., Prolaz Marije Krucifikse Kozulić 3, 51000 Rijeka, Croatia,
info@intechopen.com or visit our website at intechopen.com.

Meet the editor

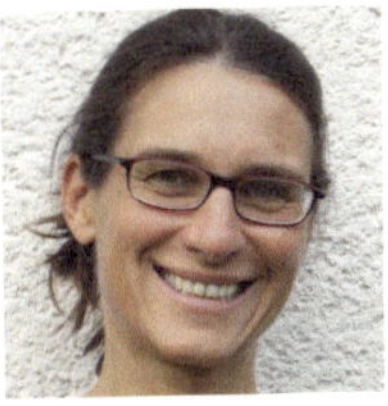

Helena Lenasi is an assistant professor of Physiology employed at the Institute of Physiology, Faculty of Medicine, University of Ljubljana, Slovenia. She obtained her MD title in 1996 and her PhD in 2003, both at the University of Ljubljana. Her working activities mainly include teaching and education. She gives lectures in Physiology for pre- and postgraduate students at the Faculty of Medicine and Faculty of Sport at the University of Ljubljana. Her main research interests are cardiovascular and exercise physiology with a focus on human microcirculation in health and disease. She is a member of the Slovenian Physiological Society as part of the Federation of European Physiological Societies, the Medical Chamber of Slovenia, and the European Society for Microcirculation. She is an editor of the *Slovenian Medical Journal* and *Southeastern European Medical Journal* and has served as a reviewer and author of scientific papers and textbook chapters.

Contents

Preface

The endothelium, the inner vascular layer, is far from being solely a mechanical barrier because it enables communication between blood and tissues. In many ways, including its metabolic, secretory, permeability, and vascular tone regulatory roles, it has been implicated as a highly active organ, importantly contributing to cardiovascular homeostasis. Because tissues depend on proper vascularization, the endothelium could indeed be considered as one of the main determinants of tissue perfusion. It actually exhibits immense heterogeneity, which could partly expain its many different functions and roles.

An immense expansion of knowledge on endothelial structure and function was achieved by the discovery of electron microscopy combined with various labeling techniques. Nevertheless, there are many obscurities regarding *in vivo* studies, even more so in humans. Respectively, it is not always easy to extrapolate the observations obtained in animal or cell culture studies to humans, leaving a number of unanswered questions.

Exposed to instantanously changing environments and influences, the endothelium is susceptible to noxious stimuli, which may lead to endothelial dysfunction. The latter is imminently connected also to normal aging and has nowadays been recognized as the leading cause of atherosclerosis development predisposing to cardiovascular diseases. Therefore, an insight into molecular mechanisms of endothelial activity is crucial from a clinical point of view because early detection of endothelial dysfunction might postpone the development of disease. Currently, clinical evaluation of endothelial dysfunction remains to be accomplished, appropriate clinical methods to timely and accurately detect endothelial dysfunction are lacking, and only more or less robust estimations are available. It is therefore essential to pursue investigations into endothelial function and dysfunction. Accordingly, this book presents recent findings on certain aspects of endothelial (dys)function and the mechanisms involved, as well as potential therapeutic targets involving endothelium and surrogate markers for estimation of endothelial (dys)function.

The book consists of 17 chapters written by reputed authors; because it is impossible to cover all aspects of endothelial function, the chapters present only selected topics. It starts with an introduction by the editor briefly presenting basic characteristics of endothelial structure and function relevant for subsequent chapters. The chapter written by Claudio Aguayo and coauthors follows, addressing genetic aspects with a focus on the Hox gene family directing endothelial differentiation and angiogenesis. The process of endothelial cell senescence as one of the main causes of the development of endothelial dysfunction is presented by Carracedo, while the chapter written by Wang and coauthors extensively exposes the regulation and function of the longevity regulator sirtuin, proposing also its potential role as an antiaging regulator. Subsequent chapters comprehensively present endothelial elements involved in shear stress sensing, such as the endothelial cilium, described by Escudero and coauthors, and the glycocalyx by Ziganshina and coauthors, and some pathologies associated with their malfunctioning. The mechanisms of the von Willebrand factor action and its involvement in thrombotic and inflammatory diseases is outlined in the chapter written by Rusu and Minshall. It has long been appreciated that hyperglycemia adversely impacts the endothelium; accordingly, the chapters by Domokos and Alvarez and coauthors extensively describe the hyperglycemia-associated mechanisms that lead to endothelial dysfunction and expose an important role of oxidative stress. Some altered endothelial metabolic pathways in diabetes and their link to atherosclerosis are also covered in the chapter by Sena and coauthors. The chapter by Korybalska deals with the impact of caloric restriction on endothelial dysfunction focusing on angiogenesis in adipose tissue. Peculiarities of pulmonary endothelium and endothelial dysfunction associated with respiratory diseases are outlined in the chapters by Gonzales and Verin and Nevzorova and coauthors, the latter focusing on their connection to smoking. The chapter by Sousa and Diniz presents important crosstalk between the endothelium and the sympathetic nervous system. The mechanisms of HIV-1-infected cells in sustaining an aberrant endothelial cell function are outlined by Caccuri and coauthors followed by the chapter by Aerts and coauthors who extensively describe the impact of ionizing radiation on the endothelium. The last chapter by Drenjančević and coauthors exposes some potential markers for clinical evaluation of endothelial activation and dysfunction.

I would like to express my gratitude to all authors for their excellent and dedicated reviews, which readers will hopefully enjoy as much as I did. Finally, I'd like to thank the publishing process managers, Mrs Renata Sliva and Mrs Lada Božić, for their help and patience, and InTech publishers for inviting me to be the editor of this book.

I hope that the chapters will be useful for anyone interested in recapitulating endothelial (patho)physiology and expanding the knowledge of molecular mechanisms involved in endothelial function and dysfunction, and will hopefully uncover additional questions for further, potentially more clinically oriented, investigations.

Helena Lenasi, MD, PhD
Assistant Professor of Physiology
University of Ljubljana
Faculty of Medicine
Institute of Physiology
Ljubljana, Slovenia

Chapter 1

Endothelium at a Glance

Helena Lenasi

Additional information is available at the end of the chapter

http://dx.doi.org/10.5772/intechopen.81286

Abstract

Exposed to the blood milieu and variable hemodynamic forces, endothelial cells of different vessels exhibit significant heterogeneity, directing also the variety of endothelial functions. Endothelial cells are actively involved in many physiological processes, including vascular tone regulation, fluid filtration and reabsorption processes, maintenance of blood fluidity and proper hemostasis, leucocyte trafficking, tissue repair, and angiogenesis; accordingly, healthy endothelium is crucial for vascular homeostasis. On the other hand, many exo- and endogenous harmful factors can cause endothelial dysfunction, associated with inflammation, thrombosis, pathological vascular wall remodeling, and predisposing to the development of cardiovascular and other diseases. In order to design accurate clinical and pharmacological strategies to postpone or ameliorate endothelial dysfunction, endothelial dysfunction should firstly be recognized. Therefore, understanding endothelial physiology is crucial for clinical measures to be timely taken. The review briefly outlines some basic concepts of endothelial structure and function, focusing on endothelial barrier function and endothelium-dependent vasodilation, and addressing some potential therapeutic targets. Additional specific concepts of endothelial (dys)function, with particular emphasis on its involvement in inflammation, hemostasis, and its (mal)adaptation to environmental challenges are extensively described in the following book chapters.

Keywords: endothelium, endothelial cells, endothelial dysfunction, vascular tone regulation, nitric oxide, capillary permeability, cardiovascular diseases, oxidative stress

1. Introduction: general concepts

Endothelium, composed of approximately one trillion endothelial cells and extending over an area of 300 m^2 [1, 2], is a monolayer cell lining covering the luminal surface of blood and lymphatic vessels, and the heart. Its strategic position, being in a direct contact with the blood on one side and with the underlying tissues on the other, enables its communication with blood elements and the adjacent cells. Developmentally, it arises from mesoderm via the differentiation of hemangioblasts and angioblasts [3]. However, other cell lineages, such as adipose lineage and mesenchymal cells, can transdifferentiate into endothelial cells even in adulthood [4, 5].

Besides presenting a mechanical barrier between the blood and the tissues, the endothelium is actively involved in various processes, including the regulation of vascular tone, maintaining blood fluidity, and enabling proper hemostasis when needed, in leucocyte trafficking, inflammation, wound repair, and angiogenesis, and, therefore, is of crucial importance for vascular homeostasis. As it metabolizes and releases many physiologically active substances that by acting in auto-, para-, and endocrine manner, govern the above physiological processes, it might justified be called an endocrine organ.

1.1. Endothelial heterogeneity

Although stemming from the same ontogenetic origin, to fulfill different metabolic and functional demands of tissues, the endothelial cells of different tissues exhibit distinct phenotypic and morphologic characteristics, accounting for its huge molecular and functional heterogeneity.

Endothelial heterogeneity could also be explained by the diversity of the vessel networks it is part of, namely arteries, veins, and capillaries which all serve different functions. While the endothelium of arteries and veins forms a continuous layer, it can be continuous, fenestrated, or discontinuous in capillaries, directing endothelial permeability and thus the degree of the filtration and reabsorption in the corresponding tissue. The representative tissues with the continuous non-fenestrated type of endothelium include the brain, the skin, the lung, and the heart; the continuous fenestrated type is found in tissues exhibiting extensive transcapillary transport: exo- and endocrine glands, the intestine mucosa, and the kidney glomeruli, whereas the prototype of the discontinuous endothelium are sinusoids in the liver and bone marrow vascular beds [1]. Endothelial cells of certain capillary beds, concomitantly with the adjacent tissue cells form specialized structures such as the blood-brain barrier composed of the brain capillary endothelial cells and the adjacent astrocytes, or special communications between maternal endothelial cells of the spiral arteries and fetal trophoblast cells in placenta [6].

While the thin capillary walls (of 0.2 μm order of magnitude) are composed only of endothelial cells anchored in their basal lamina (and surrounded by pericytes), in larger vessels, endothelium is part of the much thicker vascular wall. The latter comprises also the beneath lying vascular smooth muscle cells (VSMC) of arteries and veins, respectively, and the perivascular cells including macrophages and mesenchymal cells from the vessel adventitia.

It has been appreciated that the endothelial lining of arteriolar vascular beds primarily affects vascular tone and thus vascular resistance regulation, adjusted to tissue demands. Capillary endothelium in turn mainly determines water and solute passage into the tissues, whereas the one in the postcapillary venules directs vascular permeability and blood cell trafficking, being more involved in immune and inflammatory processes governing tissue repair and angiogenesis [7]. Therefore, apart from inter-endothelial cell junctions influencing capillary permeability, mutual communication of endothelial cells with other elements of the vascular wall importantly contributes to vascular homeostasis [8].

The vast heterogeneity of the endothelium of arteries and veins could additionally be explained by significantly different physiological and physical conditions to which endothelial cells of various vascular beds are exposed, such as blood pressure, shear stress, and pulsatility. Hemodynamic forces significantly impact endothelial structure and function: compared to ellipsoid morphology and coaxial alignment under the conditions of laminar flow, cell morphology and alignment change drastically in the settings of turbulent flow and at vessel bifurcations, all predisposing to atherogenicity [9, 10].

Endothelial cells therefore exhibit a wide range of plasticity, from alterations in the expression of various membrane receptors and adhesion molecules, changes in their morphology and shape, their mitogenic potential and even their potential to migrate or transit into different cell types (endothelial-to-mesenchymal transition) [3, 11].

1.2. Endothelial dysfunction

Being directly exposed to intravascular milieu, it is obvious that the composition of blood and the (patho)physiological conditions strongly affect endothelial cells, in terms of mediating signals which directly target their surface and activate numerous intracellular signaling pathways. During our life span, we are exposed to a variety of risk factors and toxic and noxious stimuli from the external environment (including air pollutants, tobacco smoke, chemicals from food, radiation, different eating habits in terms of high salt, sugar or saturated fatty acids intake, etc.) which strongly impact endothelial cells and their functions. As such, endothelial cells are constantly being challenged by changing internal environment to which they adapt more or less successfully. As long as their adaptive capacity in terms of maintaining homeostasis between vasoconstrictors and vasodilators reflecting vascular tone regulation; anti- and procoagulant activity reflecting hemostatic processes; anti- and pro-inflammatory mediators affecting the inflammatory response, and pro- and antiangiogenic factors affecting new vessel formation, remains in physiological limits, one might consider the endothelium to be healthy. However, the delineation between health and disease is not easy to define. When the maladaptive patterns overweigh, endothelial dysfunction issues what leads to disease [12].

Although the mostly exposed clinical sign of endothelial dysfunction is impaired endothelium-dependent vasodilation, endothelial dysfunction on a broader scale encompasses a pro-inflammatory, proadhesive, procoagulant, and proliferative state predisposing to atherosclerosis [13]. Multiple mechanisms have been involved in the development of endothelial dysfunction, connected to alterations in glucose and lipid metabolism, insulin resistance, obesity, dyslipidemia, hyperhomocysteinemia, altered hormone and cytokine secretion, imbalance in the autonomic nervous system activity, arterial hypertension, etc. Oxidative stress is acknowledged to play a central role in the development of endothelial dysfunction; moreover, oxidative stress has been appreciated as one of the main factors involved in normal aging, which imminently is also associated with endothelial dysfunction [14]. Although the severity of endothelial dysfunction might differ between vascular beds, independent studies have shown correlations between endothelial dysfunction in different vascular beds [13, 15]. Therefore, endothelial dysfunction can be regarded as a systemic disorder: as tissues and organs depend on proper vascularization and an adequate supply of nutrients and removal of waste products, the dysfunctional endothelium not only predisposes to the development of cardiovascular diseases (atherosclerosis, hypertension, peripheral arterial disease, stroke, etc.) but also to a wide range of other diseases, including metabolic (diabetes, obesity), inflammatory, rheumatoid, oncology, and degenerative diseases, and in the worst scenario, culminates in organ failure.

Accordingly, understanding the physiology of the endothelium is of crucial clinical importance, and there is an ongoing search for potential strategies to postpone or at least ameliorate endothelial dysfunction and disease progression, either in terms of drugs application or avoiding the known risk factors; even more, when timely treated, endothelial dysfunction might be reversible [13]. To this end, additional methodological tools have to be accomplished in order to timely detect potential endothelial dysfunction. In spite of huge effort put in mechanistic studies performed on animal models and cell cultures, the exact tool to specifically reveal endothelial dysfunction clinically is missing and, at the moment, is far from being optimal. Various molecules have been used as surrogate markers of endothelial function, including soluble vascular adhesion molecule-1 (sVCAM-1), von Willebrand factor (vWF), angiopoietin-2 [16], adipocytokines [17], microparticles [18], and several more; yet, they mostly lack the sensitivity and specificity, and are often too robust to detect subtle preclinical changes. Also functional studies to assess endothelium, such as measurement of arterial intima-media thickness or flow-mediated dilation (FMD), offer just a raw estimation of endothelial function. As proper organ functioning strongly depends on microcirculation, particular attention should be given to this vascular bed also in the clinics. An interesting observation when tracing the microcirculation *in vivo* is that it exhibits typical oscillations of distinct frequencies [19, 20]. It has been suggested that each of them could reflect particular aspect of vascular tone regulation: low frequency oscillations have shown good correlations with the endothelial component of vascular tone regulation and therefore could be used as a marker of microvascular endothelial function [19].

Endothelium represents a therapeutic potential: many newer drugs targeting endothelium—either its surface and the corresponding membrane receptors, or intracellular targets affecting various signaling or metabolic pathways or directly its genome, are being developed and tested on the level of preclinical and clinical studies. In addition, independent studies have also shown that many classical cardiovascular drugs, such as angiotensin receptor antagonists, calcium (Ca^{2+}) antagonists, angiotensin converting enzyme (ACE) inhibitors, and beta adrenergic blockers, and other drugs (antidiabetic agents, sulfonylurea, etc.) apart from acting via their established mechanisms also exert positive actions connected directly or indirectly to endothelium [21–23]. Yet, keeping in mind the huge heterogeneity of endothelial cell phenotype, one must not forget that therapy affecting endothelium should be targeted to specific vascular beds. In the last time, endothelium-targeted nanomedicine has evolved as a promising new model to deliver drugs directly into the endothelial cells [24]. Last but not least, exercise has long been appreciated as one of the most efficient measures to improve endothelial (dys)function in various ways: increasing nitric oxide (NO) bioavailability; induction of reactive oxygen species (ROS) scavenging enzymes [25]; affecting the sympathetic nervous system; and increasing the number of endothelial progenitor cells (EPCs) to list just a few.

In the subsequent sections of the chapter, basic concepts of endothelial (patho)physiology, relevant for the book, will briefly be addressed. More detailed information on endothelial (dys) function, with particular emphasis on its genetic background and senescence, its involvement in inflammation and hemostasis, and its adaptation to various environmental challenges are extensively given in the following book chapters.

2. Endothelial function depends on its structural and molecular characteristics

Electron microscopy combined with various labeling techniques has enabled an insight into the endothelial structure. Along the arterial tree, the shape of endothelial cells varies from predominantly flat in arteries and capillaries to even cuboidal in high endothelial venules, a special type of postcapillary venules [1, 7]. As endothelial cells are challenged by diverse extracellular stimuli from their environment on a spatial and temporal basis, various signaling pathways finally culminate in (post)transcriptional modifications and thus marked alterations of the phenotype. In addition, some site-specific properties of endothelium are epigenetically determined. Using DNA microarray analysis, distinct gene patterns between large vessel and microvascular endothelial cells, as well as between blood and lymphatic endothelial cells have been shown [26]. While large vessels express several genes involved in the biosynthesis and remodeling of extracellular matrix (fibronectin, various collagens, osteonectin), microvascular endothelial cells abundantly express genes coding for basement membrane proteins (laminin, various integrins, CD36). In addition, microvascular endothelial cells were shown to express higher levels of transcripts encoding proteins involved in trafficking of circulating blood cells and pathogens which enables pathogens and immune cells to migrate to target tissues [26]. Interestingly, data suggest that the artery-vein identities of endothelial cells are established before blood circulation begins [26]. Recent findings on the organotypical differentiation of microvascular beds are extensively presented elsewhere [3, 27].

2.1. On endothelial permeability, inter-endothelial cell junctions, and caveolae

Given the pivotal role of the microvascular endothelium in supplying tissues with nutrients and oxygen, endothelial integrity is crucial for tissue-fluid homeostasis. While basal permeability mainly governs water and solutes transport across the capillary wall of a healthy endothelium, the term inducible (or induced) permeability refers to alterations in endothelial permeability associated with inflammation and occurs predominantly at the site of postcapillary venules [1]. The latter occurs as a consequence of endothelial cell retraction and intercellular gap formation by a variety of agonists (histamine, serotonin, bradykinin, substance P, vascular endothelial growth factor (VEGF)) [28], or according to more recent speculations, due to transcellular vascular leakage of macromolecules [29].

In general, microvascular endothelial structure directs the capillary dynamics: fluids and small solutes (less than 3 nm) move passively across the endothelium mainly via paracellular transport mechanisms or transcellularly by simple diffusion (nonpolar substances and gases) whereas larger macromolecules are transported by transcellular mechanisms, including receptor-dependent and receptor-independent transcytosis [30].

Paracellular transport pathways across the capillary wall depend on endothelial permeability. Permeability is mainly determined by the integrity of endothelial glycocalyx and two types of inter-endothelial cell junctions, the distribution of which depends on the capillary network: tight junctions (TJs) and adherens junctions (AJs). The main component of AJs are cadherins (cadherin-VE being the most abundant), which belong to adhesion molecules and are also connected to actin cytoskeleton [31, 32]. Changes in VE-cadherin dynamics at AJs can lead to disassembly of AJs, increasing the junctional permeability; chronic vascular leakage that occurs in tumor vessels is associated with downregulation of VE-cadherin expression [33]. Interestingly, endothelial NO synthase (eNOS) hyperactivation in response to vascular endothelial growth factor (VEGF) or platelet aggregating factor (PAF) triggers S-nitrosylation of VE-cadherin, thereby causing destabilization of AJs, and leading to endothelial hyperpermeability [34]. In addition, ROS have been implicated in junctions disorganization [35]. As altered Ca^{2+} signaling has been implicated in inducing endothelial hyperpermeability, activation of transient receptor potential (TRP) channels which regulate Ca^{2+} entry has been associated with hyperpermeability states and transendothelial migration of leukocytes [31]. In addition, the integrity of AJs depends on small RhoGTPases that have been intensively investigated as potential drug targets [31]. Interestingly, statins (simvastatin) have been shown to prevent vascular injury associated with hyperpermeability and inflammation by affecting the RhoA- and Rac1-mediated cytoskeletal arrangements [36].

Transcellular transport mechanisms are accomplished by membrane-bound vesicular carriers, such as caveolae and vesiculo-vacuolar organelles. Caveolae are plasma-membrane invaginations composed of lipids and caveolins, scaffolding proteins that are involved in transmembrane signaling. Caveolin has been used as molecular marker for the isolation of caveolae-enriched membranes from *in vitro* cultured cells [37].

With reference to endothelial heterogeneity, there are significant differences in the number of caveolae in endothelium along the vascular tree reaching up to 10,000 per cell in the capillaries [1]. Besides being involved in transcellular trafficking, caveolar network in endothelial cells affects many other endothelial functions. Caveolin can modulate signal transduction: G-protein-coupled receptors and receptor tyrosine kinases are localized into caveolae and interact with caveolin [37]. Caveolins have also been involved in cell migration, angiogenesis, and cancer [38]. VEGF is an important proangiogenic factor that promotes angiogenesis by increasing vascular permeability, endothelial cell migration, and the release of proteolytic matrix metalloproteinases (MMPs). VEGF receptors have been localized in caveolae and interact with caveolin-1 [39]. VEGF disrupts the interaction between the VEGF receptor (VEGFR)-2 and caveolin-1, thereby activating the downstream signaling [39]. Silencing caveolin-1 has been shown to affect MMPs activity and VEGF-induced angiogenesis [40]; moreover, it induced morphological alterations of endothelial cells, and reduced cell migration and tubulogenesis induced by VEGF, pointing to an important role of caveolae in angiogenesis. Additional evidence on the involvement of caveolae in vasculogenesis comes from studies showing that the recruitment of EPCs [41], which are now widely recognized as one of the key mechanisms in adult vasculogenesis, to the peripheral blood is dependent on the expression of VEGFR2 [42]. Finally, one should not forget one of the main effects of caveolin, namely inhibition of eNOS [43, 44]. As caveolin also interferes with adenosine receptor trafficking and the role of adenosine has been implicated in ischemia and inflammation, caveolar network may represent a potential therapeutic target [45].

http://dx.doi.org/10.5772/intechopen.81286

In addition, being part of the mechanosensory complex, caveolae and AJs are involved in mechanosensing [31, 46]: exposure of endothelial cells to shear stress has been shown to affect the number and distribution of caveolae [47, 48].

2.2. On endothelial barrier and mechanosensing

Mechanosensing is accomplished by a complex mechanism involving parts of endothelial cells, which convey the mechanic signals sensed by surface cellular elements in the transduction intracellular signaling pathways, finally adjusting the endothelial response to alterations of shear-stress. Mechanosensing complex, located in AJs, is composed of endothelial glycocalyx and endothelial cilium, VE-cadherins, VEGFR2 and platelet endothelial cell adhesion molecules (PECAM-1 or CD31), and various ion channels: the role of Ca^{2+}-dependent potassium channels (K^{+}_{Ca}) and TRP channels has extensively been investigated [10, 48]. However, certain predilection sites are prone to the generation of characteristic spatiotemporal shear-stress patterns favoring atherogenesis [9, 10, 48, 49].

Glycocalyx, a 50–100 μm thick structure anchored in the endothelial plasma membrane and composed of carbohydrate-rich proteoglycans, is located at the luminal surface of the endothelium [2, 30, 50]. It is importantly involved in mechanosensing, in the regulation of permeability, and inflammatory response [32, 48, 50] and has also been investigated as a potential therapeutic target [51, 52]. It prevents leucocyte and platelet adhesion [53] and mediates shear-stress-induced NO release, thus exerting vasculoprotective effects and contributing to vascular homeostasis [10, 54]. Besides being susceptible to pathological alterations in blood flow, other environmental alterations affect its composition and thus function, e.g., high glucose has been shown to be involved in glycocalyx degradation contributing to lower NO bioavailability in hyperglycemia [55, 56]. Recent concept has confirmed the existence of an additional thicker (0.5–1 μm) layer on the luminal endothelial surface (termed endothelial surface layer, ESL) which significantly impacts hemodynamic conditions, oxygen transport, vascular control, coagulation, inflammation, and atherosclerosis [2].

Endothelial cilium is a single hair-shaped projection from the cellular surface of endothelial cells. Besides being involved in sensing hemodynamic forces, it coordinates cell migration and division [30, 57]. Impaired function of the primary cilium, either genetically or due to environmental factors, results in developmental disorders or endothelial dysfunctions, respectively. The main components of the primary cilium are various membrane receptors (specific receptor tyrosine kinases, as platelet-derived growth factor (PDGF) receptor α, fibroblast growth factor receptor; insulin-like growth factor 1 (IGF-1) receptor; G-protein coupled receptors), channel proteins (polycystin-1 and -2), and special arrangement of the microtubules [30, 57]. Both polycystin proteins are importantly involved in intracellular signaling: polycystin-2, in turn, belongs to the TRP channel family which, by interacting with polycystin-1, increases intracellular Ca^{2+} leading to the activation of ryanodine receptors on the endoplasmic reticulum. The released Ca^{2+} subsequently activates a number of signaling pathways, among others the shear-stress induced activation of eNOS and an increase in NO production [57, 58]. Alterations in the patterns and magnitude of biomechanical forces induce disorganization in cilia structure: prolonged exposure to increased shear stress induces disassembly of cilia, rearrangement of cytoskeleton, and increased acetylation of microtubules [59]. Dysfunctional cilia have been implicated in kidney disease, hypertension, and the development of atherosclerosis [60].

In addition to being part of endothelial cilium, microtubules polymerized with heterodimers of alpha- and beta-tubulins are important cytoskeletal proteins in endothelial cells. They regulate numerous cellular functions, including cell shape, adhesion, intracellular transport, mitosis, and migration and thus contribute to endothelial integrity [35, 61]. Increased level of tubulin acetylation has been shown to increase cell migration [62]. On the other hand, cyclic stretch and angiotensin II (AngII) have been shown to increase tubulin deacetylation and tubular reorganization, predisposing to the development of cardiovascular diseases [63]; potential role on the AngII type 1 receptor antagonist in positively affecting endothelial microtubular organization has been implicated [63]. The longevity regulator sirtuin 1 (SIRT1), a potential therapeutic target [64], has been implicated in tubulin deacetylation and the regulation of microtubule function [63].

Disturbed flow patterns and increase of shear-stress have been acknowledged to affect the above targets, thus contributing to endothelial dysfunction in many ways, including increased generation of ROS, promoting cytoskeletal disassembly, increasing cellular permeability, expression of adhesion molecules and inflammation, as well as inducing mitogenic signaling pathways through extracellular signal-regulated kinase (ERK) and Jun kinase (JNK) involved in vascular remodeling which all favor atheroma formation [65]. Moreover, there is ample evidence that nonlaminar flow can result in gene expression of pro-inflammatory molecules in the vascular wall [49, 65].

2.3. On endothelium and inter-cellular communication

As mentioned, endothelial homeostasis involves mutual communication with other cells.

Gap junctions in turn enable a direct transmission of electrical and chemical signals and thus exchange of ions and other small molecules between endothelial cells, VSMC, and pericytes [8, 30, 66]. The main components of endothelial gap junctions are connexins (Cx) which have been shown to be defective in diseased states and thus represent a potential therapeutical target. A total of 21 connexins have been identified in humans displaying cellular specificity [67]. Healthy endothelium mainly expresses Cx-37 and Cx-40 [67, 68]. Alterations in connexin expression might be associated with endothelial dysfunction and increased susceptibility to atherosclerosis: altered expression of Cx-37 was shown to decrease NO bioavailability by decreasing eNOS activity [69], whereas endothelial-specific deletion of Cx-40 was reported to increase CD73-dependent leukocyte adhesion to endothelium [70].

Pericytes are contractile cells that wrap around the endothelial cells of capillaries and venules by sharing their basement membrane [71, 72]. As there is a considerable paracrine signaling between both cell lineages (via the release of transforming growth factor, angiopoietins, PDGF, sphingosine-1-phosphate), pericytes have been implicated in the regulation of capillary blood flow, and in the maturation and survival of endothelial cells by modulating apoptosis, and promoting angiogenesis [71–73]. Disturbance in pericyte-endothelial communication induces various pathological processes, associated with increased proneness to hemorrhage, apoptosis, impaired (tumor) angiogenesis, and endothelial hyperplasia [73].

An important communication exists between the *perivascular adipose tissue* (PVAT), endothelial cells, and VSMCs: PVAT secretes a number of adipokines (tumor necrosis factor, TNFα, interleukin-6, IL-6, resistin, irisin) with various pro- and antiatherogenic properties [8, 11]. The level of adipocytokines has been suggested as an independent predictor of endothelial dysfunction in healthy subjects [17]. In a healthy individual, PVAT importantly influences metabolism [74] and inflammatory response and modifies vascular tone regulation by secreting protective adipokines which exert paracrine actions directly and indirectly by stimulating the release of endothelial vasodilators on VSMC [75, 76]. Moreover, healthy PVAT has been shown to enhance insulin-induced vasodilation by releasing adipokines [77], as well as prostacyclin (PGI_2) [74]. Adiponectin, the most abundant adipokine, has been shown to decrease tissue inflammation [78]. However, these anti-contractile and anti-inflammatory properties of PVAT are blunted in disease, such as obesity, and hypertension where an imbalance of secreted adipokines from PVAT and alterations in metabolism predispose to inflammation and the development of endothelial dysfunction [79]. Hypoxia is one of the main mechanisms increasing the release of inflammatory cytokines (IL-6 and TNFα) from PVAT [80], and inducing macrophage activation which all favors a pro-inflammatory and pro-contractile state [81]. Moreover, in response to vascular injury [82] or high fat diet [83], PVAT has been shown to express pro-inflammatory phenotype and a significant reduction of adiponectin levels leading to atherosclerosis. Interestingly, the inflammatory profile of PVAT has been shown to differ between distinct fat depots [84]. Independent human studies have proven beneficial effects of exercise and diet on PVAT, and consequently also on endothelial dysfunction [85, 86].

Endothelial and VSMC are abundantly innervated with the fibers of *the sympathetic nervous system*, and there is a considerable and complex cross talk between various neurotransmitters released from these fibers and endothelial autacoids [87–89]. Besides noradrenaline, that binds on various adrenoceptors on endothelial cells and VSMC, other transmitters (such as adenosine triphosphate (ATP), calcitonin gene-related peptide (CGRP) acetylcholine (ACh), and neuropeptide Y) are released from nerve varicosities, thereby profoundly modulating endothelial function. Noradrenaline was shown to activate β_3-adrenergic receptors on endothelium, thereby increasing NO production [89, 90], while the co-transmitted ATP mediates endothelial hyperpolarization by acting on endothelial purinoceptors (P2Y) [88]; both effects finally induce vasorelaxation and, respectively, modulate the "classical" sympathetic vasoconstrictor effects on VSMC. Moreover, NO affects neurotransmission at the level of blood vessels, acting on presynaptic α_2-adrenergic receptors, and it also interferes with the sympathetic neurotransmission in the central nervous system [87].

Endothelial dysfunction and autonomic nervous system imbalance often coexist in the development of cardiovascular diseases [88]. Indeed, an inverse relationship between markers of endothelial function and the sympathetic activity in healthy conditions is well known: in young adults, acute increase of the sympathetic activity, as assessed by measuring the plasma noradrenaline concentration, has been shown to impair endothelium-dependent dilation [91, 92]. Sympathetic nervous system activity is also proposed to be an important factor contributing to endothelial dysfunction with age [92].

2.4. Other endothelial functions: involvement in hemostasis, inflammation, and angiogenesis

Endothelium maintains blood fluidity, preventing intravascular coagulation and thrombus formation, respectively; endothelial cells express a variety of intraluminal surface proteins (such as thrombomodulin) and secrete molecules with anticoagulant and antithrombotic properties: ectonucleotidases and protein C and S as well as substances which inhibit platelet adhesion and aggregation (PGI_2 and NO).

On the other hand, endothelium enables *hemostasis* when needed through the expression of specific membrane glycoproteins which enable adhesion of platelets to the damaged vascular wall (i.e., subendothelial matrix); and secretion of diverse substances, such as vWF, thrombin, tissue factor, and many others. Additionally, endothelium plays a crucial role in the fibrinolytic system. Nevertheless, prothrombotic, procoagulation, and antifibrinolitic states are associated with thrombi formation and cardiovascular events.

Endothelium is importantly involved in *inflammatory processes* and tissue repair as it adjusts changes in vascular reactivity and permeability in response to various cytokines and autacoids, increasing plasma extravasation and larger molecules trafficking as well as the adhesion and recruitment of leucocytes across the vessel walls, mainly of the postcapillary venules to the site of injury/inflammation. It itself produces many substances involved in inflammation and subsequent tissue repair, i.e., VEGF and various cytokines (e.g., IL-1, TNF-α). Moreover, cytokines released from endothelium in an autocrine manner augment the inflammatory response by affecting intracellular signaling pathways which activate various transcription factors, especially the transcription factor NF-kB, to finally increase the expression of proadhesive and procoagulant genes. In addition, cytokines and VEGF also promote endothelial and VSMC proliferation [93]. In response to inflammation, endothelial cells increase the expression of a variety of adhesion molecules, belonging to three gene families, namely selectins, integrins, and the immunoglobulin (Ig) superfamily (comprising VCAM, intercellular adhesion molecules (ICAM), and PECAM-1) on their surface which enable leucocytes to recognize the affected sites, adhere to endothelium and cross the vessel wall. As the level of circulating adhesion molecules is increased in diseases, they have been used as a marker of endothelial dysfunction. Inappropriate regulation of inflammatory processes has been acknowledged as an early step in the development of atherosclerosis as well as other pathological processes [94].

Endothelium is crucial for vasculo- and *angiogenesis*. Postnatally, endothelial cells are relatively quiescent and the growth of new vessels (neoangiogenesis) in healthy adults only occurs in uterine cycle, reproduction (i.e., placenta formation), and wound healing, as well as in response to repeated exercise and endurance training in myocardium and skeletal muscles. Neoangiogenesis requires a fine orchestrated interplay between endothelial cells, VSMC, pericytes, and a variety of signaling molecules, including growth factors [95], chemokines, angiopoietins, semaphorins, angiogenic enzymes, adhesion molecules, ephrins, and MMPs [93]. Neoangiogenesis involves many interdependent processes; in brief, upon stimulation by various angiogenic growth factors, endothelial cells get activated and release protease to degrade and invade basal lamina and the underlaying extracellular matrix. Endothelial cells then migrate into the interstitial space, where they proliferate and differentiate to form solid sprouts connecting neighboring vessels [38, 93, 96]. The role of VEGF and angiopoietins and the involvement of caveolae have shortly been mentioned above. In addition, circulating EPCs have also been shown to play a role in angiogenesis as they can differentiate to mature endothelial cells and replace injured or senescent endothelial cells [41, 97]. The number of circulating EPCs has been shown to be increased in cancer [98]. One of the most important (patho)physiological stimuli for neoangiogenesis in adult period is hypoxia which modifies gene expression dependent on the activation of hypoxia-inducible factor-1 (HIF-1) and, among others, it triggers endothelial cells to get activated [99]. Excessive angiogenesis in adult period also occurs in many pathological conditions, such as cancerogenesis, tumor growth, and metastasis. To this end, the processes connected to angiogenesis represent an important therapeutic niche: on one side, antiangiogenic drugs are targeted against tumor growth [100], and on the other, proangiogenic drugs have to be designed to augment the angiogenic potential [101].

Endothelial cells also express enzymes for degradation of other autacoids, and enzymes which convert humoral factors to attend their full activity, as, e.g., ACE.

Endothelium, therefore, is a highly metabolic organ. Energy supply for its pleiotropic functions is derived mainly from glucose by anaerobic metabolism although endothelium is directly exposed to blood with high oxygen partial pressure (pO_2); therefore, enough O_2 to be transported to other cells may be conserved [102]. Fatty acids represent another potential fuel for endothelial cells; yet, as they have relatively few mitochondria, fatty acids have been proposed to only modestly contribute to total ATP generation [102]. Glucose is transported into endothelial cells via insulin-independent GLUT-1 transporter [103]; respectively, endothelial cells, particularly the microvascular ones [104], are susceptible to adverse effects of hyperglycemia which in multiple ways increases the level of oxydative stress. The mechanism involves mitochondrial hyperpolarization, which affects ROS production [105, 106]. However, ROS should not only be regarded as a foe: in recent years, they have been acknowledged as important players in endothelial homeostasis, modulating endothelium-dependent vasodilation, permeability, and angiogenesis [105, 106]. On the other hand, dysfunctional mitochondria have been implicated in endothelial dysfunction and vascular aging [107–109] and as such represent a potential therapeutic target [109]. Moreover, mitochondria might be regarded as oxygen sensors since in hypoxic conditions, the generation of ROS is increased and connected to hypoxia-mediated responses, such as increased permeability, changes in cell surface adhesion molecules, cell proliferation, and angiogenesis [110]. Exercise and diet have been shown to beneficially impact mitochondria dysfunction [108, 111]. Caloric restriction has also been connected with SIRT1: decreased ATP level activates AMP-activated protein kinase (AMPK), the main cellular energy sensor which in turn activates SIRT1 [112].

3. Endothelium and vascular tone regulation: endothelial vasodilators

One of the main functions of endothelium is its involvement in vascular tone regulation. In response to mechanical and pharmacological (ACh, histamine, bradykinin, VEGF, various hormones as estrogen, CGRP, substance P, insulin, and platelets products (serotonin, ADP)) stimuli, endothelium releases a number of vasoactive mediators which, by affecting VSMC, regulate vascular tone and thus help to adjust blood flow to tissue demands. There is a considerable and complex interplay between endothelial and other humoral vasoactive substances, as well as the sympathetic nervous system. Mostly investigated endothelial vasodilators are NO, PGI_2, and endothelium-derived hyperpolarizing factor(s) (EDHF), whereas the main constrictors include endothelin, thromboxane, AngII, the cytochrome P450

(CYP)-hydroxylase-derived 20-hydroxyeicosatetraenoic acids (20-HETE) [113, 114], and constrictor prostanoids [115]. In a healthy state, vasodilators predominate whereas in endothelial dysfunction, reduced vasodilator bioavailability, in particular NO and an excessive release of vasoconstrictors result in an increased vascular tone. Moreover, in the settings of endothelial dysfunction, other vasodilators may compensate for the reduced NO bioavailability [116–118].

Endothelial vasodilators mediate the endothelium-dependent vasodilation. Yet, it must be noted that the contribution of each to the regulation of vascular tone differs between the vascular beds: while NO has mainly been implicated in the regulation of larger vessels, other vasodilators seem to play the prominent role in microcirculation [116, 117, 119].

FMD denotes endothelium-dependent decrease of vascular tone in response to increased blood flow, which is noted down—as well as upstream of the vessel tree, and has been used as a surrogate marker of endothelial function in the clinics. It is mostly tested by performing a transient occlusion of a distal (or proximal) artery to induce local ischemia and assessing blood flow increase after reperfusion. The phenomenon of postocclusive hyperemia (PORH) is a good example to explain the mechanism of FMD: endothelium-dependent vasodilation elicited by increased shear stress due to increased flow as a consequence of the vasorelaxant effect of locally accumulated metabolites additionally increases the flow to meet tissue metabolic demands and simultaneously oppose the pressure-induced myogenic vasoconstrictory response [116].

3.1. Nitric oxide exerts many vasoprotective functions

NO is constantly being formed from the amino acid L-arginine by constitutively expressed eNOS. It can also be produced by other isoforms of NOS, namely inducible (iNOS) and neuronal (nNOS), present in various cell types (endothelial cells, platelets, neurons and VSMC, macrophages, polymorphonucleated leukocytes) which are important in the settings of endothelial activation and/or dysfunction [43]. eNOS is a calmodulin-dependent enzyme requiring cofactors as Ca^{2+}, tetrahydrobiopterin (BH_4), nicotinamide adenine dinucleotide phosphate (NADP), etc. Its activity is regulated by complex interactions of the endothelial microdomain proteins whereby its association with the heat-shock protein increases and with the caveolin-1 decreases its activity [44]. Moreover, it is modulated posttranslationally in a Ca^{2+}-dependent way through the activation of various Ca^{2+}-channels on the cell membrane and by Ca^{2+}-independent way which is the main mechanism of shear-stress-induced eNOS activation. The Ca^{2+}-independent pathway mainly affects the phosphorylation of eNOS by Akt kinase, Ca^{2+}/calmodulin-dependent protein kinase II (CaMKII), protein kinase A (PKA), or AMPK, depending on the stimulus; a variety of stimuli, including hormones, growth factors, purines, histamine, bradykinin, serotonin, noradrenaline, etc., affect G-protein-coupled receptors and finally activate the corresponding target to subsequently phosphorylate eNOS and increase its activity [43]. On the other hand, hyperglycemia has been suggested to adversely affect eNOS phosphorylation thus attenuating NO production [120]. Another common post-translational modification of eNOS activity is acetylation/deacetylation: for example, SIRT-1, a class III histone deacetylase enhances the ACh- and shear-stress-induced-NO production by deacetylating eNOS, thereby enhancing its binding to calmodulin [121]. Moreover, aspirin has been shown to enhance eNOS activation by acetylating eNOS, independently of its effect on cyclooxygenase inhibition [122].

Of note is the dual role of eNOS: when the bioavailability of its substrates and/or cofactors is reduced and in conditions of increased oxidative stress, eNOS can get uncoupled and produces superoxide anion (O^{2-}) instead of NO; O^{2-} is a highly reactive radical which forms peroxynitrite ($ONOO^-$) with NO, and in this way, it additionally decreases the bioavailability of NO and contributes to endothelial dysfunction [43, 44, 90].

Besides directly inducing vascular relaxations by activating the soluble guanylate cyclase (sGC) in VSMC, NO importantly modulates other endothelial autacoids (e.g., PGI_2, EDHF, endothelin) affecting vascular tone [123, 124], and interferes with the sympathetic neurotransmission pre- and postsynaptically [89].

NO exerts other effects: it inhibits platelet aggregation (interestingly, activated-platelet-derived substances increase the activity of eNOS, thus producing more NO) and the adhesion of leucocytes to the vascular wall by decreasing the expression of adhesion molecules on endothelial surface [90]. Moreover, it interferes with cellular metabolism [125] by modulating mitochondrial function, and oxygen metabolism [106, 126]. As stated, NO forms ROS ($ONOO^-$) with increased levels of O^{2-} which, among others, impairs the mitochondrial respiratory chain [127]. On the other hand, the depolarization of mitochondrial membrane induced by mitochondrial K_{ATP}-channel activators has been reported to increase the activity of eNOS in rat cerebral arteries [128]. Other gaseous mediators involved in vascular tone regulation have also been proposed to interfere with the mitochondrial function [127].

In the settings of hypoxia, NO could alternatively be derived from the reduction of $ONOO^-$ which may partly compensate for reduced eNOS activity [129].

A number of factors have been known to exert beneficial vasoprotective effects by interfering with eNOS activity and consequently increasing NO bioavailability, including female sex hormones (the protecting effects of estrogens have long been appreciated), insulin, glucagon-like peptide, thyroid hormones, erythropoietin, high density lipoproteins, etc., as well as endothelial exposure to repetitive increases in shear stress as occurs in exercise [25, 130].

On the other hand, many factors negatively impact eNOS or scavenge NO, thereby reducing the beneficial effects of NO: ROS, reduced availability of BH_4 or arginine, due to increased levels of arginase, asymmetric dimethylarginine (ADMA), an endogenous inhibitor of eNOS, cortisol, aldosterone, and numerous others. Moreover, environmental factors, such as smoking, radiation, increased salt intake or hyperglycemia, as well as other metabolic disturbances, such as insulin resistance and metabolic syndrome, hypercholesterolemia and obesity, homocysteinemia, uric acid, diminish the NO-dependent vasodilation and other NO-associated effects [130]. The latter settings predispose to endothelial dysfunction and the development of diseases, such as hypertension and atherosclerosis, and increase the risk for cardiovascular events.

Therefore, the biosynthetic pathways of NO and its downstream targets might all represent potential therapeutic targets [90, 131].

Increased levels of ROS could be regarded as a common denominator of reduced NO bioavailability resulting in endothelial dysfunction. Fortunately, the endogenous ROS-scavenging enzymes convert O^{2-} to hydrogen peroxide (H_2O_2) which is proposed as one of important endothelial factors inducing VSMC hyperpolarization and vasodilation, respectively [75, 132, 133].

The bad ROS are turned into the good ones thus ameliorating their damaging effects [133]. Indeed, increased levels of H_2O_2 have also been suggested to overtake the role of NO in the settings of reduced NO bioavailability also in humans [134].

3.2. Endothelium-dependent relaxations beyond NO: hyperpolarization

Shear stress and various agonists also stimulate the production of other vasodilators, among which the derivatives of arachidonic acid (AA) play an important role.

AA is liberated from membrane phospholipids by the action of Ca^{2+}-stimulated phospholipase A_2, and subsequently metabolized into biologically active eicosanoids with a variety of functions. Three main complex enzymatic pathways of AA metabolism are the cyclooxygenase pathway, the cytochrome (CYP)-P450 pathway, and the lipoxygenase pathway; however, AA can be transformed into isoprostanes nonenzymatically by ROS [135]. Regarding vascular tone regulation, AA metabolites include a number of vasodilators and vasoconstrictors [113–115, 135–138].

One of the most investigated AA metabolites is PGI_2, formed by prostacyclin synthase, which belongs to the CYP-450 family and is highly expressed in endothelial cells and associated with cyclooxygenase (COX)-2 [115, 135–137]. Its vasodilator effects mainly involve binding to prostacyclin (IP) receptors and activation of adenylate cyclase increasing cAMP level in VSMC and subsequent relaxation. Yet, the role of PGI_2 as endogenous mediator of endothelium-dependent vasodilation *in vivo* has often been questioned and its other effects, such as inhibition of platelet adhesion and aggregation, and reduction of oxidative stress [135, 139] might rather account for its vasculoprotective effects. Moreover, COX-2-derived PGI_2 might play a compensatory role for the decreased NO bioavailability [117, 118]. To this end, it must be noted that other prostanoids from the COX metabolic pathways also affect vascular tone: due to various metabolic pathways as well as various prostaglandin receptors coupled to different signaling pathways, they might either induce vasoconstriction or vasodilation [115, 135, 137–139]. It is the delicate balance between vasoconstrictors and vasodilators which enables normal functioning of healthy endothelium; in endothelial dysfunction, the effect of vasoconstrictive prostanoids predominates, predisposing to the development of hypertension, atherosclerosis, and various other diseases.

Besides NO and PGI_2, endothelial hyperpolarization (EDH) accounts for endothelium-dependent, flow-mediated vasodilation; by blocking eNOS (by L-NMMA) and COX (by more or less specific COX inhibitors), the role of non-NO-non-PGE-dependent vasodilation has unequivocally been confirmed not only in *in vitro* assays and in animal models but also *in vivo* in various human vessels during resting [140–143] and exercise [144].

Many of endothelial mediators and signals are known to induce the hyperpolarization of VSMC [8, 130, 135, 136, 145, 146]: epoxyeicosatrienoic acids (EETs) produced in the CYP-450-dependent metabolism of AA [135, 136]; the above mentioned H_2O_2 [133, 140], potassium ions released from the endothelial cells via K_{ca} channels, and direct transmission of endothelial cell hyperpolarization by myoendothelial gap junctions. Thus, EDHF comprises a variety of factors which activate various potassium channels: small (SK_{Ca}), intermediate, and large-conductance K_{ca} channels; inward rectifier K^+ channels (K_{IR}) [147], and TRPV4 channels [148] have been implicated in finally inducing EDH. To this end, the corresponding channels have been investigated as potential targets to affect EDH [147, 149]. Endothelial hyperpolarization can spread via myoendothelial gap junctions to directly induce VSMC hyperpolarization: the role of gap junctions has been implicated also in humans *in vitro* and *in vivo* as carbenoxolone, a nonspecific gap junction blocker, diminished conducted vasodilation in isolated human coronary arterioles [150], and, moreover, reduced FMD in the brachial artery of healthy volunteers [151]. The term conducted dilation has been used to denote electrotonic transmission of local hyperpolarization, and may spread several mm upstream independent of alterations in shear stress [116, 119, 152]. It reflects the involvement of gap junctions and enables a coordinated adjustment of vascular resistance in larger and smaller arterioles and capillaries [153].

Age and gender might affect the EDHF-mediated response as male animals were reported to exhibit smaller EDHF-mediated endothelium-dependent relaxation compared to females; similarly, aging affected EDH. A reduced SK_{Ca} activity and a reduced expression of gap junction proteins, Cx-40 and Cx-43, have been suggested to account for these differences [154]. Moreover, 17b-estradiol has been proposed to activate AMPK and/or SIRT1, both implicated to be involved in increasing the EDHF-mediated signaling [154]. Alteration of the EDH contributes to endothelial dysfunction observed in various pathologies [145, 154].

Finally, other endothelium-derived vasodilators should be listed: adenosine and purines, various peptides, including CGRP, C-type natriuretic peptide (CNP), adrenomedullin, endocannabinoids, and gaseous transmitters other than NO, namely hydrogen sulfide (H_2S), and carbon monoxide (CO) which have been suggested to compensate for decreased NO bioavailability [127, 155, 156]. Adenosine, one of the most potent vasodilators (exerting also other vasculoprotective effects) is mainly formed from extracellular nucleotides (ATP, AMP) by the action of ectonucleotidases, expressed in endothelial cells and also investigated as potential therapeutic targets [157]. Interestingly, circulating ATP itself has been proposed to mediate vasodilation in humans *in vivo* by inducing vascular hyperpolarization via activation of K_{IR} channels [158].

4. Conclusion

By spreading throughout the vascular system and exerting pleiotropic functions, the endothelium could be regarded as one of the main players in cardiovascular physiology. The integrity of endothelium is crucial for vascular homeostasis and health. On the other hand, endothelial cells are susceptible to changes in blood composition and hemodynamic forces and as such vulnerable to developing endothelial dysfunction. Endothelial dysfunction nowadays is acknowledged a key initiating event in atherosclerosis, and connected to several pathological conditions and cardiovascular events. Accordingly, understanding endothelial function and dysfunction is crucial for recognition and treatment, or, optimally, for prevention of the development of cardiovascular diseases, the leading cause of death worldwide. To this end, it should be emphasized that the mechanistic studies on isolated vessels or on animal models cannot always be extrapolated directly to humans. Therefore, in spite of intensive investigations, additional studies to elucidate mechanisms of endothelial function and dysfunction are necessary to accomplish endothelium-targeted interventions.

Author details

Helena Lenasi

Address all correspondence to: helena.lenasi.ml@mf.uni-lj.si

Institute of Physiology, Faculty of Medicine, University of Ljubljana, Ljubljana, Slovenia

References

[1] Aird WC. Phenotypic heterogeneity of the endothelium: I. Structure, function and mechanisms. Circulation Research. 2007;**100**:158-173. Review

[2] Pries AR, Kuebler WM. Normal endothelium. Handbook of Experimental Pharmacology. 2006;**176**(Pt 1):1-40. Review

[3] Augustin HG, Koh GY. Organotypic vasculature: From descriptive heterogeneity to functional pathophysiology. Science. 2017;**357**(6353):pii: eaal2379. DOI: 10.1126/science.aal2379. Review

[4] Gao X, Xu C, Asada N, Frenette PS. The hematopoietic stem cell niche: From embryo to adult. Development. 2018;**145**(2):pii: dev139691. DOI: 10.1242/dev.139691. Review

[5] Planat-Benard V, Silvestre JS, Cousin B, et al. Plasticity of human adipose lineage cells toward endothelial cells: Physiological and therapeutic perspectives. Circulation. 2004;**109**:656-663

[6] Rai A, Cross JC. Development of the hemochorial maternal vascular spaces in the placenta through endothelial and vasculogenic mimicry. Developmental Biology. 2014;**387**(2):131-141. DOI: 10.1016/j.ydbio.2014.01.015. Review

[7] Aird WC. Phenotypic heterogeneity of the endothelium: II. Representative vascular beds. Circulation Research. 2007;**100**(2):174-190. Review

[8] Triggle CR, Samuel SM, Ravishankar S, et al. The endothelium: Influencing vascular smooth muscle in many ways. Canadian Journal of Physiology and Pharmacology. 2012;**90**(6):713-738. DOI: 10.1139/y2012-073. Review

[9] Gimbrone MA Jr, García-Cardeña G. Vascular endothelium, hemodynamics, and the pathobiology of atherosclerosis. Cardiovascular Pathology. 2013;**22**(1):9-15. DOI: 10.1016/j.carpath.2012.06.006. Review

[10] Chistiakov DA, Orekhov AN, Bobryshev YV. Effects of shear stress on endothelial cells: Go with the flow. Acta Physiologica (Oxford, England). 2017;**219**(2):382-408. DOI: 10.1111/apha.12725. Review

[11] Awgulewitsch CP, Trinh LT, Hatzopoulos AK. The vascular wall: A plastic hub of activity in cardiovascular homeostasis and disease. Current Cardiology Reports. 2017;**19**(6):51. DOI: 10.1007/s11886-017-0861-y. Review

[12] Liao JK. Linking endothelial dysfunction with endothelial cell activation. The Journal of Clinical Investigation. 2013;**123**(2):540-541. DOI: 10.1172/JCI66843

[13] Bonetti PO, Lerman LO, Lerman A. Endothelial dysfunction: A marker of atherosclerotic risk. Arteriosclerosis, Thrombosis, and Vascular Biology. 2003;**23**(2):168-175. Review

[14] Cai H, Harrison DG. Endothelial dysfunction in cardiovascular diseases: The role of oxidant stress. Circulation Research. 2000;**87**(10):840-844. Review

[15] Targonski PV, Bonetti PO, Pumper GM, et al. Coronary endothelial dysfunction is associated with an increased risk of cerebrovascular events. Circulation. 2003;**107**(22):2805-2809

[16] Zhang J, Defelice AF, Hanig JP, Colatsky T. Biomarkers of endothelial cell activation serve as potential surrogate markers for drug-induced vascular injury. Toxicologic Pathology. 2010;**38**(6):856-871. DOI: 10.1177/0192623310378866

[17] Solini A, Stea F, Santini E, Bruno RM, et al. Adipocytokine levels mark endothelial function in normotensive individuals. Cardiovascular Diabetology. 2012;**11**:103. DOI: 10.1186/1475-2840-11-103

[18] Baron M, Boulanger CM, Staels B, Tailleux A. Cell-derived microparticles in atherosclerosis: Biomarkers and targets for pharmacological modulation? Journal of Cellular and Molecular Medicine. 2012;**16**(7):1365-1376. DOI: 10.1111/j.1582-4934.2011.01486.x. Review

[19] Kvandal P, Stefanovska A, Veber M, et al. Regulation of human cutaneous circulation evaluated by laser Doppler flowmetry, iontophoresis, and spectral analysis: Importance of nitric oxide and prostaglandines. Microvascular Research. 2003;**65**(3):160-171

[20] Paparde A, Plakane L, Circenis K, Aivars JI. Effect of acute systemic hypoxia on human cutaneous microcirculation and endothelial, sympathetic and myogenic activity. Microvascular Research. 2015;**102**:1-5. DOI: 10.1016/j.mvr.2015.07.005

[21] Steven S, Münzel T, Daiber A. Exploiting the pleiotropic antioxidant effects of established drugs in cardiovascular disease. International Journal of Molecular Sciences. 2015;**16**(8):18185-18223. DOI: 10.3390/ijms160818185. Review

[22] Brown NJ. Blood pressure reduction and tissue-type plasminogen activator release. Hypertension. 2006;**47**(4):648-649

[23] Lenasi H, Kohlstedt K, Fichtlscherer B, Mülsch A, et al. Amlodipine activates the endothelial nitric oxide synthase by altering phosphorylation on Ser1177 and Thr495. Cardiovascular Research. 2003;**59**(4):844-853

[24] Shuvaev VV, Brenner JS, Muzykantov VR. Targeted endothelial nanomedicine for common acute pathological conditions. Journal of Controlled Release. 2015;**219**:576-595. DOI: 10.1016/j.jconrel.2015.09.055 Review

[25] Davies KJA. Cardiovascular adaptive homeostasis in exercise. Frontiers in Physiology. 2018;**9**:369. DOI: 10.3389/fphys.2018.00369

[26] Chi JT, Chang HY, Haraldsen G, et al. Endothelial cell diversity revealed by global expression profiling. Proceedings of the National Academy of Sciences of the United States of America. 2003;**100**(19):10623-10628

[27] Potente M, Mäkinen T. Vascular heterogeneity and specialization in development and disease. Nature Reviews. Molecular Cell Biology. 2017;**18**(8):477-494. DOI: 10.1038/nrm.2017.36 Review

[28] McDonald DM, Thurston G, Baluk P. Endothelial gaps as sites for plasma leakage in inflammation. Microcirculation. 1999;**6**:7-22

[29] Feng D, Nagy JA, Dvorak HF, Dvorak AM. Ultrastructural studies define soluble macromolecular, particulate, and cellular transendothelial cell pathways in venules, lymphatic vessels, and tumor-associated microvessels in man and animals. Microscopy Research and Technique. 2002;**57**(5):289-326. Review

[30] Mehta D, Malik AB. Signaling mechanisms regulating endothelial permeability. Physiological Reviews. 2006;**86**(1):279-367. Review

[31] Komarova YA, Kruse K, Mehta D, Malik AB. Protein interactions at endothelial junctions and signaling mechanisms regulating endothelial permeability. Circulation Research. 2017;**120**(1):179-206. DOI: 10.1161/CIRCRESAHA.116.306534. Review

[32] Curry FR, Adamson RH. Tonic regulation of vascular permeability. Acta Physiologica (Oxford, England). 2013;**207**(4):628-649. DOI: 10.1111/apha.12076. Review

[33] Hashizume H, Baluk P, Morikawa S, et al. Openings between defective endothelial cells explain tumor vessel leakiness. The American Journal of Pathology. 2000;**156**:1363-1380. DOI: 10.1016/S0002-9440(10)65006-7

[34] Thibeault S, Rautureau Y, Oubaha M, et al. S-nitrosylation of beta-catenin by eNOS-derived NO promotes VEGF-induced endothelial cell permeability. Molecular Cell. 2010;**39**(3):468-476. DOI: 10.1016/j.molcel.2010.07.01

[35] Hirase T, Node K. Endothelial dysfunction as a cellular mechanism for vascular failure. American Journal of Physiology. Heart and Circulatory Physiology. 2012;**302**(3):H499-H505. DOI: 10.1152/ajpheart.00325.2011. Review

[36] van Nieuw Amerongen GP, Vermeer MA, Nègre-Aminou P, et al. Simvastatin improves disturbed endothelial barrier function. Circulation. 2000;**102**:2803-2809

[37] Filippini A, Sica G, D'Alessio A. The caveolar membrane system in endothelium: From cell signaling to vascular pathology. Journal of Cellular Biochemistry. 2018;**119**(7):5060-5071. DOI: 10.1002/jcb.26793

[38] Schmidt T, Carmeliet P. Blood-vessel formation: Bridges that guide and unite. Nature. 2007;**465**:697-699

[39] Federico G, Francesca A, Ahmad S, et al. Vascular endothelial growth factor receptor-3 activity is modulated by its association with caveolin-1 on endothelial membrane. Biochemistry. 2007;**46**:3998-3905

[40] Madaro L, Antonangeli F, Favia A, et al. Knock down of caveolin 1 affects morphological and functional hallmarks of human endothelial cells. Journal of Cellular Biochemistry. 2013;**114**:1843-1851

[41] Hill JM, Zalos G, Halcox JP, et al. Circulating endothelial progenitor cells, vascular function, and cardiovascular risk. The New England Journal of Medicine. 2003;**348**:593-600

[42] Losordo DW, Dimmeler S. Therapeutic angiogenesis and vasculogenesis for ischemic disease. Part I: Angiogenic cytokines. Circulation. 2004;**109**:2487-2491

[43] Förstermann U, Sessa WC. Nitric oxide synthases: Regulation and function. European Heart Journal. 2012;**33**(7):829-37, 837a-837d. DOI: 10.1093/eurheartj/ehr304. Review

[44] Fleming I. Molecular mechanisms underlying the activation of eNOS. Pflügers Archiv. 2010;**459**(6):793-806. DOI: 10.1007/s00424-009-0767-7. Review

[45] Sands WA, Palmer TM. Adenosine receptors and the control of endothelial cell function in inflammatory disease. Immunology Letters. 2005;**101**:1-11

[46] TzimaE, Irani-Tehrani M, Kiosses WB, et al. A mechanosensory complex that mediates the endothelial cell response to fluid shear stress. Nature. 2005;**437**:426-431

[47] Sinha B, Koster D, Ruez R, et al. Cells respond to mechanical stress by rapid disassembly of caveolae. Cell. 2010;**144**:402-413

[48] Davies PF. Hemodynamic shear stress and the endothelium in cardiovascular pathophysiology. Nature Clinical Practice. Cardiovascular Medicine. 2009;**6**:16-26

[49] Brooks AR, Lelkes PI, Rubanyi GM. Gene expression profiling of vascular endothelial cells exposed to fluid mechanical forces: Relevance for focal susceptibility to atherosclerosis. Endothelium. 2004;**11**(1):45-57

[50] Tarbell JM, Cancel LM. The glycocalyx and its significance in human medicine. Journal of Internal Medicine. 2016;**280**:97-113

[51] Drake-Holland AJ, Noble MI. Update on the important new drug target in cardiovascular medicine—The vascular glycocalyx. Cardiovascular & Hematological Disorders Drug Targets. 2012;**12**:76-81

[52] Meuwese MC, Mooij HL, Nieuwdorp M, et al. Partial recovery of the endothelial glycocalyx upon rosuvastatin therapy in patients with heterozygous familial hypercholesterolemia. Journal of Lipid Research. 2009;**50**:148-153

[53] Lipowsky HH. The endothelial glycocalyx as a barrier to leukocyte adhesion and its mediation by extracellular proteases. Annals of Biomedical Engineering. 2012;**40**(4):840-848. DOI: 10.1007/s10439-011-0427-x

[54] Zeng L, Zhang Y, Chien S, et al. The role of p53 deacetylation in p21Waf1 regulation by laminar flow. The Journal of Biological Chemistry. 2003;**278**:24594-24599

[55] Lopez-Quintero SV, Cancel LM, Pierides A, et al. High glucose attenuates shear-induced changes in endothelial hydraulic conductivity by degrading the glycocalyx. PLoS One. 2013;**8**:e78954

[56] Nieuwdorp M, van Haeften TW, Gouverneur MC, et al. Loss of endothelial glycocalyx during acute hyperglycemia coincides with endothelial dysfunction and coagulation activation in vivo. Diabetes. 2006;**55**(2):480-486

[57] Nauli SM, Kawanabe Y, Kaminski JJ, et al. Endothelial cilia are fluid shear sensors that regulate calcium signaling and nitric oxide production through polycystin-1. Circulation. 2008;**117**(9):1161-1171. DOI: 10.1161/CIRCULATIONAHA.107.710111

[58] Abou-Alaiwi WA, Takahashi M, Mell BR, et al. Ciliary polycystin-2 is a mechanosensitive calcium channel involved in nitric oxide signaling cascades. Circulation Research. 2009;**104**(7):860-869. DOI: 10.1161/CIRCRESAHA.108.192765

[59] Sanchez I, Dynlacht BD. Cilium assembly and disassembly. Nature Cell Biology. 2016;**18**(7):711-717. DOI: 10.1038/ncb3370

[60] Van der Heiden K, Hierck BP, Krams R, et al. Endothelial primary cilia in areas of disturbed flow are at the base of atherosclerosis. Atherosclerosis. 2008;**196**(2):542-550. DOI: 10.1016/j.atherosclerosis.2007.05.030

[61] Lee TY, Gotlieb AI. Microfilaments and microtubules maintain endothelial integrity. Microscopy Research and Technique. 2003;**60**:115-127

[62] Tran AD, Marmo TP, Salam AA, et al. HDAC6 deacetylation of tubulin modulates dynamics of cellular adhesions. Journal of Cell Science. 2007;**120**:1469-1479

[63] Hashimoto-Komatsu A, Hirase T, Asaka M, Node K. Angiotensin II induces microtubule deorganization mediated by a deacetylase SIRT2 in endothelial cells. Hypertension Research. 2011;**34**:949-956

[64] Russomanno G, Corbi G, Manzo V, et al. The anti-ageing molecule sirt1 mediates beneficial effects of cardiac rehabilitation. Immunity & Ageing. 2017;**14**:7. DOI: 10.1186/s12979-017-0088-1. eCollection 2017

[65] Cunningham KS, Gotlieb AI. The role of shear stress in the pathogenesis of atherosclerosis. Laboratory Investigation. 2005;**85**(1):9-23. Review

[66] Herve JC, Derangeon M. Gap-junction-mediated cell-to-cell communication. Cell and Tissue Research. 2013;**352**(1):21-31

[67] Laird DW. Life cycle of connexins in health and disease. The Biochemical Journal. 2006;**394**(Pt 3):527-543

[68] Wong CW, Christen T, Roth I, et al. Connexin37 protects against atherosclerosis by regulating monocyte adhesion. Nature Medicine. 2006;**12**(8):950-954

[69] Pfenniger A, Derouette JP, Verma V, et al. Gap junction protein Cx37 interacts with endothelial nitric oxide synthase in endothelial cells. Arteriosclerosis, Thrombosis, and Vascular Biology. 2010;**30**(4):827-834

[70] Chadjichristos CE, Scheckenbach KE, van Veen TA, et al. Endothelial-specific deletion of connexin40 promotes atherosclerosis by increasing CD73-dependent leukocyte adhesion. Circulation. 2010;**121**(1):123-131

[71] Birbrair A, Zhang T, Wang ZM, et al. Pericytes at the intersection between tissue regeneration and pathology. Clinical Science (London, England). 2015;**128**(2):81-93. DOI: 10.1042/CS20140278. Review

[72] Winkler EA, Bell RD, Zlokovic BV. Central nervous system pericytes in health and disease. Nature Neuroscience. 2011;**14**(11):1398-1405. DOI: 10.1038/nn.2946

[73] Armulik A, Abramsson A, Betsholtz C. Endothelial/pericyte interactions. Circulation Research. 2005;**97**(6):512-523. Review

[74] Chang L, Villacorta L, Li R, Hamblin M, et al. Loss of perivascular adipose tissue on peroxisome proliferator-activated receptor-gamma deletion in smooth muscle cells impairs intravascular thermoregulation and enhances atherosclerosis. Circulation. 2012;**126**:1067-1078

[75] Gao YJ, Lu C, Su LY, et al. Modulation of vascular function by perivascular adipose tissue: The role of endothelium and hydrogen peroxide. British Journal of Pharmacology. 2007;**151**:323-331

[76] Yudkin JS, Eringa E, Stehouwer CD. "Vasocrine" signalling from perivascular fat: A mechanism linking insulin resistance to vascular disease. Lancet. 2005;**365**:1817-1820

[77] Meijer RI, Serné EH, Korkmaz HI, van der Peet DL, de Boer MP, Niessen HW, et al. Insulin-induced changes in skeletal muscle microvascular perfusion are dependent upon perivascular adipose tissue in women. Diabetologia. 2015;**58**(8):1907-1915. DOI: 10.1007/s00125-015-3606-8

[78] Sena CM, Pereira A, Fernandes R, et al. Adiponectin improves endothelial function in mesenteric arteries of rats fed a high-fat diet: Role of perivascular adipose tissue. British Journal of Pharmacology. 2017;**174**:3514-3526

[79] Omar A, Chatterjee TK, Tang Y, Hui DY, Weintraub NL. Proinflammatory phenotype of perivascular adipocytes. Arteriosclerosis, Thrombosis, and Vascular Biology. 2014;**34**:1631-1636

[80] Greenstein AS, Khavandi K, Withers SB, et al. Local inflammation and hypoxia abolish the protective anticontractile properties of perivascular fat in obese patients. Circulation. 2009;**119**(12):1661-1670. DOI: 10.1161/CIRCULATIONAHA

[81] Withers SB, Agabiti-Rosei C, Livingstone DM, et al. Macrophage activation is responsible for loss of anticontractile function in inflamed perivascular fat. Arteriosclerosis, Thrombosis, and Vascular Biology. 2011;**31**(4):908-913. DOI: 10.1161/ATVBAHA.110.221705

[82] Takaoka M, Suzuki H, Shioda S, et al. Endovascular injury induces rapid phenotypic changes in perivascular adipose tissue. Arteriosclerosis, Thrombosis, and Vascular Biology. 2010;**30**:1576-1582

[83] Chatterjee TK, Stoll LL, Denning GM, et al. Proinflammatory phenotype of perivascular adipocytes: Influence of high-fat feeding. Circulation Research. 2009;**104**:541-549

[84] Kranendonk ME, Van Herwaarden JA, Stupkova T, et al. Inflammatory characteristics of distinct abdominal adipose tissue depots relate differently to metabolic risk factors for cardiovascular disease: Distinct fat depots and vascular risk factors. Atherosclerosis. 2015;**239**:419-427

[85] Boa BCS, Yudkin JS, van Hinsbergh VWM, et al. Exercise effects on perivascular adipose tissue: Endocrine and paracrine determinants of vascular function. British Journal of Pharmacology. 2017;**174**(20):3466-3481. DOI: 10.1111/bph.13732. Review

[86] Korybalska K, Swora-Cwynar E, Luczak J, et al. Association of endothelial proliferation with the magnitude of weight loss during calorie restriction. Angiogenesis. 2016;**19**:407-419. DOI: 10.1007/s10456-016-9516-7

[87] Bruno RM, Ghiadoni L, Seravalle G, Dell'oro R, Taddei S, Grassi G. Sympathetic regulation of vascular function in health and disease. Frontiers in Physiology. 2012;**3**:284. DOI: 10.3389/fphys.2012.00284. eCollection 2012

[88] Amiya E, Watanabe M, Komuro I. The relationship between vascular function and the autonomic nervous system. Annals of Vascular Diseases. 2014;**7**(2):109-119. DOI: 10.3400/avd.ra.14-00048. Review

[89] Conti V, Russomanno G, Corbi G, et al. Adrenoreceptors and nitric oxide in the cardiovascular system. Frontiers in Physiology. 2013;**4**:321. DOI: 10.3389/fphys.2013.00321. Review

[90] Forte M, Conti V, Damato A, et al. Targeting nitric oxide with natural derived compounds as a therapeutic strategy in vascular diseases. Oxidative Medicine and Cellular Longevity. 2016;**2016**:7364138. DOI: 10.1155/2016/7364138. Review

[91] Hijmering ML, Stroes ESG, Olijhoek J, Hutten BA, Blankestijn PJ, Rabelink TJ. Sympathetic activation markedly reduces endothelium dependent, flow-mediated vasodilation. Journal of the American College of Cardiology. 2002;**39**:683-688

[92] Kaplon RE, Walker AE, Seals DR. Plasma norepinephrine is an independent predictor of vascular endothelial function with aging in healthy women. Journal of Applied Physiology. 2011;**111**:1416-1421

[93] Michiels C. Endothelial cells functions. Journal of Cellular Physiology. 2003;**193**:430-443. DOI: 10.1002/jcp.10333

[94] Mestas J, Ley K. Monocyte-endothelial cell interactions in the development of atherosclerosis. Trends in Cardiovascular Medicine. 2008;**18**:228-232

[95] Tammela T, Enholm B, Alitalo K, Paavonen K. The biology of vascular endothelial growth factors. Cardiovascular Research. 2005;**65**(3):550-563. Review

[96] Michaelis UR. Mechanisms of endothelial cell migration. Cellular and Molecular Life Sciences. 2014;**71**(21):4131-4148. DOI: 10.1007/s00018-014-1678-0. Review

[97] Melero-Martin JM, Khan ZA, Picard A, et al. In vivo vasculogenic potential of human blood-derived endothelial progenitor cells. Blood. 2007;**109**:4761-4768

[98] Nowak K, Rafat N, Belle S, et al. Circulating endothelial progenitor cells are increased in human lung cancer and correlate with stage of disease. European Journal of Cardio-Thoracic Surgery. 2010;**37**:758-763

[99] Germain S, Monnot C, Muller L, Eichmann A. Hypoxia driven angiogenesis: Role of tip cells and extracellular matrix scaffolding. Current Opinion in Hematology. 2010;**17**:245-251

[100] Hlatky L, Hahnfeldt P, Folkman J. Clinical application of antiangiogenic therapy: Microvessel density, what it does and doesn't tell us. Journal of the National Cancer Institute. 2002;**94**(12):883-893. Review

[101] Folkman J. Angiogenic therapy of the human heart. Circulation. 1998;**97**(7):628-629

[102] Eelen G, de Zeeuw P, Simons M, Carmeliet P. Endothelial cell metabolism in normal and diseased vasculature. Circulation Research. 2015;**116**(7):1231-1244. DOI: 10.1161/CIRCRESAHA.116.302855

[103] Artwohl M, Brunmair B, Fürnsinn C, et al. Insulin does not regulate glucose transport and metabolism in human endothelium. European Journal of Clinical Investigation. 2007;**37**(8):643-650

[104] Gero D, Szabo C. Glucocorticoids suppress mitochondrial oxidant production via upregulation of uncoupling protein 2 in hyperglycemic endothelial cells. PLoS One. 2016;**11**(4):e0154813

[105] Kluge MA, Fetterman JL, Vita JA. Mitochondria and endothelial function. Circulation Research. 2013;**112**(8):1171-1188

[106] Zhang DX, Gutterman DD. Mitochondrial reactive oxygen species mediated signaling in endothelial cells. American Journal of Physiology. Heart and Circulatory Physiology. 2007;**292**:H2023-H2031

[107] Trifunovic A, Larsson NG. Mitochondrial dysfunction as a cause of ageing. Journal of Internal Medicine. 2008;**263**(2):167-178. DOI: 10.1111/j.1365-2796.2007.01905.x

[108] Conley KE, Jubrias SA, Amara CE, Marcinek DJ. Mitochondrial dysfunction: Impact on exercise performance and cellular aging. Exercise and Sport Sciences Reviews. 2007;**35**:43-49

[109] Yu E, Mercer J, Bennett M. Mitochondria in vascular disease. Cardiovascular Research. 2012;**95**(2):173-182. DOI: 10.1093/cvr/cvs111. Review

[110] Chandel NS, Schumacker PT. Cellular oxygen sensing by mitochondria: Old questions, new insight. Journal of Applied Physiology. 2000;**88**:1880-1889

[111] Schiff M, Benit P, Coulibaly A, et al. Mitochondrial response to controlled nutrition in health and disease. Nutrition Reviews. 2011;**69**:65-75

[112] Houtkooper RH, Pirinen E, Auwerx J. Sirtuins as regulators of metabolism and healthspan. Nature Reviews. Molecular Cell Biology. 2012;**13**(4):225-238

[113] Fleming I. Vascular cytochrome p450 enzymes: Physiology and pathophysiology. Trends in Cardiovascular Medicine. 2008;**18**(1):20-25. DOI: 10.1016/j.tcm.2007.11.002. Review. 20-

[114] Wu CC, Gupta T, Garcia V, et al. HETE and blood pressure regulation: Clinical implications. Cardiology in Review. 2014;**22**(1):1-12. DOI: 10.1097/CRD.0b013e3182961659

[115] Félétou M, Huang Y, Vanhoutte PM. Endothelium-mediated control of vascular tone: COX-1 and COX-2 products. British Journal of Pharmacology. 2011;**164**(3):894-912. DOI: 10.1111/j.1476-5381.2011.01276.x. Review

[116] Pohl U, De Wit C, Gloe T. Large arterioles in the control of blood flow: Role of endothelium-dependent dilation. Acta Physiologica Scandinavica. 2000;**168**(4):505-510. Review

[117] Szerafin T, Erdei N, Fülöp T, et al. Increased cyclooxygenase-2 expression and prostaglandin-mediated dilation in coronary arterioles of patients with diabetes mellitus. Circulation Research. 2006;**99**:e12-e17

[118] Ward NC, Croft KD, Blacker D, et al. Cytochrome P450 metabolites of arachidonic acid are elevated in stroke patients compared with healthy controls. Clinical Science (London, England). 2011;**121**(11):501-507

[119] Bagher P, Segal SS. Regulation of blood flow in the microcirculation; role of conducted vasodilation. Acta Physiologica. 2011;**202**:271-284

[120] Du XL, Edelstein D, Dimmeler S, et al. Hyperglycemia inhibits endothelial nitric oxide synthase activity by posttranslational modification at the Akt site. The Journal of Clinical Investigation. 2001;**108**:1341-1348

[121] Mattagajasingh I, Kim CS, Naqvi A, et al. SIRT1 promotes endothelium-dependent vascular relaxation by activating endothelial nitric oxide synthase. Proceedings of the National Academy of Sciences of the United States of America. 2007;**104**:14855-14860

[122] Jung SB, Kim CS, Naqvi A, et al. Histone deacetylase 3 antagonizes aspirin-stimulated endothelial nitric oxide production by reversing aspirin-induced lysine acetylation of endothelial nitric oxide synthase. Circulation Research. 2010;**107**:877-887

[123] Nishikawa Y, Stepp DW, Chilian WM. Nitric oxide exerts feedback inhibition on EDHF-induced coronary arteriolar dilation in vivo. American Journal of Physiology. Heart and Circulatory Physiology. 2000;**279**:H459-H465

[124] Mitsutomi N, Akashi C, Odagiri J, Matsumara Y. Effects of endogenous and exogenous nitric oxide on endothelin-1 production in cultured vascular endothelial cells. European Journal of Pharmacology. 1999;**364**:65-73

[125] Heinonen I, Saltin B, Kemppainen J, et al. Effect of nitric oxide synthase inhibition on the exchange of glucose and fatty acids in human skeletal muscle. Nutrition & Metabolism (London). 2013;**10**(1):43-10

[126] Trochu JN, Bouhour JB, Kaley G, Hintze TH. Role of endothelium-derived nitric oxide in the regulation of cardiac oxygen metabolism: Implications in health and disease. Circulation Research. 2000;**87**(12):1108-1117. Review

[127] Hartmann C, Nussbaum B, Calzia E, et al. Gaseous mediators and mitochondrial function: The future of pharmacologically induced suspended animation? Frontiers in Physiology. 2017;**8**:691. DOI: 10.3389/fphys.2017.00691. eCollection 2017

[128] Katakam PV, Wappler EA, Katz PS, et al. Depolarization of mitochondria in endothelial cells promotes cerebral artery vasodilation by activation of nitric oxide synthase. Arteriosclerosis, Thrombosis, and Vascular Biology. 2013;**33**(4):752-759. DOI: 10.1161/ATVBAHA.112.300560

[129] Jaitovich A, Jourd'heuil D. A brief overview of nitric oxide and reactive oxygen species signaling in hypoxia-induced pulmonary hypertension. Advances in Experimental Medicine and Biology. 2017;**967**:71-81. DOI: 10.1007/978-3-319-63245-2_6. Review

[130] Vanhoutte PM, Shimokawa H, Feletou M, Tang EH. Endothelial dysfunction and vascular disease—A 30th anniversary update. Acta Physiologica (Oxford, England). 2017;**219**(1):22-96. DOI: 10.1111/apha.12646. Review

[131] Li H, Forstermann U. Pharmacological prevention of eNOS uncoupling. Current Pharmaceutical Design. 2014;**20**(22):3595-3606. Review

[132] Cai H. Hydrogen peroxide regulation of endothelial function: Origins, mechanisms, and consequences. Cardiovascular Research. 2005;**68**:26-36. DOI: 10.1016/j.cardiores.2005.06.021

[133] Chidgey J, Fraser PA, Aaronson PI. Reactive oxygen species facilitate the EDH response in arterioles by potentiating intracellular endothelial Ca(2+) release. Free Radical Biology & Medicine. 2016;**97**:274-284. DOI: 10.1016/j.freeradbiomed.2016.06.010

[134] Phillips SA, Hatoum OA, Gutterman DD. The mechanism of flow-induced dilation in human adipose arterioles involves hydrogen peroxide during CAD. American Journal of Physiology. Heart and Circulatory Physiology. 2007;**92**:H93-H100

[135] Drenjančević I et al. The metabolites of arachidonic acid in microvascular function. In: Lensi H, editor. Microcirculation Revisited: From Molecules to Clinical Practice. Rijeka: InTech; 2016. pp. 101-133. DOI: 10.5772/61893

[136] Campbell WB, Fleming I. Epoxyeicosatrienoic acids and endothelium-dependent responses. Pflügers Archiv. 2010;**459**(6):881-895. DOI: 10.1007/s00424-010-0804-6. Review

[137] Sandoo A, van Zanten JJ, Metsios GS, et al. The endothelium and its role in regulating vascular tone. Open Cardiovascular Medicine Journal. 2010;**4**:302-312

[138] Cavka A, Cosic A, Jukic I, et al. The role of cyclo-oxygenase-1 in high-salt diet-induced microvascular dysfunction in humans. The Journal of Physiology. 2015;**593**(24):5313-5324. DOI: 10.1113/JP271631

[139] Egan K, FitzGerald GA. Eicosanoids and the vascular endothelium. Handbook of Experimental Pharmacology. 2006;**176**(Pt1):189-211. DOI: 10.1007/3-540-32967-6

[140] Miura H, Bosnjak JJ, Ning G, et al. Role for hydrogen peroxide in flow-induced dilation of human coronary arterioles. Circulation Research. 2001;**92**:e31-e40

[141] Bellien J, Joannides R, Iacob M, et al. Evidence for a basal release of a cytochrome-related endothelium-derived hyperpolarizing factor in the radial artery in humans. American Journal of Physiology. Heart and Circulatory Physiology. 2006;**290**:H1347-HH352. DOI: 10.1152/ajpheart.01079.2005

[142] Inokuchi K, Hirooka Y, Shimokawa H, et al. Role of endothelium-derived hyperpolarizing factor in human forearm circulation. Hypertension. 2003;**42**(5):919-924

[143] Lenasi H, Strucl M. The effect of nitric oxide synthase and cyclooxygenase inhibition on cutaneous microvascular reactivity. European Journal of Applied Physiology. 2008;**103**(6):719-726. DOI: 10.1007/s00421-008-0769-8

[144] Heinonen I, Saltin B, Kemppainen J, et al. Skeletal muscle blood flow and oxygen uptake at rest and during exercise in humans: A pet study with nitric oxide and cyclooxygenase inhibition. American Journal of Physiology. Heart and Circulatory Physiology. 2011;**300**(4):H1510-H1517. DOI: 10.1152/ajpheart.00996.2010

[145] Félétou M, Vanhoutte PM. EDHF: An update. Clinical Science (London, England). 2009;**117**(4):139-155. DOI: 10.1042/CS20090096. Review

[146] Quyyumi AA, Ozkor M. Vasodilation by hyperpolarization: Beyond NO. Hypertension. 2006;**48**(6):1023-1025

[147] Goto K, Ohtsubo T, Kitazono T. Endothelium-dependent hyperpolarization (EDH) in hypertension: The role of endothelial ion channels. International Journal of Molecular Sciences. 2018;**19**(1):pii: E315. DOI: 10.3390/ijms19010315. Review

[148] Filosa JA, Yao X, Rath G. TRPV4 and the regulation of vascular tone. Journal of Cardiovascular Pharmacology. 2013;**61**(2):113-119. DOI: 10.1097/FJC.0b013e318279ba42. Review

[149] Mathew John C, Khaddaj Mallat R, George G, et al. Pharmacologic targeting of endothelial Ca^{2+}-activated K^{+} channels: A strategy to improve cardiovascular function. Channels (Austin, Tex.). 2018;**12**(1):126-136. DOI: 10.1080/19336950.2018.1454814

[150] Feher A, Broskova Z, Bagi Z. Age-related impairment of conducted dilation in human coronary arterioles. American Journal of Physiology. Heart and Circulatory Physiology. 2014;**306**:H1595-H1601

[151] Lan WR, Hou CJ, Yen CH, et al. Effects of carbenoxolone on flow-mediated vasodilatation in healthy adults. American Journal of Physiology-Heart and Circulatory Physiology. 2011;**301**(3):H1166-H1172. DOI: 10.1152/ajpheart.00967.2010

[152] Dora KA. Endothelial-smooth muscle cell interactions in the regulation of vascular tone in skeletal muscle. Microcirculation. 2016;**23**(8):626-630. DOI: 10.1111/micc.12322. Review

[153] de Wit C. Different pathways with distinct properties conduct dilations in the microcirculation in vivo. Cardiovascular Research. 2010;**85**:604-613

[154] Leung SW, Vanhoutte PM. Endothelium-dependent hyperpolarization: Age, gender and blood pressure, do they matter? Acta Physiologica (Oxford, England). 2017;**219**(1):108-123. DOI: 10.1111/apha.12628. Epub 2015 Dec 1. Review

[155] Cacanyiova S, Berenyiova A, Kristek F. The role of hydrogen sulphide in blood pressure regulation. Physiological Research. 2016;**65**(Suppl. 3):S273-S289. Review

[156] Kajimura M, Fukuda R, Bateman RM, et al. Interactions of multiple gas-transducing systems: Hallmarks and uncertainties of CO, NO, and H2S gas biology. Antioxidants & Redox Signaling. 2010;**13**:157-192. DOI: 10.1089/ars.2009.2657

[157] Zukowska P, Kutryb-Zajac B, Toczek M, et al. The role of ecto-5′-nucleotidase in endothelial dysfunction and vascular pathologies. Pharmacological Reports. 2015;**67**(4):675-681. DOI: 10.1016/j.pharep.2015.05.002. Review

[158] Crecelius AR, Kirby BS, Luckasen GJ, et al. ATP-mediated vasodilatation occurs via activation of inwardly rectifying potassium channels in humans. The Journal of Physiology. 2012;**590**:5349-5359

Chapter 2

Hox Genes in Adult Tissues and Their Role in Endothelial Cell Differentiation and Angiogenesis

Estefanía Nova-Lampeti, Valeria Aguilera, Katherine Oporto, Paula Guzmán, Valeska Ormazábal, Felipe Zúñiga, Carlos Escudero and Claudio Aguayo

Additional information is available at the end of the chapter

http://dx.doi.org/10.5772/intechopen.76745

Abstract

HOX genes belong to a family of transcription factors characterized by a 183 bp DNA sequence called homeobox, which code for a 61-amino-acid domain defined as the homeodomain. These genes play a central role during embryonic development by controlling body organization, organogenesis, and stem cell differentiation. They can also play a role in adult processes such as embryo implantation, hematopoiesis, and endothelial differentiation. Since endothelial cell differentiation is one of the main steps to initiate vasculogenesis and angiogenesis, we analyzed the role of several Hox genes in the regulation of these two processes. In this chapter, we summarized the evidence to support the function of Hox genes in adult tissues, specifically in endothelial cell differentiation, by studying their mechanism of action and how their target genes regulate vasculogenesis and angiogenesis. Understanding the cellular and molecular mechanisms triggered by Hox biological effects is pivotal for designing new drugs or therapies for high prevalent pathologies, such as cardiovascular diseases.

Keywords: Hox genes, endothelial cell differentiation, angiogenesis, vasculogenesis, embryonic development

1. Overview

Hox genes are responsible for the expression of a large family of transcriptional factors that play a key role in embryonic development, organogenesis, and anteroposterior body orientation

[1, 2]. Even though the main function of these genes is well known during embryogenesis, their role in adults remains under investigation. Several studies have linked Hox genes with adult processes such as vascularization, hematopoiesis, tumor angiogenesis, and cell differentiation [3]. In this chapter, we will focus our attention on the origin and main role of Hox genes in adult tissues, especially on endothelial cell differentiation, neovasculogenesis, and angiogenesis.

2. Origin of the Hox gene cluster

The Hox genes were discovered in 1915 by Calvin Bridges in a mutant *Drosophila melanogaster* named Bithorax, which showed a partial duplication of the thorax [4]. Years later, another mutation in the Hox genes was identified resulting in a mutant fly exhibiting legs instead of antenna named Antennapedia [5]. The Hox genes were then grouped into these two complexes (Bithorax and Antennapedia), which are located on chromosome 3 and play a key role in conferring the identity along the anteroposterior axis of the body. The role of these genes in establishing the anteroposterior axis is highly conserved in vertebrates [5, 6]; however, the Hox gene cluster has changed during its evolution, evidenced by different numbers of clusters between species (**Figure 1**). For example, whereas invertebrates typically possess a single cluster, vertebrates such as mice and humans possess four gene clusters coding for the three different axes: cervical, thoracic, and lumbosacral [2, 6]. Despite these differences, Hox genes have been identified in all species, which reflects the important role of these genes in the regulation of body structure [1, 7]. In humans, the 39 mammalian Hox genes are grouped into four chromosomal clusters named *HOXA*, *HOXB*, *HOXC*, and *HOXD*, located on chromosomes 7p14, 17q21, 12q13, and 2q31, respectively [8]. This large family encodes homeodomain transcription factors that share highly conserved DNA sequence formed by 183 bp called "homeobox," which encodes a polypeptide core of 61 amino acids formed by three alpha helices known as the homeodomain. Most homeodomains recognize highly conserved DNA elements that

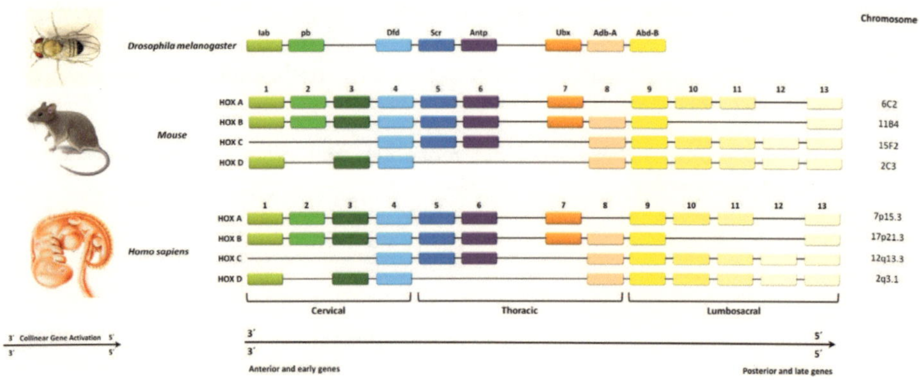

Figure 1. The composition and evolutionary differences of the HOX gene cluster between *Drosophila melanogaster*, mouse, and *Homo sapiens*. The HOX gene clusters and their chromosomal location were compared between *Drosophila melanogaster*, mouse, and *Homo sapiens*. Genes were grouped according to the distribution of the three axes corresponding to the anteroposterior part of the body (cervical, thoracic, lumbosacral).

serve as a promoter for many genes (motif TAAT) being a T in the direction 5′ determinant for this coupling acknowledgment [9]. Hox transcription factors are well known for playing a key role during cell and tissue differentiation in developing embryos; however, other studies have shown that these homeotic genes also play a role in adult process such as hematopoiesis and embryo implantation by promoting neovasculogenesis and angiogenesis [10].

3. Hox genes in adult-related processes

3.1. Endometrial tissue

Hox genes are crucial during endometrium redevelopment and corpus luteum formation because they regulate cell growth and differentiation during each reproductive cycle [10]. Expression of HoxA10 in human epithelial and stromal endometrial cells has been significantly higher in the intermediate and late phase of the menstrual cycle, suggesting that it could favor the implantation of the embryo [11–13]. Mechanistically, the protein encoded by this gene regulates the expression of several proteins related to endometrial development such as Emx2/EMX2, integrin β3, insulin-like growth factor-binding protein-1 (IGFBP-1), cyclin inhibitors, Wnt family genes, and the prostaglandin receptors EP-3 and EP-4 [14, 15].

Endometrium development is regulated by estrogen and progesterone; thus, any regulation of Hox genes by these hormones suggests that these genes play a role in the growth and development of the endometrium. For example, 17β-estradiol and progesterone significantly increased the expression of HoxA10 in endometrial cells [16] and primary culture of stromal endometrial cells, respectively, with a higher response induced by progesterone compared to 17β-estradiol [17] and even higher when both hormones were used in combination [17, 18].

HOXA11 is another hox gene from the A cluster that has been closely associated with morphological alterations [19]. During the development of the female reproductive tract, *HOXA11* is normally expressed in the cervix and lower uterine segment. When the expression of this gene is impaired, it promotes aberrant epithelial cell differentiation leading to epithelial ovarian neoplasia [20, 21]. In addition, $HOXA11^{-/-}$ mice exhibit reduced development of the stroma in the glandular tissue and decidua during pregnancy [18, 22], suggesting a role in myometrium preparation to implantation.

More recently, Yim et al. suggested that *HOXA11* promotes metastasis by regulating the expression of gene coding for metastasis-related proteins [23]. These findings indicate that *HOXA11* plays a role in the aggressive nature of ovarian cancer cells through *HOXA11*-mediated expression of target genes such as matrix metalloproteinase (MMP) and VEGF.

3.2. Implantation

Implantation is a series of sequential biological events triggered after fertilization in which the blastocyst migrates from the fallopian tube into the uterus. The fertilized egg is then attached to the uterine wall and subsequently implanted in the endometrium. Implantation occurs only in a very specific time period and place during the mid-secretory phase of the uterine cycle [24]. During this period, the uterus becomes more receptive by promoting a series of cellular and molecular events favoring the implantation of the embryo. In this stage, the role of several intercellular mediators has been implicated, which include specific cytokines, growth factors, adhesion molecules, lipid mediators, steroid hormones, and Hox transcription factors [25]. Like in endometrial tissue, *HOXA10* also plays a role during embryo implantation as it has been shown that despite the fact that *HOXA10*-deficient mice (*HOXA10*$^{-/-}$) exhibited normal ovulation cycle, the implantation did not occur. Interestingly, implantation was restored when embryos from *HOXA10*$^{-/-}$ were transferred to wild-type mice; however, wild-type embryos were not implanted in *HOXA10*$^{-/-}$ female mice [18], suggesting that *HOXA10* is required to have an adequate implantation environment. Moreover, *HOXA10*$^{-/-}$ and *HOXA11*$^{-/-}$ mice also exhibit poor implantation due to insufficient development of stromal glandular tissue and decidua during pregnancy [26]. In humans, the expression of both *HOXA10* and *HOXA11* genes rises gradually during the proliferative phase of the menstrual cycle, showing a peak of expression in mid-cycle, when implantation typically occurs [13, 27]. Interestingly, this peak of expression was not observed in women with endometriosis or in mice with induced endometriosis [13, 27], suggesting that HoxA10 and HoxA11 peaks require a healthy endometrium to support and continue with the implantation process. Several studies have shown that Hox10 not only promotes implantation directly but also inhibits detrimental factors such as empty spiracles homeobox 2 (EMX2), P300/CBP-associated factor (P/CAF), and gamma-aminobutyric acid (GABA). Studies by Taylor and colleagues demonstrated that HoxA10 repressed EMX2 expression, which in turn inhibited the proliferation of endometrial cells [28], suggesting that HoxA10 is a pro-proliferative and pro-implantation factor in these cells. Zhu and colleagues demonstrated that HoxA10 repressed the promoter activity of P/CAF, which impairs endometrial receptivity and embryo implantation by downregulating integrin β3 [29]. Recent studies have also shown that HoxA10 decreased mRNA levels and protein translocation of GABA receptor [30], which plays a role in the generation of uterine contractions and labor [31]. Thus, the quiescent uterus is required for adequate implantation and embryo development, along with reduced expression or activity of GABA receptor.

3.3. Hematopoiesis

Hox genes are highly expressed in hematopoietic stem cells (HSC) and immature progenitor cells [32]; however, this expression is gradually decreased upon cell differentiation. Moreover, overexpression of genes from the *HOXA* cluster impairs B and T lymphocyte differentiation, affects erythropoiesis, and reduces stem cell bone marrow homing, favoring the induction of myeloproliferative disorders and leukemias [33]. In fact, overexpression of *HOXA1*, *HOXA4*, and *HOXA6* genes has been shown to favor the generation of permanent cell lines [34]. Studies by Wang et al. showed increased proliferation and higher self-growth and self-renewal of hematopoietic stem progenitor cells (HSC) (Line 9 and Line H1) when HoxA6 was overexpressed compared to normal conditions [34]. The authors observed that overexpression of this gene sustained HSC self-renewal and multipotency by promoting mature erythroid lineage cells and partial apoptosis of erythroid progenitors.

Another gene involved in this process is *HOXA5*. Overexpression of HoxA5 in HSC isolated from umbilical cord blood, bone marrow [35], or mice [36] promotes a significant shift toward myeloid differentiation in relation to erythroid differentiation when compared to respective control cells [35, 36]. Then, the authors evaluated genes affected by HoxA5, and they observed downregulation of several genes involved in cell proliferation, differentiation, and metabolism [35, 36].

HOXA9 has also been associated with the regulation of myeloid cell differentiation. The activation of HoxA9 complex favors the recruitment of CREB-binding protein (CBP/p300), histone acetylation, and activation of a number of transcription factors and proto-oncogenes, including Erg, FLT3, and SOX4 Myb, which regulate hematopoiesis [37].

Another Hox gene family member linked to hematopoiesis is *HOXA10*. The expression of this gene is high in myeloid progenitor cells, and it decreases during cell maturation [38]. Bei et al. [39] studied the expression of HoxA10 in bone marrow from patients with human acute myeloid leukemia (AML), and they observed increased expression of this gene in patients with poor prognosis. Then, they developed a HoxA10-overexpresing mouse model identifying *CDX4*, a caudal gene that contain homeodomain and code for transcription factor that plays an important role in hematopoiesis, as a *HOXA10* target gene [39]. Overall, their results demonstrated that *HOXA10* was contributing to AML pathogenesis via CDX4-positive feedback. Other groups demonstrated that HoxA13 was associated with the development of monocytes and macrophages, and its expression was observed more often in monocytic leukemia cell lines in comparison with other types of leukemia [40]. Moreover, the expression of genes *HOXB3* and *HOXB4* has been found to be altered in patients with AML with poor prognosis [41].

4. Hox genes in vascularity and angiogenesis

The development of the vascular system involves two processes called vasculogenesis and angiogenesis [42]. During vasculogenesis, angioblasts derived from different sources, including mesodermal embryonic layer or bone marrow, differentiate into endothelial cells and subsequently form a primitive network of tubular structures called blood vessels [43]. Vasculogenesis occurs largely during embryonic development; however, the presence of a population of circulating endothelial progenitor cells (EPCs) derived from the bone marrow in adults strongly suggests that this process may occur in the postnatal period [44]. In contrast, angiogenesis refers to the formation of new blood vessels from preexisting vessels by cell migration and remodeling of the primitive vascular network [45]. Vasculogenesis and angiogenesis are involved in the development of the functional vascular system in the embryo and the formation of blood vessels in the postnatal period. Both vasculogenesis and angiogenesis are under the regulation of several growth factors, which include vascular endothelial growth factor (VEGF), fibroblast growth factor 2 (FGF2), platelet-derived growth factor (PDGF), and transforming growth factor β1 (TGF-β1), among others [45]. Interestingly, different research groups have found that Hox genes regulate the expression of these growth factors and, in turn, endothelial cell differentiation. In the next section, we will describe supporting evidence about the role of Hox genes in endothelial differentiation, vasculogenesis, and angiogenesis (**Figure 2**).

4.1. HOXA3

The *HOXA3* gene is required for modeling the anterior body plan during embryogenesis, but they can also play a role in promoting angiogenesis [46, 47]. It has been shown that activation of *HOXA3* favors the migration of endothelial cells and keratinocytes, associated with increased expression of urokinase-type plasminogen activator receptor (uPAR) in

Figure 2. HOX genes modulate the expression of crucial target genes to promote the differentiation of mature endothelial cells. Hox genes promote the differentiation of endothelial progenitor cells, which exhibit an immature phenotype ($CD70^+CD34^+Oct\text{-}4^+$), into mature endothelial cells that express endothelial nitric oxide synthase (eNOS), vascular endothelial growth factor receptor 2 (VEGFR2 or KDR), CD31, von Willebrand factor (vWF), and the lectin-type oxidized LDL receptor 1 (LOX-1). To promote this phenotype, some Hox genes upregulate crucial genes such as fetal liver kinase 1 (Flk1), angiopoietin 2 (ANG2), ephrin type-B receptor 4 (EphB4), and FI3K receptor, whereas other Hox genes downregulate other factors such as hypoxia-induced factor type 1α (HIF1α), cyclooxygenase-2 (cox-2), ephrin type-a receptor 1 (EphwA1), and VEGFR2.

both in vitro and in vivo studies using mice [46, 47]. Similar results were demonstrated by Hansen et al. who confirmed that *HOXA3* is a potent inducer of angiogenesis in vivo and also promotes direct keratinocyte migration [48]. These results suggest that *HOXA3* potentiates two key processes involved in efficient wound repair: angiogenesis and reepithelialization [46, 48]. Gene transfer studies of *HOXA3* suggest that this gene also functions as a potent inducer of wound repair in genetically modified diabetic animals. A single application of protein HoxA3 resulted in complete healing of wounds after 42 days, while wounds treated with the control plasmid without *HOXA3* (β gal) required 77 days for complete tissue repair. In addition, it was demonstrated that secreted protein HoxA3 or HoxA5, coming from respective genes and derived from composite skin constructs, exhibits decreased expression of CCL-2 and CxCL-12 inflammatory mediators, which play a key role in the attraction of monocytes, macrophages, and other wound immune cells [48]. Thus, reduced recruitment of leukocytes mediated by *HOXA3* may contribute to the prolonged integrity and viability of the composite skin constructs expressing *HOXA3*, by reducing inflammation during wound healing process. Taken together, the combined actions of HoxA3 on endothelial cells and keratinocytes lead to increased angiogenesis, normal epidermal differentiation, reduced expression of inflammatory mediators, and reduced graft contraction. These effects suggest that HoxA3 may have therapeutic benefits in wound repair by improving the integrity of composite skin grafts.

4.2. HOXA9

The *HOXA9* gene code for two different proteins, HA-9A and HA-9B isoform A (HA-9A) and HoxA9 protein isoform B (HA-9B) [49] that share a common homeodomain [15]. The expression of HA-9A has been observed exclusively during fetal development, whereas the HA-9B has been found not only in fetal but also in adult organism and specifically in endothelial cells [49, 50].

In 2004, Bruhl et al. showed that *HOXA9* was able to regulate angiogenesis [51]. These authors using human umbilical vein endothelial cells (HUVECs) with sense/antisense oligonucleotides or siRNA for this gene observed that *HOXA9* expression was essential for endothelial cell migration and tube formation. Also, they evaluated the regulation of ephrin type-B (Eph) receptor B4

(EphB4) by *HOXA9*, since previous reports [52, 53] showed that Eph receptors were homeobox protein potential targets. Then, they decided to study EphB4 since it was specifically associated with angiogenesis and cell migration processes [54, 55]. After elegant experimentation and analysis, they conclude that HoxA9 regulated endothelial cell migration and tube formation by promoting the expression of EphB4. Later in 2012, Zhang and colleagues established that HoxA9 was essential for postnatal neovascularization in vivo. In addition, they found that HoxA9 was able to regulate the expression of endothelial genes such as endothelial nitric oxide synthase (eNOS), vascular endothelial growth factor receptor 2 (VEGFR2), and VE-cadherin in vitro in mature endothelial cells exposed to "shear stress" [56]. Furthermore, the *HOXA9*$^{-/-}$ mouse model showed a reduced number of circulating endothelial progenitor cells (EPCs) as well as reduced overall postnatal neovascularization after ischemia compared to wild-type mice. Altogether, these results demonstrated that HoxA9 is critical for postnatal neovascularization [57].

4.3. HOXA13

The central function of the placenta is to allow the formation of a vascular labyrinth, a juxtaposed series of finely branched blood vessels and trophoblast that regulate the exchange of nutrients and residues while maintaining the separation of maternal and fetal blood supplies. The study by Shaut et al. showed a morphological alteration in the labyrinth endothelial cells, branching of the vessels, and in the integrity of the vessels when *HOXA13* was dysfunctional [58, 59]. These findings suggest that *HOXA13* regulates a number of genes in the vascular endothelium required for vessel adhesion and branching, providing a functional explanation of the mean gestational lethality exhibited by *HOXA13* mutant mice. The same authors identified that EphA6 and EphA7 were direct transcriptional targets of *HOXA13* in the genital tubercle vascular endothelia [59]. Altogether, these findings provide a new genetic pathway to consider when placental pathologies or placental evolutionary ontogeny are characterized. Evidence for this coordination is observed in the labyrinth endothelium, where the genes required for cell adhesion and vascular branching are affected concomitantly by the loss of *HOXA13* function, including Neuropilin-1, Enpp2, Lyve1, Caveolin-1, Foxf1, and Tie2, resulting in reduced levels of provascular factors required for the vascular development of the labyrinth [58].

Besides HoxA genes, the HoxB and HoxD loci have also been involved in endothelial and angiogenesis regulation processes [60]. HUVECs, for example, express several genes from these loci [7], and it has been shown that some of these genes inhibit in vitro proliferation of HUVECs, whereas others have been associated with increased capillary morphogenesis and vasculogenesis [61].

4.4. HOXB1

Previous studies have revealed an overlap between HoxA1 and HoxB1 functions during the specification of the rhombomeres, a transiently divided segment of the developing neural tube, from which neural crest cells emerge. It has been demonstrated that both HoxA1 and HoxB1 functions are required for the heart development [62, 63]. HoxB1$^{-/-}$ embryos were previously described as embryos with normal pharyngeal arch arteries and cardiac neural crest-derived tissue remodeling [64]. However, more recently, Roux et al. observed one HoxB1 mutant embryo with an aortic arch artery defect, which is characteristic of a developmental failure of the left pharyngeal arch arteries (PAA) [65]. These data suggest that *HOXB1* is important for PAA formation, and the authors provide a novel model to study the molecular origin of great artery defects, which are often observed in human patients.

4.5. HOXB3

The function of the *HOXB3* gene was studied after finding the function of its paralogous gene, *HOXD3*. While *HOXD3* is required for mediating the invasive and migratory behavior of endothelial cells during the early stages of neovascularization, *HOXB3* is required for the morphogenesis of new capillary tubes, suggesting that these paralogous Hox genes may perform complementary functions [53]. The authors also found that the capillary morphogenesis induced by *HOXB3* was mediated by ephrin A1 ligand (EFNA1) [53].

4.6. HOXB5

The *HOXB5* gene, also known as Hox-2.1, codes for a potent transcriptional regulator present in several adult tissues. Similar to *HOXA9*, *HOXB5* has been associated with vascular alterations. In this regard, studies have shown that *HOXB5* homeobox protein regulates the expression of VEGFR2, the earliest marker of endothelial precursors, by direct binding to the *HOXB5*-binding element (HBE) in the VEGFR2 gene [66]. They also found that overexpression of HoxB5 increased the number of angioblasts during embryonic stem cell differentiation and the number of mature endothelial cells, which in turn have been associated with high expression of platelet endothelial cell adhesion molecule (PECAM) and the formation of primitive blood vessels [66]. Years later, the same research group investigated the in vivo role of HoxB5 in angiogenesis using the chick (*Gallus gallus*) chorioallantoic membrane assay. They concluded that HoxB5 exerted an activating effect on angiopoietin 2 (ANG2), which was essential for endothelial cell sprouting and vascular growth [60]. More recently, the same group investigated the role of HoxB5 overexpression during revascularization in ischemic disease using femoral artery ligation in C57BL/6 mice. They observed that HoxB5 enhanced perfusion restoration and increased capillary density in vivo via monocyte chemotactic protein-1 (MCP-1) and interleukin-6 (IL-6) upregulation and increased endothelial cell migration [67].

Furthermore, other studies have shown that HoxB5 is a transactivator of the promoter of VEGFR2, an early marker of endothelial precursors [66], which might be involved in the differentiation of mesoderm-derived precursors toward an endothelial phenotype [66, 68]. In fact, it has been described that overexpression of HoxB5 leads to differentiation of mesoderm-derived precursors toward the endothelial phenotype, which in turn lead to high expression of angiopoietin 2 (ANG2) and therefore enhance vascularization in a model of fertilized white Leghorn chicken eggs [68].

4.7. HOXB7

HOXB7 has been associated with tumor progression and angiogenesis [61]. Care et al. in 2001 provided evidence that HoxB7 promotes tumor-associated angiogenesis by increasing the expression of VEGF, melanoma growth stimulatory activity/growth-related oncogene alpha, interleukin-8, and angiopoietin 2 (ANG2) in SkBr3 cells [69]. The authors concluded that HoxB7 acted as a key factor in a tumor-associated angiogenic switch [69]. In 2008, Murthi et al. identified differences in the expression of HoxB7 between micro- and macrovascular endothelial cells [70]. They observed higher expression of HoxB7 in macrovascular HUVECs and placenta compared to microvascular endothelial cells such as human placental endothelial cell (HPEC) line, human microvascular endothelial cells (HMVEC), and freshly isolated placental microvascular endothelial cells (PLEC). Storti et al. found that HoxB7 was expressed in 10 out of 22 multiple myeloma patients analyzed at the diagnosis related to high bone marrow angiogenesis [61]. They also found that HoxB7 was overexpressed in about 40% of myeloma cell lines compared with normal plasma cells [61]. Furthermore, they observed that HoxB7 overexpression in multiple myeloma cells significantly modified their transcriptional and angiogenic profile by upregulating VEGF, fibroblast growth factor 2 (FGF2), metalloproteinase-2 (MMP-2), platelet-derived growth factor A (PDGFA), and WNT5a, while HoxB7 also downregulates thrombospondin-2, an inhibitor of angiogenesis [61]. Finally, the homeobox gene HoxB7 is overexpressed across a range of cancers and promotes tumorigenesis by inducing cell proliferation, survival, invasion, and tumor angiogenesis in pancreatic adenocarcinoma [71], cervical cancer [72], glioblastoma tumors [73], and breast cancer [74].

4.8. HOXD1

HOXD1 is specifically expressed in mature endothelial cells compared to early-stage EPC [62, 75]. However, not only HoxD1 is expressed in these cells, but also microarray studies have revealed that several Hox genes from the cluster on chromosome 2 such as *HOXD1, HOXD3, HOXD4, HOXD8,* and *HOXD9* were highly expressed in blood-derived endothelial cells [62]. In particular, *HOXD1* regulates endothelial cell migration and cell adhesion on fibronectin by targeting integrin β1 (ITGβ1) in mature endothelial cells [75].

4.9. HOXD3

HOXD3 is a member of the *HOXD* cluster on chromosome 2, and it can be induced by extracellular matrix protein, Del-1, and integrin alphavbeta5 interaction on resting endothelium. Del-1 is a protein that accumulates around angiogenic blood vessels and promotes angiogenesis in the absence of exogenous growth factors [76]. Zhong et al. showed that Del-1 initiates angiogenesis by binding to integrin alphavbeta5 on the resting endothelium, resulting in expression of HoxD3 [76]. HoxD3 was then promoting angiogenesis by inducing the expression of the pro-angiogenic molecule integrin alphavbeta3 (integrin β3) [76]. These findings provide evidence for an angiogenic switch that can be initiated in the absence of exogenous growth factors indicating that the angiogenic matrix protein Del-1 may be a useful tool for the therapy of ischemic disease [76]. A year later, Chen and Ruley demonstrated the role of HoxD3 expression in human brain vessels [52]. They showed that HoxD3 expression significantly induced cerebral angiogenesis, increased focal cerebral blood flow, and reduced vascular leakage by inducing integrin β3. These data suggest that HoxD3 plays an important role in regulating angiogenesis. Other studies reported that HoxD3 mediates the basic fibroblast growth factor (bFGF)-induced expression of integrin β3 and urokinase plasminogen activator (uPA) in HUVECs [77] and promotes angiogenesis in in vivo models [78, 79]. Furthermore, *HOXD3* has been shown to be involved in cerebral angiogenesis in mice [52].

4.10. Hox genes with anti-angiogenic effects

As previously described, several transcription factors encoded by Hox genes contribute to anti-angiogenic activity such as *HOXA5*, *HOXC9*, and *HOXD10* [79].

4.11. HOXA5

It has been shown that the presence of HoxA5 was associated with the upregulation of thrombospondin-2 (TSP-2), a naturally occurring inhibitor of angiogenesis. In addition, HoxA5 expression was also associated with downregulation of pro-angiogenic genes such as Ephrin A1 (Efna1), VEGFR2, hypoxia-inducible 1α (HIF1α), and cyclooxygenase-2 (COX-2) [80].

4.12. HOXC9

HOXC9 is a transcription factor expressed in blood vessels in mice [81] and in the cardinal vein of zebrafish [82]. Kroll's group investigated this transcription factor in human vascular endothelial cells and zebrafish, and they observed that this protein was a negative regulator of circulating endothelial cells. They found that HoxC9 was highly expressed in resting endothelial cells; however, its expression was downregulated under hypoxic conditions, and overexpression of this factor inhibited endothelial migration, tube formation, and endothelial cell proliferation by targeting IL-8 transcription [82]. Finally, using a zebrafish model, they observed in vivo that HoxC9 overexpression inhibited the development of their vascular structure; this defect was rescued with exogenous IL-8. This data suggests that HoxC9 plays a negative role in the induction of endothelial cell growth by inhibiting IL-8 production [81, 82].

4.13. HOXD10

HOXD10 is another negative regulator gene for angiogenesis as its overexpression inhibited dermal microvascular endothelial cell migration in vitro [53]. In addition, it has been shown that HoxD10 reduces the expression of GATA-binding protein transcription factor, a family of transcription factors that contain two zinc finger motifs and bind to the DNA sequence (A/T) GATA(A/G), from where it acquires its name. HoxD10 via those transcription factors is able to regulate expression of VEGFR1 and VEGFR2 in differentiated endothelial cells [83]. Therefore,

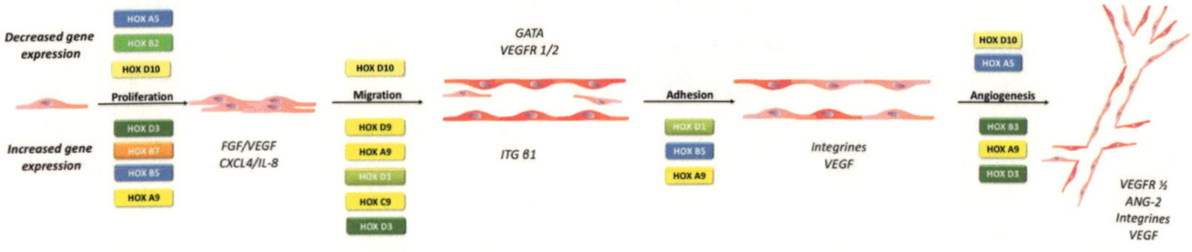

Figure 3. HOX genes regulate angiogenesis. Differential expression of Hox genes tightly regulates endothelial cell proliferation, migration, adhesion, and blood vessel formation (angiogenesis) by activating or silencing relevant target genes, such as fibroblast growth factor (FGF), vascular endothelial growth factor (VEGF), platelet factor 4 (PF4) or chemokine (C-X-C motif) ligand 4 (CXCL4), interleukin-8 (IL-8), integrin beta 1 (ITGβ1), and both vascular endothelial growth factor receptors 1 and 2 (VEGFR1/VEGFR2).

these observations suggest that there is an overlapping and complementary role between Hox genes to maintain a balance between pro-angiogenic and anti-angiogenic states (**Figure 3**).

5. Hox genes and adult stem cells

Hox genes act as transcriptional regulators, which have been involved in the differentiation of stem cells into several lineages and different cell types. One of the main steps to initiate vasculogenesis and angiogenesis is the differentiation to endothelial lineage from pluripotent stem cells. Studies have suggested that Hox genes contribute to the differentiation of EPCs into mature endothelial cells (**Table 1**). In the next section, we will present the evidence for the role of Hox genes in the differentiation of adult stem cell.

5.1. Endothelial progenitor cells

Several members of the Hox family play an important role in the embryonic development of the cardiovascular system and regulate angiogenesis in adults [84]. In addition, some Hox transcription factors such as HoxD3, HoxC6, and HoxC8 modulate the expression of proteins in mature endothelial cells, whereas HoxB5 appears to be involved in the in vitro differentiation of embryonic precursor cells toward endothelial lineage [66, 81]. *HoxA9* is important for myeloid, erythroid, and lymphoid hematopoiesis [88, 89] and stem cell expansion [90]. It is also essential for the migration and tube-forming capacity of mature endothelial cells [51] and could serve as a switch toward endothelial commitment during progenitor cell maturation. The *HOXD3* gene is also involved in the differentiation of EPC to endothelial cell. The expression of *HOXD3* retained endothelial cells in an invasive state and prevented vessel maturation leading to vascular malformations and vascular tumors. Therefore, HoxD3 regulates endothelial cell gene expression associated with the invasive stage of angiogenesis. The expression

Cellular type	**Hox genes**	**Period of expression**	**Target gene**	**Regulation**	**Functions**	**Reference**
Pro-angiogenic						
Endothelial cells of the human dermal microvasculature	HoxA3	Late embryogenesis and wound healing	uPAR	+	Endothelial cell migration	[47]
			MMP-14	+		
HUVECs	HoxA9	Post birth neovasculogenesis	EphrinB4	+	Angiogenesis	[51]
			eNOS	+	Endothelial cell proliferation	[84]
			VEGFR2	+	Endothelial cell activation	
Cellular line (MDA-MB-231, T47D, MTLn3)	HoxB2					
Endothelial cells of the human dermal microvasculature	HoxB3	Neovascularization	Ephrin A1	+	Endothelial cell vessel formation	[53]

Cellular type	Hox genes	Period of expression	Target gene	Regulation	Functions	Reference
Angioblasts (rat)	HoxB5	Neovascularization	VEGFR2	+	Endothelial cell activation	[66]
HUVECs	HoxD3	Neovascularization	Collagen1A1	+	Adhesion and migration of endothelial cells	[77]
Human microvasculature endothelial cells			Integrin-α	+		[78]
Murine embryonic stem cells	HoxA13	Postnatal neovascularization	EphA4	+	Organización células endoteliales y formación de vasos	[54]
			EphA7	+		
Vascular smooth muscle cells	Prx1	Late embryogenesis	TN-C	+	Proliferation of smooth muscle cells	[85]
			α-Actin	+		[65]
Vascular smooth muscle cells	Prx2	Late embryogenesis	TN-C	+	Proliferation of smooth muscle cells	[85]
Human pulmonary endothelial cells	Hhex	Vascular insult	Myh10	+	Plasticity smooth muscle cells	[84]
Human brain endothelial cells	Meox2	Postnatally	MLL77	—	Endothelial cell apoptosis	[66]
Anti-angiogenic						
HUVECs	HoxA5	Postnatally	VEGFR2	–	Endothelial cell activation	[86]
			Ephrin A1	–	Endothelial cell migration	[87]
Human endothelial cells	HoxD10	Postnatally	Integrin-α	—	Endothelial cell migration	[53]

uPAR, urokinase receptor; MMP-14, matrix metalloproteinase-14; EhB4, ephrin type-B receptor 4; eNOS, endothelial nitric oxide synthase; VEGFR2, vascular endothelial growth factor receptor 2; Myh10, myosin heavy chain 10; MLL, histone-lysine N-methyltransferase; HUVEC, human umbilical vein endothelial cell.

Table 1. Regulation of the Hox genes in vascular cells.

of HoxD genes has been shown to be temporally regulated as the expression of HoxD10 is maximal 3 days after stimulation with angiogenic factors, whereas the expression of HoxD3 increases after 3 days, indicating that the differentiation and maturation of endothelial cells work alongside with changes in the expression of Hox genes [90].

6. Conclusions

Hox genes have been traditionally recognized as genes involved in the embryonic development; however, further research showed that homeobox genes also play a role as master regulators of tissue and organ patterning in adults. These genes can regulate cell differentiation, proliferation, and migration to tissues exposed to constant turnover, such as vasculature, endometrium, and bone marrow. Thus, it has been shown that Hox genes can play a role in defining an endothelial phenotype and/or promoting neovascularization; however, other genes from the Hox family can also play an anti-angiogenic role by preventing angiogenesis. These genes regulate different processes by targeting key proteins related to angiogenesis such as VEGF, IL-8, Efna1, and TSP-2 among other gene targets.

Since Hox genes play a role in the regulation of stem cell differentiation into endothelium, angiogenesis, and vasculogenesis, the manipulation of these genes could lead to a useful gene therapy in patients with vascular damage. A better understanding of the cellular and molecular mechanisms related to the biological effects of Hox genes is essential for designing new drugs and treatment to treat worldwide prevalent diseases such as cancer and cardiovascular disease.

Acknowledgements

We would like to thank the research staff of the Vascular Physiology Laboratory, the Group of Investigation in Tumor Angiogenesis (GIANT) from the University of Bio Bio, and the Group of Research and Innovation in Vascular Health (GRIVAS Health) for the outstanding discussion of the ideas presented in this manuscript.

Source of funding

C.A. is funded by PCI N° PII20150053, and Dirección de Investigación, Universidad de Concepcion (DIUC 211.072.034-1.0), Chile, and Convenio de Desempeño, Universidad de Concepcion, UCO1201. C.E. is funded by Fondecyt Regular 1140586, Fondequip EQM140104, DIUBB 166709 3/R, and GI 171709/VC. E.N-L. is funded by CONICYT—Fondecyt de Iniciacion (Grant Number: 11170610) and Programa de Atracción e Inserción (Grant Number: 79170073).

Author details

Estefanía Nova-Lampeti[1], Valeria Aguilera[1], Katherine Oporto[1], Paula Guzmán[1], Valeska Ormazábal[2], Felipe Zúñiga[1], Carlos Escudero[3,4] and Claudio Aguayo[1,4*]

*Address all correspondence to: caguayo@udec.cl

1 Department of Clinical Biochemistry and Immunology, Faculty of Pharmacy, University of Concepcion, Chile

2 Department of Pharmacology, Faculty of Biological Sciences, University of Concepcion, Concepcion, Chile

3 Vascular Physiology Laboratory, Group of Investigation in Tumor Angiogenesis (GIANT), Department of Basic Sciences, University of Bio-Bio, Chillan, Chile

4 Group of Research and Innovation in Vascular Health (GRIVAS Health), Chillan, Chile

References

[1] Rux DR, Wellik DM. Hox genes in the adult skeleton: Novel functions beyond embryonic development. Developmental Dynamics: An Official Publication of the American Association of Anatomists. 2017;**246**(4):310-317

[2] Wagner GP, Amemiya C, Ruddle F. Hox cluster duplications and the opportunity for evolutionary novelties. Proceedings of the National Academy of Sciences of the United States of America. 2003;**100**(25):14603-14606

[3] Hrycaj SM, Wellik DM. Hox genes and evolution. F1000Research. 2016;**5**:1-7

[4] Bender W, Akam M, Karch F, Beachy PA, Peifer M, Spierer P, Lewis EB, Hogness DS. Molecular genetics of the Bithorax complex in Drosophila melanogaster. Science. 1983;**221**(4605):23-29

[5] Burke AC, Nelson CE, Morgan BA, Tabin C. Hox genes and the evolution of vertebrate axial morphology. Development. 1995;**121**(2):333-346

[6] Mallo M, Wellik DM, Deschamps J. Hox genes and regional patterning of the vertebrate body plan. Developmental Biology. 2010;**344**(1):7-15

[7] Kachgal S, Mace KA, Boudreau NJ. The dual roles of homeobox genes in vascularization and wound healing. Cell Adhesion & Migration. 2012;**6**(6):457-470

[8] McGinnis W, Krumlauf R. Homeobox genes and axial patterning. Cell. 1992;**68**(2):283-302

[9] Phelan ML, Sadoul R, Featherstone MS. Functional differences between HOX proteins conferred by two residues in the homeodomain N-terminal arm. Molecular and Cellular Biology. 1994;**14**(8):5066-5075

[10] Zanatta A, Rocha AM, Carvalho FM, Pereira RM, Taylor HS, Motta EL, Baracat EC, Serafini PC. The role of the Hoxa10/HOXA10 gene in the etiology of endometriosis and its related infertility: A review. Journal of Assisted Reproduction and Genetics. 2010;**27**(12):701-710

[11] Arici A, Oral E, Bukulmez O, Duleba A, Olive DL, Jones EE. The effect of endometriosis on implantation: Results from the Yale University in vitro fertilization and embryo transfer program. Fertility and Sterility. 1996;**65**(3):603-607

[12] Simon C, Gutierrez A, Vidal A, de los Santos MJ, Tarin JJ, Remohi J, Pellicer A. Outcome of patients with endometriosis in assisted reproduction: Results from in-vitro fertilization and oocyte donation. Human Reproduction. 1994;**9**(4):725-729

[13] Taylor HS, Bagot C, Kardana A, Olive D, Arici A. HOX gene expression is altered in the endometrium of women with endometriosis. Human Reproduction. 1999;**14**(5):1328-1331

[14] Daftary GS, Taylor HS. Endocrine regulation of HOX genes. Endocrine Reviews. 2006; **27**(4):331-355

[15] Kim JJ, Taylor HS, Lu Z, Ladhani O, Hastings JM, Jackson KS, Wu Y, Guo SW, Fazleabas AT. Altered expression of HOXA10 in endometriosis: Potential role in decidualization. Molecular Human Reproduction. 2007;**13**(5):323-332

[16] Daftary GS, Troy PJ, Bagot CN, Young SL, Taylor HS. Direct regulation of beta3-integrin subunit gene expression by HOXA10 in endometrial cells. Molecular Endocrinology. 2002;**16**(3):571-579

[17] Kulak J Jr, Ferriani RA, Komm BS, Taylor HS. Tissue selective estrogen complexes (TSECs) differentially modulate markers of proliferation and differentiation in endometrial cells. Reproductive Sciences. 2013;**20**(2):129-137

[18] Satokata I, Benson G, Maas R. Sexually dimorphic sterility phenotypes in Hoxa10-deficient mice. Nature. 1995;**374**(6521):460-463

[19] Gross S, Krause Y, Wuelling M, Vortkamp A. Hoxa11 and Hoxd11 regulate chondrocyte differentiation upstream of Runx2 and Shox2 in mice. PLoS One. 2012;**7**(8):e43553

[20] Chen Y, Xu B, Arderiu G, Hashimoto T, Young WL, Boudreau N, Yang GY. Retroviral delivery of homeobox D3 gene induces cerebral angiogenesis in mice. Journal of Cerebral Blood Flow and Metabolism: Official Journal of the International Society of Cerebral Blood Flow and Metabolism. 2004;**24**(11):1280-1287

[21] Kelly ZL, Michael A, Butler-Manuel S, Pandha HS, Morgan RG. HOX genes in ovarian cancer. Journal of Ovarian Research. 2011;**4**:16

[22] Hsieh-Li HM, Witte DP, Weinstein M, Branford W, Li H, Small K, Potter SS. Hoxa 11 structure, extensive antisense transcription, and function in male and female fertility. Development. 1995;**121**(5):1373-1385

[23] Yim GW, Kim HJ, Kim LK, Kim SW, Kim S, Nam EJ, Kim YT. Long non-coding RNA HOXA11 antisense promotes cell proliferation and invasion and predicts patient prognosis in serous ovarian cancer. Cancer Research and Treatment: Official Journal of Korean Cancer Association. 2017;**49**(3):656-668

[24] Hewitt SC, Harrell JC, Korach KS. Lessons in estrogen biology from knockout and transgenic animals. Annual Review of Physiology. 2005;**67**:285-308

[25] Edwards RG. Implantation, interception and contraception. Human Reproduction. 1994;**9**(6):985-995

[26] Gendron RL, Paradis H, Hsieh-Li HM, Lee DW, Potter SS, Markoff E. Abnormal uterine stromal and glandular function associated with maternal reproductive defects in Hoxa-11 null mice. Biology of Reproduction. 1997;**56**(5):1097-1105

[27] Taylor HS, Arici A, Olive D, Igarashi P. HOXA10 is expressed in response to sex steroids at the time of implantation in the human endometrium. The Journal of Clinical Investigation. 1998;**101**(7):1379-1384

[28] Troy PJ, Daftary GS, Bagot CN, Taylor HS. Transcriptional repression of peri-implantation EMX2 expression in mammalian reproduction by HOXA10. Molecular and Cellular Biology. 2003;**23**(1):1-13

[29] Zhu LH, Sun LH, Hu YL, Jiang Y, Liu HY, Shen XY, Jin XY, Zhen X, Sun HX, Yan GJ. PCAF impairs endometrial receptivity and embryo implantation by down-regulating beta3-integrin expression via HOXA10 acetylation. The Journal of Clinical Endocrinology and Metabolism. 2013;**98**(11):4417-4428

[30] Sadeghi H, Taylor HS. HOXA10 regulates endometrial GABAA {pi} receptor expression and membrane translocation. American Journal of Physiology Endocrinology and Metabolism. 2010;**298**(4):E889-E893

[31] Yotova I, Hsu E, Do C, Gaba A, Sczabolcs M, Dekan S, Kenner L, Wenzl R, Tycko B. Epigenetic alterations affecting transcription factors and signaling pathways in stromal cells of endometriosis. PLoS One. 2017;**12**(1):e0170859

[32] Fischbach NA, Rozenfeld S, Shen W, Fong S, Chrobak D, Ginzinger D, Kogan SC, Radhakrishnan A, Le Beau MM, Largman C, Lawrence HJ. HOXB6 overexpression in murine bone marrow immortalizes a myelomonocytic precursor in vitro and causes hematopoietic stem cell expansion and acute myeloid leukemia in vivo. Blood. 2005;**105**(4):1456-1466

[33] van Oostveen J, Bijl J, Raaphorst F, Walboomers J, Meijer C. The role of homeobox genes in normal hematopoiesis and hematological malignancies. Leukemia. 1999;**13**(11):1675-1690

[34] Wang L, Menendez P, Shojaei F, Li L, Mazurier F, Dick JE, Cerdan C, Levac K, Bhatia M. Generation of hematopoietic repopulating cells from human embryonic stem cells independent of ectopic HOXB4 expression. The Journal of Experimental Medicine. 2005;**201**(10):1603-1614

[35] Crooks GM, Fuller J, Petersen D, Izadi P, Malik P, Pattengale PK, Kohn DB, Gasson JC. Constitutive HOXA5 expression inhibits erythropoiesis and increases myelopoiesis from human hematopoietic progenitors. Blood. 1999;**94**(2):519-528

[36] Yang D, Zhang X, Dong Y, Liu X, Wang T, Wang X, Geng Y, Fang S, Zheng Y, Chen X, Chen J, Pan G, Wang J. Enforced expression of Hoxa5 in haematopoietic stem cells leads to aberrant erythropoiesis in vivo. Cell Cycle. 2015;**14**(4):612-620

[37] Huang Y, Sitwala K, Bronstein J, Sanders D, Dandekar M, Collins C, Robertson G, MacDonald J, Cezard T, Bilenky M, Thiessen N, Zhao Y, Zeng T, Hirst M, Hero A, Jones S, Hess JL. Identification and characterization of Hoxa9 binding sites in hematopoietic cells. Blood. 2012;**119**(2):388-398

[38] Sugimura R, Jha DK, Han A, Soria-Valles C, da Rocha EL, Lu YF, Goettel JA, Serrao E, Rowe RG, Malleshaiah M, Wong I, Sousa P, Zhu TN, Ditadi A, Keller G, Engelman AN, Snapper SB, Doulatov S, Daley GQ. Haematopoietic stem and progenitor cells from human pluripotent stem cells. Nature. 2017;**545**(7655):432-438

[39] Bei L, Huang W, Wang H, Shah C, Horvath E, Eklund E. HoxA10 activates CDX4 transcription and Cdx4 activates HOXA10 transcription in myeloid cells. The Journal of Biological Chemistry. 2011;**286**(21):19047-19064

[40] Bach C, Buhl S, Mueller D, Garcia-Cuellar MP, Maethner E, Slany RK. Leukemogenic transformation by HOXA cluster genes. Blood. 2010;**115**(14):2910-2918

[41] Qu X, Davison J, Du L, Storer B, Stirewalt DL, Heimfeld S, Estey E, Appelbaum FR, Fang M. Identification of differentially methylated markers among cytogenetic risk groups of acute myeloid leukemia. Epigenetics. 2015;**10**(6):526-535

[42] Eberhard A, Kahlert S, Goede V, Hemmerlein B, Plate KH, Augustin HG. Heterogeneity of angiogenesis and blood vessel maturation in human tumors: Implications for antiangiogenic tumor therapies. Cancer Research. 2000;**60**(5):1388-1393

[43] Risau W. Mechanisms of angiogenesis. Nature. 1997;**386**(6626):671-674

[44] Asahara T, Murohara T, Sullivan A, Silver M, van der Zee R, Li T, Witzenbichler B, Schatteman G, Isner JM. Isolation of putative progenitor endothelial cells for angiogenesis. Science. 1997;**275**(5302):964-967

[45] Neufeld G, Cohen T, Gengrinovitch S, Poltorak Z. Vascular endothelial growth factor (VEGF) and its receptors. FASEB Journal: Official Publication of the Federation of American Societies for Experimental Biology. 1999;**13**(1):9-22

[46] Kuo JH, Cuevas I, Chen A, Dunn A, Kuri M, Boudreau N. Secreted HoxA3 promotes epidermal proliferation and angiogenesis in genetically modified three-dimensional composite skin constructs. Advances in Wound Care. 2014;**3**(10):605-613

[47] Mace KA, Hansen SL, Myers C, Young DM, Boudreau N. HOXA3 induces cell migration in endothelial and epithelial cells promoting angiogenesis and wound repair. Journal of Cell Science. 2005;**118**(Pt 12):2567-2577

[48] Hansen SL, Myers CA, Charboneau A, Young DM, Boudreau N. HoxD3 accelerates wound healing in diabetic mice. The American Journal of Pathology. 2003;**163**(6):2421-2431

[49] Borrow J, Shearman AM, Stanton VP Jr, Becher R, Collins T, Williams AJ, Dube I, Katz F, Kwong YL, Morris C, Ohyashiki K, Toyama K, Rowley J, Housman DE. The t(7,11)(p15;p15) translocation in acute myeloid leukaemia fuses the genes for nucleoporin NUP98 and class I homeoprotein HOXA9. Nature Genetics. 1996;**12**(2):159-167

[50] Patel CV, Sharangpani R, Bandyopadhyay S, DiCorleto PE. Endothelial cells express a novel, tumor necrosis factor-alpha-regulated variant of HOXA9. The Journal of Biological Chemistry. 1999;**274**(3):1415-1422

[51] Bruhl T, Urbich C, Aicher D, Acker-Palmer A, Zeiher AM, Dimmeler S. Homeobox A9 transcriptionally regulates the EphB4 receptor to modulate endothelial cell migration and tube formation. Circulation Research. 2004;**94**(6):743-751

[52] Chen J, Ruley HE. An enhancer element in the EphA2 (Eck) gene sufficient for rhombomere-specific expression is activated by HOXA1 and HOXB1 homeobox proteins. The Journal of Biological Chemistry. 1998;**273**(38):24670-24675

[53] Myers C, Charboneau A, Boudreau N. Homeobox B3 promotes capillary morphogenesis and angiogenesis. The Journal of Cell Biology. 2000;**148**(2):343-351

[54] Fuller T, Korff T, Kilian A, Dandekar G, Augustin HG. Forward EphB4 signaling in endothelial cells controls cellular repulsion and segregation from ephrinB2 positive cells. Journal of Cell Science. 2003;**116**(Pt 12):2461-2470

[55] Palmer A, Zimmer M, Erdmann KS, Eulenburg V, Porthin A, Heumann R, Deutsch U, Klein R. EphrinB phosphorylation and reverse signaling: Regulation by Src kinases and PTP-BL phosphatase. Molecular Cell. 2002;**9**(4):725-737

[56] Zhang N, Gong L, Zhang H, Cao C. High glucose-induced dysfunction of endothelial cells can be restored by HoxA9EC. Annals of Vascular Surgery. 2012;**26**(7):1002-1010

[57] Bandyopadhyay S, Ashraf MZ, Daher P, Howe PH, DiCorleto PE. HOXA9 participates in the transcriptional activation of E-selectin in endothelial cells. Molecular and Cellular Biology. 2007;**27**(12):4207-4216

[58] Shaut CA, Keene DR, Sorensen LK, Li DY, Stadler HS. HOXA13 is essential for placental vascular patterning and labyrinth endothelial specification. PLoS Genetics. 2008;**4**(5):e1000073

[59] Shaut CA, Saneyoshi C, Morgan EA, Knosp WM, Sexton DR, Stadler HS. HOXA13 directly regulates EphA6 and EphA7 expression in the genital tubercle vascular endothelia. Developmental Dynamics: An Official Publication of the American Association of Anatomists. 2007;**236**(4):951-960

[60] Wellik DM. Hox patterning of the vertebrate axial skeleton. Developmental Dynamics: An Official Publication of the American Association of Anatomists. 2007;**236**(9):2454-2463

[61] Storti P, Donofrio G, Colla S, Airoldi I, Bolzoni M, Agnelli L, Abeltino M, Todoerti K, Lazzaretti M, Mancini C, Ribatti D, Bonomini S, Franceschi V, Pistoia V, Lisignoli G, Pedrazzini A, Cavicchi O, Neri A, Rizzoli V, Giuliani N. HOXB7 expression by myeloma cells regulates their pro-angiogenic properties in multiple myeloma patients. Leukemia. 2011;**25**(3):527-537

[62] Bertrand N, Roux M, Ryckebusch L, Niederreither K, Dolle P, Moon A, Capecchi M, Zaffran S. Hox genes define distinct progenitor sub-domains within the second heart field. Developmental Biology. 2011;**353**(2):266-274

[63] Roux M, Laforest B, Capecchi M, Bertrand N, Zaffran S. Hoxb1 regulates proliferation and differentiation of second heart field progenitors in pharyngeal mesoderm and genetically interacts with Hoxa1 during cardiac outflow tract development. Developmental Biology. 2015;**406**(2):247-258

[64] Gaufo GO, Flodby P, Capecchi MR. Hoxb1 controls effectors of sonic hedgehog and Mash1 signaling pathways. Development. 2000;**127**(24):5343-5354

[65] Roux M, Laforest B, Eudes N, Bertrand N, Stefanovic S, Zaffran S. Hoxa1 and Hoxb1 are required for pharyngeal arch artery development. Mechanisms of Development. 2017;**143**:1-8

[66] Wu Y, Moser M, Bautch VL, Patterson C. HoxB5 is an upstream transcriptional switch for differentiation of the vascular endothelium from precursor cells. Molecular and Cellular Biology. 2003;**23**(16):5680-5691

[67] Fessner A, Esser JS, Bluhm F, Grundmann S, Zhou Q, Patterson C, Bode C, Moser M. The transcription factor HoxB5 stimulates vascular remodelling in a cytokine-dependent manner. Cardiovascular Research. 2014;**101**(2):247-255

[68] Winnik S, Klinkert M, Kurz H, Zoeller C, Heinke J, Wu Y, Bode C, Patterson C, Moser M. HoxB5 induces endothelial sprouting in vitro and modifies intussusceptive angiogenesis in vivo involving angiopoietin-2. Cardiovascular Research. 2009;**83**(3):558-565

[69] Care A, Felicetti F, Meccia E, Bottero L, Parenza M, Stoppacciaro A, Peschle C, Colombo MP. HOXB7: A key factor for tumor-associated angiogenic switch. Cancer Research. 2001;**61**(17):6532-6539

[70] Murthi P, Hiden U, Rajaraman G, Liu H, Borg AJ, Coombes F, Desoye G, Brennecke SP, Kalionis B. Novel homeobox genes are differentially expressed in placental microvascular endothelial cells compared with macrovascular cells. Placenta. 2008;**29**(7):624-630

[71] Nguyen Kovochich A, Arensman M, Lay AR, Rao NP, Donahue T, Li X, French SW, Dawson DW. HOXB7 promotes invasion and predicts survival in pancreatic adenocarcinoma. Cancer. 2013;**119**(3):529-539

[72] How C, Hui AB, Alajez NM, Shi W, Boutros PC, Clarke BA, Yan R, Pintilie M, Fyles A, Hedley DW, Hill RP, Milosevic M, Liu FF. MicroRNA-196b regulates the homeobox B7-vascular endothelial growth factor axis in cervical cancer. PLoS One. 2013;**8**(7):e67846

[73] Milanovic D, Sticht C, Rohrich M, Maier P, Grosu AL, Herskind C. Inhibition of 13-cis retinoic acid-induced gene expression of reactive-resistance genes by thalidomide in glioblastoma tumours in vivo. Oncotarget. 2015;**6**(30):28938-28948

[74] Heinonen H, Lepikhova T, Sahu B, Pehkonen H, Pihlajamaa P, Louhimo R, Gao P, Wei GH, Hautaniemi S, Janne OA, Monni O. Identification of several potential chromatin binding sites of HOXB7 and its downstream target genes in breast cancer. International Journal of Cancer. 2015;**137**(10):2374-2383

[75] Toshner M, Dunmore BJ, McKinney EF, Southwood M, Caruso P, Upton PD, Waters JP, Ormiston ML, Skepper JN, Nash G, Rana AA, Morrell NW. Transcript analysis reveals a specific HOX signature associated with positional identity of human endothelial cells. PLoS One. 2014;**9**(3):e91334

[76] Zhong J, Eliceiri B, Stupack D, Penta K, Sakamoto G, Quertermous T, Coleman M, Boudreau N, Varner JA. Neovascularization of ischemic tissues by gene delivery of the extracellular matrix protein Del-1. The Journal of Clinical Investigation. 2003;**112**(1):30-41

[77] Boudreau N, Andrews C, Srebrow A, Ravanpay A, Cheresh DA. Induction of the angiogenic phenotype by Hox D3. The Journal of Cell Biology. 1997;**139**(1):257-264

[78] Boudreau NJ, Varner JA. The homeobox transcription factor Hox D3 promotes integrin alpha5beta1 expression and function during angiogenesis. The Journal of Biological Chemistry. 2004;**279**(6):4862-4868

[79] Mujahid S, Nielsen HC, Volpe MV. MiR-221 and miR-130a regulate lung airway and vascular development. PLoS One. 2013;**8**(2):e55911

[80] Cuevas I, Layman H, Coussens L, Boudreau N. Sustained endothelial expression of HoxA5 in vivo impairs pathological angiogenesis and tumor progression. PLoS One. 2015;**10**(3):e0121720

[81] Politz O, Gratchev A, McCourt PA, Schledzewski K, Guillot P, Johansson S, Svineng G, Franke P, Kannicht C, Kzhyshkowska J, Longati P, Velten FW, Johansson S, Goerdt S.

Stabilin-1 and -2 constitute a novel family of fasciclin-like hyaluronan receptor homologues. The Biochemical Journal. 2002;**362**(Pt 1):155-164

[82] Stoll SJ, Bartsch S, Augustin HG, Kroll J. The transcription factor HOXC9 regulates endothelial cell quiescence and vascular morphogenesis in zebrafish via inhibition of interleukin 8. Circulation Research. 2011;**108**(11):1367-1377

[83] An N, Luo X, Zhang M, Yu R. MicroRNA-376b promotes breast cancer metastasis by targeting Hoxd10 directly. Experimental and Therapeutic Medicine. 2017;**13**(1):79-84

[84] Gorski DH, Walsh K. The role of homeobox genes in vascular remodeling and angiogenesis. Circulation Research. 2000;**87**(10):865-872

[85] Jones FS, Holst BD, Minowa O, De Robertis EM, Edelman GM. Binding and transcriptional activation of the promoter for the neural cell adhesion molecule by HoxC6 (Hox-3.3). Proceedings of the National Academy of Sciences of the United States of America. 1993;**90**(14):6557-6561

[86] Rhoads K, Arderiu G, Charboneau A, Hansen SL, Hoffman W, Boudreau N. A role for Hox A5 in regulating angiogenesis and vascular patterning. Lymphatic Research and Biology. 2005;**3**(4):240-252

[87] Cheng W, Liu J, Yoshida H, Rosen D, Naora H. Lineage infidelity of epithelial ovarian cancers is controlled by HOX genes that specify regional identity in the reproductive tract. Nature Medicine. 2005;**11**(5):531-537

[88] Izon DJ, Rozenfeld S, Fong ST, Komuves L, Largman C, Lawrence HJ. Loss of function of the homeobox gene Hoxa-9 perturbs early T-cell development and induces apoptosis in primitive thymocytes. Blood. 1998;**92**(2):383-393

[89] Lawrence HJ, Christensen J, Fong S, Hu YL, Weissman I, Sauvageau G, Humphries RK, Largman C. Loss of expression of the Hoxa-9 homeobox gene impairs the proliferation and repopulating ability of hematopoietic stem cells. Blood. 2005;**106**(12):3988-3994

[90] Thorsteinsdottir U, Mamo A, Kroon E, Jerome L, Bijl J, Lawrence HJ, Humphries K, Sauvageau G. Overexpression of the myeloid leukemia-associated Hoxa9 gene in bone marrow cells induces stem cell expansion. Blood. 2002;**99**(1):121-129

Chapter 3

Endothelial Cell Senescence in the Pathogenesis of Endothelial Dysfunction

Julia Carracedo, Rafael Ramírez-Carracedo,
Matilde Alique and Rafael Ramírez-Chamond

Additional information is available at the end of the chapter

http://dx.doi.org/10.5772/intechopen.73024

Abstract

Aging is the main risk factor for cardiovascular diseases (CVD), and senescence in endothelial cells seems to be an initial step in the cascade of events that will culminate with the development of these pathologies. In this chapter, we examine the pathophysiological mechanism(s) involved in endothelial senescence, leading to CVD as well as the biochemical and cellular pathways that may explain the activation and development of the process of endothelial senescence, and we discuss new hypotheses supported by experimental results which suggest that the senescent endothelial cell may induce a general process of vascular senescence. This process is probably induced either by soluble molecules secreted by these senescent cells and/or by intercellular signals transported in cellular vesicles that may be useful as biomarkers and as potential therapeutic targets in endothelial senescence.

Keywords: aging, biomarkers, cardiovascular disease, endothelium, microvesicles

1. Introduction

The term "cardiovascular diseases" (CVD) refers to a group of pathologies that share a common nexus, as they are preceded by process of damage and endothelial dysfunction. The imbalance of oxidative stress within the endothelium promotes the activation of cellular senescence processes, altering the biological functions of endothelial cells [1] and favoring CVD development. Indeed, chronologic aging or premature senescence (caused by pathologic environment) is significantly associated with CVD development [2].

Cellular senescence is an irreversible biological phenomenon triggered by potentially harmful stimuli which can damage the cell genome. During this process, the cell interrupts the division process, entering a state of cell cycle arrest and becoming quiescent. Senescence is a protective mechanism which affects the major part of the cells within the organism, including the vascular cells [3, 4]. It is considered indispensable to prevent tumor development, although turns to be pathologic when senescent cells extensively accumulate in tissues as a consequence of aging.

Cell senescence can be triggered prematurely due to aging-associated pathologies such as CVD or chronic kidney disease (CKD). In fact, several studies confirm that CKD patients manifest premature aging in several tissues, including those in the cardiovascular system [5]. This is partly explained because CKD patients show "classic" cardiovascular risk factors (age, lifestyle, left ventricular hypertrophy, dyslipidemia, hypertension and diabetes mellitus). Kidney failure leads to the accumulation of circulating uremic toxins in the blood of those patients, causing stress and damage to the endothelium and activating endothelial cells senescence. Furthermore, CKD patients often show subclinical chronic inflammation associated with an immunosenescence process, which seems to be induced by the uremic toxins and other factors [6]. The renal replacement therapies may have a significant role in this process, as they induce the activation of immunocompetent cells [7].

Taken together, these concepts show that blood circulating toxins cause endothelial cells to become senescent leading to the appearance of several CVD. For example, some studies have proved that, at least in atherosclerotic processes, the pathogenic basis by which the CVD is developed is endothelial senescence [8, 9]. When endothelial cells become senescent, their imbalanced functionality may lead to the loss of the vascular structure. Moreover, the senescent endothelium cannot regulate correctly the repairing and regenerative activity of endothelial progenitor cells (EPCs), which increases the harmful effect in the vascular bed [10]. It is easy to understand in this context that endothelial senescence acts as the first element in the development of CVD.

Recently, microvesicles (MVs) have been proposed as endothelial response elements that can take part both in damaging and repairing processes in the endothelium [10–12]. There is certain knowledge, yet scarce, about the mechanisms underlying the participation of MVs in endothelial homeostasis, although the implication of those MVs in endothelial senescence remains an unresolved question.

Therefore, to understand and characterize the mechanisms by which the senescent endothelial cells show an imbalanced functionality, it is necessary to identify early biomarkers and to design therapeutic targets for CVD.

2. Endothelial dysfunction as the first step in the development of vascular disease

Endothelial dysfunction is an earlier pathophysiologic stage in CVD development. Ross in 1976 published his theory of response to damage, where he hypothesized that the initial event in atherogenesis is the endothelial injury, followed by the proliferation of smooth muscle cells [13]. Over the past years, this theory has been consolidated as endothelial damage is shown to be decisive in the promotion of vascular diseases. Indeed, diverse pharmacologic and dietetic interventions are intended to prevent the imbalance of the endothelial function, trying to interfere with the development of atherosclerosis and its clinical consequences [14, 15].

The endothelium is a thin monocellular layer that covers the inner surface of blood vessels, separating the circulating blood from the interstitial fluid [16]. The endothelium is not an inert organ, as it can respond to physical or chemical stimuli by liberating the adequate regulatory substance to keep the correct vasomotor equilibrium and homeostasis [17]. The endothelium acts as an autocrine, paracrine and endocrine gland. Endothelial cells produce vasodilating, antiproliferative, antithrombotic and antiadherent mediators, like nitric oxide (NO), prostacyclin, the endothelium-derived hyperpolarizing factor (EDHF) and the natriuretic peptide, type C (CNP). The actions of those molecules are compensated by the release of substances with the opposing effect, as endothelin 1, thromboxane A2, prostaglandin H2 and the superoxide anion. Thus, endothelium regulates the tone of the smooth muscle cells of the vessel wall, causing its relaxation or contraction and conditioning the vasodilation or vasoconstriction processes. Also, it regulates hemostasis by controlling the production of prothrombotic or antithrombotic molecules, as well as fibrinolytic and antifibrinolytic substances. Endothelium takes part in inflammatory and immune processes by regulating proliferation and cell migration, as well as adherence and leukocytes activation. It is capable of producing cytokines and adhesion molecules that regulate the inflammatory process, contributing to the defensive function of the organism by the activation of neutrophils and macrophages [18].

Cardiovascular risk factors provoke an oxidative stress which alter the function of the endothelial cells and provoke endothelial dysfunction by reducing the ability of the endothelium to maintain the homeostasis and concluding with the development of vascular diseases [19]. The term "endothelial dysfunction" has been used to define diverse syndromes which include a change of the endothelial phenotype from a "basal" to an active state. It is a complex disorder which includes alterations in the vasomotor and antithrombotic responses, in the vascular permeability, the leukocytes recruitment and the proliferation of endothelial cells [20, 21]. In the progress of endothelial dysfunction, the presence of pathologic conditions can contribute accelerating CVD development [22, 23].

Among the cardiovascular risk factors, the age arises as a critical factor. It is associated with damage and endothelial dysfunction, as well with atherosclerosis development which will lead to vascular pathologies [24]. Epidemiologic studies have demonstrated that aging is the most important risk factor for the development of CVD, mainly atherosclerotic [23]. During the gradual aging, the incidence and prevalence of atherothrombotic and coronary diseases and cerebrovascular accidents increases. For that reason, there must be a causal relationship between the age-associated changes and vascular damage. It has been demonstrated that, during aging, the vasculature of healthy subjects suffers several changes, as endothelial dysfunction [21], the arterial wall thickening and remodeling [25], angiogenesis alterations, incorrect vascular repair [26] and increased atherosclerosis prevalence [27]. The relationship between the development of these disorders and the aging process remain poorly understood, but it is possible that throughout the physiologic aging of the organisms some similar changes occur, comparable to those in the vascular diseases and sharing common cellular mechanisms.

3. Endothelial cellular senescence as pathophysiological mechanism of vascular pathology

One of the mechanisms that have been postulated as a possible pathophysiological participant is the cellular senescence of the endothelium. Cellular senescence is an irreversible process typical for all cells in which cells leave the cycle division as a consequence of the cellular damage associated with diseases [28] and aging [29]. Cell senescence processes appear to be involved in physiological processes of control such as cancer protection, biological developmental processes, tissue repair in aging situations and age-related disorders. Although their involvement in the aging process was postulated by Shay and Wright (Hayflick limit) [30], the absence of specific markers of senescence has hampered efforts to characterize senescent cells that accumulate *in vivo* in tissues and organs. Nowadays, the process of cell senescence is becoming better known due to the availability of new techniques to determine and quantify the senescent characteristics. In general, the main characteristic of the senescent phenotype is that cells decline in DNA replication until they cease to proliferate associated with the molecular changes of elements related to the cell cycle [31]. In general, senescent cells exhibit an upregulation and secretion of growth factors, proinflammatory cytokines, and also they release extracellular matrix-degrading proteins, the overall contribution constitutes the senescence-associated secretory phenotype (SASP) [32] and cells lose the ability to divide at the end of replicative lifespan and decrease their ability to migrate [33]. At a phenotypic level, senescent cells acquire the typical flattened and enlarged morphology [34] (**Figure 1**). Aforementioned

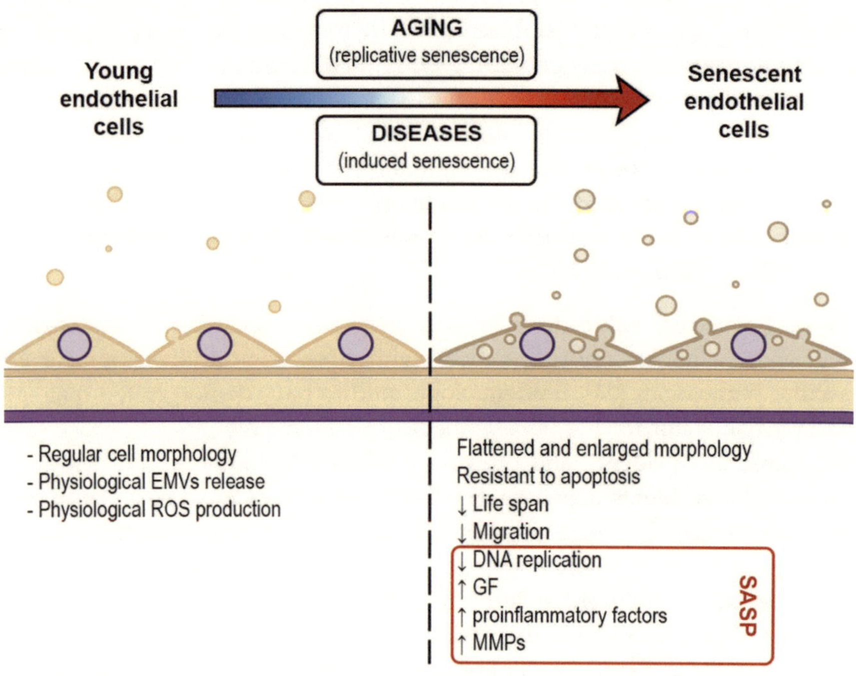

Figure 1. Mechanisms by which endothelial cells become senescent and their characteristics. GF, growth factors; MMPs, matrix metalloproteinases; SASP, senescence-associated secretory phenotype; EMVs, endothelial microvesicles; ROS, reactive oxidative species.

cells undergo distinctive phenotypic alterations, including profound chromatin and secretome changes, telomere shortening, genomic and epigenomic damage, unbalanced mitogenic signals and tumor-suppressor activation [28, 29]. Also, in human replicative senescence, telomere lengths decline with each cell cycle [35]. Most of these cells are resistant to some apoptosis signals, therefore, they become senescent [31]. Senescence and apoptosis are responses to cellular stress, and both are important in the activation of tumor suppressors [36], but senescence avoids the damage in the stressed cells. To date, some senescence markers have been described (**Table 1**) that are involved in cellular senescence, most of which participate in cell cycle control and DNA repair [31]. Further analysis has highlighted that many common

Characteristics	Markers	Regulation	Techniques	References
DNA replication (senescent cells decline in DNA replication)	BrdU	↓	Fluorescence microscope	[31]
	^{3}H-dT	↓	Incorporation of radioactivity	
	PCNA	↓	Immunostaining/Western blot	
	Ki-67	↓	Immunostaining/Western blot	
SA-β-gal activity (the SA-β-gal derives from the lysosomal β-galactosidase and reflects the increased lysosomal biogenesis)	X-gal substrate	↑	Light microscopy (production of blue precipitate)	[41, 42]
	C_{12}FDG (fluorogenic substrate)	↑	Fluorescence microscopy (production of green fluorogenic color)	
Cell cycle arrest proteins (early markers of DNA damage-induced senescence)	p16	↑	Western blot/immunostaining	[43–45]
	p21			[29, 46]
	p53			
	Cyclin D1			[38]
	Lamin B1	↓		[39]
SAHFs (reorganization of chromatin into discrete foci)	DNA dyes: DAPI	↑ Presence of certain heterochromatin-associated histone modifications	Fluorescence microscopy	[31, 47]
SDF (different DNA repair proteins)	γ-H2AX: marker of DNA double strand breaks and genomic instability	↑	Fluorescence microscopy/Western blot	[31]
	53BP1: protein associated with DNA damage	↑	Fluorescence microscopy	

BrdU, 5-bromodeoxyuridine; ^{3}H-dT, ^{3}Hthymidine; PCNA, Proliferating cell nuclear antigen; SA-β-gal, Senescence-associated β-galactosidase; X-gal substrate, 5-bromo-4-chloro-3-indolyl-D-galactoside; C_{12}FDG, 5-dodecanoylaminofluorescein di-β-D-galactopyranoside; SAHFs, senescence-associated heterochromatin foci; DAPI, 4′,6-diamidino-2-phenylindole; SDF, senescence-associated DNA damage foci; γ-H2AX; phosphorylated histone H2AX; 53BP1, p53-binding protein-1.

Table 1. Senescence markers.

cellular markers of senescence (upregulation of senescence-associated (SA)-β-galactosidase (gal) and p16) [29] are not robust and might overestimate the numbers of senescent cells that are present at low frequencies [37]. Thus, other cellular markers, such as cyclin D1 and lamin B1 [38, 39], are considered more reliable markers of senescence.

The use of all these elements to define senescent cells has provided convincing evidence that these senescent cells accumulate in tissues of humans, primates and rodents with advanced age, as well as in sites of tissue injury and remodeling. The most prominent feature of the senescent cells is a cell cycle arrest, which permanently withholds replication and the resistance to apoptosis. An important fact to note is that the cells with senescent characteristics are found in damaged tissues of patients with chronic diseases such as osteoarthritis, pulmonary fibrosis, atherosclerosis, Alzheimer's disease or CKD [40].

4. Chronic kidney disease, a model of chronic pathology that accelerates endothelial aging

CKD is known to promote cellular senescence and an accelerated aging. It is caused by the accumulation of toxins in the internal medium, and the consequence is the development of elderly associated pathologies, mainly CVD [48]. CKD-associated CVD show similar characteristics to the natural CVD in elderly, and for this reason, several authors propose that the biggest challenge in the treatment of CVD may be to understand why CKD promote the premature aging of the cardiovascular system [49].

Even though the progress in the last few years in the renal replacement therapy is substantial, the mortality of terminal CKD patients remains excessively high, with an incidence between 10 and 20-fold over the general population [50].

Uremic patients have higher rates of cardiovascular morbidity and mortality than would be predicted by Framingham risk factors [50–52]. However, the presence of those factors is not enough to explain the significant increment of the cardiovascular risk in those patients. CKD patients show additional factors associated with uremia that could explain this increased CVD risk [53]. The presence of microalbumin and uremic toxins in blood, hyperhomocysteinemia, anemia, the abnormal calcium/phosphate metabolism, parathyroid hormone (PTH) level alterations, the treatment with vitamin D derived substances, the volume overload, the electrolytic imbalance, oxidative stress, inflammation, malnutrition, thrombogenic factors and the imbalance of NO/endothelin are risk factors intrinsically associated to CKD [54]. The valuation and modulation of those factors are of high importance in CKD patients, as some are variable and the correct treatment may prevent the progression of the pathology.

In CKD patients, the endothelium is exposed to an additional stress because of the presence of factors related to the uremic state. This state can be modified depending on the conservative treatment or renal transplantation, but it has been demonstrated that it relies on a persistent microinflammatory state directly related to endothelial damage, partaking in atherosclerosis processes [7, 55, 56]. Under this hostile uremic-associated state, the endothelium loses its integrity. Some damage substances and molecules will be released as a reflection of the harmful stimuli [56, 57].

Among several inflammatory factors, the subpopulation of monocytes habitually augmented in elderly, increases in the peripheral blood. The contribution of monocytes in inflammation and the CVD development has been widely studied by several groups, including ours [58]. Peripheral blood monocytes show a significant heterogeneity, reflected by the differential expression of the lipopolysaccharide binding receptor (CD14) at their surface and the low-affinity receptor Fc, FcγRIII (CD16). In the last years, monocytes have been divided into three populations or subsets based on the intensity of CD14 and CD16 expression (cell surface marker phenotype) being functionally differentiated in: classical monocytes (CD14++/CD16−), present mainly in healthy patients; intermediate monocytes (CD14++/CD16+) and non-classical monocytes (CD14+/CD16++). A possible causal role in the development of atherosclerosis in general population and CKD patients has been attributed to intermediate monocytes (CD14++/CD16+) [59]. CD14+/CD16++ monocytes are inflammatory senescent cells characterized by their increased capacity to produce proinflammatory cytokines and because of their strong function as dendritic cells [60]. CD14+/CD16++ can be differentiated *in vitro* from CD14++/CD16− monocytes by a cellular senescence process. CD14+/CD16++ show senescent cells characteristics, such as an increased content of the enzyme β-gal or a shortened telomere length in comparison to monocytes CD14++/CD16−, and they accumulate in peripheral blood of elderly or CKD patients as a result of their resistance to apoptosis [7, 61]. Intermediate monocytes (CD14++/CD16+) are a developmental step between the classical monocytes (CD14++/CD16−) and non-classical (CD14+/CD16++) and whose activity is related to CVD [62, 63]. Moreover, non-classical CD14+/CD16++ monocytes appear to be involved in the endothelial damage which is usually by elderly people and CKD or others chronic inflamed patients [62, 63] leading to endothelial cells from the neighborhood achieve senescence status. Also, high frequency of CD14+/CD16++ ("non-classical") monocytes is associated with increased vascular superoxide production and apoptosis in endothelial cells [64, 65]. In normal states, the vascular endothelium does not allow the adhesion of leukocytes and prevents their passage. When hemodynamic conditions are altered monocytes, adopt a peripheral position along the endothelial surface producing adhesion of monocytes to the activated endothelium. The injury of endothelial cells is associated with the senescence of endothelial cell [66].

In vitro studies performed with CD14+/CD16++ in mature endothelial cells cultures, we found that those monocytes express high levels of vascular adhesion molecules, have a high adhesion capability to endothelial cells, produce chemokines, angiogenic factors and induce the production of vascular damage-associated MVs [7, 56]. MVs may contain molecules such as proteins, nucleic acids and lipids, which could contribute to the CVD development and also the profile of these molecules, are specific of the cell type of origin [67]. Thus, the accumulation of CD14+/CD16++ monocytes in peripheral blood not only can play a crucial role in the induction and can be responsible for prolonging the inflammatory response in elderly and CKD patients but can be directly related to CVD development. In CKD patients, we found that inflammatory monocytes are increased, mostly in those patients subjected to hemodialysis [68]. Proinflammatory or non-classical monocytes have a high binding affinity for endothelial cells conferred by their high expression of adhesion molecules. As a consequence, CD16-positive monocytes might preferentially adhere to the activated endothelium, enabling the propagation of further vascular damage by secretion of proinflammatory mediators [59].

In addition to the activity of the immune cells in endothelial damage, some other factors could be involved, as some specific molecules are known to be increased in the peripheral blood of CKD. In different models, it has been shown that endothelial cells activated pathologically with uremic serum or uremic toxins enter into a premature senescent state. Also, they reduce their proliferative capability and show shortened telomeres, augmenting the expression of β-gal [69]. Another possible factor in the development of the CKD-associated CVD is the incorrect repair of the damaged endothelium by EPCs. This failure occurs mainly due to two factors: a decreased number of EPCs or their imbalanced function. In our studies, we demonstrated that in CKD patients there is a decrease in the number of EPCs and that this number is considerably lower in severe patients with, for example, vascular calcifications [10, 70]. Also, it has been demonstrated that EPCs lose their angiogenic capability, generally needed in the process of regeneration of harmed vascular structures (vasculogenesis). In this regard, the association between some diseases such as CKD-associated CVD and both number and function of EPCs, accelerate the processes of EPCs senescence and therefore damage in endothelial cells harboring.

5. Microvesicles and endothelium

The endothelial MVs (EMVs) are extracellular vesicles produced by endothelial cells whose essential role is to act as a signaling system between the elements involved in the function and homeostasis of the vessel [71].

In general, the extracellular vesicles can be found in many body fluids, including plasma and urine. They have a variable size, between 0.05 and 5 μm [71], and are involved in physiological and pathophysiological processes, participating as mediators in intercellular communication. They can act directly on the target cells by binding to ligands, cell surface receptors and/or membrane-associated enzymes, delivering or releasing their contents directly into the cytoplasm. Extracellular vesicles are elevated in patients with neurodegenerative, metabolic, pulmonary, autoimmune and vascular diseases, chronic inflammation and cancer [72]. The use of extracellular vesicles as markers for the prediction, diagnosis and prognosis of the disease is increasingly interesting, as well as their potential as new therapeutic targets [73]. There are several types of extracellular vesicles: exosomes, the MVs or microparticles and the apoptotic bodies, which are produced by different mechanisms [65]. The MVs are a heterogeneous population of up 2 μm diameter, which are formed from the cell membrane in a regulated active process, dependent on enzyme activity and calcium.

Recently, it has been demonstrated that MVs may play an essential role in cellular senescence processes [74] since they have been proposed as elements of an endothelial response that can participate in the damaging and repair processes of the endothelium [10–12]. MVs generated from different cell types can induce endothelial dysfunction because they are responsible for increasing oxidative stress, reducing the bioavailability of NO and producing cardiovascular inflammation. The knowledge about their formation and release represent an attractive therapeutic goal to limit MVs levels, but the mechanisms underlying the release are not fully elucidated. On the other hand, a direct or indirect inhibition of the effect of MVs is a more effective proposal [75]. The effect of certain drugs that are used to decrease cardiovascular risk have been shown to affect the MVs plasma levels, suggesting that the beneficial effects of these drugs could, at least in part, be mediated through a reduction of the concentration of MVs [76]. Moreover, different authors have highlighted the importance of diet on MVs release, being perhaps one of the mechanisms involved in the role of diet in the development of CVD [14, 77]. The process of identification and separation of extracellular vesicles is complicated due to their extensive variability. In fact, currently, the absolute separation of exosomes, apoptotic bodies and MVs is not possible because their size ranges may overlap. The most common method for the separation and isolation of extracellular vesicles is the serial centrifugation. In the majority of the studies, a first centrifugation is performed at 200–1500 × g to remove cells and cell debris. Extracellular vesicles more than 100 nm are pelleted at 10,000–20,000 × g and small vesicles of 100 nm at 100,000–200,000 × g [78]. Following these protocols, we can obtain EMVs from supernatants of mature endothelial cells cultures, cellular debris and exosomes-free. The EMVs might also be obtained from plasma by similar processes, but would be found mixed with other MVs derived from other circulating cells.

The most common methods to study single MVs are flow cytometry (FC), tunable resistive pulse sensing (TRPS), dynamic light scattering (DLS) and nanoparticle tracking analysis (NTA) [79]. To date, FC is the method most used to establish the cellular origin and the phenotype of the MVs and is based on the detection of light scatter and fluorescence intensity of the labeled MVs [80–82]. To characterize their cellular origin, different antigens expressed on the membrane of the MVs are identified. For this purpose, monoclonal antibodies (mAb) labeled with different fluorochromes that define the phenotype are used. To identify EMVs, specific fluorescent antibodies against endothelial cell can be used to characterize the phenotype. Some markers used to describe EMVs are CD144, CD105 and CD146. Moreover, the phospholipids are a class of lipids that are a major component of all biological membranes and in MVs are externalized. For this reason, these phospholipids present in the MVs membrane have also been used for EMVs detection and characterization [83]. The combination of several mAb simultaneously can facilitate the identification of the origin and the state of activation or apoptosis of the cell from which the MVs originate [84]. The EMVs determination protocol includes some preliminary steps designed to identify sizes, with beads that allow adjustments to the equipment, before the introduction of the samples. However, this method has limitations in identifying the smallest MVs that are below the detection limit of conventional FC equipment (diameter size lower 300 nm) [79]. Recent studies have shown that FC equipment with high sensitivity can amplify the forward scatter parameter capacity, which is used to identify the size of the MVs [85]. On the other hand, it is very helpful to provide information regarding functional activity of the extracellular vesicles [86–89].

In this regard, novel instruments including NTA or DLS have shown their advantages in the analysis of extracellular vesicles. NTA measures the distribution of the absolute size of the vesicles that range from 50 nm to 1 μm [90]. The vesicles in suspension are illuminated by a laser that produces light scattering or fluorescence. A microscope determines the position of individual vesicles, which are continuously moving due to Brownian motion [91]. When a fluorescent marker is used, NTA can also be used to determine the size of a subgroup of vesicles [92]. The principal advantage of this method is the detection of particles below 100 nm in diameter. In contrast, the limitation of this technique, the low resolution, therefore, NTA is incapable of distinguishing MVs from particles in suspension (debris) with the same size [79]. DLS, also known as photon correlation spectroscopy, measures the size distribution of vesicles between 1 nm and 6 μm. However, the absolute concentration of the vesicles cannot be determined by DLS because the average amplitude of the signal depends on the diameter, concentration and the refractive index of the vesicles [93–95].

The last method TRPS consists in the movement of the MVs through tunable nanopores which are capable of registering MVs between 80 and 1000 nm [96]. Particles passing the pore generate a change in the electric resistance, thus providing information on diameter, surface charge and concentration of single particles. The major disadvantage of TRPS is that it cannot distinguish between MVs and similarly sized particles [79]. Independently of the method used to study of the MVs, it has been recommended to confirm the presence of MVs by measuring them at least with two different techniques.

In addition, enzyme-linked immunosorbent assay (ELISA), Western blot or quantitative real-time PCR (qPCR) are useful tools for the detection of proteins or RNA in preparations of purified MVs. Electron microscopy can provide information concerning the vesicular morphology, size and the presence of markers. Moreover, proteomic analysis and profiles of RNA/microRNA (miRNA) may help to determine the composition of the MVs.

In the absence of pathology, the EMVs are involved in the maintenance of vascular homeostasis, participating in the metabolism of the vascular environment [97]. The EMVs can act on the vascular wall, at the endothelial level, and on smooth muscle cells [98], regulating both vasomotor reactivity and angiogenesis. In fact, the formation of EMVs and their elimination seems to reflect a balance between activation and cell damage, cell survival/apoptosis and angiogenesis. Endothelial responses may be immediate; releasing various factors or can be delayed, modulating the expression of genes involved in regulating the structure and function of the vascular system (**Figure 2**). In *in vitro* models, endothelial cell cultures produce EMVs in a meager percentage without additional stimulus. However, in response to activation

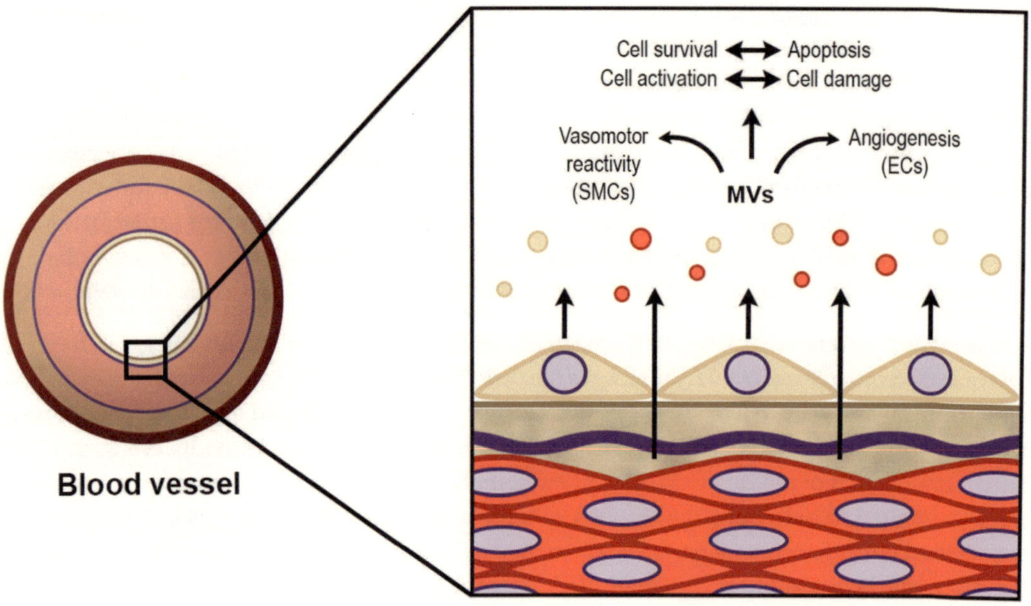

Figure 2. Mechanisms of endothelial microvesicles (MVs) action upon target cells. SMCs, smooth muscle cells; ECs, endothelial cells.

processes and/or apoptosis, the number of EMVs increases significantly. Physiological blood levels of EMVs present in healthy individuals are between 10^3 and 10^4 EMVs/mL and pathological concentrations (present in individuals with CVD) are 10^5 EMVs/mL [99]. Several authors have found that mature endothelial cells in culture, exposed to activation by cytokines, released more EMVs [100, 101].

MVs concentration in blood from healthy subjects is clinically irrelevant. However, in patients with cardiovascular risk factors and after cardiovascular events, EMVs concentrations are increased significantly [10, 102]. In fact, in patients with CVD, an association between the number of circulating EMVs and the Framingham risk score has been shown [72]. In particular, high levels of EMVs in diseases associated with vascular injury seem to reflect an inflammatory and prothrombotic process. EMVs may participate in the development and amplification of CVD through both cardiac and vascular cells. On the other hand, numerous studies have emphasized the effect of cardioprotective drugs on reducing concentrations of extracellular vesicles [73] which reinforces the evidence about the possible correlation of EMVs and vascular injury.

EMVs, and in general all extracellular vesicles, carry a specific load that is capable of delivering to other cells, even in remote locations. Extracellular vesicles share characteristics with their parental cells such as cell surface receptors, integral membrane proteins, cytosolic molecules, organelles, mRNAs, miRNAs or small amounts of DNA and proteins, including transcription factors, cytokines and growth factors [103]. Cell receptors and transmembrane proteins can help in the identification of EMVs, and also are indicative of the ability of vesicles to interact directly with receptors on the surface of target cells, resulting in an intracellular signal transmission. In addition to its effect on specific receptors, it has been shown that EMVs may be fused to the target cell and transfer its contents directly inside as a vehicle for transfer of genetic information [11, 67, 104, 105]. Extracellular vesicles are considered as the main source of miRNAs, released into the bloodstream during cell activation or apoptosis [106]. In fact, most miRNAs are associated with extracellular vesicles and only small amounts of them can be found free in plasma. It is thought that extracellular vesicles are necessary to protect circulating miRNAs from degradation by RNases, transferring safely functional miRNAs from the parental cells receptor cells. miRNAs act as regulatory molecules in endothelial cells, vascular smooth muscle cells, platelets and inflammatory cells that contribute to modulate the initiation and progression of atherosclerosis. It is known that the release of miRNAs does not occur randomly but they are produced and released by controlled mechanisms [107, 108]. It has been described that there are several miRNAs involved in the regulation of vascular function and repair. It is expected that in the future, a better understanding of these molecules provides new options both diagnostic and therapeutic in the vascular pathology.

The MVs from different sources such as endothelial cells, monocytes and lymphocytes can promote oxidative stress in the endothelium through processes that may involve several enzymatic systems [109]. The MVs can regulate the production of reactive oxygen species (ROS), although there are some discrepancies regarding ROS generation systems affected. These contradictory results may be due to the fact that MVs populations studied are from different sources or produced by different stimuli [105, 110]. From the biological point of view, these differences in the production of MVs have a significant for the potential to define MVs populations with different biological activities.

One of the best-provided properties of MVs is its ability to promote coagulation [98]. In fact, the MVs are elevated in hypercoagulative disorders probably as a result of their active participation [98]. It is not clear how far MVs contribute to the *in vivo* coagulation, but there are several *in vitro* studies that demonstrate their procoagulant role. This capacity has been extensively studied in platelet-derived MVs, but the fact is that the MVs have two specific and common physical characteristics that may be responsible for this procoagulant activity: firstly, the externalization of phosphatidylserine as coagulation promoter and secondly, the expression of tissue factor, which is a critical component of the early stages of coagulation [11]. Indeed, tissue factor is not expressed under physiological conditions in circulating and endothelial cells, but it is expressed in pathological conditions.

Chronic inflammation is a crucial factor in the development of atherosclerosis, and the effects of EMVs in inflammatory processes have been the subject of numerous studies since they may represent both a cause and a consequence of inflammation [12]. The MVs isolated from human atherosclerotic plaques can transfer intercellular adhesion molecule-1 (ICAM-1) to endothelial cells and could increase the ability to recruit inflammatory cells in a manner dependent of phosphatidylserine, which may increase the progression of the atherosclerotic plaque. The most conclusive evidence of a proinflammatory role for EMVs is that the administration of exogenous EMVs to rats is associated with acute lung injury, with increased levels of proinflammatory cytokines (IL-1β and TNF-α) and neutrophil infiltration on histological lesion perivascular space [111].

Different studies have described a role of MVs in the regulation of angiogenesis [112]. Platelet-derived MVs were first involved in the angiogenesis process since platelets contain at least 20 factors that regulate angiogenesis. Platelet-derived MVs stimulate proliferation, survival, migration, and formation of capillary-like structures in endothelial cells *in vitro*. Furthermore, injection of platelet-derived MVs increases myocardial post-ischemic capillary density in rats [113]. Subsequent studies have shown that MVs isolated from atherosclerotic plaques are involved in the formation of new blood vessels and in the progression of the plaques to rupture. Endothelial cells in the culture containing MVs that release matrix metalloproteinases (MMP-2 and MMP-9) and promote matrix degradation and the formation of new blood vessels.

In addition to being a potent stimulus for the formation of MVs, apoptosis can also be a consequence of MVs signaling [112]. Monocyte, erythrocytes, platelets and endothelial cells-derived MVs contain caspase-3. It is thought that the content of caspases may be a mechanism directed to control the apoptosis, suggesting that MVs could release caspase-3 into the target cells, participating in the induction of apoptosis. In addition, caspase-3 is implicated in numerous cellular processes, so the release of this protein could have an even more significant impact on the target cell.

The MVs contain proteolytic enzymes, and then some of its effects could be attributed to alterations in the extracellular matrix or proteolytic cleavage of various signaling molecules. For example, the microvasculature-derived EMVs containing MMP-1, MMP-2, MMP-13 and MMP-7, which degrade fibronectin *in vitro* [114]. Moreover, MVs isolated from human atherosclerotic plaques contain an active form of ADAM17 (metallopeptidase domain 17), an enzyme with a role in the control of inflammation and tissue regeneration. This enzyme could contribute to the release of cytokines and the development of alterations mediated by MVs in the extracellular environment [115].

Initially, proliferation and migration of adjacent endothelial cells have been identified as a factor of endothelial repair, and subsequent studies have shown that the maintenance of the endothelial structure is associated with EPCs and their ability to differentiate and repair damaged endothelial tissue. Due to the importance of this repair mechanism in the maintenance of vascular homeostasis, it is logical to think about the existence of close communication between damaged endothelial cells and EPCs. Previous studies performed by our group suggest that plasma EMVs, both of healthy subjects and patients with CKD; participate in the activity of the EPCs [10]. Our hypothesis is that EMVs can be an essential and necessary physiological mechanism of signaling to initiate the recruitment of EPCs from bone marrow. In *in vitro* models, we have shown that EMVs may be the key element in the regeneration and maintenance of vascular homeostasis, acting on EPCs [116]. Indeed, in response to different stimuli, the endothelial cells can induce EMV with different membrane characteristics, miRNA and other molecules in your content that reduce the ability of EPC to regenerate and participate in the signaling pathways involved in apoptosis and oxidative stress [117]. These specific mechanisms may constitute therapeutic objectives in future studies.

Vascular calcification is an increasingly constant process in developed countries and can contribute significantly to increased cardiovascular risk. The processes and mechanisms involved in the formation of vascular calcifications are poorly understood and are needed to develop new therapeutic strategies to prevent or avoid calcification. Patients CKD have a higher incidence of vascular calcification, and our group has shown that EMVs are increased in patients with an elevated degree of calcification [10]. In *in vitro* studies, EMVs produced in an inflammatory environment or obtained from patients with CKD promoted the calcification of smooth muscle cells, as assessed by some calcification markers (bone morphogenetic protein-2 (BMP-2) and alkaline phosphatase (ALP)) and the phenolsulfonephthalein method [100]. Other authors have also described a role of the MVs in the mineralization of vascular smooth muscle cells [118].

MVs have also been associated with endothelial senescence. As we said before, senescent cells release characteristic molecules and substances composing the SASP. However, some of those substances which are known to be part of this SASP cannot be released as soluble molecules due to their nature, as some transmembrane proteins [119]. It is known that the premature induction of cellular senescence *in vitro* increases the release of extracellular vesicles [120]. Those concepts suggest the contribution of MVs as part of the SASP, which have two important consequences: (1) SASP MVs can be the mechanism by which those insoluble proteins are released and (2) the carrier molecules can activate signaling processes in the target cells. Nevertheless, the specific mechanisms underlying MVs releasing from the senescent cells are still unresolved. It has been described that p53, a tumor-suppressor protein, remarkably upregulated in senescence, modulates the release of extracellular vesicles [121]. Also, p53 takes part in the transcription of some molecules implicated in extracellular vesicles biogenesis, partly explaining how senescence and MVs releasing activation can be related [122–124]. Moreover, the content within those MVs may be necessary in the induction of senescence in the target cells, as it has been shown that some miRNAs can regulate the p53 and pRB pathways [125–127]. Loss of pRB results in deregulated cell proliferation and apoptosis, whereas loss of p53 desensitizes cells to checkpoint signals, including apoptosis [128]. Thus, the presence of those miRNAs in MVs may be associated with hormonal changes driving aging (endocrine senescence induction) playing a critical role in the aging process and adding a new perspective on the mechanisms involved in aging.

6. Conclusions and perspectives

CVD seem to begin as a consequence of a damaging process and endothelial dysfunction, and there are pieces of evidence implying cellular senescence in the functional imbalance of the endothelium. Cellular senescence is a physiological mechanism which occurs as a consequence of aging, but

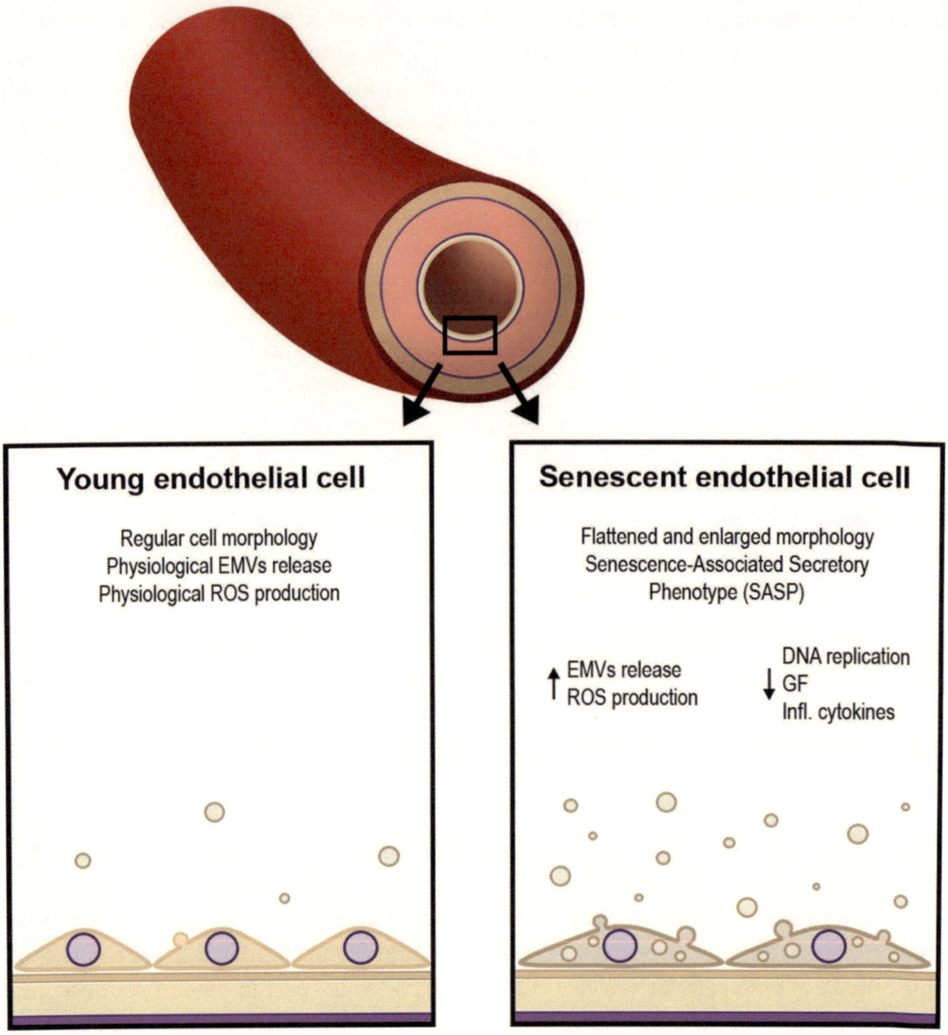

Figure 3. Different characteristics of young and senescent endothelial cells. Senescent cells undergo distinctive phenotypic, morphological alterations and senescence-associated secretory phenotype (SASP). The number of endothelial microvesicles (EMVs) of the senescent cells is greater than those derived from young cells. Also, the reactive oxygen species (ROS) production is higher in senescent endothelial cells compared with young endothelial cells. Moreover, the secretion of growth factors (GF) and proinflammatory cytokines (infl. cytokines) from senescent endothelial cells are reduced.

under different pathologic conditions, its regulation is modified, as in CVD or CKD. Senescent endothelial cells change their morphological and functional characteristics (**Figure 3**) and cannot correctly regulate the repairing and regenerative activity of EPCs. In the endothelial senescence context, the role of EMVs appears to be important. EMVs are considered as biomarkers of endothelial injury and are associated with an inflammatory and prothrombotic state. However, the perspectives of their study are beyond their role as biomarkers, as they are capable of transmitting biologic information in several physiologic and physiopathologic processes. EMVs are increased in elderly, but also in patients with CVD and CKD. Many questions remain unresolved to understand the role of EMVs in the endothelial function and damage. To comprehend and characterize the mechanisms by which the senescent endothelial cells show an imbalanced functionality is of great interest, opening new perspectives to increase our knowledge and to identify useful biomarkers in the timely diagnostics and to design therapeutic objectives in CVD.

Acknowledgements

This work was supported by Plan Nacional Proyectos de Investigación en Salud of Instituto de Salud Carlos III (ISCIII) Fondos Feder European Grants (PI14/00806 and PI17/01029); Red de Investigación Renal (REDinREN; RD16/0009/0034) Junta de Andalucía Grants, P12-CTS-7352 and Santander Universidad Complutense de Madrid PR41/17-20964. Matilde Alique is a fellow of the program "Ayuda Postdoctoral Programa Propio" from Universidad de Alcalá, Madrid, Spain. Rafael Ramírez-Carracedo is a fellow of the program FPI (Formación de Personal Universitario) from Universidad Francisco de Vitoria, Madrid, Spain".

Author details

Julia Carracedo[1]*, Rafael Ramírez-Carracedo[2], Matilde Alique[3] and
Rafael Ramírez-Chamond[3]

*Address all correspondence to: julcar01@ucm.es

1 Department of Genetic, Physiology and Microbiology, Faculty of Biology, Complutense University/Instituto de Investigación Sanitaria Hospital 12 de Octubre (imas12), Madrid, Spain

2 Cardiovascular Joint Research Unit, University Francisco de Vitoria/University Hospital Ramon y Cajal Research Unit (IRYCIS), Madrid, Spain

3 Biology Systems Department, Physiology, Alcala University, Alcala de Henares, Madrid, Spain

References

[1] Widlansky ME, Gokce N, Keaney JF, Vita JA. The clinical implications of endothelial dysfunction. Journal of the American College of Cardiology. 2003;**42**(7):1149-1160

[2] Donato AJ, Morgan RG, Walker AE, Lesniewski LA. Cellular and molecular biology of aging endothelial cells. Journal of Molecular and Cellular Cardiology. 2015;**89**(Pt B):122-135

[3] Seals DR, Jablonski KL, Donato AJ. Aging and vascular endothelial function in humans. Clinical Science (London, England). 2011;**120**(9):357-375

[4] López-Otín C, Blasco MA, Partridge L, Serrano M, Kroemer G. The hallmarks of aging. Cell. 2013;**153**(6):1194-1217

[5] Stenvinkel P, Larsson TE. Chronic kidney disease: A clinical model of premature aging. American Journal of Kidney Diseases. 2013;**62**(2):339-351

[6] Kooman J, Dekker M, Usvyat LA, Kotanko P, Van der Sande F, Schalkwijk CG, et al. Inflammation and premature aging in advanced chronic kidney disease. American Journal of Physiology-Renal Physiology. 2017;**313**(4):F938-F950. DOI: 10.1152/ajprenal.00256.2017

[7] Merino A, Buendia P, Martin-Malo A, Aljama P, Ramirez R, Carracedo J. Senescent CD14+CD16+ monocytes exhibit proinflammatory and proatherosclerotic activity. Journal of Immunology. 2011;**186**(3):1809-1815

[8] Minamino T, Miyauchi H, Yoshida T, Ishida Y, Yoshida H, Komuro I. Endothelial cell senescence in human atherosclerosis: Role of telomere in endothelial dysfunction. Circulation. 2002;**105**(13):1541-1544

[9] Childs BG, Baker DJ, Wijshake T, Conover CA, Campisi J, van Deursen JM. Senescent intimal foam cells are deleterious at all stages of atherosclerosis. Science. 2016;**354**(6311):472-477

[10] Soriano S, Carmona A, Triviño F, Rodriguez M, Alvarez-Benito M, Martín-Malo A, et al. Endothelial damage and vascular calcification in patients with chronic kidney disease. American Journal of Physiology. Renal Physiology. 2014;**307**(11):F1302-F1311

[11] Liu ML, Williams KJ. Microvesicles: Potential markers and mediators of endothelial dysfunction. Current Opinion in Endocrinology, Diabetes, and Obesity. 2012;**19**(2):121-127

[12] Schiro A, Wilkinson FL, Weston R, Smyth JV, Serracino-Inglott F, Alexander MY. Endothelial microparticles as conveyors of information in atherosclerotic disease. Atherosclerosis. 2014;**234**(2):295-302

[13] Ross R, Glomset JA. The pathogenesis of atherosclerosis (first of two parts). The New England Journal of Medicine. 1976;**295**(7):369-377

[14] Marin C, Ramirez R, Delgado-Lista J, Yubero-Serrano EM, Perez-Martinez P, Carracedo J, et al. Mediterranean diet reduces endothelial damage and improves the regenerative capacity of endothelium. The American Journal of Clinical Nutrition. 2011;**93**(2):267-274

[15] Edirisinghe I, Burton-Freeman BM. Age associated endothelial dysfunction: Role of oxidative stress, inflammation and Western diet. Nutrition and Aging. 2014;**2**:197-211

[16] Lüscher TF, Barton M. Biology of the endothelium. Clinical Cardiology. 1997;**20**(11 Suppl 2): II-3-10

[17] El Assar M, Angulo J, Vallejo S, Peiró C, Sánchez-Ferrer CF, Rodríguez-Mañas L. Mechanisms involved in the aging-induced vascular dysfunction. Frontiers in Physiology. 2012;**3**:132

[18] Al-Soudi A, Kaaij MH, Tas SW. Endothelial cells: From innocent bystanders to active participants in immune responses. Autoimmunity Reviews. 2017;**16**:951-962

[19] Félétou M, Vanhoutte PM. Endothelial dysfunction: A multifaceted disorder (the Wiggers award lecture). American Journal of Physiology. Heart and Circulatory Physiology. 2006;**291**(3):H985-1002

[20] Liao JK. Linking endothelial dysfunction with endothelial cell activation. The Journal of Clinical Investigation. 2013;**123**(2):540-541

[21] Celermajer DS, Sorensen KE, Spiegelhalter DJ, Georgakopoulos D, Robinson J, Deanfield JE. Aging is associated with endothelial dysfunction in healthy men years before the age-related decline in women. Journal of the American College of Cardiology. 1994;**24**(2):471-476

[22] Badimon L, Badimon JJ, Penny W, Webster MW, Chesebro JH, Fuster V. Endothelium and atherosclerosis. Journal of Hypertension. Supplement. 1992;**10**(2):S43-S50

[23] Laina A, Stellos K, Stamatelopoulos K. Vascular ageing: Underlying mechanisms and clinical implications. Experimental Gerontology. 2017

[24] Regina C, Panatta E, Candi E, Melino G, Amelio I, Balistreri CR, et al. Vascular ageing and endothelial cell senescence: Molecular mechanisms of physiology and diseases. Mechanisms of Ageing and Development. 2016;**159**:14-21

[25] Lakatta EG, Levy D. Arterial and cardiac aging: Major shareholders in cardiovascular disease enterprises: Part I: Aging arteries: A "set up" for vascular disease. Circulation. 2003;**107**(1):139-146

[26] Weinsaft JW, Edelberg JM. Aging-associated changes in vascular activity: A potential link to geriatric cardiovascular disease. The American Journal of Geriatric Cardiology. 2001;**10**(6):348-354

[27] Erusalimsky JD, Kurz DJ. Cellular senescence in vivo: Its relevance in ageing and cardiovascular disease. Experimental Gerontology. 2005;**40**(8-9):634-642

[28] Cellular BDG. Senescence, ageing and disease. Age (Dordrecht, Netherlands). 2009;**31**(1):1-9

[29] Campisi J. Aging, cellular senescence, and cancer. Annual Review of Physiology. 2013;**75**:685-705

[30] Shay JW, Wright WE. Hayflick, his limit, and cellular ageing. Nature Reviews. Molecular Cell Biology. 2000;**1**(1):72-76

[31] Campisi J, d'Adda di Fagagna F. Cellular senescence: When bad things happen to good cells. Nature Reviews. Molecular Cell Biology. 2007;**8**(9):729-740

[32] Coppé JP, Desprez PY, Krtolica A, Campisi J. The senescence-associated secretory phenotype: The dark side of tumor suppression. Annual Review of Pathology. 2010;**5**:99-118

[33] Ruiz-Torres A, Lozano R, Melón J, Carraro R. Age-dependent decline of in vitro migration (basal and stimulated by IGF-1 or insulin) of human vascular smooth muscle cells. The Journals of Gerontology. Series A, Biological Sciences and Medical Sciences. 2003;**58**(12):B1074-B1077

[34] Georgakopoulou EA, Tsimaratou K, Evangelou K, Fernandez Marcos PJ, Zoumpourlis V, Trougakos IP, et al. Specific lipofuscin staining as a novel biomarker to detect replicative and stress-induced senescence. A method applicable in cryo-preserved and archival tissues. Aging (Albany NY). 2013;**5**(1):37-50

[35] Tchkonia T, Morbeck DE, Von Zglinicki T, Van Deursen J, Lustgarten J, Scrable H, et al. Fat tissue, aging, and cellular senescence. Aging Cell. 2010;**9**(5):667-684

[36] Green DR, Evan GI. A matter of life and death. Cancer Cell. 2002;**1**(1):19-30

[37] Lawless C, Wang C, Jurk D, Merz A, Zglinicki T, Passos JF. Quantitative assessment of markers for cell senescence. Experimental Gerontology. 2010;**45**(10):772-778

[38] Burton DG, Sheerin AN, Ostler EL, Smith K, Giles PJ, Lowe J, et al. Cyclin D1 overexpression permits the reproducible detection of senescent human vascular smooth muscle cells. Annals of the New York Academy of Sciences. 2007;**1119**:20-31

[39] Freund A, Laberge RM, Demaria M, Campisi J. Lamin B1 loss is a senescence-associated biomarker. Molecular Biology of the Cell. 2012;**23**(11):2066-2075

[40] Childs BG, Gluscevic M, Baker DJ, Laberge RM, Marquess D, Dananberg J, et al. Senescent cells: An emerging target for diseases of ageing. Nature Reviews. Drug Discovery. 2017;**16**:718-735

[41] Lee BY, Han JA, Im JS, Morrone A, Johung K, Goodwin EC, et al. Senescence-associated beta-galactosidase is lysosomal beta-galactosidase. Aging Cell. 2006;**5**(2):187-195

[42] Debacq-Chainiaux F, Erusalimsky JD, Campisi J, Toussaint O. Protocols to detect senescence-associated beta-galactosidase (SA-betagal) activity, a biomarker of senescent cells in culture and in vivo. Nature Protocols. 2009;**4**(12):1798-1806

[43] Krishnamurthy J, Torrice C, Ramsey MR, Kovalev GI, Al-Regaiey K, Su L, et al. Ink4a/Arf expression is a biomarker of aging. The Journal of Clinical Investigation. 2004;**114**(9):1299-1307

[44] Beauséjour CM, Krtolica A, Galimi F, Narita M, Lowe SW, Yaswen P, et al. Reversal of human cellular senescence: Roles of the p53 and p16 pathways. The EMBO Journal. 2003;**22**(16):4212-4222

[45] Itahana K, Zou Y, Itahana Y, Martinez JL, Beausejour C, Jacobs JJ, et al. Control of the replicative life span of human fibroblasts by p16 and the polycomb protein Bmi-1. Molecular and Cellular Biology. 2003;**23**(1):389-401

[46] Campisi J. Senescent cells, tumor suppression, and organismal aging: Good citizens, bad neighbors. Cell. 2005;**120**(4):513-522

[47] Narita M, Nũnez S, Heard E, Lin AW, Hearn SA, Spector DL, et al. Rb-mediated heterochromatin formation and silencing of E2F target genes during cellular senescence. Cell. 2003;**113**(6):703-716

[48] London G, Covic A, Goldsmith D, Wiecek A, Suleymanlar G, Ortiz A, et al. Arterial aging and arterial disease: Interplay between central hemodynamics, cardiac work, and organ flow-implications for CKD and cardiovascular disease. Kidney International Supplements. 2011;**1**(1):10-12

[49] Gekle M. Kidney and aging—A narrative review. Experimental Gerontology. 2017;**87** (Pt B):153-155

[50] Parfrey PS, Foley RN. The clinical epidemiology of cardiac disease in chronic renal failure. Journal of the American Society of Nephrology. 1999;**10**(7):1606-1615

[51] McClellan WM, Chertow GM. Beyond Framingham: Cardiovascular risk profiling in ESRD. Journal of the American Society of Nephrology. 2005;**16**(6):1539-1541

[52] Foley RN, Parfrey PS, Sarnak MJ. Epidemiology of cardiovascular disease in chronic renal disease. Journal of the American Society of Nephrology. 1998;**9**(12 Suppl):S16-S23

[53] Cases A, Vera M, López Gómez JM. Cardiovascular risk in patients with chronic renal failure. Patients in renal replacement therapy. Nefrología. 2002;**22**(Suppl 1):68-74

[54] Pannier B, Guerin AP, Marchais SJ, Metivier F, Safar ME, London GM. Postischemic vasodilation, endothelial activation, and cardiovascular remodeling in end-stage renal disease. Kidney International. 2000;**57**(3):1091-1099

[55] Merino A, Portolés J, Selgas R, Ojeda R, Buendia P, Ocaña J, et al. Effect of different dialysis modalities on microinflammatory status and endothelial damage. Clinical Journal of the American Society of Nephrology. 2010;**5**(2):227-234

[56] Ramírez R, Carracedo J, Merino A, Soriano S, Ojeda R, Alvarez-Lara MA, et al. CD14+CD16+ monocytes from chronic kidney disease patients exhibit increased adhesion ability to endothelial cells. Contributions to Nephrology. 2011;**171**:57-61

[57] Carracedo J, Buendía P, Merino A, Soriano S, Esquivias E, Martín-Malo A, et al. Cellular senescence determines endothelial cell damage induced by uremia. Experimental Gerontology. 2013;**48**(8):766-773

[58] Merino A, Nogueras S, García-Maceira T, Rodríguez M, Martin-Malo A, Ramirez R, et al. Bacterial DNA and endothelial damage in haemodialysis patients. Nephrology, Dialysis, Transplantation. 2008;**23**(11):3635-3642

[59] Heine GH, Ortiz A, Massy ZA, Lindholm B, Wiecek A, Martínez-Castelao A, et al. Monocyte subpopulations and cardiovascular risk in chronic kidney disease. Nature Reviews. Nephrology. 2012;**8**(6):362-369

[60] Ziegler-Heitbrock L, Ancuta P, Crowe S, Dalod M, Grau V, Hart DN, et al. Nomenclature of monocytes and dendritic cells in blood. Blood. 2010;**116**(16):e74-e80

[61] Ramírez R, Carracedo J, Soriano S, Jiménez R, Martín-Malo A, Rodríguez M, et al. Stress-induced premature senescence in mononuclear cells from patients on long-term hemodialysis. American Journal of Kidney Diseases. 2005;**45**(2):353-359

[62] Li G, Kim YJ, Mantel C, Broxmeyer HE. P-selectin enhances generation of CD14+CD16+ dendritic-like cells and inhibits macrophage maturation from human peripheral blood monocytes. Journal of Immunology. 2003;**171**(2):669-677

[63] Ramirez R, Carracedo J, Merino A, Nogueras S, Alvarez-Lara MA, Rodríguez M, et al. Microinflammation induces endothelial damage in hemodialysis patients: The role of convective transport. Kidney International. 2007;**72**(1):108-113

[64] Urbanski K, Ludew D, Filip G, Filip M, Sagan A, Szczepaniak P, et al. CD14(+)CD16(++) "nonclassical" monocytes are associated with endothelial dysfunction in patients with coronary artery disease. Thrombosis and Haemostasis. 2017;**117**(5):971-980

[65] Ziegler-Heitbrock L. The CD14+ CD16+ blood monocytes: Their role in infection and inflammation. Journal of Leukocyte Biology. 2007;**81**(3):584-592

[66] Fenyo IM, Gafencu AV. The involvement of the monocytes/macrophages in chronic inflammation associated with atherosclerosis. Immunobiology. 2013;**218**(11):1376-1384

[67] Lawson C, Vicencio JM, Yellon DM, Davidson SM. Microvesicles and exosomes: New players in metabolic and cardiovascular disease. The Journal of Endocrinology. 2016;**228**(2):R57-R71

[68] Carracedo J, Merino A, Nogueras S, Carretero D, Berdud I, Ramírez R, et al. On-line hemodiafiltration reduces the proinflammatory CD14+CD16+ monocyte-derived dendritic cells: A prospective, crossover study. Journal of the American Society of Nephrology. 2006;**17**(8):2315-2321

[69] Carracedo J, Buendía P, Merino A, Madueño JA, Peralbo E, Ortiz A, et al. Klotho modulates the stress response in human senescent endothelial cells. Mechanisms of Ageing and Development. 2012;**133**(11-12):647-654

[70] Ramirez R, Carracedo J, Nogueras S, Buendia P, Merino A, Cañadillas S, et al. Carbamylated darbepoetin derivative prevents endothelial progenitor cell damage with no effect on angiogenesis. Journal of Molecular and Cellular Cardiology. 2009;**47**(6):781-788

[71] Minciacchi VR, Freeman MR, Di Vizio D. Extracellular vesicles in cancer: Exosomes, microvesicles and the emerging role of large oncosomes. Seminars in Cell & Developmental Biology. 2015;**40**:41-51

[72] Amabile N, Cheng S, Renard JM, Larson MG, Ghorbani A, McCabe E, et al. Association of circulating endothelial microparticles with cardiometabolic risk factors in the Framingham Heart Study. European Heart Journal. 2014;**35**(42):2972-2979

[73] Yin M, Loyer X, Boulanger CM. Extracellular vesicles as new pharmacological targets to treat atherosclerosis. European Journal of Pharmacology. 2015;**763**(Pt A):90-103

[74] Lei Q, Liu T, Gao F, Xie H, Sun L, Zhao A, et al. Microvesicles as potential biomarkers for the identification of senescence in human mesenchymal stem cells. Theranostics. 2017;**7**(10):2673-2689

[75] Martinez MC, Tual-Chalot S, Leonetti D, Andriantsitohaina R. Microparticles: Targets and tools in cardiovascular disease. Trends in Pharmacological Sciences. 2011;**32**(11):659-665

[76] Baron M, Boulanger CM, Staels B, Tailleux A. Cell-derived microparticles in atherosclerosis: Biomarkers and targets for pharmacological modulation? Journal of Cellular and Molecular Medicine. 2012;**16**(7):1365-1376

[77] Marin C, Delgado-Lista J, Ramirez R, Carracedo J, Caballero J, Perez-Martinez P, et al. Mediterranean diet reduces senescence-associated stress in endothelial cells. Age (Dordrecht, Netherlands). 2012;**34**(6):1309-1316

[78] Szatanek R, Baran J, Siedlar M, Baj-Krzyworzeka M. Isolation of extracellular vesicles: Determining the correct approach (review). International Journal of Molecular Medicine. 2015;**36**(1):11-17

[79] Ridger VC, Boulanger CM, Angelillo-Scherrer A, Badimon L, Blanc-Brude O, Bochaton-Piallat ML, et al. Microvesicles in vascular homeostasis and diseases. Position paper of the European Society of Cardiology (ESC) working group on atherosclerosis and vascular biology. Thrombosis and Haemostasis. 2017;**117**(7):1296-1316

[80] van der Pol E, Coumans FA, Sturk A, Nieuwland R, van Leeuwen TG. Refractive index determination of nanoparticles in suspension using nanoparticle tracking analysis. Nano Letters. 2014;**14**(11):6195-6201

[81] Lacroix R, Robert S, Poncelet P, Kasthuri RS, Key NS, Dignat-George F, et al. Standardization of platelet-derived microparticle enumeration by flow cytometry with calibrated beads: Results of the international society on thrombosis and haemostasis SSC collaborative workshop. Journal of Thrombosis and Haemostasis. 2010;**8**(11):2571-2574

[82] Lacroix R, Da Silva S, Gaig MV, Rousseau R, Délia ML, Bergel A. Modelling potential/current distribution in microbial electrochemical systems shows how the optimal bioanode architecture depends on electrolyte conductivity. Physical Chemistry Chemical Physics. 2014;**16**(41):22892-22902

[83] Erdbrügger U, Le TH. Extracellular vesicles in renal diseases: More than novel biomarkers? Journal of the American Society of Nephrology. 2016;**27**(1):12-26

[84] Alique M, Ruíz-Torres MP, Bodega G, Noci MV, Troyano N, Bohórquez L, et al. Microvesicles from the plasma of elderly subjects and from senescent endothelial cells promote vascular calcification. Aging (Albany NY). 2017;**9**:778-789

[85] Robert S, Lacroix R, Poncelet P, Harhouri K, Bouriche T, Judicone C, et al. High-sensitivity flow cytometry provides access to standardized measurement of small-size microparticles—Brief report. Arteriosclerosis, Thrombosis, and Vascular Biology. 2012;**32**(4):1054-1058

[86] Erdbrügger U, Rudy CK, Etter ME, Dryden KA, Yeager M, Klibanov AL, et al. Imaging flow cytometry elucidates limitations of microparticle analysis by conventional flow cytometry. Cytometry. Part A. 2014;**85**(9):756-770

[87] Headland SE, Jones HR, D'Sa AS, Perretti M, Norling LV. Cutting-edge analysis of extracellular microparticles using ImageStream(X) imaging flow cytometry. Scientific Reports. 2014;**4**:5237

[88] Vallhov H, Gutzeit C, Johansson SM, Nagy N, Paul M, Li Q, et al. Exosomes containing glycoprotein 350 released by EBV-transformed B cells selectively target B cells through CD21 and block EBV infection in vitro. Journal of Immunology. 2011;**186**(1):73-82

[89] Zuba-Surma EK, Kucia M, Abdel-Latif A, Lillard JW, Ratajczak MZ. The ImageStream system: A key step to a new era in imaging. Folia Histochemica et Cytobiologica. 2007;**45**(4):279-290

[90] Lytvyn Y, Xiao F, Kennedy CR, Perkins BA, Reich HN, Scholey JW, et al. Assessment of urinary microparticles in normotensive patients with type 1 diabetes. Diabetologia. 2017;**60**(3):581-584

[91] Dragovic RA, Gardiner C, Brooks AS, Tannetta DS, Ferguson DJ, Hole P, et al. Sizing and phenotyping of cellular vesicles using nanoparticle tracking analysis. Nanomedicine. 2011;**7**(6):780-788

[92] Braeckmans K, Buyens K, Bouquet W, Vervaet C, Joye P, De Vos F, et al. Sizing nanomatter in biological fluids by fluorescence single particle tracking. Nano Letters. 2010;**10**(11):4435-4442

[93] Chan MY, Dowling QM, Sivananthan SJ, Kramer RM. Particle sizing of nanoparticle adjuvant formulations by dynamic light scattering (DLS) and nanoparticle tracking analysis (NTA). Methods in Molecular Biology. 2017;**1494**:239-252

[94] Dieckmann Y, Cölfen H, Hofmann H, Petri-Fink A. Particle size distribution measurements of manganese-doped ZnS nanoparticles. Analytical Chemistry. 2009;**81**(10):3889-3895

[95] Gardiner C, Shaw M, Hole P, Smith J, Tannetta D, Redman CW, et al. Measurement of refractive index by nanoparticle tracking analysis reveals heterogeneity in extracellular vesicles. Journal of Extracellular Vesicles. 2014;**3**:25361

[96] Coumans FA, van der Pol E, Böing AN, Hajji N, Sturk G, van Leeuwen TG, et al. Reproducible extracellular vesicle size and concentration determination with tunable resistive pulse sensing. Journal of Extracellular Vesicles. 2014;**3**:25922

[97] Gaceb A, Martinez MC, Andriantsitohaina R. Extracellular vesicles: New players in cardiovascular diseases. The International Journal of Biochemistry & Cell Biology. 2014;**50**:24-28

[98] Meziani F, Tesse A, Andriantsitohaina R. Microparticles are vectors of paradoxical information in vascular cells including the endothelium: Role in health and diseases. Pharmacological Reports. 2008;**60**(1):75-84

[99] França CN, Izar MC, Amaral JB, Tegani DM, Fonseca FA. Microparticles as potential biomarkers of cardiovascular disease. Arquivos Brasileiros de Cardiologia. 2015;**104**(2): 169-174

[100] Buendía P, Montes de Oca A, Madueño JA, Merino A, Martín-Malo A, Aljama P, et al. Endothelial microparticles mediate inflammation-induced vascular calcification. The FASEB Journal. 2015;**29**(1):173-181

[101] Fernandez-Martínez AB, Torija AV, Carracedo J, Ramirez R, de Lucio-Cazaña FJ. Microparticles released by vascular endothelial cells increase hypoxia inducible factor expression in human proximal tubular HK-2 cells. The International Journal of Biochemistry & Cell Biology. 2014;**53**:334-342

[102] Noci MV, Ramírez R, Lluch M, Rodríguez M, Carracedo J. Changes in endothelial microparticles and endothelial progenitor cells in obese patients in response to surgical stress. The Journal of Bone and Joint Surgery. American Volume. 2015;**97**(5):353-358

[103] Moldovan L, Batte K, Wang Y, Wisler J, Piper M. Analyzing the circulating microRNAs in exosomes/extracellular vesicles from serum or plasma by qRT-PCR. Methods in Molecular Biology. 2013;**1024**:129-145

[104] Quesenberry PJ, Aliotta J, Deregibus MC, Camussi G. Role of extracellular RNA-carrying vesicles in cell differentiation and reprogramming. Stem Cell Research & Therapy. 2015;**6**:153

[105] Greening DW, Xu R, Gopal SK, Rai A, Simpson RJ. Proteomic insights into extracellular vesicle biology—defining exosomes and shed microvesicles. Expert Review of Proteomics. 2017;**14**(1):69-95

[106] Menghini R, Stöhr R, Federici M. MicroRNAs in vascular aging and atherosclerosis. Ageing Research Reviews. 2014;**17**:68-78

[107] Goettsch C, Hutcheson JD, Aikawa E. MicroRNA in cardiovascular calcification: Focus on targets and extracellular vesicle delivery mechanisms. Circulation Research. 2013;**112**(7):1073-1084

[108] Sohel MH. Extracellular/circulating MicroRNAs: Release mechanisms, functions and challenges. Achievements in the Life Sciences. 2016:175-186

[109] Brodsky SV, Zhang F, Nasjletti A, Goligorsky MS. Endothelium-derived microparticles impair endothelial function in vitro. American Journal of Physiology. Heart and Circulatory Physiology. 2004;**286**(5):H1910-H1915

[110] Larson MC, Hillery CA, Hogg N. Circulating membrane-derived microvesicles in redox biology. Free Radical Biology & Medicine. 2014;**73**:214-228

[111] Zhu YG, Feng XM, Abbott J, Fang XH, Hao Q, Monsel A, et al. Human mesenchymal stem cell microvesicles for treatment of *Escherichia coli* endotoxin-induced acute lung injury in mice. Stem Cells. 2014;**32**(1):116-125

[112] Burger D, Schock S, Thompson CS, Montezano AC, Hakim AM, Touyz RM. Microparticles: Biomarkers and beyond. Clinical Science (London, England). 2013;**124**(7):423-441

[113] Brill A, Dashevsky O, Rivo J, Gozal Y, Varon D. Platelet-derived microparticles induce angiogenesis and stimulate post-ischemic revascularization. Cardiovascular Research. 2005;**67**(1):30-38

[114] Lozito TP, Tuan RS. Endothelial cell microparticles act as centers of matrix metalloproteinsase-2 (MMP-2) activation and vascular matrix remodeling. Journal of Cellular Physiology. 2012;**227**(2):534-549

[115] Canault M, Leroyer AS, Peiretti F, Lesèche G, Tedgui A, Bonardo B, et al. Microparticles of human atherosclerotic plaques enhance the shedding of the tumor necrosis factor-alpha converting enzyme/ADAM17 substrates, tumor necrosis factor and tumor necrosis factor receptor-1. The American Journal of Pathology. 2007;**171**(5):1713-1723

[116] Luna C, Carmona A, Alique M, Carracedo J, Ramirez R. TNF alpha-damaged-HUVECs microparticles modify endothelial progenitor cell functional activity. Frontiers in Physiology. 2015;**6**:395

[117] Carmona A, Guerrero F, Buendia P, Obrero T, Aljama P, Carracedo J. Microvesicles derived from indoxyl sulfate treated endothelial cells induce endothelial progenitor cells dysfunction. Frontiers in Physiology. 2017;**8**:666

[118] Kapustin AN, Davies JD, Reynolds JL, McNair R, Jones GT, Sidibe A, et al. Calcium regulates key components of vascular smooth muscle cell-derived matrix vesicles to enhance mineralization. Circulation Research. 2011;**109**(1):e1-12

[119] Urbanelli L, Buratta S, Sagini K, Tancini B, Emiliani C. Extracellular vesicles as new players in cellular senescence. International Journal of Molecular Sciences. 2016;**17**(9):1408

[120] Lehmann BD, Paine MS, Brooks AM, McCubrey JA, Renegar RH, Wang R, et al. Senescence-associated exosome release from human prostate cancer cells. Cancer Research. 2008;**68**(19):7864-7871

[121] Yu X, Harris SL, Levine AJ. The regulation of exosome secretion: A novel function of the p53 protein. Cancer Research. 2006;**66**(9):4795-4801

[122] Lespagnol A, Duflaut D, Beekman C, Blanc L, Fiucci G, Marine JC, et al. Exosome secretion, including the DNA damage-induced p53-dependent secretory pathway, is severely compromised in TSAP6/Steap3-null mice. Cell Death and Differentiation. 2008;**15**(11):1723-1733

[123] Yu X, Riley T, Levine AJ. The regulation of the endosomal compartment by p53 the tumor suppressor gene. The FEBS Journal. 2009;**276**(8):2201-2212

[124] Feng Z. p53 regulation of the IGF-1/AKT/mTOR pathways and the endosomal compartment. Cold Spring Harbor Perspectives in Biology. 2010;**2**(2):a001057

[125] Yamakuchi M, Lowenstein CJ. MiR-34, SIRT1 and p53: The feedback loop. Cell Cycle. 2009;**8**(5):712-715

[126] Grillari J, Hackl M, Grillari-Voglauer R. miR-17-92 cluster: Ups and downs in cancer and aging. Biogerontology. 2010;**11**(4):501-506

[127] Ugalde AP, Ramsay AJ, de la Rosa J, Varela I, Mariño G, Cadiñanos J, et al. Aging and chronic DNA damage response activate a regulatory pathway involving miR-29 and p53. The EMBO Journal. 2011;**30**(11):2219-2232

[128] Hickman ES, Moroni MC, Helin K. The role of p53 and pRB in apoptosis and cancer. Current Opinion in Genetics & Development. 2002;**12**(1):60-66

Chapter 4

Targeting Endothelial SIRT1 for the Prevention of Arterial Aging

Yumeng Guo and Yu Wang

Additional information is available at the end of the chapter

http://dx.doi.org/10.5772/intechopen.73019

Abstract

Cardiovascular diseases are the leading cause of morbidity and mortality in the elderly population all over the world. Arterial aging is the earliest manifestation and a key risk factor for age-induced cardiovascular abnormalities. The longevity regulator Sirtuin 1 (SIRT1) is abundantly expressed in the endothelium of the arteries and elicits potent protective functions against arterial aging. Targeting endothelial SIRT1 represents a promising approach for the prevention and treatment of cardiovascular diseases. This chapter provides an overview of SIRT1's regulation and function in endothelial cells and discusses the potential applications of targeting endothelial SIRT1 for arterial aging-related cardiovascular diseases.

Keywords: sirtuins, endothelium, cellular senescence, vasodilatation, arterial remodeling, hypertension, atherosclerosis

1. Arterial aging

Chronological age is associated with a progressive alteration of arterial structure and function, herein referred to as arterial aging, which contributes to the development of a wide range of cardiovascular diseases including hypertension, atherosclerosis, heart failure, and stroke [1–3]. Arterial system is composed of three types of arteries including large elastic or conduit arteries, medium-sized muscular arteries, and small arteries referred to resistance arteries. Arterial aging is characterized by endothelial dysfunction and arterial remodeling, indicating a decline in arterial elasticity/distensibility, decreased arterial compliance, and increased arterial stiffness. Physiological alterations of the vascular wall are dynamic and occur throughout life [4]. During aging, gradual thickening of the arterial wall, changes in wall composition (i.e., elastin fragmentation and collagen deposition), and an increase of artery diameter are observed in conduit arteries [2]. Increased intimal-to-media thickness (IMT) is a valid indicator of arterial aging supported by the finding that the IMT of the carotid artery increases twofold to threefold between 20 and 90 years of age [4]. Pulse wave velocity (PWV) is a noninvasive measure of vascular stiffness. Stiffening of the conduit arteries leads to increased aortic pulse pressure and increased PWV, which occurs in both sexes along aging [5].

The endothelium, a monolayer of flattened, polygonal cells lining the inner surface of arteries, plays an important role in regulating arterial structure and function. The endothelium can respond to pathophysiological signals by producing various factors that regulate vascular tone, cellular adhesion, thromboresistance, smooth muscle cell proliferation, and inflammation. During arterial aging, senescence, activation, and dysfunction of endothelial cells (ECs) represent the earliest abnormalities that lead to an impaired endothelium-dependent vasodilatation and adverse arterial wall remodeling [6]. Senescent ECs undergo permanent growth arrest, get enlarged and flattened in morphology, and also display positive staining for senescence-associated β-galactosidase (SA-β-gal) [7]. There are mainly two types of senescence. One is caused by successive cell duplication as a kind of natural aging process termed as "replicative senescence" and characterized by shortening of telomere [8]. The other is called "premature senescence" and induced by several stress conditions such as oxidative stress, radiations, and exposure to oncogenes [9]. Endothelial activation is defined as the initial event in atherogenesis. Circulating proinflammatory molecules including cytokines (i.e., tumor necrosis factor-α (TNF-α)) or modified lipoproteins (i.e., oxidized low-density lipoprotein (oxLDL)) activates ECs to express chemokines, cytokines, and adhesion molecules, thus attracting and recruiting inflammatory cells such as macrophages and T cells. Both endothelial senescence and activation can induce endothelial dysfunction which is reflected by impairment of endothelium-dependent vasorelaxation caused by a loss of nitric oxide (NO) bioavailability in the vessel wall and altered anticoagulant and anti-inflammatory properties of the endothelium. Impaired endothelium-dependent vasodilation in the coronary circulation of humans has profound prognostic implications in that it predicts adverse cardiovascular events and long-term outcomes [1, 2, 10, 11].

Age-related loss of arterial functions has been demonstrated, and underlying mechanisms were studied in human studies. Reduced NO bioavailability in older age was reported by observing diminished forearm vasoconstrictor response to infusion of NO-synthase inhibitor L-NMMA in resistance arteries [12]. In older adults, supplementation of NO precursor, L-arginine, improves coronary artery blood flow response to acetylcholine [13] and skin blood flow response to whole body heating [14]. Moreover, age-related decline in synthesis of tetrahydrobiopterin, a co-factor in NO production, provides further evidence for impairment of vasodilation NO-pathway during aging [15]. In the aspect of vasoconstrictor pathways, a greater lower limb vasodilatation response to endothelin (ET)-receptor blockade in old men was reported [16]. A small but significant age-related impairment in vascular smooth muscle function was also observed in conduit and resistance arteries in a meta-analysis [17].

2. SIRT1 in endothelial cells: expression and regulation

Sirtuin 1 (SIRT1) is the mammalian orthologue of the yeast longevity regulator Sir2 [18]. Members of the Sirtuin family share a highly conserved core domain to catalyze deacetylation,

ADP-ribosyltransferation, desuccinylation, and demalonylation [19]. Sirtuins regulate energy homeostasis, stress resistance, circadian rhythmicity, mitochondrial functions, and embryonic development, which in turn contribute to increased lifespan [20].

Human SIRT1 gene is located at chromosome 10q21.3 containing 11 exons with a total length of 33,715 base pair [21]. SIRT1 is composed of 747 amino acids including a core catalytic domain consisting of 275 amino acids and both N- and C-terminal extensions spanning about 240 amino acids [22]. There are two nuclear localization signals and two nuclear exportation signals located in the extensions whose balanced functionality determines the presence of SIRT1 in either the nucleus or cytoplasm and explains the distinct location of SIRT1 among different cell lines and tissues [23].

Regulation of SIRT1 enzymatic activity occurs at various levels including post-translational modification, protein complex formation, transcriptional regulation, and concentrations of enzymatic substrates [19, 24]. Phosphorylation of SIRT1 represents the major form of post-translational modifications. Independent studies report multiple phosphorylation sites by distinct proteins, including c-Jun N-terminal kinase 1 (Ser27/47), cyclin B/cyclin-dependent kinase 1 (Thr530, Ser540), casein kinase 2 (Ser659/661), and adenosine 5′-monophosphate-activated protein kinase (AMPK) (Thr344) [25–28]. Additional post-translational modifications include methylation by SET7/9 [29], nitrosylation by glyceraldehyde-3-phosphate dehydrogenase [30], and sumoylation by sentrin-specific protease 1 [31]. In addition, several endogenous protein-binding partners of SIRT1 are found to regulate its function via forming protein complex. For example, the active regulator of SIRT1 can bind to amino acids 114–217 in the N-terminus of SIRT1 and stimulate deacetylation of p53 in vivo [32]. On transcriptional level, SIRT1 was reported that nicotinamide phosphoribosyltransferase (NAMPT) upregulated the expression of SIRT1 and SIRT1 antisense long noncoding RNA, thus regulating senescence, proliferation, and migration of endothelial progenitor cells (EPCs) [33]. SIRT1 activity is also thought to be affected by the levels of intracellular co-substrate nicotinamide adenine dinucleotide (NAD+) and its product nicotinamide [34].

With age, SIRT1 expression in ECs is progressively downregulated. Overexpression of SIRT1 in the endothelium prevents cellular senescence, enhances vasodilatory responses, and attenuates aging-induced vascular damages [35–37]. The subsequent review will summarize the recent progresses related to the molecular regulation of SIRT1 expression in ECs and the anti-vascular aging effects of SIRT1 by focusing on endothelial dysfunction and arterial remodeling.

3. SIRT1 in endothelial cells: molecular targets and biological functions

Apart from histones, SIRT1 can mediate the deacetylation of various signaling substrates to exert vasoprotective functions. SIRT1 is abundant in ECs mediating postnatal blood vessel growth via Foxo1 and helps to maintain endothelial function [38]. In vitro experiments showed that downregulation of SIRT1 using small interfering RNA (siRNA) uniquely inhibited endothelial sprout formation via a three-dimensional assay, while other mammalian sirtuin family members (SIRT2–SIRT7) could not [38]. In addition, the reduction of matrix metalloproteinase-14

(MMP-14), a membrane-anchored MMP essential for tip cell activity during sprouting angiogenesis, was found in siRNA-SIRT1-treated endothelial sprouts [39]. Decreased expression of SIRT1 either by mRNA silencing or pharmacological inhibition could induce premature-senescence-like phenotypes in ECs [40, 41]. SIRT1 displays anti-senescence activity in ECs by inducing the deacetylation of diversified signaling substrates [42]. For example, SIRT1 can deacetylate tumor suppressor protein p53 to downregulate its stability and activity as to promote cell survival in response to cellular stress [43]. SIRT1 also plays an important role in enhancing the endothelial NO synthase (eNOS) transcription and translation by deacetylating eNOS on lysine 496 and 506 to generate more NO, thus enhancing vessel dilatation, mediating vessel tone regulation, and providing athero-protective effects [44, 45]. Recent study demonstrated that SIRT1 activation could help reduce traction forces and reorganize actin localization (increased peripheral actin) in aged ECs, which is also a sign of anti-senescent effect [46]. Moreover, while senescent porcine aortic ECs (PAECs) showed decreased expression of SIRT1 compared to young PAECs, the protein level of liver kinase B1 (LKB1), a serine/threonine kinase and tumor suppressor, was dramatically increased as well as the phosphorylation of its downstream target AMPK (Thr172). In this case, SIRT1 can antagonize LKB1-dependent AMPK activation by promoting the deacetylation, ubiquitination, and proteasome-mediated degradation in order to retard PAEC senescence which also correlated with the Akt survival signaling pathway [41]. Furthermore, it was reported that SIRT1 can bind to the DOC domain of HERC2 [HECT and RLD domain containing E3 ubiquitin protein ligase 2] and then ubiquitinate LKB1 in the nuclear compartment of ECs [37]. SIRT1 can also negatively modulate Notch signaling in ECs via deacetylation of the Notch1 intracellular domain (NICD), in which loss of endothelial SIRT1 activity leads to impaired growth and sprout elongation [47]. Intracellular NAMPT-NAD+-SIRT1 cascade was shown to improve post-ischemic neovascularization through modulation of Notch signaling pathway [48]. Adapter protein p66Shc which can directly stimulate mitochondrial reactive oxygen species (ROS) generation was discovered downregulated by SIRT1 in mice with hyperglycemia-induced endothelial dysfunction [49]. Moreover, in vitro experiments using human aortic ECs (HUVECs) demonstrated that SIRT1 can deacetylate RelA/p65 to diminish tissue factor expression and suppress nuclear factor-κB (NF-κB) signaling, thus preventing atherothrombosis [50]. In EPCs, SIRT1 was implicated to protect against oxidative stress-induced apoptosis by inhibiting Foxo3a via ubiquitination and degradation [36]. microRNA-34a (miR-34a), regulated by p53 and able to control cell cycle arrest, has been reported to promote cardiac, endothelial, and EPC senescence via down-regulation of SIRT1 [51]. Also, visfatin (an adipocytokine closely associated with human cell senescence) was reported to attenuate the oxLDL-induced senescence of EPCs by upregulating SIRT1 expression through the PI3K/Akt/ERK pathway [52].

4. Endothelial SIRT1 prevents arterial aging

Various animal studies demonstrated that SIRT1 plays a vital role in anti-endothelial senescence and anti-atherogenesis. Infiltration of monocyte-derived macrophages into the subendothelial space is a crucial step in atherogenesis [53]. SIRT1 can decrease cholesterol uptake especially oxLDL and prevent macrophage foam cell formation via suppressing the expression of scavenger receptor Lox-1 [54] and reducing the expression of various pro-inflammatory molecules including TNF-α, monocyte chemotactic protein-1, and interleukins [55]. A recent discovery showed that treatment of the SIRT1 activator SRT3025 decreased plasma levels of LDL cholesterol and total cholesterol and attenuated atherosclerosis, owing to reduced secretion of hepatic Pcsk9 and enhanced protein expression of LDL receptor in apolipoprotein E-deficient ($ApoE^{-/-}$) mice [56]. In the meantime, SIRT1 was demonstrated to promote reverse cholesterol (mainly HDLs) transport into macrophages by directly deacetylating and subsequently regulating the transcriptional activity of liver X receptors, which play a significant role in lipid homeostasis and inflammation and can help express ATP-binding cassette transporter 1 that transport cholesterol into pre-βHDL particles [57].

Some studies regarding upstream regulators of SIRT1 including cathepsin, caspase-1, and cyclin-dependent kinase 5 (CDK5) elucidate beneficial roles of SIRT1 in anti-endothelial senescence and anti-atherogenesis [58–60]. The cysteine cathepsins belong to the leaked lysosomal contents with the viability in cleavage and degradation of SIRT1, which lead to stress-induced premature senescence [58]. Studies on $ApoE^{-/-}$/caspase-$1^{-/-}$ double knockout mice have shown promising evidences that early hyperlipidemia promoted endothelial activation via a Caspase-1-SIRT1 pathway [59]. In this case, researchers found that inhibition of caspase-1 resulted in SIRT1 accumulation in the $ApoE^{-/-}$ mouse aorta and $ApoE^{-/-}$/caspase-$1^{-/-}$ mice had attenuated early atherosclerosis, decreased aortic expression of proinflammatory cytokines, and reduced aortic monocyte recruitment, as well as decreased endothelial activation [59]. Another upstream regulator of SIRT1 is CDK5, which was proved to increase the phosphorylation of SIRT1 especially at S47 during cellular senescence [60]. In this study, replacing S47 with nonphosphorable alanin (S47A) elevated, while mutation of S47 to phospho-mimicking aspartic acid (S47D) abolished the beneficial effects of SIRT1 such as anti-senescence, growth promotion, and downregulation of LKB1 expression [60]. Interaction between SIRT1 and telomeric repeat-binding factor 2-interacting protein 1 was abolished when S47 was phosphorylated. NF-κB signaling pathway is activated to induce endothelial inflammation and leads to endothelial senescence and atherosclerosis. Downregulation of CDK5 by either knockdown (by siRNA) or inhibition (by roscovitine) reduced percentage of senescent ECs and attenuated inflammatory gene expression. Meanwhile, long-term treatment of $ApoE^{-/-}$ mice with the CDK5 inhibitor, roscovitine, resulted in attenuated atherosclerosis in aortae [60]. As CDK5R1(p35/p25) is the crucial activator mediating the kinase activity of CDK5 [60, 61], further research will be conducted to unveil the underlying mechanism of CDK5-p35/p25-SIRT1 pathway in ECs.

Limited information is available concerning the role of endothelial SIRT1 in vascular remodeling. In eNOS-deficient mice, overexpression of endothelial SIRT1 prevents hypertension and age-related adverse arterial remodeling [37].

Laminar shear stress is an important stimulus for the endothelium-dependent control of vascular tone and of vascular remodeling processes. In cultured ECs, laminar flow increases both the expression and activity of SIRT1, whereas oscillating flow decreases SIRT1 expression [62]. In mouse arteries, the formation of neointima is accompanied by a progressive downregulation of SIRT1 expression [63]. SIRT1 inhibition in ECs increases the expressions of p53 and its downstream target, plasminogen activator inhibitor-1 (PAI-1), which promotes the formation of neointima and vascular remodeling in response to vascular injury [40].

Loss of vascular smooth muscle cell (VSMC) function is an alarming sign of vascular disease. During the aging process, VSMCs undergo increased dysregulation, apoptosis, and senescence [64]. In VSMCs, SIRT1 can act as a modulator of neointima formation (associated with repression of activator protein-1 (AP-1) activity [63]) and protect against DNA damage. Aging-related loss of SIRT1 expression correlates with lower capacity for vascular repair, abolished stress response, and elevated senescence [63].

Decreased expression of SIRT1 in VSMCs exerts its proatherogenic effects by the failure to deacetylate histones in DNA repair, response to oxidant stress and LDL, and therefore leads to VSMC senescence and apoptosis [63, 65]. As to atherosclerotic plaques, SIRT1 activity has been suggested to deacetylate the regulatory factor for X-box (RFX5) and antagonized repression of collagen type I (COL1A2) transcription in VSMCs, consequently stabilizing the plaque and avoiding rupture [66]. Another most recent finding relevant to destabilization of atherosclerotic plaque is that SIRT1 participated in downregulation of platelet-activating factor receptor (PAFR) in VSMCs through β-arrestin 2-mediated internalization and degradation, resulting in the inhibition of PAF-induced matrix metalloproteinase (MMP-2) generation [67]. In addition, inhibition of miR-138 was found to increase SIRT1 expression in VSMCs separated from diabetic (db/db) mice and in SMC lines C-12511 in recent study, which indicated miR-138 as another potential inhibitory target to attenuate the proliferation and migration of VSMCs and cure atherosclerosis [68]. Furthermore, SIRT1 was also found to inhibit angiotensin II-induced VSMC hypertrophy in rat embryonic aortic VSMCs [69]. Later on, SIRT1 demonstrated antihypertensive activity in transgenic mice with selective overexpression of SIRT1 in VSMCs (SV-Tg). Alleviated vascular remodeling in mouse thoracic and renal aortae induced by angiotensin II is observed, along with significantly decreased transforming growth factor-β1 (TGF-β1) expression, ROS generation, vascular inflammation, and collagen formation in the arterial wall of SV-Tg mice [70]. Similar to contribution in ECs, overexpression of miR-34a can upregulate p21 level and inflammation through SIRT1 downregulation and cause senescence-associated secretory phenotype factors induction (including proinflammatory molecules such as cytokines, chemokines, proteases, growth factors, soluble receptors, etc.), promoting VSMC senescence and leading to arterial dysfunction [71].

5. Targeting endothelial SIRT1 for the prevention of arterial aging

Slowing down the vascular aging requires early intervention, lifelong treatment, and site-specific approaches. To reduce arterial stiffness, pharmacological agents, including angiotensin-converting enzyme inhibitors, angiotensin II type 1 blockers, aldosterone antagonists, and statins, are currently available and in clinical use [35]. The evident vasoprotective effects of SIRT1 definitely pose great opportunities and challenges for drug discovery targeting endothelial dysfunction. So far, a few natural and synthetic substances have been demonstrated as SIRT1 activators to promote vascular health. The first potent activator of SIRT1 is resveratrol, a small polyphenol discovered in red wine, which could protect ECs against inflammation, apoptosis, and oxidative stress [72]. It was found to dramatically lower the incidence of cardiovascular diseases in spite of high saturated fat diet, which was termed as "French paradox" [73]. Several natural ingredients extracted from various traditional Chinese herbs were also found to activate SIRT1. Tetramethylpyrazine is proved to reverse high-glucose-induced endothelial dysfunction via SIRT1 [74]. Polydatin can attenuate hemorrhagic shock by upregulating SIRT1 [75]. Quercetin is capable of inhibiting oxidized LDL-induced EC damage by SIRT1 activation [76]. Some other natural polyphenols including fisetin and butein can also activate SIRT1 [77]. Vitamin D protects ECs from irradiation-induced senescence and apoptosis by modulating MAPK/SirT1 axis [78]. On the other hand, a series of SIRT1 activators like SRT2183, SRT1460, SRT1720, SRT2379, SRT501, SRT2104, SRT3025, and BMT0-512 have been synthesized and developed as potential drugs to protect against vascular aging [77, 79].

Despite the fact that SIRT1 is as an optimal therapeutical target for cardiovascular diseases, the dosage of upregulation of SIRT1 should be considered seriously and titrated cautiously in clinical practice. It was reported that 2.5- to 7-fold overexpression of SIRT1 prevented heart from oxidative stress via SIRT1/FOXO, while 12.5-fold overexpression of SIRT1 increased apoptosis and hypertrophy and decreased cardiac function, suggesting that only low to moderate doses of SIRT1 can exert beneficial effects [80]. The aforementioned findings call for more careful evaluation of dosage and possible adverse effects in drug development targeting endothelial SIRT1.

In light of all the above studies, there have already been several potential drugs to target the anti-vascular aging effects of endothelial SIRT1. The entry of SIRT1 activators into human trials is exciting but also highlights the necessity to better understand the SIRT1 specificity, clinical effects, and side effects of these promising activators in vivo.

Acknowledgements

This work was financially supported by Hong Kong Health and Medical Research Fund 13142651.

Conflict of interest

No interest of conflict was declared.

Author details

Yumeng Guo and Yu Wang*

*Address all correspondence to: yuwanghk@hku.hk

Department of Pharmacology and Pharmacy, The University of Hong Kong, Hong Kong

References

[1] Benjamin EJ, Blaha MJ, Chiuve SE, Cushman M, Das SR, Deo R, de Ferranti SD, Floyd J, Fornage M, Gillespie C, Isasi CR, Jimenez MC, Jordan LC, Judd SE, Lackland D, Lichtman JH, Lisabeth L, Liu S, Longenecker CT, Mackey RH, Matsushita K, Mozaffarian D, Mussolino ME, Nasir K, Neumar RW, Palaniappan L, Pandey DK, Thiagarajan RR, Reeves MJ, Ritchey M, Rodriguez CJ, Roth GA, Rosamond WD, Sasson C, Towfighi A, Tsao CW, Turner MB, Virani SS, Voeks JH, Willey JZ, Wilkins JT, Wu JH, Alger HM, Wong SS, Muntner P. American Heart Association Statistics, and S. Stroke Statistics. Heart disease and stroke statistics-2017 update: A report from the American Heart Association. Circulation. 2017;**135**(10):e146-e603

[2] Thijssen DH, Carter SE, Green DJ. Arterial structure and function in vascular ageing: Are you as old as your arteries? The Journal of Physiology. 2016;**594**(8):2275-2284

[3] Rubio-Ruiz ME, Perez-Torres I, Soto ME, Pastelin G, Guarner-Lans V. Aging in blood vessels. Medicinal agents FOR systemic arterial hypertension in the elderly. Ageing Research Reviews. 2014;**18**:132-147

[4] Lakatta EG. The reality of aging viewed from the arterial wall. Artery Research. 2013;**7**(2):73-80

[5] Nilsson PM, Khalili P, Franklin SS. Blood pressure and pulse wave velocity as metrics for evaluating pathologic ageing of the cardiovascular system. Blood Pressure. 2014; **23**(1):17-30

[6] Eckers A, Haendeler J. Endothelial cells in health and disease. Antioxidants & Redox Signaling. 2015;**22**(14):1209-1211

[7] Bai B, Wang Y. Methods to investigate the role of SIRT1 in endothelial senescence. Methods in Molecular Biology. 2013;**965**:327-339

[8] Wang Y, Liang Y, Vanhoutte PM. SIRT1 and AMPK in regulating mammalian senescence: A critical review and a working model. FEBS Letters. 2011;**585**(7):986-994

[9] Kuilman T, Michaloglou C, Mooi WJ, Peeper DS. The essence of senescence. Genes & Development. 2010;**24**(22):2463-2479

[10] Takumi T, Yang EH, Mathew V, Rihal CS, Gulati R, Lerman LO, Lerman A. Coronary endothelial dysfunction is associated with a reduction in coronary artery compliance and an increase in wall shear stress. Heart. 2010;**96**(10):773-778

[11] Curcio S, Garcia-Espinosa V, Arana M, Farro I, Chiesa P, Giachetto G, Zocalo Y, Bia D. Growing-related changes in arterial properties of healthy children, adolescents, and young adults nonexposed to cardiovascular risk factors: Analysis of gender-related differences. International Journal of Hypertension. 2016;**2016**:4982676

[12] Taddei S, Galetta F, Virdis A, Ghiadoni L, Salvetti G, Franzoni F, Giusti C, Salvetti A. Physical activity prevents age-related impairment in nitric oxide availability in elderly athletes. Circulation. 2000;**101**(25):2896-2901

[13] Chauhan A, More RS, Mullins PA, Taylor G, Petch MC, Schofield PM. Aging-associated endothelial dysfunction in humans is reversed by L-arginine. Journal of the American College of Cardiology. 1996;**28**(7):1796-1804

[14] Holowatz LA, Thompson CS, Kenney WL. L-arginine supplementation or arginase inhibition augments reflex cutaneous vasodilatation in aged human skin. The Journal of Physiology. 2006;**574**(Pt 2):573-581

[15] Pierce GL, Larocca TJ. Reduced vascular tetrahydrobiopterin (BH4) and endothelial function with ageing: Is it time for a chronic BH4 supplementation trial in middle-aged and older adults? The Journal of Physiology. 2008;**586**(11):2673-2674

[16] Thijssen DH, Rongen GA, van Dijk A, Smits P, Hopman MT. Enhanced endothelin-1-mediated leg vascular tone in healthy older subjects. Journal of Applied Physiology. 2007;**103**(3):852-857

[17] Montero D, Pierce GL, Stehouwer CD, Padilla J, Thijssen DH. The impact of age on vascular smooth muscle function in humans. Journal of Hypertension. 2015;**33**(3):445-453; discussion 453

[18] Wang Y, Xu C, Liang Y, Vanhoutte PM. SIRT1 in metabolic syndrome: Where to target matters. Pharmacology & Therapeutics. 2012;**136**(3):305-318

[19] Feldman JL, Dittenhafer-Reed KE, Denu JM. Sirtuin catalysis and regulation. Journal of Biological Chemistry. 2012;**287**(51):42419-42427

[20] Cencioni C, Spallotta F, Mai A, Martelli F, Farsetti A, Zeiher AM, Gaetano C. Sirtuin function in aging heart and vessels. Journal of Molecular and Cellular Cardiology. 2015

[21] Alcaín FJ, Villalba JM. Sirtuin inhibitors. Expert Opinion on Therapeutic Patents. 2009; **19**(3):283-294

[22] Huhtiniemi T, Wittekindt C, Laitinen T, Leppänen J, Salminen A, Poso A, Lahtela-Kakkonen M. Comparative and pharmacophore model for deacetylase SIRT1. Journal of Computer-Aided Molecular Design. 2006;**20**(9):589-599

[23] Canto C, Auwerx J. Targeting sirtuin 1 to improve metabolism: All you need is NAD(+)? Pharmacological Reviews. 2012;**64**(1):166-187

[24] Flick F, Luscher B. Regulation of sirtuin function by posttranslational modifications. Frontiers in Pharmacology. 2012;**3**:29

[25] Sasaki T, Maier B, Koclega KD, Chruszcz M, Gluba W, Stukenberg PT, Minor W, Scrable H. Phosphorylation regulates SIRT1 function. PLoS One. 2008;**3**(12):e4020

[26] Lee CW, Wong LL, Tse EY, Liu HF, Leong VY, Lee JM, Hardie DG, Ng IO, Ching YP. AMPK promotes p53 acetylation via phosphorylation and inactivation of SIRT1 in liver cancer cells. Cancer Research. 2012;**72**(17):4394-4404

[27] Nasrin N, Kaushik VK, Fortier E, Wall D, Pearson KJ, de Cabo R, Bordone L. JNK1 phosphorylates SIRT1 and promotes its enzymatic activity. PLoS One. 2009;**4**(12):e8414

[28] Zschoernig B, Mahlknecht U. Carboxy-terminal phosphorylation of SIRT1 by protein kinase CK2. Biochemical and Biophysical Research Communications. 2009;**381**(3):372-377

[29] Liu X, Wang D, Zhao Y, Tu B, Zheng Z, Wang L, Wang H, Gu W, Roeder RG, Zhu WG. Methyltransferase Set7/9 regulates p53 activity by interacting with Sirtuin 1 (SIRT1). Proceedings of the National Academy of Sciences of the United States of America. 2011;**108**(5):1925-1930

[30] Kornberg MD, Sen N, Hara MR, Juluri KR, Nguyen JV, Snowman AM, Law L, Hester LD, Snyder SH. GAPDH mediates nitrosylation of nuclear proteins. Nature Cell Biology. 2010;**12**(11):1094-1100

[31] Yang Y, Fu W, Chen J, Olashaw N, Zhang X, Nicosia SV, Bhalla K, Bai W. SIRT1 sumoylation regulates its deacetylase activity and cellular response to genotoxic stress. Nature Cell Biology. 2007;**9**(11):1253-1262

[32] Kim EJ, Kho JH, Kang MR, Um SJ. Active regulator of SIRT1 cooperates with SIRT1 and facilitates suppression of p53 activity. Molecular Cell. 2007;**28**(2):277-290

[33] Ming GF, Wu K, Hu K, Chen Y, Xiao J. NAMPT regulates senescence, proliferation, and migration of endothelial progenitor cells through the SIRT1 AS lncRNA/miR-22/SIRT1 pathway. Biochemical and Biophysical Research Communications. 2016;**478**(3):1382-1388

[34] Jackson MD, Schmidt MT, Oppenheimer NJ, Denu JM. Mechanism of nicotinamide inhibition and transglycosidation by Sir2 histone/protein deacetylases. The Journal of Biological Chemistry. 2003;**278**(51):50985-50598

[35] Guo Y, Xu A, Wang Y. SIRT1 in endothelial cells as a novel target for the prevention of early vascular aging. Journal of Cardiovascular Pharmacology. 2016;**67**(6):465-473

[36] Wang YQ, Cao Q, Wang F, Huang LY, Sang TT, Liu F, Chen SY. SIRT1 protects against oxidative stress-induced endothelial progenitor cells apoptosis by inhibiting FOXO3a via FOXO3a ubiquitination and degradation. Journal of Cellular Physiology. 2015;**230**(9):2098-2107

[37] Bai B, Man AW, Yang K, Guo Y, Xu C, Tse HF, Han W, Bloksgaard M, De Mey JG, Vanhoutte PM, Xu A, Wang Y. Endothelial SIRT1 prevents adverse arterial remodeling by facilitating HERC2-mediated degradation of acetylated LKB1. Oncotarget. 2016;**7**(26):39065-39081

[38] Potente M, Ghaeni L, Baldessari D, Mostoslavsky R, Rossig L, Dequiedt F, Haendeler J, Mione M, Dejana E, Alt FW. SIRT1 controls endothelial angiogenic functions during vascular growth. Genes & Development. 2007;**21**(20):2644-2658

[39] Yana I, Sagara H, Takaki S, Takatsu K, Nakamura K, Nakao K, Katsuki M, Taniguchi SI, Aoki T, Sato H. Crosstalk between neovessels and mural cells directs the site-specific expression of MT1-MMP to endothelial tip cells. Journal of Cell Science. 2007;**120**(9):1607-1614

[40] Ota H, Akishita M, Eto M, Iijima K, Kaneki M, Ouchi Y. Sirt1 modulates premature senescence-like phenotype in human endothelial cells. Journal of Molecular and Cellular Cardiology. 2007;**43**(5):571-579

[41] Zu Y, Liu L, Lee MY, Xu C, Liang Y, Man RY, Vanhoutte PM, Wang Y. SIRT1 promotes proliferation and prevents senescence through targeting LKB1 in primary porcine aortic endothelial cells. Circulation Research. 2010;**106**(8):1384-1393

[42] Bai B, Vanhoutte PM, Wang Y. Loss-of-SIRT1 function during vascular ageing: Hyperphosphorylation mediated by cyclin-dependent kinase 5. Trends in Cardiovascular Medicine. 2014;**24**(2):81-84

[43] Luo J, Nikolaev AY, Imai SI, Chen D, Su F, Shiloh A, Guarente L, Gu W. Negative control of p53 by Sir2α promotes cell survival under stress. Cell. 2001;**107**(2):137-148

[44] Wallerath T, Li H, Gödtel-Ambrust U, Schwarz PM, Förstermann U. A blend of polyphenolic compounds explains the stimulatory effect of red wine on human endothelial NO synthase. Nitric Oxide. 2005;**12**(2):97-104

[45] Mattagajasingh I, Kim CS, Naqvi A, Yamamori T, Hoffman TA, Jung SB, DeRicco J, Kasuno K, Irani K. SIRT1 promotes endothelium-dependent vascular relaxation by activating endothelial nitric oxide synthase. Proceedings of the National Academy of Sciences of the United States of America. 2007;**104**(37):14855-14860

[46] Cheung TM, Yan JB, Fu JJ, Huang J, Yuan F, Truskey GA. Endothelial cell senescence increases traction forces due to age-associated changes in the Glycocalyx and SIRT1. Cellular and Molecular Bioengineering. 2015;**8**(1):63-75

[47] Guarani V, Deflorian G, Franco CA, Kruger M, Phng LK, Bentley K, Toussaint L, Dequiedt F, Mostoslavsky R, Schmidt MH, Zimmermann B, Brandes RP, Mione M, Westphal CH, Braun T, Zeiher AM, Gerhardt H, Dimmeler S, Potente M. Acetylation-dependent regulation of endothelial notch signalling by the SIRT1 deacetylase. Nature. 2011;**473**(7346):234-238

[48] Wang P, Du H, Zhou CC, Song J, Liu X, Cao X, Mehta JL, Shi Y, Su DF, Miao CY. Intracellular NAMPT-NAD+-SIRT1 cascade improves post-ischaemic vascular repair by modulating notch signalling in endothelial progenitors. Cardiovascular Research. 2014;**104**(3):477-488

[49] Chen HZ, Wan YZ, Liu DP. Cross-talk between SIRT1 and p66Shc in vascular diseases. Trends in Cardiovascular Medicine. 2013;**23**(7):237-241

[50] Breitenstein A, Stein S, Holy EW, Camici GG, Lohmann C, Akhmedov A, Spescha R, Elliott PJ, Westphal CH, Matter CM. Sirt1 inhibition promotes in vivo arterial thrombosis and tissue factor expression in stimulated cells. Cardiovascular Research. 2010;**89**(2):464-472

[51] Xu Q, Seeger FH, Castillo J, Iekushi K, Boon RA, Farcas R, Manavski Y, Li YG, Assmus B, Zeiher AM. Micro-RNA-34a contributes to the impaired function of bone marrow-derived mononuclear cells from patients with cardiovascular disease. Journal of the American College of Cardiology. 2012;**59**(23):2107-2117

[52] Ming GF, Tang YJ, Hu K, Chen Y, Huang WH, Xiao J. Visfatin attenuates the ox-LDL-induced senescence of endothelial progenitor cells by upregulating SIRT1 expression through the PI3K/Akt/ERK pathway. International Journal of Molecular Medicine. 2016;**38**(2):643-649

[53] Stein S, Matter CM. Protective roles of SIRT1 in atherosclerosis. Cell Cycle. 2011;**10**(4):640-647

[54] Stein S, Lohmann C, Schäfer N, Hofmann J, Rohrer L, Besler C, Rothgiesser KM, Becher B, Hottiger MO, Borén J. SIRT1 decreases Lox-1-mediated foam cell formation in atherogenesis. European Heart Journal. 2010;**31**(18):2301-2309

[55] Schug TT, Xu Q, Gao H, Peres-da-Silva A, Draper DW, Fessler MB, Purushotham A, Li X. Myeloid deletion of SIRT1 induces inflammatory signaling in response to environmental stress. Molecular and Cellular Biology. 2010;**30**(19):4712-4721

[56] Miranda MX, Van Tits LJ, Lohmann C, Arsiwala T, Winnik S, Tailleux A, Stein S, Gomes AP, Suri V, Ellis JL. The Sirt1 activator SRT3025 provides atheroprotection in Apoe−/− mice by reducing hepatic Pcsk9 secretion and enhancing Ldlr expression. European Heart Journal. 2015;**36**(1):51-59

[57] Kim HJ, Park KG, Yoo EK, Kim YH, Kim YN, Kim HS, Kim HT, Park JY, Lee KU, Jang WG. Effects of PGC-1α on TNF-α-induced MCP-1 and VCAM-1 expression and NF-κB activation in human aortic smooth muscle and endothelial cells. Antioxidants & Redox Signaling. 2007;**9**(3):301-307

[58] Chen J, Xavier S, Moskowitz-Kassai E, Chen R, Lu CY, Sanduski K, Spes A, Turk B, Goligorsky MS. Cathepsin cleavage of sirtuin 1 in endothelial progenitor cells mediates stress-induced premature senescence. The American Journal of Pathology. 2012; **180**(3):973-983

[59] Yin Y, Li X, Sha X, Xi H, Li YF, Shao Y, Mai J, Virtue A, Lopez-Pastrana J, Meng S. Early hyperlipidemia promotes endothelial activation via a Caspase-1-Sirtuin 1 pathway. Arteriosclerosis, Thrombosis, and Vascular Biology. 2015;**35**(4):804-816

[60] Bai B, Liang Y, Xu C, Lee MY, Xu A, Wu D, Vanhoutte PM, Wang Y. Cyclin-dependent kinase 5–mediated hyperphosphorylation of Sirtuin-1 contributes to the development of endothelial senescence and atherosclerosis. Circulation. 2012;**126**(6):729-740

[61] Ko J, Humbert S, Bronson RT, Takahashi S, Kulkarni AB, Li E, Tsai LH. p35 and p39 are essential for cyclin-dependent kinase 5 function during neurodevelopment. The Journal of Neuroscience. 2001;**21**(17):6758-6771

[62] Chen Z, Peng IC, Cui X, Li YS, Chien S, Shyy JY. Shear stress, SIRT1, and vascular homeostasis. Proceedings of the National Academy of Sciences of the United States of America. 2010;**107**(22):10268-10273

[63] Li L, Zhang HN, Chen HZ, Gao P, Zhu LH, Li HL, Lv X, Zhang QJ, Zhang R, Wang Z. SIRT1 acts as a modulator of neointima formation following vascular injury in mice. Circulation Research. 2011;**108**(10):1180-1189

[64] Thompson AM, Wagner R, Rzucidlo EM. Age-related loss of SirT1 expression results in dysregulated human vascular smooth muscle cell function. American Journal of Physiology-Heart and Circulatory Physiology. 2014;**307**(4):H533-H541

[65] Gorenne I, Kumar S, Gray K, Figg N, Yu H, Mercer J, Bennett M. Vascular smooth muscle cell sirtuin 1 protects against DNA damage and inhibits atherosclerosis. Circulation. 2013;**127**(3):386-396

[66] Xia J, Wu X, Yang Y, Zhao Y, Fang M, Xie W, Wang H, Xu Y. SIRT1 deacetylates RFX5 and antagonizes repression of collagen type I (COL1A2) transcription in smooth muscle cells. Biochemical and Biophysical Research Communications. 2012;**428**(2):264-270

[67] Kim YH, Bae JU, Lee SJ, Park SY, Kim CD. SIRT1 attenuates PAF-induced MMP-2 production via down-regulation of PAF receptor expression in vascular smooth muscle cells. Vascular Pharmacology. 2015;**72**:35-42

[68] Xu J, Li L, Yun HF, Han YS. MiR-138 promotes smooth muscle cells proliferation and migration in db/db mice through down-regulation of SIRT1. Biochemical and Biophysical Research Communications. 2015;**463**(4):1159-1164

[69] Li L, Gao P, Zhang H, Chen H, Zheng W, Lv X, Xu T, Wei Y, Liu D, Liang C. SIRT1 inhibits angiotensin II-induced vascular smooth muscle cell hypertrophy. Acta Biochimica Et Biophysica Sinica. 2010;**43**(2):103-109

[70] Gao P, Xu TT, Lu J, Li L, Xu J, Hao DL, Chen HZ, Liu DP. Overexpression of SIRT1 in vascular smooth muscle cells attenuates angiotensin II-induced vascular remodeling and hypertension in mice. Journal of Molecular Medicine. 2014;**92**(4):347-357

[71] Badi I, Burba I, Ruggeri C, Zeni F, Bertolotti M, Scopece A, Pompilio G, Raucci A. MicroRNA-34a induces vascular smooth muscle cells senescence by SIRT1 downregulation and promotes the expression of age-associated pro-inflammatory secretory factors. The Journals of Gerontology. Series A, Biological Sciences and Medical Sciences. 2014;**70**(11):1304-1311

[72] Kopp P. Resveratrol, a phytoestrogen found in red wine. A possible explanation for the conundrum of the 'French paradox'? European Journal of Endocrinology. 1998; **138**(6):619-620

[73] Catalgol B, Batirel S, Taga Y, Ozer NK. Resveratrol: French paradox revisited. Frontiers in Pharmacology. 2012;**3**(141):1-18

[74] Xu Q, Xia P, Li X, Wang W, Liu Z, Gao X. Tetramethylpyrazine ameliorates high glucose-induced endothelial dysfunction by increasing mitochondrial biogenesis. PLoS One. 2014;**9**(2):e88243

[75] Zhang W, Huang Q, Zeng Z, Wu J, Zhang Y, Chen Z. Sirt1 inhibits oxidative stress in vascular endothelial cells. Oxidative Medicine and Cellular Longevity. 2017;**2017**:7543973

[76] Hung CH, Chan SH, Chu PM, Tsai KL. Quercetin is a potent anti-atherosclerotic compound by activation of SIRT1 signaling under oxLDL stimulation. Molecular Nutrition & Food Research. 2015;**59**(10):1905-1917

[77] Milne JC, Lambert PD, Schenk S, Carney DP, Smith JJ, Gagne DJ, Jin L, Boss O, Perni RB, Vu CB, Bemis JE, Xie R, Disch JS, Ng PY, Nunes JJ, Lynch AV, Yang H, Galonek H, Israelian K, Choy W, Iffland A, Lavu S, Medvedik O, Sinclair DA, Olefsky JM, Jirousek MR, Elliott PJ, Westphal CH. Small molecule activators of SIRT1 as therapeutics for the treatment of type 2 diabetes. Nature. 2007;**450**(7170):712-716

[78] Marampon F, Gravina GL, Festuccia C, Popov VM, Colapietro EA, Sanita P, Musio D, De Felice F, Lenzi A, Jannini EA, Di Cesare E, Tombolini V. Vitamin D protects endothelial cells from irradiation-induced senescence and apoptosis by modulating MAPK/SirT1 axis. Journal of Endocrinological Investigation. 2016;**39**(4):411-422

[79] Villalba JM, Alcaín FJ. Sirtuin activators and inhibitors. BioFactors. 2012;**38**(5):349-359

[80] Alcendor RR, Gao S, Zhai P, Zablocki D, Holle E, Yu X, Tian B, Wagner T, Vatner SF, Sadoshima J. Sirt1 regulates aging and resistance to oxidative stress in the heart. Circulation Research. 2007;**100**(10):1512-1121

Chapter 5

Sensing Fluid-Shear Stress in the Endothelial System with a Special Emphasis on the Primary Cilium

Meriem Rezgaoui, Andres Rodriguez,
Kurt Herlitz and Carlos Escudero

Additional information is available at the end of the chapter

http://dx.doi.org/10.5772/intechopen.73134

Abstract

Fluid shear stress (FSS) is able to generate phenotypic changes in the cells in direct contact with the strain force. In order to detect and transduce FSS into intracellular pathways, biological systems use a specific set of sensors, called mechanosensors. The process involves the conversion of the mechanical force into a chemical or electrical signal. Primary cilium is a non-motile organelle that emanates from the cell surface of most mammalian cell types that act as a mechanosensor. Increasing evidence suggests that primary cilia are key coordinators of signaling pathways in tissue homeostasis and when defective may cause human diseases and developmental disorders. Here, we will describe the endothelial primary cilium as a mechanotransductory organelle sensing FSS. To fulfill this function, primary cilium requires the localization of mechanoproteins, polycystin-1 and -2, in their membrane and the structural gene product, polaris. Physiologically, deflection of primary cilium increases the intracellular calcium concentration triggering a signaling pathway that leads to nitric oxide (NO) formation and vasodilation. Additionally, ciliopathies, such as polycystic kidney disease and atherosclerosis, will also be discussed. We also analyze available information regarding a trio of membrane receptors involved in FSS sensing and transducing such as vascular endothelial growth factor receptors (VEGFRs) and its coreceptor neuropilin (NRP), as well as purinergic receptors (P2Y2). Whether or not they modulate, the primary cilium role in sensing FSS is poorly understood. This chapter highlights the main relevance of primary cilium in sensing blood flow, although exact mechanisms are not fully known yet.

Keywords: shear stress, endothelial dysfunction, primary cilium, nitric oxide, reactive oxygen species, neuropilin, purinergic receptors

1. Introduction

Blood, urine and air are primary examples of biological fluids. Biophysically, fluids can be classified into four basic types: ideal fluid, real fluid, Newtonian fluid and non-Newtonian fluid. Among them, biological fluids are classified only as Newtonian and non-Newtonian. Blood and urine belong to non-Newtonian biofluids since their viscosity is not a constant with respect to the rate of shearing stress; moreover, the removal of the stress causes them to return to their initial viscosity state [1].

In order to regulate blood flow, vascular smooth muscle cells (VSMC) induce changes in blood vessel diameter by contraction and relaxation mechanism. Smooth muscle contraction is regulated by central neuronal as well as by local control mechanisms. In particular, the local control, also termed autoregulation, is an important mechanism of vascular tone regulation, maintaining the immediate control of the amount of blood flow within a specific region. Vessel diameter decreases by a sudden increase of transmural pressure and increases by faster flow or high shear stress [2]. Flow shear stress (FSS) is one of the important blood flow-induced hemodynamic forces (**Table 1**) acting on the blood vessel and is determined by the velocity of blood flow, fluid viscosity and vessel geometry [2–5]. An important determinant of shear stress is the viscosity of blood; shear stress is the energy transferred to the vessel wall due to interaction with a fluid in motion [6]. Shear stress forces are imposed directly to the endothelium and modulate endothelial structure and function through local mechanotransduction mechanisms [5, 7]. FSS is crucial for vascular homeostasis [5].

In a normal homeostatic mechanism and steady laminar shear stress, endothelial cells respond promptly with an increase in the cytosolic calcium (Ca^{2+}), activation of endothelial nitric oxide synthase (eNOS) and nitric oxide (NO) production [4, 8] and with the ultimate gene modulation [3, 5, 8]. However, besides laminar flow, oscillatory and turbulent flow patterns are also imposed to the endothelium, which has then to continuously fine-tune its activities as a response [5].

Several structures and processes have been implicated in FSS mechanotransduction into specific biochemical signals, intracellular signaling pathways and gene modulation [5]. Among those structures implicated, the primary cilium emerges as a key sensor of FSS under physiological conditions [9]. Nevertheless, in vascular injury occurring as a result of hypertension for example, normal homeostatic mechanisms are disturbed and vessel wall becomes dysfunctional associated with impaired formation and/or function of primary cilium [5, 10]. Moreover,

Hemodynamic forces	Generated by	Force name
Distention force	Surrounding muscle	Stretch force
Contractile force	Differential pressure along the vascular system	Compression force
Pulsatile force	Turbulent flow of blood	Cyclic strain
Systolic force on intima surface (endothelial cells)	Blood flow	Pressure force
Drag force on intima surface (endothelial cells)	Blood flow	Shear stress

Table 1. Various types of hemodynamic forces acting on the blood vessel wall.

http://dx.doi.org/10.5772/intechopen.73134

ciliopathies or ciliary dysfunctions can lead to a series of disorders such as PKD, hypertension and atherosclerotic lesions [9].

Physiologically, the primary cilium, a solitary non-motile microtubule-based organelle, protrudes from the surface of mammalian cells [11] into the surrounding tube (vessel/tubule) lumen. Primary cilia work as a chemo- and mechanosensors responding to diverse stimuli, including FSS [12, 13].

Since the importance of the primary cilium as a sensor of FSS has been described mainly in the kidney and in the blood vessels, it is worth to describe in brief some aspects of the renal system.

During the process of urine formation, the flow of the ultrafiltrate through the proximal tubule (PT) is pulsatile, with variable oscillations due to the heart rate and to tubuloglomerular feedback mechanism mediated by the *macula densa*. This ultrafiltration mechanism exposes kidney epithelial cells to a constant FSS in a similar way that mimics vascular endothelial cells [14]. Changes in urinary flow through the nephron depend on short-term variations in glomerular filtration rate, tubuloglomerular feedback and fluid absorption along the nephron as well as on long-term factors such as high salt or high protein diet, hypertension and early stages of diabetes [15]. Variations in luminal urinary flow alter the mechanical forces (shear stress, stretch and pressure), which in turn affect epithelial cells in the nephron. Thus, kidney epithelial cells exhibit a highly differentiated brush border composed by microvilli, glycocalyx and primary cilium in order to sense apical shear stress [14]. Tubular flow acts as potent modulator of epithelial kidney cell phenotype by affecting the organization of the cytoskeleton and the brush border, changing cell polarity and modifying various cellular functions such as solute reabsorption and extracellular matrix remodeling.

Recently, several reports showed that an alteration of primary cilia length and function is associated with acute and chronic kidney disease [12, 13, 16–21]. However, the underlying mechanisms behind these associations are still unclear. The main scope of this chapter focuses on the role of primary cilium as one of the multiple mechanotransduction machineries in sensing FSS in the endothelial vascular and epithelial renal system.

In the blood vessels, endothelial cells exhibit cilia that have been involved in blood vessel autoregulation [9], as well as in the pathogenesis of hypertension [9] and atherosclerotic lesions [22, 23].

In this chapter, we will present the physiological role of the endothelial primary cilium as a sensor of FSS. We will make a short review about potential implication of reactive oxygen species (ROS), vascular endothelial growth factor (VEGF) and purinergic signaling as modulators of the function of primary cilium. Finally, implication of the primary cilium dysfunction in the kidney and atherosclerotic lesions will be overviewed.

2. Structure of the primary cilium

Primary cilia differ from motile cilia in both structure and function and are usually classified as non-motile organelles, which were first described in 1867 by Alexander Kowalesky in vertebrate cells [24]. Motile cilia contain microtubules (MT) arranged in a (9 + 2) manner consisting of a nine doublets MT ring surrounding a central pair of MT and presenting protein spokes and dynein inner and outer arms necessary for movement. In contrast the primary cilium shows (9 + 0) organization with nine pairs of MT at the periphery lacking the central pair of MTs, as well as the protein spoke and the dynein arms (**Figure 1**). In both cases, MT extend from a basal body originating from "mother" centriole of the centrosome [25]. The structure and maintenance of the primary cilium are regulated by intraflagellar transport (IFT) particles [26].

In physiological conditions, nearly all quiescent differentiated mammalian cells exhibit a primary cilium, which emanates from the surface as a single long hair-shaped projection [27]. Therefore, primary cilia are found in a large number of mammalian cells including stem cells, epithelial and endothelial cells [19]. Their presence was demonstrated in adult vascular system (reviewed in [2]), developing chicken endocardium [4], embryonic mouse aortic endothelium [9], cultured human umbilical vein endothelial cells (HUVECs) [28, 29] and epithelial cells including *macula densa* [30] or tubular epithelial cells [20]. Nevertheless, alteration in the number, length and structural features has been implicated in pathological conditions such as polycystic kidney disease, atherosclerosis and hypertension, among others [18, 23, 31].

Depending on structural and functional features, five distinct domains were described in the primary cilium [2] (**Figure 1**):

1. The ciliary membrane housing many sensory receptors and channels supporting sensory function of cilia.

2. The soluble compartment or cilioplasm constituting the fluid between the ciliary membrane and the axoneme and where IFT machinery is located to assemble and maintain the cilia.

3. The axoneme composed of tubulin that supports ciliary transport. It is composed of nine pairs of MTs.

4. The ciliary tip is the distal part of the axoneme where specialized proteins localize whose function is still unclear.

5. The basal body, the network foundation from which the primary cilium emanates.

3. Primary cilium sensing fluid-shear depends on mechanoproteins polycystins and structural polaris

3.1. Intraflagellar transport

IFT is required for assembly and maintenance of cilia. Briefly, ciliogenesis is initiated in the apical cytoplasm at the basal body. Proteins involved in cilium formation concentrate and assemble into complexes that migrate along the cilia axonemal microtubules through a process called IFT. The anterograde movement of particles from the cell body to the tip of the flagella/cilia is driven by

http://dx.doi.org/10.5772/intechopen.73134

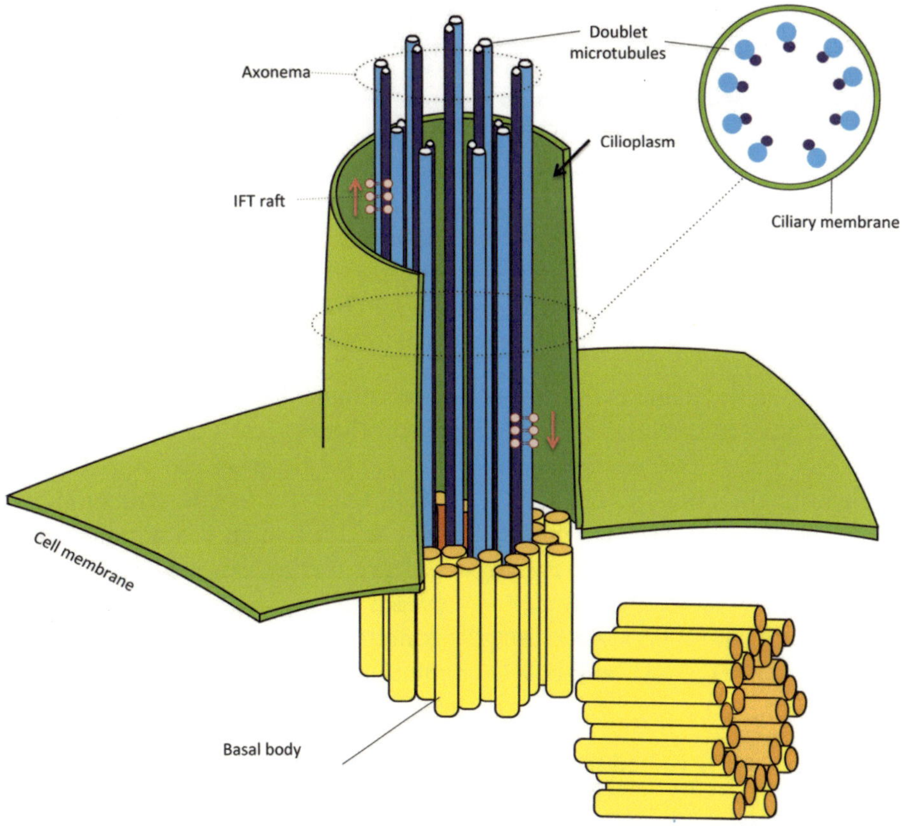

Figure 1. Scheme of the primary cilium. Longitudinal section showing the axoneme with the nine doublets of microtubules originating from the basal body. The right part of the figure shows transversal sections of motile and non-motile primary cilia. Note the absence of the central pair of microtubules and dynein arms in the primary cilium. Figure adapted with permission of [90].

kinesin II [26], whereas the retrograde movement from the tip back to the cell body is driven by cytoplasmic dynein [32]. The protein polaris is the gene product of the IFT particle 88 (*ift88*) that in mammalis is homologous to the gene *Tg737*. This protein is localized to the basal body [26, 33] and is required for ciliogenesis.

3.2. Polycystin-1, polycystin-2 and polaris

Among sensory molecules housing into the primary cilium, both polycystin-1 (PKD1) and polycystin-2 (PKD2) have been described. These are membrane integral proteins. Experimental data show that they are highly expressed in human endothelial and epithelial cells and are required for normal physiological cilia function (reviewed in [2]). The importance of these proteins has been highlighted due to the finding that mutations in *pkd1* or *pkd2* genes result in polycystic kidney disease, hence their name [9].

PKD1 is a 3327 amino acids long transmembrane protein with 11 membrane-spanning domains. Its long extracellular N-terminus has a mechanosensory function, while its short intracellular

C-terminus is involved in intracellular signaling and interaction with PKD2 [34, 35]. PKD1 has been shown to mediate fluid-shear sensing in epithelial and endothelial cells [9, 36].

PKD2, a 968 amino acids long protein, is a non-selective Ca^{2+} permeable transient receptor potential (TRP) channel consisting of six membrane-spanning domains and intracellular C- and N-terminal domains [37]. The sensory function of PKD2 depends on PKD1 and has to be localized to endothelial primary cilia [38]. Accordingly, PKD2 functioning as a Ca^{2+} channel [29] allows extracellular Ca^{2+} influx into the cilioplasm in response to FSS [39]. Thus, mechanistically, PKD1 and PKD2 interact through their C-terminus [29, 34, 35] and localized to the ciliary membrane; they are able to detect extracellular FSS and to increase cytosolic Ca^{2+}. This turns on a signaling cascade leading to the production of NO [9, 38, 40].

A series of mutation and deletion experiments demonstrated that besides PKD1 and PKD2, the protein polaris also orchestrates FSS sensing. The physiological Ca^{2+} and NO increase in response to FSS is abolished when the *pkd1*, *pkd2* and *polaris* genes are mutated or knocked out [29]. Interestingly, mutations or deletion of *polaris* seem to affect the structural integrity of cilia through the PKD1 and PKD2 mislocalization, which remain concentrated at the basal body [9, 29, 32, 41]. Together these findings evidence that polaris mediates the PKD1 and PKD2 primary cilium localization, implying a polaris cilium sensory function regulation. In order to achieve a proper fluid-shear sensing by endothelial cells and an adequate response, all three components, PKD1, PKD2 and polaris, are thus indispensable.

3.3. Molecular cascade involved in shear stress-induced calcium and NO signaling

FSS leads to cilia bending leading to PKD2-mediated increase of intracellular Ca^{2+} that leads to activation of ryanodine receptors (RyR) and inositol 1,4,5-triphosphate receptor (InsP3R) present in the endoplasmic reticulum, which then releases its stores of Ca^{2+} enhancing the intracellular levels of Ca^{2+} [42, 43]. Subsequently, Ca^{2+} activates several intracellular signaling pathways, including the activation of the eNOS-bound calmodulin, thus increasing the production of NO that diffuses from endothelial cells to neighboring VSMC inducing vasodilatation [2, 29]. This particular pathway is summarized in **Figure 2**.

The works of AbouAlaiwi et al. [29] have helped to elucidate this last mechanism. In order to prove that FSS-dependent primary cilia bending induces extracellular Ca^{2+} influx, they used Ca^{2+} chelator EGTA (ethylene glycol-bis (β-aminoethyl ether)-N,N,N′,N′-tetraacetic acid). In these experiments, EGTA abolished both Ca^{2+} and NO increases. In addition, the inhibitor of the eNOS, N^G-nitro-L-arginine methyl ester (L-NAME) blocked the FSS-induced NO release without affecting Ca^{2+} increase. The same effect was shown after blocking calcium-dependent mechanisms of NO production using calphostin C as an inhibitor of protein kinase C (PKC) or W7 as antagonist of calmodulin. Similarly, inhibiting protein kinase B (PKB)/Akt abolished NO release without altering Ca^{2+} increase. Inhibiting IP_3 kinase using LY-294002 did not alter neither Ca^{2+} nor NO increase. These findings indicate that calmodulin, PKC and Akt/PKB are downstream of the calcium pathway and that they are necessary for NO release during primary cilium-mediated FSS signaling [29] (**Figure 2**).

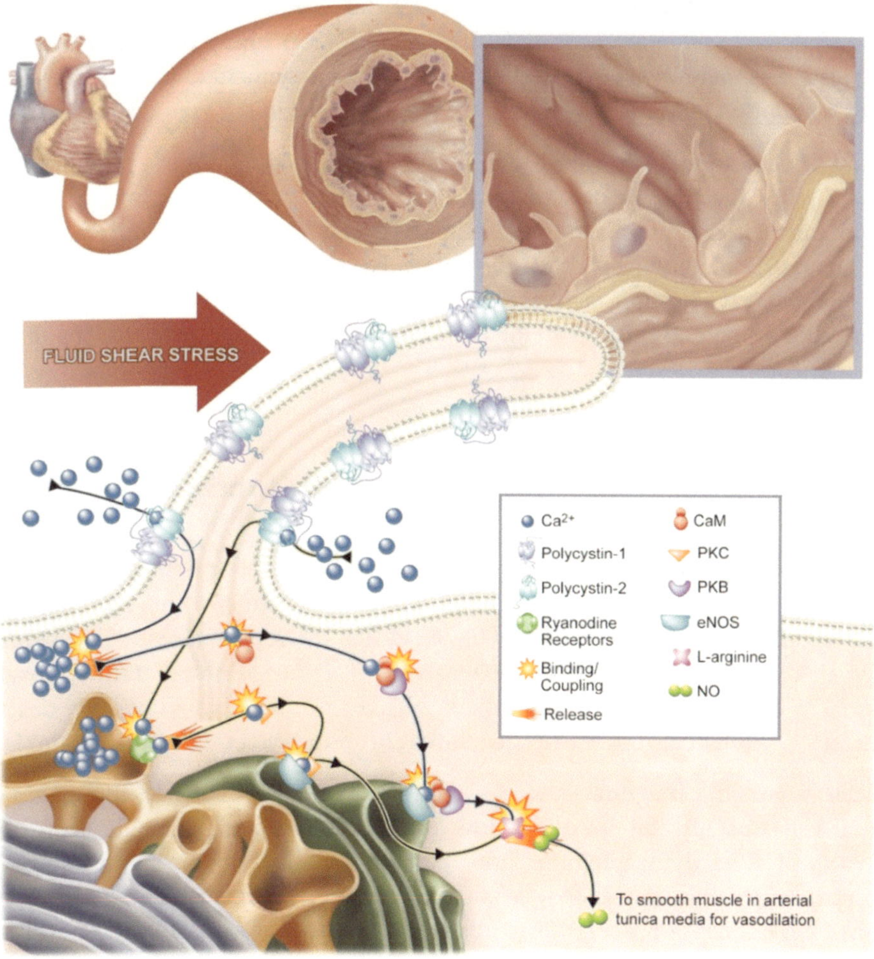

Figure 2. Mechanotransduction of FSS at the endothelial primary cilium. Extracellular FSS leads to cilia bending and activation of polycycstin-1/-2 complex, conducing to extracellular calcium influx. Calcium binds to ryanodine receptors and an efflux of intracellular organelle calcium. This is followed by activation of calmodulin (CaM), protein kinase C (PKC), protein kinase B (PKB/Akt), eNOs and NO production. Figure reproduced with permission [38].

4. The regulation of ciliary function

Changes in fluid patterns generate differential biomechanical forces, which lead to alteration of cilia function or structure [2]. Indeed, almost all blood vessels possess cilia [4, 23]. Particularly, arteries with low FSS or high fluid turbulence have cilia [2]. A prolonged exposure of endothelial cells to high FSS induces the disassembly of cilia [28] and inactivation of PKD1 by proteolytic cleavage [9], suggesting that primary cilia may not be required only to sense high shear stress [2].

The process of disassembly observed here involves the termination of IFT and the inability of the oldest centriole to maintain or initiate the assembly of primary cilia under laminar shear stress [28]. The disassembly of cilia parallels a major rearrangement of the cytoskeleton and an increase of acetylation of MT [18, 44].

In the renal system, tubular flow and ROS act as potent modulators of epithelial kidney cell phenotype also by affecting the organization of the cytoskeleton and the brush border, changing cell polarity and modifying various cellular functions such as solute reabsorption and extracellular matrix remodeling [17]. Under oxidative stress, ROS directly induce the breakdown of the cell cytoskeleton, activate various cell death-associated signals and regulate elongation, shortening and release of cilia [45]. The mechanism and implications of this regulation are still unclear.

5. Reactive oxygen species, shear stress and cilia function

ROS and NO have been implicated in sensing FSS in both vascular homeostasis and diseases [46]. ROS include collective oxygen (O_2) radicals such as superoxide, $O_2^{\cdot -}$ and hydroxyl radical, OH, and non-radical derivatives of O_2, including hydrogen peroxide (H_2O_2) and ozone (O_3). Several sources of ROS have been extensively described in the literature, in which the nicotidamine adenine dinucleotide phosphate (NADP) oxidase (Nox) has been described as one of the main cellular sources of ROS generation in endothelial cells under FSS [47].

Flow patterns and the magnitude of shear determine the amount of ROS produced by endothelial cells, usually an irregular flow pattern (disturbed or oscillatory) producing higher levels of ROS than a regular flow pattern (steady laminar or pulsatile) [48]. In addition to flow pattern, endothelial cells exposed to a prolonged laminar shear stress for more than 24 h display a reduced $O_2^{\cdot -}$ formation and ROS levels [49]. ROS production is closely linked to NO generation: elevated levels of ROS lead to low NO bioavailability, as is often observed in endothelial cells exposed to irregular flow patterns [48]. The low NO bioavailability is partially provoked by ROS reaction with NO to form peroxynitrite ($ONOO^-$), a key molecule that is implicated in oxidative and nitrosative damage [50]. NO can also take part in redox signaling by modifying proteins and lipids via cysteine S-nitrosation and fatty acid nitration, respectively [51], in this respect affecting the regulation of the vascular system [52].

5.1. Free radical signaling and primary cilia

Information related to primary cilium and free radical signaling emerges mainly from kidney research area. However, how ROS can regulate this mechanosensory organelle is not well described in the literature [17, 30, 53]. It is known that renal primary cilia protrude from the epithelial cell surface into the lumen detecting fluid flow and responding to diverse stimuli [12]. Indeed, several reports show that an alteration of primary cilia length is associated with acute and chronic kidney disease [16].

Information about primary cilia acting as an upstream regulator of ROS comes primarily from *in vitro* experiments, in which immortalized *macula densa* cell line (MMDD1) exposed to an increment in shear stress shows augmented NO production, this effect was blunted by silencing polaris protein in primary cilia using si-RNA methodology [54]. In addition, in isolated perfused juxtaglomerular apparatus preparations incubated with the diuretic furosemide (an inhibitor of Na-K-Cl cotransporter), an increase in tubular flow-induced NO production was observed. This suggests that the NO stimulatory effect is independent of Na^+ concentration in the tubular fluid, as well as volume changes, suggesting a direct FSS-dependent regulation [30]. Also, the results elucidate that FSS can stimulate NO production independently of NaCl delivery to the *macula densa*. Therefore, these results indicate that the primary cilium acts as a mechanosensory organelle for FSS inside the nephron tubule via NO.

The opposite mechanism in which free radical species can regulate primary cilia function is showed mainly in renal ischemia/reperfusion (I/R) experiments. I/R setting is characterized by an increase in free radical species production [55]. Acute tubular necrosis induced by I/R on mice model resulted in changes in primary cilium length. Thus, primary cilium was shortened after 4 h and 1 day of ischemia versus non-ischemic control cells, an effect that was blunted after 16 days [16]. The oxidative stress from I/R derived injury is able to break down cell cytoskeleton and activate various cell death-associated signals, like cell autophagy [45]. As presented by Kim et al. [53], the treatment with the antioxidant molecule Mn(III) tetrakis (1-methyl-4-pyridyl) porphyrin (MnTMPyP) during the reperfusion (i.e., recovery) period of damaged kidneys accelerated the normalization of cilia length in experiments of I/R. Concomitantly, they also showed that MnTMPyP decrease oxidative stress and recover nephron tubule morphology, indicating that the ROS signals are an integral part of cilium length regulation. In addition, cultured kidney cells treated with H_2O_2 released a ciliary fragment into the extracellular medium. MnTMPyP treatment inhibited this deciliation process [17, 53]. Moreover, the extracellular signal-regulated kinase (ERK) inhibitor U0126 blocked the cilium elongation of normal and H_2O_2-treated cells [53]. Taken together, these observations show that primary cilia length can be regulated, at least in part, by H_2O_2 through an ERK-dependent pathway. Similar results were found related in acute kidney injury after hepatic I/R from liver transplantation or resection experiments in the kidney [56]. In particular, transient hepatic ischemia caused functional and histological kidney damage, including brush border loss of tubular epithelial cells and tubule atrophy. This cellular damage also induces a shortening and deciliation of kidney primary cilia via ROS/oxidative stress, suggesting that the presence of ciliary proteins in the urine could be a potential indication of kidney injury [17]. Therefore, remote organ injury model can increase the content of O_2^-, and H_2O_2 subsequently shortening the primary cilium length in several nephron sections [56]. These data confirm that free radical species can modulate the primary cilium length, at least in the kidney, but the mechanism and functional implications of such modulation remain unclear.

6. Vascular endothelial growth factor and shear stress

VEGFs are a complex family of glycoproteins that are structurally related to platelet-derived growth factor (PDGF) [57]. Through alternative RNA splicing, VEGF family is constituted by several isoforms, including $VEGF_{165}$, which has been named VEGF-A or VEGF, the isoform involved in many of the functions attributed to the VEGF family. All members of the VEGF family activate tyrosine kinase receptors known as VEGF receptors (VEGFRs), which include VEGFR-1 (also known as fms-like tyrosine kinase 1 or Flt-1), VEGFR-2 (or kinase insert-domain containing receptor, KDR) and VEGFR-3 [58, 59]. Activation of VEGFRs has been implicated in several vascular functions, including angiogenesis, vascular tone regulation and endothelial cell survival, among others [59–61].

Importantly, VEGF and VEGFRs have also been associated with sensing FSS. High expression of VEGF [62] and the activation of VEGFR2 [63, 64] have been linked to the FSS sensing. Moreover, the activation of VEGFRs generally leads to NO synthesis in many kinds of cells, including endothelial cells [58]. Therefore, it is not surprising that VEGFR2 triggers NO-dependent flow regulation. Jin et al. [63] showed that FSS leads to VEGFR2 activation in a ligand-independent manner and leads to eNOS activation in cultured endothelial cells. Intra-cellular downstream pathway associated with NO synthesis due to FSS-stimulated VEGFR2 activation included phosphoinositide 3-kinase (PI3K) and PKB/Akt. Interestingly, contrary to PKB/Akt, the PI3K pathway has not been associated to endothelial primary cilium FSS sensory function [29]. Also, *in vivo* experiments confirmed that VEGFR2 is a key mechanotransducer that activates eNOS in response to blood flow [63]. Despite these evidences, as far as we known there is no information related to VEGFRs present in the primary cilium as potential regulator of FSS sensing.

7. Neuropilins and the primary cilium

VEGF can also bind to neuropilins (NRP), a family of transmembrane glycoproteins that play key role in axonal guidance, angiogenesis, tumorigenesis and immunological response [65]. NRPs have been characterized as co-receptors for VEGFRs and plexins, the receptors of the extracellular secreted ligands, belonging to class III semaphorins [60]. In turn, semaphorins are a class of secreted and membrane proteins that were originally identified as axonal growth cone guidance molecules. At least two neuropilin genes, NRP1 and NRP2, have been identified [66]. Genetic studies in mice have confirmed that NRPs are key components of vasculogenesis, angiogenesis and lymphangiogenesis [65, 66]. Nevertheless, NRPs can bind to growth factors such as VEGF, placental growth factor (PlGF), hepatocyte growth factor (HGF) and fibroblast growth factor (FGF), among others. And due to VEGF binding, NRPs can also modulate blood flow [65].

In endothelial cells, NRPs are thought to increase signaling through the VEGFRs acting as a co-receptor of VEGF and by stabilizing the VEGF/VEGFR complexes and therefore enhancing VEGF activity. Thus, the interaction of VEGF-A_{165} with NRP1 is required for stable binding of VEGF-A_{165} to VEGFR-2, full activation of VEGFR-2 and downstream signaling and biological responses [65, 67].

Limited information about the localization of NRP in primary cilium is available. Before presenting those evidences, we should give some information about hedgehog (HH) signaling. Briefly, HH signaling is essential for tissue patterning and organ formation during embryonic and postnatal development, as well as in cancer development and tissue homeostasis renewal and repair in adult animals [68]. The HH pathway acts via activation of transcriptional effectors, such as the glioblastoma (Gli) proteins, a family of transcription factors whose target genes remain enigmatic. The Gli protein family includes Gli1, Gli2 and Gli3 [69].

Referring to the primary cilium, studies conducted by Pinskey et al. [68] found that NRP1 and NRP2 promote the activation of Gli transcription factor. Interestingly, the authors found that a conserved 12 amino acid region of the NRP1 cytoplasmic domain between amino acids 890 and 902 is responsible for the HH-signal promotion. Considering that an intact primary cilium is a main component of the HH signaling, they also looked for the localization of NRP1 in this subcellular compartment and showed the unique evidence until now about the localization of NRP1, but not NRP2, in the primary cilium [68]. Despite the fact that the localization of NRP1 in the primary cilium was not required for HH signaling promotion, it is intriguing why NRP1 is present in primary cilium and what would be its physiological relevance there. This observation is important considering that NRP1, as indicated previously, may interact with growth factors, such as VEGF, PlGF, HGF and FGF, among others, regulating their action. Still more questions than answers emerge and more investigation is required to lighten these intriguing possibilities.

8. Purinergic receptors and the primary cilium

Since early 1970s [70], adenosine triphosphate (ATP) has been recognized as an extracellular signaling molecule activating a pathway defined as "purinergic signaling" where ATP, ADP and adenosine are involved. The signaling pathway starts with the activation of a family of membrane receptors. At this moment, separate families for adenosine purinergic (P1) and ATP and ADP purinergic (P2) receptors have been characterized. Briefly, adenosine receptor or P1 family includes at least four members of G-protein-coupled receptor subtypes identified as A_1, A_{2A}, A_{2B} and A_3. In contrast, the P2 family encompasses seven members of purinergic receptor type X (P2X), a family of ion channels receptor subtypes (P2X1–7) and at least eight members of P2Y G-protein-coupled receptor subtypes ($P2Y_1$, $P2Y_2$, $P2Y_4$, $P2Y_6$, $P2Y_{11}$, $P2Y_{12}$, $P2Y_{13}$ and $P2Y_{14}$) [71]. $P2Y_1$, $P2Y_2$, $P2Y_4$ and $P2Y_6$ are associated with the intracellular calcium (iCa^{2+}) signaling pathway, whereas $P2Y_2$, $P2Y_{13}$ and $P2Y_{14}$ are associated with cyclic adenosine monophosphate (cAMP) signaling. In contrast, $P2Y_{11}$ has been shown to be associated with both iCa^{2+} and cAMP signaling [71].

ATP is released by almost all cell types after gentle mechanical stimulation and acts in an autocrine or paracrine manner [72]. Living cells under stressful conditions (i.e., hypoxia) or dying cells release ATP [72]. Interestingly, purinergic signaling parallel to flow sensor activity of the primary cilium [73]. Purinergic signaling associated with flow sensing was detected in several structures such as kidney tubules [20], intrahepatic bile ducts [74, 75], endothelial cells [31], among other lining cells. Therefore, deflection of the primary cilium has been related with ATP release leading to autocrine or paracrine activation of purinergic receptors.

The relationship between ATP, purinergic signaling and primary cilium has been studied in the kidney tubular system [73]. The main physiological area that established a relationship between these three elements is related to urinary flow sensor, where a flow-stimulated increase of iCa^{2+} has been characterized. Initial investigation suggested that deflecting the cilium releases a paracrine factor, such as ATP that can activate a G-protein-coupled receptor and generate inositol triphosphate (IP_3) leading to iCa^{2+} increase throughout the cytosol due to the release of Ca^{2+} from the intracellular stores. Also, increasing the tubular flow triggered an increase in iCa^{2+}. The same experiments were also performed in renal tubules from mice lacking $P2Y_2$ receptors or cells lacking the primary cilium. In those experiments, the response to tubular flow was markedly reduced only in those cells lacking the $P2Y_2$ [76]. These results strongly suggested that tubular flow triggers ATP release, followed by auto- and paracrine activation of epithelial P2 receptors. However, a direct link to the primary cilium could not be established in these experiments. Despite that, information regarding how purinergic signaling can be associated or not to function of primary cilia is missing.

9. Ciliopathies: an insight into some clinical consequences of impaired ciliary function

9.1. Polycystic kidney disease

As indicated above, the relevance of the primary cilium function has been well established in the kidney, as evidenced in polycystic kidney disease [37, 77, 78]. Also, previous reports suggest that the outcome of I/R in kidneys is associated with the change of primary cilia length [17]. Physiologically, urinary flow through the nephron is a highly variable process. In the short term, flow changes can be caused by variations in glomerular filtration rate [79], tubuloglomerular feedback [80] and fluid absorption along the nephron [79]. In the long term, urinary flow fluctuations can be caused by a high salt [81] or high protein diet [82], as well as due to hypertension [83] or early stages of diabetes [84]. Variations in luminal urinary flow alter the mechanical forces (shear stress, stretch and pressure) that affect epithelial cells in the nephron.

Polycystic kidney disease is a genetic disease characterized by bilateral enlarged cystic kidneys. It is caused by mutations of genes encoding for PKD1 and PKD2 linked to polycystic kidney disease type 1 (*pkd1*) and polycystic kidney disease type 2, respectively [37, 77, 78]. The frequencies of cardiovascular complications are very high in polycystic kidney disease patients. Hypertension occurs in 50–70% of patients even before any substantial kidney disorder [85]. Polycystic kidney disease has been associated with abnormalities in FSS sensing due to primary cilia dysfunction [36]. Mechanistically, polycystic kidney disease patients exhibit impairment of endothelium-dependent relaxation and a decrease of eNOS activity, impaired release of NO and, therefore, endothelial dysfunction [86]. Furthermore, polycystic kidney disease has been associated to the inability of renal epithelia [87] or vascular endothelia [9] to induce Ca^{2+} influx in response to FSS. Endothelial cells isolated from mice and humans with polycystic kidney disease lack PKD1 and/or PKD2 in the primary cilium and fail to produce NO in response to FSS [2, 9, 29].

Abnormal PKD2 function or expression has been associated with hypertension [88]. Mutations of *pkd2* gene abolish Ca^{2+} and NO increases in endothelial cells showing that PKD2 mediates FSS sensing in endothelial cells [29]. In addition, PKD2 sensory function as a Ca^{2+} channel depends on its localization at the primary cilium and on PKD1. Thus, impaired function and expression of PKD2 are associated with endothelial dysfunction. Interestingly, prolonged exposure of endothelial cells to high FSS induces the disassembly of cilia [28] and inactivation of PKD1 by proteolytic cleavage [9], reducing the ability of endothelial cells to properly sense alterations in blood pressure.

9.2. Atherosclerosis

Initial evidence showed that primary cilia were present in the vascular beds where flow is disturbed, and related to atherosclerosis [89]. Particularly, the primary cilia were found in the endothelial cells of human aortic fatty dots and streaks, but not in those of the normal intima [89]. Moreover, recent evidences also found the primary cilium in cells exposed to laminar blood flow [27]. Regarding atherosclerotic plaque, primary cilia have been shown to be located at the atherosclerotic predilection sites, where flow is disturbed and around atherosclerotic lesions in the aortic arch in wild-type mice and apolipoprotein E-deficient mice, respectively [23]. In addition, experimentally induced pathologic turbulent flow in mice leads to induction of primary cilia, and subsequently to atherogenesis, suggesting a role of primary cilia in endothelial activation and dysfunction [23].

Contrary, another evidence found an inverse correlation between the presence of endothelial primary cilia and vascular calcified areas, although the signaling mechanisms involved remain unknown [22]. In order to analyze this phenomenon, Sanchez-Duffhues et al. [22] used the Tg737 cilium-defective mouse model and they found that non-ciliated aortic endothelial cells acquire the ability to trans-differentiate into mineralizing osteogenic cells. The mechanism for this trans-differentiation requires the presence of bone morphogenetic proteins (BMP). Therefore, these data emphasize the role of the endothelial cells in vascular calcification and generation of atherosclerosis. Whether these findings are associated or not to iCa^{2+}, eNOS activation and NO synthesis remains unclear.

Apparently, differences in blood flow patterns along the endothelium trigger abnormal vascular responses that have been associated with pathophysiological consequences, such as atherosclerosis. While endothelial cells exposed to laminar blood flow are protected from atherosclerosis formation, turbulent blood flow, which occurs at bends and bifurcations of blood vessels, facilitates the process of atherosclerosis. Primary cilia presence and function have barely been studied in both endothelial activation and dysfunction. Hence, more studies are required to better understand these issues.

10. Concluding remarks

Phenotypic cell alterations resulting from flow-induced mechanical strains and their implication in diseases are a growing field of research in many cell types such as vascular endothelial, smooth muscle, kidney epithelial cells and chondrocytes.

In the chapter, we presented the role of the primary cilium as one of the multiple physiological mechanosensors for FSS in endothelial and renal cells, where it regulates vascular homeostasis and epithelial function. To respond to FSS, a functional primary cilium requires the constitutive proteins, PKD1, PKD2 and polaris. The primary cilium is functional under normal FSS and activates the Ca^{2+} and NO signaling cascade; nevertheless, it becomes dysfunctional after prolonged exposure to high FSS analogous to a hypertensive situation present in any kind of biological fluid. Respectively, growing evidence implicates the primary cilium and the disruption of its function in many diseases such as hypertension, atherosclerotic lesions and acute and chronic kidney disease.

In this regards, we have summarized evidences implicating that polycystic kidney disease, a pathology characterized by lack of PKD1 and/or PKD2 expression, leads to impaired vascular endothelial FSS sensing. Even when the primary organ affected by the disease is the kidney, the endothelial dysfunction is a common extra renal symptom observed in polycystic kidney disease. Those patients exhibit an impairment of endothelium-dependent relaxation and a decrease of primary cilia-dependent NO production leading to hypertension.

Contrary to its physiological role in sensing FSS, it has also been described that primary cilium is related to plaque formation, since this organelle was present in the endothelial cells of human aortic fatty dots and streaks. Indeed, primary cilium has been shown to be located at the atherosclerotic predilection sites, where flow is disturbed and around atherosclerotic lesions in the aortic arch in wild-type mice and apolipoprotein E-deficient mice, respectively [31]. In addition, primary cilia have been involved in endothelial activation and dysfunction present in atherosclerosis. Despite relevance of these evidences, it is highlighted in this review that more studies are required to better understand the role of endothelial primary cilium in normal and pathological conditions, such as atherosclerosis.

We also presented examples of regulatory signals that control NO bioavailability or might participate as modulators of primary cilium. For instance, ROS can modulate cilia length and deciliation process in tubular kidney cells. Whether these effects could be extrapolated to endothelial cells is worth of more investigation.

Finally, we presented the interconnected coreceptors VEGF and VEGFRs, neuropilins, ATP, adenosine and purinergic receptors. All have been suggested to be involved in FSS sensing and/or colocalization in the primary cilium. To this respect, we can provide more questions than answers. NRP1, a VEGFR2 receptor, localizes to the primary cilium but its physiological relevance is still unknown. On the other hand, ATP and adenosine are involved in sensing FSS, in a primary cilium-independent manner. Moreover, information regarding whether or not purinergic signaling can be associated to the primary cilia function is missing.

In conclusion, these data emphasize the role of the primary cilium present in endothelial cells as a microsensory organelle transducing FSS. Impairment in the ciliogenesis, cilia length and intracellular pathways can be involved in cardiovascular diseases. The participation of ROS, VEGF and purinergic signaling pathways is being described, but more research is required to elucidate their participation in the primary cilium-mediated sensing of FSS in normal and pathological conditions, such as hypertension, atherosclerosis or polycystic kidney disease.

Acknowledgements

We would like to thank the research staff of the Vascular Physiology Laboratory; the Group of Investigation in Tumor Angiogenesis (GIANT) from the Universidad del Bío-Bío; Group of Research and Innovation in Vascular Health (GRIVAS Health) group for the outstanding discussion of the ideas presented in this manuscript.

Conflict of interest

None.

Source of funding

This study was supported by Fondecyt Regular 1140586; Fondequip EQM140104; DIUBB 166709 3/R and GI 171709/VC.

Financial disclosure

None.

Abbreviations

eNOS	Endothelial nitric oxide synthase
ERK	Extracellular signal-regulated Kinase
FGF	Fibroblast growth factor
FSS	Fluid shear stress
Gli	Glioblastoma transcription factors
HH	Hedgehog signaling pathway
HGF	Hepatocyte growth factor
HUVECs	Human umbilical vein endothelial cells
MMDD1	Immortalized macula densa cell line

InsP3R	Inositol 1,4,5-triphosphate receptor
IP_3	Inositol triphosphate
iCa^{2+}	Intracellular calcium
ift88 or Tg737	Intraflagellar transport particle 88
IFT	Intraflagellar transport particles
I/R	Ischemia/reperfusion
MT	Microtubules
MnTMPyP	Mn(III) tetrakis (1-methyl-4-pyridyl) porphyrin
NRP	Neuropilins
L-NAME	N^G-nitro-L-arginine methyl ester
Nox	Nicotidamine adenine dinucleotide phosphate oxidase
NO	Nitric Oxide
$ONOO^-$	peroxynitrite
PI3K	Phosphoinositide 3-kinase
PlGF	Placental growth factor
PDGF	Platelet-derived growth factor
PKD	Polycystic kidney disease
PKD1	Polycystin-1
PKD2	Polycystin-2
PKB	Protein kinase B
PKC	Protein kinase C
PT	Proximal tubule
ROS	Reactive oxygen species
RyR	Ryanodine receptors
siRNA	Small interference RNA
VEGF	Vascular endothelial growth factor
VSMC	Vascular smooth muscle cells
VEGFRs	VEGF receptors
VEGFR-1	Also known as fms-like tyrosine kinase 1 or Flt-1
VEGFR-2	Or kinase insert-domain containing receptor, KDR

Author details

Meriem Rezgaoui[1,2], Andres Rodriguez[1,2,3], Kurt Herlitz[2,3] and Carlos Escudero[1,2,3]*

*Address all correspondence to: cescudero@ubiobio.cl

1 Department of Basic Sciences, Universidad del Bio Bio, Chillan, Chile

2 Vascular Physiology Laboratory, Group of Investigation in Tumor Angiogenesis (GIANT), Department of Basic Sciences, Universidad del Bío-Bío, Chillán, Chile

3 Group of Research and Innovation in Vascular Health (GRIVAS Health), Pedro de Valdivia, Chillan, Chile

References

[1] Waite L, Fine J. Applied Bio Fluid Mechanics. McGraw Hill Companies, Inc; 2007

[2] Nauli SM, Jin X, Hierck BP. The mechanosensory role of primary cilia in vascular hypertension. International Journal of Vascular Medicine. Hindawi. 2011;**2011**:376281. DOI: 10.1155/2011/376281. PubMed PMID: 21748021; PubMed Central PMCID: PMCPMC3124932

[3] Groenendijk BC, Hierck BP, Gittenberger-De Groot AC, Poelmann RE. Development-related changes in the expression of shear stress responsive genes KLF-2, ET-1, and NOS-3 in the developing cardiovascular system of chicken embryos. Developmental Dynamics. 2004;**230**(1):57-68. DOI: 10.1002/dvdy.20029. PubMed PMID: 15108309

[4] Van der Heiden K, Groenendijk BC, Hierck BP, Hogers B, Koerten HK, Mommaas AM, et al. Monocilia on chicken embryonic endocardium in low shear stress areas. Developmental Dynamics. 2006;**235**(1):19-28. DOI: 10.1002/dvdy.20557. PubMed PMID: 16145662

[5] Cunningham KS, Gotlieb AI. The role of shear stress in the pathogenesis of atherosclerosis. Laboratory Investigation. 2005;**85**(1):9-23. DOI: 10.1038/labinvest.3700215. PubMed PMID: 15568038

[6] Baieth HE. Physical parameters of blood as a non-Newtonian fluid. International Journal of Biomedical Science and Engineering. 2008;**4**(4):323-329. PubMed PMID: 23675105; PubMed Central PMCID: PMCPMC3614720

[7] Buschmann I, Schaper W. The pathophysiology of the collateral circulation (arteriogenesis). The Journal of Pathology. 2000;**190**(3):338-342. DOI: 10.1002/(SICI)1096-9896(200002)190:3<338::AID-PATH594>3.0.CO;2-7. PubMed PMID: 10685067

[8] Resnick N, Yahav H, Shay-Salit A, Shushy M, Schubert S, Zilberman LC, et al. Fluid shear stress and the vascular endothelium: For better and for worse. Progress in Biophysics and Molecular Biology 2003;**81**(3):177-199. PubMed PMID: 12732261

[9] Nauli SM, Kawanabe Y, Kaminski JJ, Pearce WJ, Ingber DE, Zhou J. Endothelial cilia are fluid shear sensors that regulate calcium signaling and nitric oxide production through polycystin-1.

Circulation. 2008;**117**(9):1161-71. DOI: 10.1161/CIRCULATIONAHA.107.710111. PubMed PMID: 18285569; PubMed Central PMCID: PMCPMC3071982

[10] Della-Morte D, Rendek T. The role of shear stress and arteriogenesis in maintaining vascular homeostasis and preventing cerebral atherosclerosis. Brain Circulation. 2015; **1**(1):53-62

[11] Wheatley DN, Wang AM, Strugnell GE. Expression of primary cilia in mammalian cells. Cell Biology International. 1996;**20**(1):73-81. DOI: 10.1006/cbir.1996.0011. PubMed PMID: 8936410

[12] Praetorius HA, Spring KR. A physiological view of the primary cilium. Annual Review of Physiology. 2005;**67**:515-529. DOI: 10.1146/annurev.physiol.67.040403.101353. PubMed PMID: 15709968

[13] Praetorius HA, Spring KR. Removal of the MDCK cell primary cilium abolishes flow sensing. The Journal of Membrane Biology. 2003;**191**(1):69-76. DOI: 10.1007/s00232-002-1042-4. PubMed PMID: 12532278

[14] Raghavan V, Weisz OA. Discerning the role of mechanosensors in regulating proximal tubule function. American Journal of Physiology Renal Physiology. 2016;**310**(1):F1-F5. DOI: 10.1152/ajprenal.00373.2015. PubMed PMID: 26662200; PubMed Central PMCID: PMC4675802

[15] Carlstrom M, Wilcox CS, Arendshorst WJ. Renal autoregulation in health and disease. Physiological Reviews. 2015;**95**(2):405-511. DOI: 10.1152/physrev.00042.2012. PubMed PMID: 25834230; PubMed Central PMCID: PMC4551215

[16] Verghese E, Ricardo SD, Weidenfeld R, Zhuang J, Hill PA, Langham RG, et al. Renal primary cilia lengthen after acute tubular necrosis. Journal of the American Society of Nephrology : JASN. 2009;**20**(10):2147-2153. DOI: 10.1681/ASN.2008101105. PubMed PMID: 19608704; PubMed Central PMCID: PMC2754102

[17] Han SJ, Jang HS, Seu SY, Cho HJ, Hwang YJ, Kim JI, et al. Hepatic ischemia/reperfusion injury disrupts the homeostasis of kidney primary cilia via oxidative stress. Biochimica et Biophysica Acta. 2017;**1863**(7):1817-1828. DOI: 10.1016/j.bbadis.2017.05.004. PubMed PMID: 28495528

[18] Sanchez I, Dynlacht BD. Cilium assembly and disassembly. Nature Cell Biology. 2016; **18**(7):711-717. DOI: 10.1038/ncb3370. PubMed PMID: 27350441; PubMed Central PMCID: PMCPMC5079433

[19] Satir P, Pedersen LB, Christensen ST. The primary cilium at a glance. Journal of Cell Science. 2010;**123**(Pt 4):499-503. DOI: 10.1242/jcs.050377. PubMed PMID: 20144997; PubMed Central PMCID: PMCPMC2818190

[20] Rodat-Despoix L, Delmas P. Ciliar functions in the nephron. Pflügers Archiv. 2009;**458**(1): 179-187. DOI: 10.1007/s00424-008-0632-0. PubMed PMID: 19153764

[21] Wang L, Weidenfeld R, Verghese E, Ricardo SD, Deane JA. Alterations in renal cilium length during transient complete ureteral obstruction in the mouse. Journal of Anatomy. 2008;

213(2):79-85. DOI: 10.1111/j.1469-7580.2008.00918.x. PubMed PMID: 18537851; PubMed Central PMCID: PMCPMC2526103

[22] Sanchez-Duffhues G, de Vinuesa AG, Lindeman JH, Mulder-Stapel A, DeRuiter MC, Van Munsteren C, et al. SLUG is expressed in endothelial cells lacking primary cilia to promote cellular calcification. Arteriosclerosis, Thrombosis, and Vascular Biology. 2015;**35**(3): 616-627. DOI: 10.1161/ATVBAHA.115.305268. PubMed PMID: 25633317

[23] Van der Heiden K, Hierck BP, Krams R, de Crom R, Cheng C, Baiker M, et al. Endothelial primary cilia in areas of disturbed flow are at the base of atherosclerosis. Atherosclerosis. 2008;**196**(2):542-550. DOI: 10.1016/j.atherosclerosis.2007.05.030. PubMed PMID: 17631294

[24] Kowalewsky A. Entwicklungsgeschichte des Amphioxus Lanceolatus. Mém L'Acad Imp Sci St-Pétersboug. 1867;**11**:1-17

[25] Adams M. The primary cilium: An orphan organelle finds a home. Nature Education. 2010;**3**(9):54

[26] Kozminski KG, Johnson KA, Forscher P, Rosenbaum JL. A motility in the eukaryotic flagellum unrelated to flagellar beating. Proceedings of the National Academy of Sciences of the United States of America. 1993;**90**(12):5519-5523. PubMed PMID: 8516294; PubMed Central PMCID: PMCPMC46752

[27] Satir P, Christensen ST. Overview of structure and function of mammalian cilia. Annual Review of Physiology. 2007;**69**:377-400. DOI: 10.1146/annurev.physiol.69.040705.141236. PubMed PMID: 17009929

[28] Iomini C, Tejada K, Mo W, Vaananen H, Piperno G. Primary cilia of human endothelial cells disassemble under laminar shear stress. The Journal of Cell Biology. 2004;**164**(6):811-817. DOI: 10.1083/jcb.200312133. PubMed PMID: 15024030; PubMed Central PMCID: PMCPMC2172280

[29] AbouAlaiwi WA, Takahashi M, Mell BR, Jones TJ, Ratnam S, Kolb RJ, et al. Ciliary polycystin-2 is a mechanosensitive calcium channel involved in nitric oxide signaling cascades. Circulation Research. 2009;**104**(7):860-869. DOI: 10.1161/CIRCRESAHA.108.192765. PubMed PMID: 19265036; PubMed Central PMCID: PMCPMC3085025

[30] Cabral PD, Garvin JL. Luminal flow regulates NO and O_2^- along the nephron. American Journal of Physiology Renal Physiology. 2011;**300**(5):F1047-F1053. DOI: 10.1152/ajprenal.00724.2010. PubMed PMID: 21345976; PubMed Central PMCID: PMC3094045

[31] Dinsmore C, Reiter JF. Endothelial primary cilia inhibit atherosclerosis. EMBO Reports. 2016;**17**(2):156-166. DOI: 10.15252/embr.201541019. PubMed PMID: 26769565; PubMed Central PMCID: PMCPMC5290813

[32] Pazour GJ, Dickert BL, Vucica Y, Seeley ES, Rosenbaum JL, Witman GB, et al. Chlamydomonas IFT88 and its mouse homologue, polycystic kidney disease gene tg737, are required for assembly of cilia and flagella. The Journal of Cell Biology. 2000;**151**(3):709-718. PubMed PMID: 11062270; PubMed Central PMCID: PMCPMC2185580

[33] Taulman PD, Haycraft CJ, Balkovetz DF, Yoder BK. Polaris, a protein involved in left-right axis patterning, localizes to basal bodies and cilia. Molecular Biology of the Cell. 2001;**12**(3):589-599. PubMed PMID: 11251073; PubMed Central PMCID: PMCPMC30966

[34] Hanaoka K, Qian F, Boletta A, Bhunia AK, Piontek K, Tsiokas L, et al. Co-assembly of polycystin-1 and -2 produces unique cation-permeable currents. Nature. 2000;**408**(6815): 990-994. DOI: 10.1038/35050128. PubMed PMID: 11140688

[35] Tsiokas L, Kim E, Arnould T, Sukhatme VP, Walz G. Homo- and heterodimeric interactions between the gene products of PKD1 and PKD2. Proceedings of the National Academy of Sciences of the United States of America. 1997;**94**(13):6965-6970. PubMed PMID: 9192675; PubMed Central PMCID: PMCPMC21268

[36] Nauli SM, Zhou J. Polycystins and mechanosensation in renal and nodal cilia. BioEssays. 2004;**26**(8):844-856. DOI: 10.1002/bies.20069. PubMed PMID: 15273987

[37] Mochizuki T, Wu G, Hayashi T, Xenophontos SL, Veldhuisen B, Saris JJ, et al. PKD2, a gene for polycystic kidney disease that encodes an integral membrane protein. Science. 1996;**272**(5266):1339-1342. PubMed PMID: 8650545

[38] Abou Alaiwi WA, Lo ST, Nauli SM. Primary cilia: Highly sophisticated biological sensors. Sensors (Basel). 2009;**9**(9):7003-7020. DOI: 10.3390/s90907003. PubMed PMID: 22423203; PubMed Central PMCID: PMCPMC3290460

[39] Kathem SH, Mohieldin AM, Nauli SM. The roles of primary cilia in polycystic kidney disease. AIMS Molecular Science. 2014;**1**(1):27-46. DOI: 10.3934/molsci.2013.1.27. PubMed PMID: 25599087; PubMed Central PMCID: PMCPMC4296740

[40] Nauli SM, Jin X, AbouAlaiwi WA, El-Jouni W, Su X, Zhou J. Non-motile primary cilia as fluid shear stress mechanosensors. Methods in Enzymology. 2013;**525**:1-20. DOI: 10.1016/B978-0-12-397944-5.00001-8. PubMed PMID: 23522462; PubMed Central PMCID: PMCPMC4096622

[41] Yoder BK, Tousson A, Millican L, Wu JH, Bugg CE Jr, Schafer JA, et al. Polaris, a protein disrupted in orpk mutant mice, is required for assembly of renal cilium. American Journal of Physiology Renal Physiology. 2002;**282**(3):F541-F552. DOI: 10.1152/ajprenal.00273.2001. PubMed PMID: 11832437

[42] Anyatonwu GI, Ehrlich BE. Calcium signaling and polycystin-2. Biochemical and Biophysical Research Communications. 2004;**322**(4):1364-1373. DOI: 10.1016/j.bbrc.2004.08.043. PubMed PMID: 15336985

[43] Anyatonwu GI, Estrada M, Tian X, Somlo S, Ehrlich BE. Regulation of ryanodine receptor-dependent calcium signaling by polycystin-2. Proceedings of the National Academy of Sciences of the United States of America. 2007;**104**(15):6454-6459. DOI: 10.1073/pnas.0610324104. PubMed PMID: 17404231; PubMed Central PMCID: PMCPMC1851053

[44] Seeley ES, Nachury MV. The perennial organelle: Assembly and disassembly of the primary cilium. Journal of Cell Science. 2010;**123**(Pt 4):511-518. DOI: 10.1242/jcs.061093. PubMed PMID: 20144999; PubMed Central PMCID: PMCPMC2818191

[45] Navarro-Yepes J, Burns M, Anandhan A, Khalimonchuk O, del Razo LM, Quintanilla-Vega B, et al. Oxidative stress, redox signaling, and autophagy: Cell death versus survival. Antioxidants & Redox Signaling. 2014;**21**(1):66-85. doi: 10.1089/ars.2014.5837. PubMed PMID: 24483238; PubMed Central PMCID: PMC4048575

[46] Matlung HL, Bakker EN, VanBavel E. Shear stress, reactive oxygen species, and arterial structure and function. Antioxidants & Redox Signaling. 2009;**11**(7):1699-1709. DOI: 10.1089/ARS.2008.2408. PubMed PMID: 19186981

[47] Lassegue B, San Martin A, Griendling KK. Biochemistry, physiology, and pathophysiology of NADPH oxidases in the cardiovascular system. Circulation Research. 2012;**110**(10): 1364-1390. DOI: 10.1161/CIRCRESAHA.111.243972. PubMed PMID: 22581922; PubMed Central PMCID: PMC3365576

[48] De Keulenaer GW, Chappell DC, Ishizaka N, Nerem RM, Alexander RW, Griendling KK. Oscillatory and steady laminar shear stress differentially affect human endothelial redox state: Role of a superoxide-producing NADH oxidase. Circulation Research. 1998;**82**(10): 1094-1101. PubMed PMID: 9622162

[49] White SJ, Hayes EM, Lehoux S, Jeremy JY, Horrevoets AJ, Newby AC. Characterization of the differential response of endothelial cells exposed to normal and elevated laminar shear stress. Journal of Cellular Physiology. 2011;**226**(11):2841-2848. DOI: 10.1002/jcp.22629. PubMed PMID: 21302282; PubMed Central PMCID: PMC3412226

[50] Cai H, Harrison DG. Endothelial dysfunction in cardiovascular diseases: The role of oxidant stress. Circulation Research. 2000;**87**(10):840-844. PubMed PMID: 11073878

[51] Thomas DD, Heinecke JL, Ridnour LA, Cheng RY, Kesarwala AH, Switzer CH, et al. Signaling and stress: The redox landscape in NOS2 biology. Free Radical Biology & Medicine. 2015;**87**:204-225. DOI: 10.1016/j.freeradbiomed.2015.06.002. PubMed PMID: 26117324; PubMed Central PMCID: PMC4852151

[52] Heo KS, Fujiwara K, Abe J. Disturbed-flow-mediated vascular reactive oxygen species induce endothelial dysfunction. Circulation Journal. 2011;**75**(12):2722-2730. PubMed PMID: 22076424; PubMed Central PMCID: PMCPMC3620204

[53] Kim JI, Kim J, Jang HS, Noh MR, Lipschutz JH, Park KM. Reduction of oxidative stress during recovery accelerates normalization of primary cilia length that is altered after ischemic injury in murine kidneys. American Journal of Physiology Renal Physiology. 2013;**304**(10):F1283-F1294. DOI: 10.1152/ajprenal.00427.2012. PubMed PMID: 23515720

[54] Wang L, Shen C, Liu H, Wang S, Chen X, Roman RJ, et al. Shear stress blunts tubuloglomerular feedback partially mediated by primary cilia and nitric oxide at the macula densa. American Journal of Physiology. Regulatory, Integrative and Comparative Physiology. 2015;**309**(7):R757-R766. DOI: 10.1152/ajpregu.00173.2015. PubMed PMID: 26269519; PubMed Central PMCID: PMCPMC4666931

[55] Plotnikov EY, Kazachenko AV, Vyssokikh MY, Vasileva AK, Tcvirkun DV, Isaev NK, et al. The role of mitochondria in oxidative and nitrosative stress during ischemia/reperfusion

in the rat kidney. Kidney International. 2007;**72**(12):1493-1502. DOI: 10.1038/sj.ki.5002568. PubMed PMID: 17914353

[56] Nastos C, Kalimeris K, Papoutsidakis N, Tasoulis MK, Lykoudis PM, Theodoraki K, et al. Global consequences of liver ischemia/reperfusion injury. Oxidative medicine and cellular longevity. 2014;**2014**:906965. DOI: 10.1155/2014/906965. PubMed PMID: 24799983; PubMed Central PMCID: PMC3995148

[57] Ruiz de Almodovar C, Lambrechts D, Mazzone M, Carmeliet P. Role and therapeutic potential of VEGF in the nervous system. Physiological Reviews. 2009;**89**(2):607-648. Epub 2009/04/04. DOI: 10.1152/physrev.00031.2008. PubMed PMID: 19342615

[58] Olsson AK, Dimberg A, Kreuger J, Claesson-Welsh L. VEGF receptor signalling—In control of vascular function. Nature Reviews. Molecular Cell Biology. 2006;**7**(5):359-371. Epub 2006/04/25. DOI: 10.1038/nrm1911. PubMed PMID: 16633338

[59] Shibuya M. Differential roles of vascular endothelial growth factor receptor-1 and receptor-2 in angiogenesis. Journal of Biochemistry and Molecular Biology. 2006;**39**(5):469-478. Epub 2006/09/28. PubMed PMID: 17002866

[60] Tammela T, Enholm B, Alitalo K, Paavonen K. The biology of vascular endothelial growth factors. Cardiovascular Research. 2005;**65**(3):550-563. DOI: 10.1016/j.cardiores.2004.12.002. PubMed PMID: 15664381

[61] Shibuya M. Vascular endothelial growth factor and its receptor system: Physiological functions in angiogenesis and pathological roles in various diseases. Journal of Biochemistry. 2013;**153**(1):13-19. Epub 2012/11/23. DOI: 10.1093/jb/mvs136. PubMed PMID: 23172303; PubMed Central PMCID: PMC3528006

[62] Gee E, Milkiewicz M, Haas TL. p38 MAPK activity is stimulated by vascular endothelial growth factor receptor 2 activation and is essential for shear stress-induced angiogenesis. Journal of Cellular Physiology. 2010;**222**(1):120-126. DOI: 10.1002/jcp.21924. PubMed PMID: 19774558; PubMed Central PMCID: PMCPMC3947629

[63] Jin ZG, Ueba H, Tanimoto T, Lungu AO, Frame MD, Berk BC. Ligand-independent activation of vascular endothelial growth factor receptor 2 by fluid shear stress regulates activation of endothelial nitric oxide synthase. Circulation Research. 2003;**93**(4):354-363. DOI: 10.1161/01.RES.0000089257.94002.96. PubMed PMID: 12893742

[64] dela Paz NG, Melchior B, Frangos JA. Early VEGFR2 activation in response to flow is VEGF-dependent and mediated by MMP activity. Biochemical and Biophysical Research Communications. 2013;**434**(3):641-646. DOI: 10.1016/j.bbrc.2013.03.134. PubMed PMID: 23583373; PubMed Central PMCID: PMCPMC4074593

[65] Sulpice E, Plouet J, Berge M, Allanic D, Tobelem G, Merkulova-Rainon T. Neuropilin-1 and neuropilin-2 act as coreceptors, potentiating proangiogenic activity. Blood. 2008; **111**(4):2036-2045. DOI: 10.1182/blood-2007-04-084269. PubMed PMID: 18065694

[66] Rossignol M, Gagnon ML, Klagsbrun M. Genomic organization of human neuropilin-1 and neuropilin-2 genes: Identification and distribution of splice variants and soluble isoforms. Genomics. 2000;**70**(2):211-222. DOI: 10.1006/geno.2000.6381. PubMed PMID: 11112349

[67] Fantin A, Vieira JM, Plein A, Denti L, Fruttiger M, Pollard JW, et al. NRP1 acts cell autonomously in endothelium to promote tip cell function during sprouting angiogenesis. Blood. 2013;**121**(12):2352-2362. DOI: 10.1182/blood-2012-05-424713. PubMed PMID: 23315162; PubMed Central PMCID: PMC3606070

[68] Pinskey JM, Franks NE, McMellen AN, Giger RJ, Allen BL. Neuropilin-1 promotes hedgehog signaling through a novel cytoplasmic motif. The Journal of Biological Chemistry. 2017;**292**(37):15192-15204. DOI: 10.1074/jbc.M117.783845. PubMed PMID: 28667171

[69] Hui CC, Angers S. Gli proteins in development and disease. Annual Review of Cell and Developmental Biology. 2011;**27**:513-537. DOI: 10.1146/annurev-cellbio-092910-154048. PubMed PMID: 21801010

[70] Burnstock G. Purinergic nerves. Pharmacological Reviews. 1972;**24**(3):509-581. PubMed PMID: 4404211

[71] Burnstock G. Purine and pyrimidine receptors. Cellular and Molecular Life Sciences. 2007;**64**(12):1471-1483. DOI: 10.1007/s00018-007-6497-0. PubMed PMID: 17375261

[72] Burnstock G. Purinergic Signaling in the cardiovascular system. Circulation Research. 2017;**120**(1):207-228. DOI: 10.1161/CIRCRESAHA.116.309726. PubMed PMID: 28057794

[73] Praetorius HA, Leipziger J. Primary cilium-dependent sensing of urinary flow and paracrine purinergic signaling. Seminars in Cell & Developmental Biology. 2013;**24**(1):3-10. DOI: 10.1016/j.semcdb.2012.10.003. PubMed PMID: 23085624

[74] Masyuk AI, Gradilone SA, Banales JM, Huang BQ, Masyuk TV, Lee SO, et al. Cholangiocyte primary cilia are chemosensory organelles that detect biliary nucleotides via P2Y12 purinergic receptors. American Journal of Physiology. Gastrointestinal and Liver Physiology. 2008;**295**(4):G725-G734. DOI: 10.1152/ajpgi.90265.2008. PubMed PMID: 18687752; PubMed Central PMCID: PMCPMC2575915

[75] Masyuk AI, Masyuk TV, LaRusso NF. Cholangiocyte primary cilia in liver health and disease. Developmental Dynamics. 2008;**237**(8):2007-2012. DOI: 10.1002/dvdy.21530. Pub Med PMID: 18407555; PubMed Central PMCID: PMCPMC2574848

[76] Jensen ME, Odgaard E, Christensen MH, Praetorius HA, Leipziger J. Flow-induced $[Ca^{2+}]_i$ increase depends on nucleotide release and subsequent purinergic signaling in the intact nephron. Journal of the American Society of Nephrology. 2007;**18**(7):2062-2070. DOI: 10.16 81/ASN.2006070700. PubMed PMID: 17554149

[77] Hayashi T, Mochizuki T, Reynolds DM, Wu G, Cai Y, Somlo S. Characterization of the exon structure of the polycystic kidney disease 2 gene (PKD2). Genomics. 1997;**44**(1):131-136. DOI: 10.1006/geno.1997.4851. PubMed PMID: 9286709

[78] The polycystic kidney disease 1 gene encodes a 14 kb transcript and lies within a duplicated region on chromosome 16. The European Polycystic Kidney Disease Consortium. Cell. 1994;**78**(4):725. PubMed PMID: 8069919

[79] Leyssac PP, Karlsen FM, Holstein-Rathlou NH, Skott O. On determinants of glomerular filtration rate after inhibition of proximal tubular reabsorption. The American Journal of Physiology. 1994;**266**(5 Pt 2):R1544-R1550. PubMed PMID: 8203631

[80] Holstein-Rathlou NH, Marsh DJ. A dynamic model of the tubuloglomerular feedback mechanism. The American Journal of Physiology. 1990;**258**(5 Pt 2):F1448-F1459. PubMed PMID: 2337158

[81] Mozaffari MS, Jirakulsomchok S, Shao ZH, Wyss JM. High-NaCl diets increase natriuretic and diuretic responses in salt-resistant but not salt-sensitive SHR. The American Journal of Physiology. 1991;**260**(6 Pt 2):F890-F897. PubMed PMID: 2058709

[82] Seney FD Jr, Persson EG, Wright FS. Modification of tubuloglomerular feedback signal by dietary protein. The American Journal of Physiology. 1987;**252**(1 Pt 2):F83-F90. PubMed PMID: 3812704

[83] DiBona GF, Rios LL. Mechanism of exaggerated diuresis in spontaneously hypertensive rats. The American Journal of Physiology. 1978;**235**(5):409-416. PubMed PMID: 727292

[84] Pollock CA, Lawrence JR, Field MJ. Tubular sodium handling and tubuloglomerular feedback in experimental diabetes mellitus. The American Journal of Physiology. 1991; **260**(6 Pt 2):F946-F952. PubMed PMID: 1829330

[85] Ecder T, Schrier RW. Hypertension in autosomal-dominant polycystic kidney disease: Early occurrence and unique aspects. Journal of the American Society of Nephrology: JASN. 2001;**12**(1):194-200. PubMed PMID: 11134267

[86] Ecder T, Schrier RW. Cardiovascular abnormalities in autosomal-dominant polycystic kidney disease. Nature Reviews. Nephrology. 2009;**5**(4):221-228. DOI: 10.1038/nrneph.2009.13. PubMed PMID: 19322187; PubMed Central PMCID: PMCPMC2720315

[87] Xu C, Rossetti S, Jiang L, Harris PC, Brown-Glaberman U, Wandinger-Ness A, et al. Human ADPKD primary cyst epithelial cells with a novel, single codon deletion in the PKD1 gene exhibit defective ciliary polycystin localization and loss of flow-induced Ca^{2+} signaling. American Journal of Physiology Renal Physiology. 2007;**292**(3):F930-F945. DOI: 10.1152/ajprenal.00285.2006. PubMed PMID: 17090781; PubMed Central PMCID: PMCPMC3586432

[88] Hateboer N, Veldhuisen B, Peters D, Breuning MH, San-Millan JL, Bogdanova N, et al. Location of mutations within the PKD2 gene influences clinical outcome. Kidney International. 2000;**57**(4):1444-1451. DOI: 10.1046/j.1523-1755.2000.00989.x. PubMed PMID: 10760080

[89] Haust MD. Endothelial cilia in human aortic atherosclerotic lesions. Virchows Archiv. A, Pathological Anatomy and Histopathology. 1987;**410**(4):317-326. PubMed PMID: 3101281

[90] Ainsworth C. Cilia: Tails of the unexpected. Nature. 2007;**448**(7154):638-641. DOI: 10.1038/448638a. PubMed PMID: 17687297

Chapter 6

Endothelial Dysfunction as a Consequence of Endothelial Glycocalyx Damage: A Role in the Pathogenesis of Preeclampsia

Marina M. Ziganshina, Ekaterina L. Yarotskaya, Nicolai V. Bovin and Gennady T. Sukhikh

Additional information is available at the end of the chapter

http://dx.doi.org/10.5772/intechopen.75043

Abstract

The endothelial glycocalyx is an intravascular compartment which consists of carbohydrate part of membrane glycoconjugates, free proteoglycans and associated proteins. It is thought to play an important role in the vascular tone regulation, vascular permeability and thromboresistance. It was suggested that the leading cause of endothelial dysfunction in various cardiovascular, inflammatory, and kidney diseases is the damage of the endothelial glycocalyx. This review presents the changes in the composition and structure of the endothelial glycocalyx in the settings of damage and under systemic inflammatory response, and the impact of these changes on the functions of endothelial cells and intercellular contacts, mediating the interaction of endothelium and the immune cells. The second issue, discussed in this article is a possible role of endothelial glycocalyx in the pathogenesis of preeclampsia—a complication of pregnancy associated with hypertension, proteinuria and edema. The reviewed data contribute a new insight in the endothelial dysfunction pathogenesis.

Keywords: glycocalyx, endothelial glycome, endothelial dysfunction, glycobiology of inflammation, pregnancy, preeclampsia

1. Introduction

Preeclampsia (PE) is one of the main problems of modern obstetrics. PE develops in 2–9% of all pregnancies; it is the second most frequent cause of maternal morbidity and one of the leading causes of neonatal morbidity and mortality. PE is now regarded as a syndrome which is caused by disrupted adaptation to pregnancy and manifests with the development of complex, multiorganic and polysystemic insufficiency with clinical signs appearing after the 20th week of gestation [1, 2]. Despite of vigorous research in this area, pathogenesis of PE is still not clear. However, it is well known that the key factors of PE are immune system hyperactivation and the following excessive systemic inflammatory response (SIR), which initiate endothelium activation and cause endothelial dysfunction in cases of early onset and complicated course of the disease [3].

Inflammatory response is accompanied by cell phenotype transformation (formation of activation cell status), leading to the generation of "danger" signals (generated from products of trauma, ischemia, necrosis or oxidative stress) [4, 5], which are recognizable by the immune system. It was found that the composition of endothelial glycocalyx (eGC) changed under excessive inflammatory response. Hypoglycosylated structures which may be perceived by immune system as neoantigens, appear on the membrane of endothelial cells; also, antigens which are normally covert become apparent [6]. These events may promote autotolerance disruption and cause production of autoreactive antibodies damaging endothelial cells. In this regard, in this chapter a special attention is paid to eGC—functional layer of endothelial cells, which mediates all endothelial functions. Much evidence that under SIR, the alterations of eGC are associated with changes of cardiovascular system hemodynamics, vascular tone regulation, vascular permeability [7]—the main vectors of pathophysiological disorders in PE, and that alterations affect endothelial autoimmune phenotype formation, allow to assume that eGC may be one of the main targets of PE.

2. Endothelium: its role in homeostasis and in pathology

Vascular endothelium is a metabolically active neuroendocrine organ, which is spread in all tissues. The main functions of endothelium are: expression of receptor molecules, synthesis and secretion of biologically active molecules, vascular tone control, vascular permeability and new vessels formation, transportation of blood cells and soluble factors; homeostasis balance, participation in innate and adaptive immunity [8–10].

Supporting homeostasis, the endothelium is also subject to damage by factors, which cause endothelium pathology. Multiorganic dysfunction due to long-lasting activation under the effects of damaging factors lead to severe consequences.

Recent studies show that the homeostatic control over the cardiovascular and other systems is, among others, exerted by eGC, the outer above-membrane endothelium layer, which is formed by the sugar chains of transmembrane glycoconjugates and the associated not-anchored proteoglycans [7]. However, there is limited data on eGC composition and its alterations under inflammatory and other pathological conditions.

2.1. Endothelial glycocalyx structure and composition

Endothelium surface layer is located on the luminal surface of the endothelium (endothelial surface layer—ESL). It is formed by the glycoproteins, proteoglycans and glycosphingolipids that are anchored in the membrane, as well as by secretory proteoglycans and glycosaminoglycans (GAGs), that are not anchored and are inter-connected by non-covalent interactions [11–13]. Their carbohydrate part contains a large amount of sialo and sulpho residues, forming overall negative charge of the endothelial cell surface. The outer segment of this layer (spreading out toward the vascular lumen), formed by the carbohydrate part of glycoconjugates, is a polysaccharide gel—eGC [14], with thickness ranging 2–4.5 μm [15] in different departments of the vascular system.

The base of the eGC is formed by carbohydrate-protein conjugates—transmembrane and secretory proteins; their carbohydrate part is represented by both short (2–15 monosaccharide residues) branched oligosaccharides, often decorated with sialic acid and sulfate (in glycoproteins), and by high-molecular glycans, often ending with highly sulfated residues (in proteoglycans) [16]. The glycoproteins can contain N-linked (Asn-linked) and/or O-linked (Ser/Thr-linked) glycans of variable length and composition. Complex hybrid and high-mannose glycans are usually present in the glycoproteins [17]. The main glycoproteins of endothelial cells are cell adhesion molecules (selectins, integrins, immunoglobulin superfamily molecules, endothelial mucins and addressins) which provide homing, migration and interaction between cells in different processes, and secretory molecules associated with eGC, participating in vascular homeostasis support, fibrinolysis and coagulation (thrombomodulin, von Willebrand factor (vWF)), antithrombin III, etc.). These molecules expression depends on factors, altering endothelium activation [16]. Under inflammatory response, the glycans modification occurs, leading to alteration of intercellular contacts, hemostasis and blood rheology. Biochemical eGC composition (the main structural and associated molecules) is presented in **Tables 1** and **2** (parts I and II).

It was found that the carbohydrate part is crucially important for glycoprotein function. N-linked glycans, particularly high-mannose chains, determine specific interactions of different molecules from the intercellular adhesion molecule (ICAM) family with the receptors [17]. N-glycans of the junctional adhesion molecule-A (JAM-A) regulate leukocyte adhesion and lymphocyte function-associated antigen-1 (LFA-1) binding [22]. Platelet/endothelial cell adhesion molecule-1 (PECAM-1 or CD31), a membrane highly glycosylated protein (~30% of molecular mass), has N-linked glycans represented by neutral and sialylated glycans [51, 52]. E-selectin is heavily glycosylated protein with hybrid/complex type N-linked oligosaccharides [53]. Cadherin of the vascular endothelium (VE-cadherin, CD144)—is the main transmembrane protein of adhesion contacts; its carbohydrate part is presented mainly by sialylated biantennary N-glycans of a complex type, and sialylated hybride N-chains (~40 and 28% of all identified glycans, respectively). Branched tri- and tetraantennary N-glycans, as well as N-glycans of high-mannose type are represented in smaller quantity in N-glycans of VE-cadherin [21, 54]. In the presence of anti-inflammatory factors (such as tumor necrosis factor-α, TNF-α) the quantity of glycans ending with α2,6-sialic acid residues and fucose-α1,2-galactose-β1,4-N-acetylglucosamine increases, as well as the expression of N-glycans of high-mannose and hybrid type, which mediate intercellular contacts of monocytes with endothelium in the rolling and adhesion, particularly at the intercellular connections sites [55].

Hemostasis controlling proteins associated with outer eGC are also highly-glycosylated. VWF is a key component for maintenance of normal hemostasis, acting as the carrier protein of

Group	Members	Comments	References
Adhesion molecules	E-selectin	Contains 11 potential N-glycosylation site	[13]
	P-selectin	Contains 9 potential N-glycosylation sites	[13]
	Integrins: α1β1, α2β1, α3β1, α5β1, α6β1, α8β1, α9β1, αVβ1, αVβ3, α6β4, αVβ5	N-linked glycans	[14, 15]
	VE-cadherin	Contains 7 potential N-glycosylation sites	[16]
	JAM-1	Contains 1 N-glycosylation site	[17]
	JAM-2	Contains 2 N-glycosylation sites	[18]
	JAM-3	Contains 2 N-glycosylation sites	[19]
	ICAM-1	Contains 8 N-glycosylation sites	[13]
	ICAM-2	Contains 6 N-glycosylation sites	[20]
	VCAM-1	Contains 6 N-glycosylation sites	[13]
	PECAM-1	Contains 9 N-glycosylation sites	[13]
	ClyCAM-1	Mucin, containing predominantly O-linked carbohydrate chains (T-antigen and 6′ sulfated sialyl-Lewis-X)	[21, 22]
	CD34	Mucin, O-glycosylation sites are more abundant than N-glycosylation sites	[23]
	MadCAM-1	Mucin; contain O-linked glycans (SLe^x)	[24]
Coagulation and fibrinolysis regulators	Von Willebrand factor	Contains at least 10 potential N- and 10 O-glycosylation sites	[25, 26]
	Thrombomodulin	Contains at least 4 N- and 1 O-glycosylation sites	[27–32]
	Antithrombin III	Contains 4 potential N-glycosylation sites	[33, 34]
	Heparin cofactor II	Contains 3 potential N-glycosylation sites	[35]

MadCAM-1, mucosal addressin cell adhesion molecule-1; JAM-1, junctional adhesion molecule-1; JAM-2, junctional adhesion molecule-2; JAM-3, junctional adhesion molecule-3; ICAM-1, inter-cellular adhesion molecule-1; ICAM-2, inter-cellular adhesion molecule-2; VCAM-1, vascular cell adhesion molecule-1; PECAM-1, platelet/endothelial cell adhesion molecule-1; SLe^x, sialyl-Lewis-X.

Table 1. Biochemical composition of endothelial glycocalyx—main components (part I: glycoproteins).

the coagulant Factor VIII and mediating platelet adhesion at the sites of vascular injury [31]. VWF is heavily glycosylated by N- and O-linked oligosaccharides, and glycosylation affects many of its functions [30]. Antithrombin is a major inhibitor of the blood coagulation cascade.

Group	Members	Number/type of GAG-chains linked	Comments	Ref
Glycosaminoglycans	HA	—	Anionic, nonsulfated glycosaminoglycan; structural unit of HA is a repeating disaccharide consisting of β-D-glucuronic acid and β-N-acetyl-D-glucosamine; contains no core protein	[9]
	HS	—	The most common disaccharide unit within HS is composed of a mono-sulfated β-glucuronic acid linked to tri-sulfated α-N-acetylglucosamine	[36]
	CS	—	CS is a linear acidic polysaccharide, composed of repeating disaccharide units of β-glucuronic acid and β-N-acetyl-D-galactosamine and modified with sulfate residues at different positions	[37]
	DS	—	Backbone of DS chains is a linear polymer composed of repeating disaccharide units of α-iduronic acid and β-N-acetyl-D-galactosamine. These sugar residues can be modified by ester sulfate at various positions	[38]
	KS	—	Basic repeating disaccharide unit within keratan sulfate is units of β-D-galactose and β-N-acetyl-D-galactosamine	[39]
Proteoglycans (extracellularly secreted)	Perlecan	3/HS,CS	A large basement membrane heparan sulfate proteoglycan; protein core of approximately 500 kDa	[40]
	Versican	10-30/CS,DS	Large aggregating chondroitin sulfate proteoglycan, core protein (at >350 kDa)	[41, 42]
	Endocan	1/DS	Is a DSPG, small proteoglycan molecules (20 kDa) with a single DS chain; DS of endocan consists of about 32 disaccharide units	[43]
	Decorin	1/CS,DS	A prototype small leucine-rich proteoglycan (40 kDa); it has N-terminal attachment site for a single GAG chain of chondroitin or dermatan sulfate	[44]
	Biglycan	2/CS,DS	small leucine-rich proteoglycan (42 kDa protein core)	[45, 46]
	Mimecan	2–3/KS	Small leucine-rich proteoglycan; (12–34 kDa protein core)	[47, 48]
Proteoglycans (associated with the cell surface)	Syndecans	5/HS,CS	Transmembrane proteoglycans Family of HSPGs, the syndecan protein family has four members. Core protein of all glypicans is ranging between 198 to 346 kDa	[49]

Group	Members	Number/type of GAG-chains linked	Comments	Ref
	Glypicans	3/HS,CS	GPI-anchored proteoglycans Family of HSPGs The glypican protein family has six members core protein of all glypicans is similar in size, approximately ranging between 60 and 70 kDa	[50]

GAG, glycosaminoglycan; HA, hyaluronan; HS, heparan sulfate; CS, chondroitin sulfate; DS, dermatan sulfate; KS, keratan sulfate; DSPG, dermatan sulfate proteoglycans; HSPGs, heparan sulfate proteoglycans.

Table 2. Biochemical composition of endothelial glycocalyx—main components (part II: glycosaminoglycans and proteoglycans).

Two isoforms exist in the circulation, α-antithrombin and β-antithrombin, which differ in the glycosylation of the polypeptide chain; β-antithrombin lacks the carbohydrate present at Asn135 in α-antithrombin. Of the two forms, β-antithrombin has the higher affinity for heparin due to the conformational change that occurs upon heparin binding being sterically hindered by the presence of the additional bulky glycan in α-antithrombin [56]. The carbohydrate structures of heparin cofactor II (member of serpin superfamily) circulating in blood are complex-type biantennary and triantennary chains in a ratio of 6:1 with the galactose being >90% sialylated with α2-6-linked N-acetylneuraminic acid. About 50% of the triantennary structures contain one sialyl Le^x motif (SLe^x) [40]. Thrombomodulin (TM) is an endothelial cell surface glycoprotein (contains N- and O-linked glycans) that directly inhibits the procoagulant activities of thrombin and the TM-thrombin complex accelerates the thrombin catalyzed activation of protein C. Moreover, the GAG O-linked chains of TM contained chondroitin-4-sulfate and dermatan sulfate, which were repeated approximately 30 times. Soluble TM in urine has no GAG chain which could promote its anticoagulant activities. Studies of the rabbit recombinant TM have shown that addition of a GAG chain may increase its anticoagulant function [33, 34].

Endothelial mucins (CD34; glycosylation-dependent cell adhesion molecule-1 (GlyCAM-1); mucosal addressin cell adhesion molecule-1 (MadCAM-1)) contact leukocytes by their binding to L-selectin. This interaction facilitates leukocytes transportations from blood to lymphoid organs and inflamed tissues [28]. Major capping group in GlyCAM-1, CD34 and MadCAM-1 is the sulfated SLe^x [27, 28, 57]. For example, CD34 functions as a L-selectin ligand mediating lymphocyte extravasation only when properly glycosylated to express a sulfated carbohydrate epitope. CD34 can exist in 2 glycoforms: the L-selectin-binding (L-B-CD34) and non-binding (L-NB-CD34) glycoforms. L-B-CD34 is relatively minor compared with L-NB-CD34 and represents less than 10% of total CD34. It has been shown, that a minor glycoform of CD34 carries relatively abundant 6-sulfo SLe^x epitopes on O-glycans that are important for its recognition by L-selectin [28].

The eGC mostly consists of proteoglycans—highly glycosylated proteins (glycans account for 90–95% of the molecular mass); GAGs branches form their carbohydrate part. There are

http://dx.doi.org/10.5772/intechopen.75043

five types of GAG chains: heparan sulfate (HS), chondroitin sulfate (CS), dermatan sulfate (DS), keratan sulfate (KS), and hyaluronan (hyaluronic acid, HA). They are linear polymers of disaccharides with variable lengths that are modified by sulfation and/or (de)acetylation to a variable extent [15]. In the human body the GAGs are present in a protein bound form (i.e., in proteoglycans composition) and do not exist in a free form, except for HA. Besides playing structuring and supporting roles, proteoglycans are involved in cell signaling, regulation of cell proliferation, adhesion, migration, differentiation [55]. Key eGC glycans are heparan sulfate proteoglycans (HSPGs), which compose about 50–90% of the total amount of proteoglycans present in the eGC, and HA—the main supporting glycan [14, 15]. Main proteoglycans of the eGC and their characteristics are given in **Table 2** (part II).

Glycosphingolipids (GSLs), a class of ceramide-based glycolipids, are also a significant part of eGC. Glycosphingolipids are subclassified as neutral (no charged sugars or ionic groups), sialylated (gangliosides), or sulfated [58]. GSLs cluster with cholesterol in cell membranes to form GSL-enriched lipid raft [59]. Cultured human umbilical vein endothelial cells (HUVEC) appeared to contain complex lacto and globo series compounds (lactosylceramide, Gb_3Cer and Gb_4Cer), but the most abundant neutral GSL is lactosylceramide (LacCer, CDw17) [60]. LacCer can bind to various microorganisms, is highly expressed on the plasma membranes of human phagocytes, and forms lipid rafts containing the Src family tyrosine kinase Lyn. LacCer-enriched lipid rafts mediate immunological and inflammatory reactions, including superoxide generation, chemotaxis, and non-opsonic phagocytosis [61, 62]. Therefore, LacCer-enriched membrane microdomains are thought to function as pattern recognition receptors (PRRs), which recognize pathogen-associated molecular patterns (PAMPs) expressed on microorganisms. LacCer also serves as a signal transduction molecule for functions mediated by CD11b/CD18-integrin as well as being associated with several key cellular processes [63]. Endothelium activation by pro-inflammatory cytokines, particularly by TNF-α, affect the Gb_3Cer and Gb_4Cer [64] expression; interferon gamma (IFNγ) has a striking effect on the surface expression of GSLs; IL-1 increases the cell content of neutral and acidic GSLs but does not alter their surface expression [55]. Cytokines TNF-α and IL-1 can potentiate the toxic effect of verocytotoxin (Shiga-like toxin-produced by *Escherichia coli* and the main cause of hemolytic uremic syndrome) to human endothelial cells by inducting an increase in the Gb_3Cer synthesis in these cells [65], because Gb_3Cer (CD77) binds to the verocytotoxin and injures human endothelial cells [66].

Acidic GSLs of human endothelial cells are: monosialoganglioside or GM3—the major ganglioside of endothelial cells, and it constitutes about 90% of the whole ganglioside fraction [67], and sulfoglucuronyl paragloboside (SGPG), a minor GSL in endothelial cells, is a ligand for L-selectin [55]. Although GIyCAM-1 and CD34 constitute the major L-selectin ligand on venous endothelium, endothelial SLe^x gangliosides may also play a role, since L-selectin can also bind SLe^x GSLs under physiologic flow conditions [68].

2.2. Functions of the endothelial glycocalyx

The eGC is considered as an intravascular compartment which has various functions.

First, eGC mediates the endothelial mechanotransduction of shear stress and performs regulation of shear stress-induced nitric oxide (NO) production [69]. This is provided by the impact of tangential stress of blood flow shift primarily to eGC; the latter accepts and scatters the load, created by fluid shear stress. Local spin moment, created by fluid shear stress, affects the proteoglycans chains, and further—the core proteins (syndecans and glypicans), causing actin cytoskeleton reorganization and transmission of the signal into the cell and the cell nucleus [70, 71]. The study of Fu and Tarbell (2013) aimed to determine the eGC role in mechanosensing and transduction, and measured the flow-induced production of NO *in vitro* [7]. It was found that compared to static conditions, the application of steady flow shear stress rapidly increased NO production from the baseline in bovine aortic endothelial cells. Enzymatic treatment of the key components of eGC (HS, HA) completely blocked flow-induced NO production without affecting receptor-mediated NO production, suggesting that the eGC has a direct effect on the NO production machinery [7]. Therefore, the eGC under physiological conditions (intact eGC) transforms hemodynamic effect into cell biochemical signals, which regulate the vascular tone.

Second, the negatively charged eGC forms a polyanionic hydrated mesh on the surface of endothelial cells, which acts as a selective permeability electrostatic barrier for plasma cells and proteins and serves as a selective permeability [72]. According to Salmon and Satchell, in both continuous and fenestrated microvessels, this eGC is acting as an integral component of the multilayered barrier provided by the walls of these microvessels (i.e., acting in concert with clefts or fenestrae across endothelial cell layers, basement membranes and pericytes) [73]. Dysfunction of any of these capillary wall components, including the eGC, can disrupt normal microvascular permeability. Disruption of eGC manifests with increased systemic microvascular permeability and albuminuria in the glomerulus [73]. Evidence from the experiments on Munich-Wistar-Fromter (MWF) rats, used as a model of spontaneous albuminuric chronic kidney disease (CKD), confirm that loss of eGC could contribute to both renal and systemic vascular dysfunction in proteinuric CKD [74]. Also, in the 5/6-nephrecomized rats model with CKD a significant decrease in eGC thickness and stiffness in the blood explants of aorta endothelial cell isolated from CKD rats was demonstrated [75]. An increase of the levels of the two major components of the eGC, namely syndecan-1 (Syn-1) and HA, in the blood of patients with CKD indicated the disease progression and correlated tightly with plasma markers of endothelial dysfunction such as soluble fms-like tyrosine kinase-1 (sFlt-1), soluble vascular adhesion molecule-1 (sVCAM-1), vWF and angiopoietin-2 [75]. The study of experimental eGC degradation in mice induced by long-term hyaluronidase infusion, including evaluation of the eGC thickness and composition by immunohistochemical methods and by transmission electron microscopy for complete and integral assessment of glomerular albumin passage, showed that glomerular fenestrae were filled with dense negatively charged polysaccharide structures that were largely removed in the presence of circulating hyaluronidase, leaving the polysaccharide surfaces of other glomerular cells intact [76]. Thus, HA is a key component of the glomerular endothelial protein permeability barrier; reduction of the HA facilitates albumin passage across the endothelial layer and the glomerular basement membrane toward the epithelial compartment [76].

Regulation of selective permeability by eGC, and the role of its separate components in this, is still subject of discussion. According to Lennon and Singleton, the HA plays key role in supporting endothelial barrier function [77]. HA maintains vascular integrity through eGC modulation, caveolin-enriched microdomain regulation and interaction with endothelial HA binding proteins. Certain disease states, especially accompanied by SIR, increase hyaluronidase activity and reactive oxygen species (ROS) generation which break down high molecular weight HA to low molecular weight fragments causing damage to the eGC. Further, these HA fragments can activate specific HA binding proteins upregulated in vascular disease to promote actin cytoskeletal reorganization and inhibition of endothelial cell–cell contacts [77]. A glycocalyx-junction-break model, described by Curry and Adamson summarizes multiple studies and the role of the eGC in vascular permeability regulation [78]. According to this model, the layered structure of the endothelial barrier requires continuous activation of signaling pathways regulated by sphingosine-1-phosphate (S1P) and intracellular cAMP. These pathways modulate the adherens junction (*zonula adherens*), continuity of tight junction strands, and the balance of synthesis and degradation of eGC components [78].

Third, the eGC forms anti-inflammatory and anti-adhesive barrier at the endothelial cells. Vascular protection via inhibition of coagulation and leukocyte adhesion is provided by maintenance of the composition permanence and balance of degradation under the impact of stress shift and synthesis of eGC components [73, 79]. Total negative charge, formed by carbohydrate residues of the glycoconjugates chains on cell surface, prevents adhesive interactions of blood cells with vascular wall, biologically active molecules with anti-thrombotic action, while eGC-associated molecules provide hemostasis [80, 81]. Also eGC plays a structural role, impeding adhesion by covering adhesion molecules on the surface of the cell and by creating steric hindrance, making leukocyte binding more challenging [82]. Under the effect of damaging factors, the structure and composition of eGC change, its thickness may reduce significantly, and carbohydrate residues, normally covert and masked, become apparent. Main damaging factors, affecting the eGC *in vivo,* are: inflammation, hyperglycemia, endotoxemia, septic shock, oxidized low-density lipoproteins, cytokines, natriuretic peptides, abnormal shift stress and damage due to ischemia-reperfusion [79]. Shedding of eGC components in response to cytokines and chemoattractants occurs in all compartments of microvasculature: arterioles [83], capillaries [83, 84] and venules [84–86].

According to Lipowsky, the studies of leukocytic-endothelial adhesion in response to chemoattractants and cytokines, and shedding of constituents of the eGC, suggest that activation of extracellular proteases (matrix metalloproteases, MMPs) play a role in mediating the dynamics of leukocytes adhesion in response to inflammatory and ischemic stimuli [79]. Inhibition of MMP activation with sub-antimicrobial doses of doxycycline, or zinc chelators, have also inhibited leukocytes adhesion and shedding of glycans from the endothelial cells surface in response to the chemoattractant. Experiments by McDonald et al. have confirmed that under the enzymatic degradation of eGC with heparinase, endothelial cells developed a pro-inflammatory phenotype when exposed to uniform steady shear stress leading to an increase in leukocyte adhesion [82]. The results show an up-regulation of ICAM-1 (expression increases in 3 times) with degradation compared to non-degraded controls, and attribute this effect to a down-regulation in nuclear factor kappa-light-chain-enhancer of activated B cells (NF-κB) activity in response to flow; this suggests that eGC is not solely a physical barrier to adhesion but rather plays an important role in governing the phenotype of endothelial cells, a key determinant in leukocyte adhesion [82]. Other mechanisms also contribute to the initiation of lymphocytes adhesion to the endothelial cells after reduction of eGC layer: decrease of NO production, which is capable to inhibit leukocyte-endothelial cell adhesion [87]; appearance of eGC fragments, (such as low-molecular-weight HA), which show their pro-inflammatory properties, affecting the maturity of dendritic cells and stimulating them to produce cytokines [14, 88]; and exposure and synthesis under inflammatory response of hypoglycosylated structures, which interact with cell adhesion molecules of leukocytes [18, 89].

Modulation of eGC structure under effects of damaging factors, including inflammation, shows a thromboresistance loss [90, 91]. This occurs due to destabilization of heparin sulfate chains, the binding sites for coagulation inhibitor factors (antithrombin-III, the protein C system, and tissue factor pathway inhibition); this leads to a reduction of their local concentration at the vascular wall. In turn, a concentration gradient of protective and regulative molecules, associated with eGC (albumin, fibrinogen, orosomucoid, extracellular superoxide dismutase, fibronectin, vitronectin, collagens, thrombospondin-1 and other), and of growth factors (fibroblast growth factors, vascular endothelial growth factors, transforming growth factor-β, platelet-derived growth factors) is also decreased, facilitating pathological processes in blood vessels [80].

Therefore, the eGC is a labile structure; its composition changes under effects of damaging factors. This determines development of pathophysiological processes of endothelium activation/dysfunction with loss of vascular tone regulation, hemostasis and barrier function. Endothelium activation/dysfunction is induced by inflammation and accompanies it, thus forming a vicious cycle, which can be overcome only under normal immune system functioning. Inflammatory response of various degree accompanies not only pathologic processes, it is also observed under physiological conditions, for example, a pro-inflammatory background is shown at certain periods of normal pregnancy.

Understanding the mechanisms of disruption of maternal immunology tolerance to fetus, causes of transition of physiologic inflammatory reaction to systemic and excessive inflammatory response (as in PE), accompanied by endothelial activation/dysfunction, and revelation of the contribution of eGC damage to preeclampsia development may be subject of new discoveries in the disease pathogenesis.

3. The development of systemic inflammatory response in pregnancy

There is much experimental evidence of a so-called "physiological", controlled SIR during pregnancy. Similarly to the classic inflammatory response, physiological inflammatory response during pregnancy is a reaction to local damage (matrix remodeling, associated with implantation, placentation and angiogenesis in placenta) [92, 93] and foreign invaders (cells, microparticles and soluble factors of placental origin) [94, 95]. Humoral factors, cellular debris and subcellular particles of trophoblast are considered to be the triggers of SIR, but they can also play a role of adjuvants [95, 96]. Cells-effectors of the maternal innate immunity detect fetal products as pathogen/danger images, implementing cell and molecular protection mechanisms against allogeneic material [97]. The gene products inherited from the father can be

http://dx.doi.org/10.5772/intechopen.75043

regarded as exogenous factors, while endogenous factors are gene products, resulting from trauma, ischemia, necrosis or oxidative stress [97]. Also there are some reports on generation of various new antigens due to inflammatory response; they are variations of the "modified own"; of the neoantigens formed as a result of the post-translational proteins modification [98]; and of antigens, mobilized to membrane from cytoplasm and the inner cell compartments interacting with membrane proteins or phospholipids, and acting as images of danger [99]. The enhanced pro-inflammatory background in normal pregnancy is evidenced by an increase of the level of the soluble cell adhesion molecules (sCAM) in blood, indicating the activation of leukocytes (increase of sE-selectin, sVCAM-1, sICAM-1 levels) and endothelial cells [100, 101].

3.1. The glycan-mediated processes in inflammation

Central event of the inflammatory response is the contact between leukocytes and endothelium, with subsequent migration of immune cells to the inflammatory lesion. At early stages of inflammatory response endothelial selectins (E-selectin and P-selectin) and lymphocytic L-selectin form reversible bonds with carbohydrate counter-receptors on the partner cell, thus providing tethering and the leukocyte rolling along the vascular wall.

The counter-receptors for selectins are typically heavily glycosylated molecules, many of which bear terminal SLe^x motifs (Neu5Acα2-3Galβ1-4(Fucα1-3)GlcNAc) [102]. P- and L-selectin, but not E-selectin, bind to some forms of heparin/HS. However, each of the selectins binds with higher affinity to its specific macromolecular ligands. Many of the known ligands are mucins containing sialylated fucosylated O-glycans. The major ligand for P-selectin, named P-selectin glycoprotein ligand-1 (PSGL-1), has sulfated tyrosine residues adjacent to a core-2 based O-glycan expressing SLe^x. Also, PSGL-1 is one of the physiological ligands for E-selectin, but E-selectin can also interact with several other glycoproteins that express the SLe^x motif on either N- or O-glycans, including the E-selectin ligand-1, CD44, L-selectin (in humans), and possibly long-chain GSLs expressing the SLe^x [68, 103]. Ligands for L-selectin that occur within specialized endothelia termed high endothelial venules (HEV; HEV are specialized post-capillary venous swellings characterized by plump endothelial cells as opposed to the usual thinner endothelial cells found in regular venules. HEVs enable lymphocytes circulating in the blood to directly enter a lymph node by crossing through the HEV) contain 6-sulfo-SLe^x motif on mucin-type O-glycans and on N-glycans [104]. The ligands for E- and P-selectin are expressed on circulating leukocytes whereas L-selectin binds to ligands on both leukocytes and the endothelium [89].

At the firm adhesion stage, following the leukocyte capture stage and rolling, N-linked glycans on ICAM-1 regulate binding to its integrin ligands—macrophage-1 antigen (Mac-1) and LFA-1. Moreover, it was found that Mac-1 binds with higher avidity to molecules of ICAM-1 with smaller N-linked oligosaccharide chains, since the binding with the ligand increased after the use of α-mannosidase inhibitor deoxymannojirimicin (DMJ). In contrast, LFA-1 binds with higher affinity to glycoforms of ICAM-1, which has a more complex carbohydrate chain [89]. Also, there is experimental evidence that high-mannose ICAM-1 can function in leukocyte firm-adhesion [105]. It is speculated that some N-glycan-binding sites on ICAM-1 may be pro-adhesive, whereas the neighboring sites may be anti-adhesive, underscoring the potential breadth of how ICAM-1 function may be regulated by N-glycosylation [106]. On the stage of firm adhesion an important aspect of inflammatory response is exposure of the active epitope of integrins, provided by chemokines, which are present on the endothelial cell surface, and are bound to HS. Glycosylation of chemokine receptors also contributes to the adequate dynamics of the inflammatory reaction, thus increasing the binding affinity of the chemokine to the receptor and protecting the latter from proteolytic cleavage (reviewed in [18, 89]).

Key molecules mediating leukocyte transmigration: PECAM-1, JAM-1, ICAM-2 and VE-cadherin, are highly-glycosylated. However, carbohydrates part in leukocyte transmigration is still not clear. The recent studies show that N-glycosylation of JAM-A is required for the protein's ability to reinforce barrier function [22]; sialic acid-containing glycan of PECAM-1 reinforces dynamic endothelial cell-cell interactions by stabilizing the PECAM-1 homophilic binding interface [52]; glycosylation status of ICAM-2 (hypo- or non-glycosylated variants) significantly affects the function of this protein in cell motility assays [107]; in pro-inflammatory conditions, modification of VE-cadherin glycans is observed [55]. This obviously requires further investigations. Molecules that mediate intercellular interactions during inflammation are presented in **Table 3**.

Many studies demonstrate modification of endothelial glycome (glycome is the entire complement of sugars, whether free or present in more complex molecules, of an organism) under inflammatory response. Modeling of inflammatory response *in vitro* on endothelial cell lines showed that an enhanced α2,6-sialylation was observed after TNF stimulation [108]. Pro-inflammatory stimuli increase hypoglycosylated (namely, high-mannose/hybrid) N-glycans on the cell surface as determined by lectin histochemistry, and cause an increase in genes encoding for fucosylation and sialylation (confirmed at specific staining with relevant lectins [18]; this correlates with increased monocyte adhesion [18]. Glycosylation of the endothelium has been proposed to act as a "zip code" for directing leukocyte subtype-specific recruitment in different vascular beds in response to specific stimuli [89].

3.2. The glycobiology of immunoregulation

The carbohydrate-protein interactions not only mediate the initial stages of inflammation, but also promote many cellular contacts, which regulate innate and adaptive immune response. The main carbohydrate binding proteins are endogenous lectins [109], widely present on the immune system cells and expressed both in membrane-linked and in soluble forms. Three main classes of endogenous lectins include:

A. C-type lectins, which, depending of specificity, are:

- Specific to mannose (Man-) and/or fucose (Fuc-) terminated glycans;
- Specific to galactose (Gal-) or N-acetylgalactosamine (GalNAc-)/N-acetylglucosamine (GlcNAc-)

Lectins of C-type are present on macrophages, dendritic cells, natural killer cells, leukocytes. They act as pattern-recognition receptors and fulfill signaling and adhesion functions [110]. Glycoconjugates: bacterial lipooligosaccharides, peptidoglycans, and molecules emerged

Cell adhesion molecules (proteins)	Counter-receptors (carbohydrates)	Comments
L-selectin	1. MadCAM-1 2. CD34 3. Sgp200 4. GlyCAM-1 5. Endoglycan 6. Endomucin 7. PCLP 8. PSGL-1 9. 6-sulfo-SLe^x determinant is associated with the MECA-79 epitope	Binding L-selectin with: • peripheral node addressins (no. 1, 2, 3, 4, 5, 6, 7) mediates lymphocyte recirculation (homing); • SLe^x-containing (no. 8) and sulfated glycans (no. 9) mediates leukocyte capture and rolling
P-selectin	1. PSGL-1 (major counter-receptor) 2. heparin/heparin sulfate (binds weakly) 3. some glycoproteins (mucins containing highly clustered glycans) that bear the SLe^x determinant	Mediates: • leukocyte recruitment in both acute and chronic inflammation; • leukocyte capture and rolling
E-selectin	1. PSGL-1 2. ESL-1 3. CD44 4. L-selectin (in humans)	glycoproteins that express the SLe^x antigen on either N- or O-glycans and possibly long-chain glycosphingolipids expressing the SLe^x antigen; Mediate: • recruit leukocytes recruitment to sites of inflammation; • leukocyte capture and rolling
ICAM-1	1. LFA-1 (αLβ2-integrin) 2. Mac-1 (αMβ2-integrin)	Mediates the stage of firm adhesion of leukocytes to endothelium
VCAM-1	• VLA-4 (α4β1-integrin)	Mediates the stage of firm leucocytes adhesion of leukocytes to endothelium

MadCAM-1, mucosal addressin cell adhesion molecule-1; GlyCAM-1, glycosylation-dependent cell adhesion molecule-1; PCLP, podocalyxin-like protein; SLe^x, sialyl-Lewis X; PSGL-1, P-selectin glycoprotein ligand 1; ESL-1, E-selectin ligand-1; LFA-1, lymphocyte function-associated antigen-1; Mac-1, macrophage-1 antigen; VLA-4, very late antigen-4.

Table 3. Molecules, mediating carbohydrate-protein interactions in inflammation site [80, 91, 92].

as a result of tissue damage: HA fragments or glycosaminoglycans of the extracellular cell matrix (ECM) and eGC [111], may act as pathogen/danger images for these lectins. The best known molecules related to C-type lectins are: selectins and myeloid range receptors (mannose-binding receptors DEC-205 and mannose receptor CD206); dectin-1 and dectin-2, DC-SIGN (CD209), and langerin (CD207) [112].

B. **Galectins** are a family of 15 evolutionary conserved carbohydrate-binding proteins [89, 113], belonging to the glycoproteins and glycolipids of cell surface and ECM [114] and specifically binding mainly to N-acetyllactosamine. The main ligands are Galβ1-3GlcNAc- or Galβ1-4GlcNAc- [115]. Galectins are involved in many cell activities: cell cycle regulation, migration, cell signals transmission, effectory functions, apoptosis, immunoregulation [116]. Galectins may regulate inflammatory reaction both positively (Gal-3, Gal-8, Gal-9) and negatively (Gal-1). The endothelium may be a source of Gal-1, which then targets the neutrophils to inhibit cell recruitment, and Gal-3, Gal-8, Gal-9 promote neutrophil and eosinophil adhesion [89].

C. Siglecs are a family of 17 known lectins, which specifically bind the glycans structures with terminal sialic acid [117]. Sialyl Tn (Neu5Acα2,6GalNAcα-) is a common ligand for all members of this family. Glycan 6′ sulfated SLe^x is a ligand for Siglec-8, and is important for selectin-dependent cell adhesion [118]. The majority of this family members are inhibitory receptors as they bear an immunoreceptor tyrosine-based inhibition motif (ITIM) in their structure, and they are mainly expressed on immune cells [119]. Siglecs participate in regulation/restriction of an excessive activation response to inflammatory reaction, initiated via recognition of pathogen associated molecular patterns, and damage-associated molecular patterns, with following phagocytosis of cells, bearing these patterns [120, 121]. Siglecs regulate cell proliferation, differentiation, apoptosis, adhesion, cytokines synthesis and negative regulation of B-lymphocyte signaling [122].

Some endogenous lectins are capable, like autoantibodies, to interact with the body's unchanged antigens (glycans), so-called own self-images (SAMPs-self-associated molecular patterns) [111]. Molecular patterns, containing sialic acid and heparin/HS are supposed to act as self-images [111]. Also it is thought that interaction of lectins, recognizing SAMPs, (mainly siglecs), with ligands, inhibits the immune response to foreign/damaging effects [111, 120].

It is known that presence of terminal sialic acid is very important: this substance provides the overall negative charge of cell surface, glycoconjugates conformation stabilization, production of glycoconjugates, and cells protection from recognition and degradation. Sialylation protective properties manifest not only with sialylated structures interaction with inhibited receptors, but also with masking of sugar residues which are the antigen determinants [123, 124]. For example, at desialylation, the unmasked residues of Galβ-, GalNAc-, and mannose, interacting with lectins from galectins family and C-type lectins [120]; these interactions are important for metastasis and SIR development.

Therefore, inflammatory response regulation is implemented under direct involvement of the glycan binding proteins (endogenous lectins) and glycans; composition and structure of these vary significantly under physiological and pathophysiological conditions, providing evidence of the eGC modification at inflammation, and of formation of the carbohydrate "zip code", which acts as navigator for immune cells. Inflammatory reactions in pregnancy are initiated by pathogenic and danger images, which are formed at the fetal-mother cell contact; this activates innate and adaptive immunity. SIR may be enhanced or restricted through mechanisms based on carbohydrate-protein interaction [125–127]. Excessive SIR developing in pathologic pregnancy is characterized by compensatory reactions and development of various dysfunctions, resulting in organic or multi-organic failure [128].

http://dx.doi.org/10.5772/intechopen.75043

4. Endothelial activation and endothelial dysfunction

As a rule, in the studies dedicated to determination of endothelium role in different pathologies, the authors use terms "endothelial activation" and "endothelial dysfunction" [129]. Activation should be distinguished from activity because in its resting state, endothelium is a metabolically active organ, which produces vasodilatory substances and bears anticoagulative and antiadhesive phenotype. Activation of endothelium under various pathophysiologic processes leads to alterations of its phenotype and function. These events may be reversible, but also may cause multiorgan failure.

There are two stages in endothelial activation: endothelial stimulation (early events) and endothelial activation (later events). The latter can be subdivided in endothelial activation of types I and II, respectively [130, 131]. Endothelial activation of type I follows the stimulation stage and manifests with shedding of the adhesion molecules and molecules with antithrombotic properties, such as P-selectin, thrombin, heparin, antithrombin III and thrombomodulin, from the surface of the endothelial cells. In the same time, the endothelial cells of the venules and small veins decrease in volume, and the contacts between the cells become distorted, resulting in hemorrhages, edema, and increase of vessels permeability [131]. Endothelial activation of type II is a slightly delayed process, which depends on gene transcription activation and protein synthesis *de novo*. As a result, the genes coding for the adhesion molecules, chemokines and procoagulative factors: E-selectin, vWF, IL-8, thrombocytes activating factor [132], are activated. Also, the secretion of NO and prostacyclin increases. Morphologic changes show protrusion of the endothelial cells into the vessel lumen, cell hypertrophy and an increase of cell permeability. The result of this stage is leukocyte contact with activated endothelium through lectin-carbohydrate interactions, extravasation, transendothelial migration, and, possibly, leucocyte binding with Fc-receptors (FcR) of endothelial cells with immune complexes disposition [131]. Alterations of phenotype, accompanying endothelial cells activation, manifest also with the change of the carbohydrate composition of the molecules forming the eGC.

Therefore, endothelial activation implies an alteration of the endothelial cells phenotype under the activation factors (cytokines, endotoxins, etc.) impact, inducing shedding and modification of the vasculoprotective surface layer associated with the membrane, and expression of the activation antigens. This correlates with pro-adhesive, antigen-presenting and procoagulative properties of the endothelial cells. Activation reflects an ability of endothelial cells to perform new functions, but this status does not presume a cell damage or their uncontrolled division. Endothelium activation is a reverse process with a possibility to return to a state of active reposing cells [131].

Endothelium dysfunction, on the other hand, is a stage following the endothelium activation and manifesting with cell functional activity change; it leads to loss of the ability of endothelium to perform its function, and to a disbalance of factors, which provide homeostasis and a normal course of all processes, mediated by endothelium [8, 129, 131]. Endothelial dysfunction is a consequence of chronic, permanent endothelial activation and may lead to non-reversible damage of the endothelial cells, their apoptosis and necrosis.

5. Preeclampsia as a manifestation of excessive systemic inflammatory response, accompanied by endothelial activation/dysfunction

PE is a multisystemic pathologic condition, manifesting after the 20th week of pregnancy. PE clinical signs are: an increase of systolic blood pressure (SBP) above 140 mm Hg, diastolic blood pressure (DBP) above 90 mm Hg for the first time noted during pregnancy; proteinuria (≥0.3 g/L) in daily urine, edema, manifestation of multiorganic/polysystemic dysfunction/insufficiency [133]. Severe PE is accompanied by acute renal failure, eclampsia, pulmonary edema, HELLP (hemolysis, elevated liver enzymes, and low platelet count)-syndrome [3].

Etiology of PE is not clear; genetic, immunological and microenvironment may play a role [134–138]. Currently two phenotypic variations of PE are distinguished: early manifestation of the symptoms (before the 34th week of gestation) and later manifestation (after the 34th week of gestation) [139]. Pathophysiological mechanisms of PE development are distinguished accordingly [140]. The first—"fetal" pathway—is characterized by inadequate or microcellular invasion of trophoblast cells into the uterine spiral arteries and lack or incompleteness of the phase of substitution of placental smooth muscle elastic fibers with fibrinoid [140, 141]. In this mechanism, physiological remodeling and transformation of spiral arteries is lacking, and this affects the uterine-placentary blood flow quality [142–144]. Fetal mechanism of PE development presents with severe disease course and frequent complications in the neonate. The second pathway is "maternal", where the deficiency of uterine-placental blood flow appears as a result of spiral arteries damage due to certain maternal diseases, especially thrombophilias (genetic or acquired). In this case, the study of placental morphology testifies adequate gestational reorganization of spiral arteries. Maternal pathway usually implies later manifestation and a milder course. Some also distinguish the third (or "mixed") pathway, where the arteries are both affected and poorly reorganized [145, 146].

Disrupted trophoblast invasion initiates ischemic and hypoxic damage of placental cells and tissues, leading to increase of cell debris and microparticles of fetal origin contents in the mother's blood. These processes result in the mother's immune cells activation and inflammatory cytokines synthesis induction [147], leading to the development of generalized endothelial activation/dysfunction with development of multiorganic insufficiency [148] (**Figure 1**). Trophoblast debris was also found in the mother's is blood in a normal pregnancy and it was primarily apoptotic. Particles of trophoblast debris range from polynuclear aggregates of the syncytium cells to subcellular micro and nanoparticles. *In vitro* co-culturing of trophoblast debris, obtained from women with normal pregnancy, with macrophages and endothelial cells leads to tolerogenic M2-phenotype of macrophages [149, 150]. Trophoblast debris becomes more necrotic when *in vitro* system is supplemented with antiphospholipid antibodies or IL-6. Phagocytosis of the necrotic debris by the endothelial cells is accompanied by their activation [151]. Activation of endothelial cells is also caused by the addition of the trophoblast debris isolated from patients with preeclampsia to the culture of the endothelial cells [152].

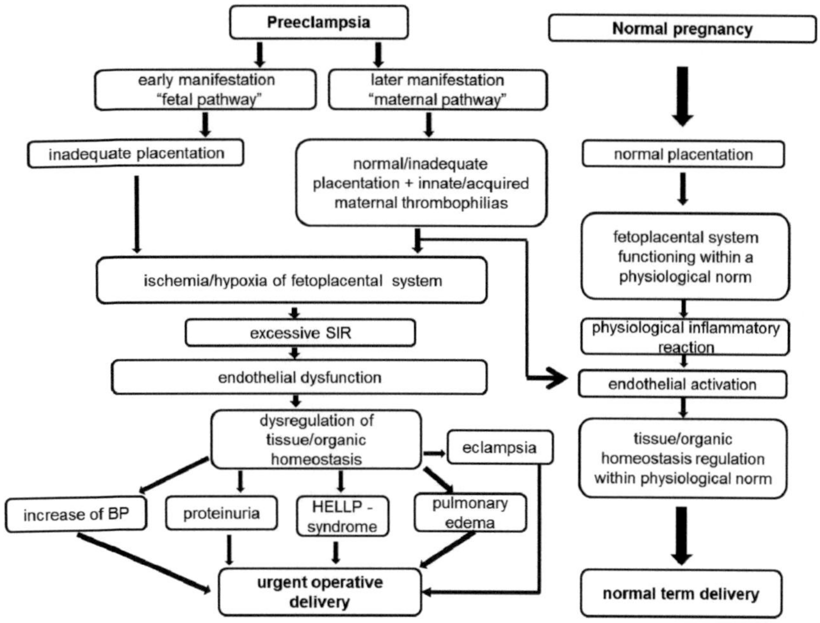

Figure 1. Modern concept of the pathogenesis of preeclampsia (PE). Two phenotypic PE variations (early onset-PE and late onset-PE) exhibit different pathophysiology and clinical outcome. Clinical manifestations of endothelial activation/dysfunction are expressed in various degree and in both forms. SIR, systemic inflammatory response; BP, blood pressure; HELLP, hemolysis, elevated liver enzymes, and low platelet count.

5.1. Endothelium activation markers in preeclampsia

Numerous studies have shown that in PE, manifestations of excessive SIR are observed due to the loss of control over the balance of production of pro/anti-inflammatory cytokines. This leads to an increase in the synthesis and expression of key molecules that mediate intercellular contacts between leukocytes and endothelium [147, 153, 154]. In this context, it has been shown that in PE, the plasma levels of sE-selectin, sVCAM-1 and sICAM-1 were significantly elevated [100, 155–157], and that cultivation of endothelial cells with the blood serum of PE women significantly increased the expression of ICAM-1 by the endothelial cells [158].

It was found that the expression of E-selectin and P-selectin in the endothelial cell culture was significantly higher after administration of trophoblast cells from the PE patients, than after cultivation of endothelial cells with trophoblast cells isolated from placental tissue of healthy women [159]. We have shown in a prospective longitudinal study that in patients with severe PE, the levels of sE-selectin, sVCAM-1 and sICAM-1 were increased from the 8th week of pregnancy until the appearance of clinical symptoms of the disease [160]. In a similar design study, it was shown that joint determination of sICAM-1 and sVCAM-1 levels measured in peripheral blood within 22–29 weeks of gestation, was of high predictive value and capable to detect up to 55% of women with a pathologic pregnancy [161]. The increased levels of sICAM-1 and sVCAM-1 in blood during PE significantly correlated with the signs of the acute phase of inflammation and PE: hypertension, proteinuria, increase of hepatic enzymes levels

[162]. Also it was noted that high levels of sVCAM-1 and sE-selectin in women with PE could result in adverse perinatal outcome and endothelial dysfunction in fetus, as confirmed by negative correlation between sVCAM-1 and endogenous NO synthesis by HUVECs, isolated from the umbilical cord after birth [163].

5.2. Alteration of endothelial glycocalyx in preeclampsia

The signs of endothelial activation are the expression of activation markers by endothelial cells and increased plasma concentrations of the soluble forms of CAMs and of the factors, regulating angiogenesis and blood clotting. However, the main feature of the evolving endothelial activation is alteration, damage and shedding of the eGC and an increase of its components concentration in blood. Currently, there are limited studies of this phenomena in PE, but available reports show significant alteration of eGC composition in the placental structures in PE [164]. The most prominent alteration of the eGC composition was found in the placentas of women with severe PE. Alterations take place also in the eGC capillaries of terminal placental villi: the content of glycans with terminal β-galactosyl and α-mannosyl residues increase, while the content of α2,3-linked sialic acids decrease in the glycome in severe PE [165]. These alterations are supposed to point to the exposure of glycans bearing the "danger signals" and being the counter-receptors for endogenous lectins; interaction with these activate maternal immune system [166, 167] (REF). Such studies, performed by immunohistochemistry of placenta after childbirth and using the lectins panel or monoclonal antibodies to carbohydrates antigens, give an idea of alterations of the placental glycome and its separate structures, including capillary endothelium, and provide evidence obtained by direct eGC visualization [165, 168]. Since direct visualization of the eGC is impossible in clinical trials where no surgical tissue sampling is implied, in these cases, an indirect assessment of the content of the degradation products of eGC is used.

Indirect methods have significant limitations, but they are the only possibility to evaluate the eGC *in vivo*. Indirect assessment of the eGC by ELISA show that in PE, the plasma content of the structural proteoglycans (endocan-1, syndecan-1, decorin and HA) and the GAGs of eGC increase [169–171]. Serum endocan concentrations were significantly elevated in women with PE versus normotensive controls, and concentrations seem to be associated with the severity of the disease [172]. Median maternal plasma endocan concentrations were higher in PE patients and lower in acute pyelonephritis with bacteremia than in uncomplicated pregnancy. No significant difference was observed in the median plasma endocan concentration between other obstetrical syndromes and uncomplicated pregnancies [173]. It is suggested that in PE, the maternal endothelium is a source of GAGs in blood, and intensive eGC shedding thus indicates a manifestation of endothelial dysfunction [169–174]. Also, patients with PE show GAGs excretion in urine; this is thought to be linked with the eGC proteoglycans alterations and with the glomerular basement membrane changes, and associated with proteinuria [175]. *In vitro* and *in vivo* experimental studies, using cell and animal models is another opportunity of indirect eGC evaluation. This approach was used to study CKD [74, 75], cardio-vascular and inflammatory diseases [13, 176], cancer [13, 176, 177]—the conditions manifestating with hypertension, proteinuria, edema, SIR, thrombosis. The results of such studies provide some keys to PE, which is less studied, but exhibits similar clinical signs. Experimental models allow to evaluate not only the degree of the eGC damage by various factors (SIR being the most significant), but also the molecular changes of the eGC composition. This moment is a crucial point because SIR is not a specific process; it accompanies almost any pathology and promotes the generation of neoantigens, acting as an adaptive response trigger and provoking autoimmune reactions.

6. Conclusion

Endothelial dysfunction represents the central link in the pathogenesis of various diseases and complications, and is a subject of intensive research. On the background of the progress in understanding the mechanisms of development, diagnosis and treatment of endothelial dysfunction, many studies in the recent years have been focused on the eGC as an early indicator of endothelial injury and a potential marker of vascular injury.

Alterations of the phenotype of endothelial cells, secretion and release of various activation markers into the bloodstream and dysfunction of the endothelium are directly related to the damage of eGC. This damage is the initiating factor and the initial stage in the development of endothelial activation/dysfunction, but this stage has for a long time been obscure due to the difficulties of eGC visualization and diagnosis.

By now, the main criteria for eGC damage assessment have been defined. In addition to the appearance of eGC components in the blood, the degree of manifestation of the SIR is also an important criterium of the damage, since endothelial inflammation and dysfunction are inseparably related processes. In this regard, the molecular mechanism of the inflammatory reaction is based on the ligand-receptor, carbohydrate-protein interaction of the immune cells and endothelium, and alteration of glycome/glycocalyx is a crucial factor in the development of inflammation and endothelial dysfunction. Therefore, the pathogenesis of endothelial activation/dysfunction should be envisioned from the point of damage of the intravascular compartment—the eGC, which regulates the functions of the endothelium.

Expanding research of the eGC role in the development of endothelial dysfunction may be a subject of new discoveries in the pathogenesis of a large group of diseases, including pregnancy pathology and PE, especially since PE is a classic example of the immune system hyperactivation, manifestation of SIR and development of endothelial dysfunction. Undoubtedly, future studies of the eGC will evoke an absolutely new insight in the development and progression of endothelial dysfunction.

Acknowledgements

We thank Alexey Komarovsky and Natalia Baranova for their help in the manuscript preparation.

Conflict of interest

The authors report no conflicts of interest.

Notes/thanks/other declarations

The study has been carried out within the State Contract (№ 116082210002) "Investigation of diagnostic and prognostic value of molecular-genetic, immunologic, epigenetic factors in pre-eclampsia."

Author details

Marina M. Ziganshina[1]*, Ekaterina L. Yarotskaya[2], Nicolai V. Bovin[3] and Gennady T. Sukhikh[1]

*Address all correspondence to: mmz@mail.ru

1 Laboratory of Clinical Immunology, Federal State Budget Institution National Medical Research Center for Obstetrics, Gynecology and Perinatology named after Academician V.I. Kulakov of the Ministry of Healthcare of Russian Federation, Moscow, Russian Federation

2 Department of International Cooperation, Federal State Budget Institution National Medical Research Center for Obstetrics, Gynecology and Perinatology named after Academician V.I. Kulakov of the Ministry of Healthcare of Russian Federation, Moscow, Russian Federation

3 Laboratory of Carbohydrates of the Shemyakin-Ovchinnikov Institute of Bioorganic Chemistry of the Russian Academy of Sciences, Russian Federation

References

[1] Valdiviezo C, Garovic VD, Ouyang P. Preeclampsia and hypertensive disease in pregnancy: Their contributions to cardiovascular risk. Clinical Cardiology. 2012;**35**:160-165. DOI: 10.1002/clc.21965

[2] Magee LA, Pels A, Helewa M, Rey E, von Dadelszen P. Diagnosis, evaluation, and management of the hypertensive disorders of pregnancy: Executive summary. Journal of Obstetrics and Gynaecology Canada. 2014;**36**:575-576. DOI: 10.1016/S1701-2163(15)30533-8

[3] Ramma W, Ahmed A. Is inflammation the cause of pre-eclampsia? Biochemical Society Transactions. 2011;**39**(6):1619-1627. DOI: 10.1042/BST20110672

[4] Kim Y, Romero R, Oh S, Kim C, Kilburn B, Armant D, Nien J, Gomez R, Mazor M, Saito S, Abrahams V, Mor G. Toll-like receptor 4: A potential link between "danger signals," the innate immune system, and preeclampsia? American Journal of Obstetrics and Gynecology. 2005;**193**(3 Pt 2):921-927. DOI: 10.1016/j.ajog.2005.07.076

[5] Bernardi F, Felisberto F, Vuolo F, Petronilho F, Souza D, Luciano T, de Souza C, Ritter C, Dal-Pizzol F. Oxidative damage, inflammation, and Toll-like receptor 4 pathway are increased in preeclamptic patients: A case-control study. Oxidative Medicine and Cellular Longevity. 2012;**2012**:636419. DOI: 10.1155/2012/636419

[6] Scott DW, Vallejo MO, Patel RP. Heterogenic endothelial responses to inflammation: Role for differential N-glycosylation and vascular bed of origin. Journal of the American Heart Association. 2013;**2**(4):e000263. DOI: 10.1161/JAHA.113.000263

[7] Fu BM, Tarbell JM. Mechano-sensing and transduction by endothelial surface glycocalyx: Composition, structure, and function. Wiley Interdisciplinary Reviews. Systems Biology and Medicine. 2013;**5**(3):381-390. DOI: 10.1002/wsbm.1211

[8] Aird WC. Endothelium in health and disease. Pharmacological Reports. 2008;**60**(1):139-143

[9] Pries AR, Kuebler WM. Normal endothelium. Handbook of Experimental Pharmacology. 2006;**176**(Pt 1):1-40

[10] Galley HF, Webster NR. Physiology of the endothelium. British Journal of Anaesthesia. 2004;**93**(1):105-113. DOI: 10.1093/bja/aeh163

[11] Schött U, Solomon C, Fries D, Bentzer P. The endothelial glycocalyx and its disruption, protection and regeneration: A narrative review. Scandinavian Journal of Trauma, Resuscitation and Emergency Medicine. 2016;**24**:48. DOI: 10.1186/s13049-016-0239-y

[12] Becker BF, Chappell D, Bruegger D, Annecke T, Jacob M. Therapeutic strategies targeting the endothelial glycocalyx: Acute deficits, but great potential. Cardiovascular Research. 2010;**87**(2):300-310. DOI: 10.1093/cvr/cvq137

[13] Tarbell JM, Cancel LM. The glycocalyx and its significance in human medicine. Journal of Internal Medicine. 2016;**280**(1):97-113. DOI: 10.1111/joim.12465

[14] Ziganshina MM, Pavlovich SV, Bovin NV, Sukhikh GT. Hyaluronic acid in vascular and immune homeostasis during normal pregnancy and preeclampsia. Acta Naturae. 2016; **8**(3):59-71

[15] Reitsma S, Slaaf DW, Vink H, van Zandvoort MA, oude Egbrink MG. The endothelial glycocalyx: Composition, functions, and visualization. Pflügers Archiv 2007;**454**(3):345-359. DOI: 10.1007/s00424-007-0212-8

[16] Maksimenko AV. Translational research into vascular wall function: Regulatory effects of systemic and specific factors. Journal of Translational Science. 2017;**3**(2):1-10. DOI: 10.15761/JTS.1000180

[17] Jiménez D, Roda-Navarro P, Springer TA, Casasnovas JM. Contribution of N-linked glycans to the conformation and function of intercellular adhesion molecules (ICAMs). The Journal of Biological Chemistry. 2005;**280**(7):5854-5861. DOI: 10.1074/jbc.M412104200

[18] Scott DW, Patel RP. Endothelial heterogeneity and adhesion molecules N-glycosylation: Implications in leukocyte trafficking in inflammation. Glycobiology. 2013;**23**(6):622-633. DOI: 10.1093/glycob/cwt014

[19] Rüegg C, Mariotti A. Vascular integrins: Pleiotropic adhesion and signaling molecules in vascular homeostasis and angiogenesis. Cellular and Molecular Life Sciences. 2003;**60**(6):1135-1157. DOI: 10.1007/s00018-003-2297-3

[20] Hang Q, Isaji T, Hou S, Zhou Y, Fukuda T, Gu J. N-glycosylation of integrin $\alpha5$ acts as a switch for EGFR-mediated complex formation of integrin $\alpha5\beta1$ to $\alpha6\beta4$. Scientific Reports. 2016;**6**:33507. DOI: 10.1038/srep33507

[21] Geyer H, Geyer R, Odenthal-Schnittler M, Schnittler HJ. Characterization of human vascular endothelial cadherin glycans. Glycobiology. 1999;**9**(9):915-925

[22] Scott DW, Tolbert CE, Graham DM, Wittchen E, Bear JE, Burridge K. N-glycosylation controls the function of junctional adhesion molecule-A. Molecular Biology of the Cell. 2015;**26**(18):3205-3214. DOI: 10.1091/mbc.E14-12-1604

[23] https://www.omim.org/entry/606870#7

[24] Arrate MP, Rodriguez JM, Tran TM, Brock TA, Cunningham SA. Cloning of human junctional adhesion molecule 3 (JAM3) and its identification as the JAM2counter-receptor. The Journal of Biological Chemistry. 2001;**276**(49):45826-45832. DOI: 10.1074/jbc.M105972200

[25] Casasnovas JM, Springer TA, Liu JH, Harrison SC, Wang JH. Crystal structure of ICAM-2 reveals a distinctive integrin recognition surface. Nature. 1997;**387**(6630):312-315. DOI: 10.1038/387312a0

[26] Imai Y, Lasky LA, Rosen SD. Sulphation requirement for GlyCAM-1, an endothelial ligand for L-selectin. Nature. 1993;**361**(6412):555-557. DOI: 10.1038/361555a0

[27] Hemmerich S, Leffler H, Rosen SD. Structure of the O-glycans in GlyCAM-1, an endothelial-derived ligand for L-selectin. Journal of Biological Chemistry. 1995;**270**(20): 12035-12047

[28] Mir GH, Helin J, Skarp KP, Cummings RD, Mäkitie A, Renkonen R, Leppänen A. Glycoforms of human endothelial CD34 that bind L-selectin carry sulfated sialyl Lewis x capped O- and N-glycans. Blood. 2009;**114**(3):733-741. DOI: 10.1182/blood-2009-03-210237

[29] Wu W, Pasternack L, Hua Huang D, Koeller KM, Lin C-C, Seitz O, Wong C-H. Structural study on O-glycopeptides: Glycosylation-induced conformational changes of O-GlcNAc, O-LacNAc, O-Sialyl-LacNAc, and O-Sialyl-Lewis-X peptides of the Mucin domain of MAdCAM-1. Journal of the American Chemical Society. 1999;**121**(11):2409-2417. DOI: 10.1021/ja983474v

[30] Solecka BA, Weise C, Laffan MA, Kannicht C. Site-specific analysis of von Willebrand factor O-glycosylation. Journal of Thrombosis and Haemostasis. 2016;**14**(4):733-746. DOI: 10.1111/jth.13260

[31] Canis K, McKinnon TA, Nowak A, Haslam SM, Panico M, Morris HR, Laffan MA, Dell A. Mapping the N-glycome of human von Willebrand factor. The Biochemical Journal. 2012;**447**(2):217-228. DOI: 10.1042/BJ20120810

[32] Koyama T, Parkinson JF, Sié P, Bang NU, Müller-Berghaus G, Preissner KT. Different glycoforms of human thrombomodulin. Their glycosaminoglycan-dependent modulatory effects on thrombin inactivation by heparin cofactor II and antithrombin II. European Journal of Biochemistry. 1991;**198**(3):563-570

[33] Edano T, Inoue K, Yoshizaki H, Yamamoto S, Komine N, Tabunoki H, Sawada H, Koshi T, Murakami A, Wada Y, Ohkuchi M. Increased anticoagulant activity of recombinant thrombomodulin modified with glycosaminoglycan. Biological & Pharmaceutical Bulletin. 1998;**21**(4):375-381

[34] Edano T, Kumai N, Mizoguchi T, Ohkuchi M. The glycosylation sites and structural characteristics of oligosaccharides on recombinant human thrombomodulin. The International Journal of Biochemistry & Cell Biology. 1998;**30**(1):77-88

[35] Nadanaka S, Kitagawa H, Sugahara K. Demonstration of the immature glycosaminoglycan tetrasaccharide sequence GlcAb1-3Galb1-3Galb1-4Xyl on recombinant soluble human a-thrombomodulin. JBC. 1998;**273**(50):33728-33734

[36] Wakabayashi H, Natsuka S, Honda M, Naotsuka M, Ito Y, Kajihara J, Hase S. Structural analysis of the sugar chains of human urinary thrombomodulin. Journal of Biochemistry. 2001;**130**(4):543-552

[37] Ito T, Maruyama I. Thrombomodulin: Protectorate god of the vasculature in thrombosis and inflammation. Journal of Thrombosis and Haemostasis. 2011;**9**(Suppl. 1):168-173. DOI: 10.1111/j.1538-7836.2011.04319.x

[38] Martínez-Martínez I, Dichiara G, Gutiérrez-Gallego R, Navarro-Fernández J, Vicente V, Corral J. Increased N-glycosylation efficiency by generation of an aromatic sequon on N135 of antithrombin. PLoS One. 2014;**9**(12):e114454. DOI: 10.1371/journal.pone.0114454

[39] Kumar A, Bhandari A, Sarde SJ, Goswami C. Sequence, phylogenetic and variant analyses of antithrombin III. Biochemical and Biophysical Research Communications. 2013;**440**(4):714-724. DOI: 10.1016/j.bbrc.2013.09.134

[40] Böhme C, Nimtz M, Grabenhorst E, Conradt HS, Strathmann A, Ragg H. Tyrosine sulfation and N-glycosylation of human heparin cofactor II from plasma and recombinant Chinese hamster ovary cells and their effects on heparin binding. European Journal of Biochemistry. 2002;**269**(3):977-988

[41] Shriver Z, Capila I, Venkataraman G, Sasisekharan R. Heparin and heparin sulfate: Analyzing structure and microheterogeneity. Handbook of Experimental Pharmacology. 2012;**207**:159-176. DOI: 10.1007/978-3-642-23056-1_8

[42] Sugiura N, Shioiri T, Chiba M, Sato T, Narimatsu H, Kimata K, Watanabe H. Construction of a chondroitin sulfate library with defined structures and analysis of molecular interactions. The Journal of Biological Chemistry. 2012;**287**(52):43390-43400. DOI: 10.1074/jbc.M112.412676

[43] Akatsu C, Mizumoto S, Kaneiwa T, Maccarana M, Malmström A, Yamada S, Sugahara K. Dermatan sulfate epimerase 2 is the predominant isozyme in the formation of the chondroitin sulfate/dermatan sulfate hybrid structure in postnatal developing mouse brain. Glycobiology. 2011;**21**(5):565-574. DOI: 10.1093/glycob/cwq208

[44] Higashi K, Takeda K, Mukuno A, Okamoto Y, Masuko S, Linhardt RJ, Toida T. Identification of keratin sulfate disaccharide at C-3 position of glucuronate of chondroitin sulfate from *Mactra chinensis*. The Biochemical Journal. 2016;**473**(22):4145-4158. DOI: 10.1042/BCJ20160655

[45] Gubbiotti MA, Neill T, Iozzo RV. A current view of perlecan in physiology and pathology: A mosaic of functions. Matrix Biology. 2017;**57-58**:285-298. DOI: 10.1016/j.matbio.2016.09.003

[46] Sotoodehnejadnematalahi F, Burke B. Structure, function and regulation of versican: The most abundant type of proteoglycan in the extracellular matrix. Acta Medica Iranica. 2013;**51**(11):740-750

[47] Kenagy RD, Plaas AH, Wight TN. Versican degradation and vascular disease. Trends in Cardiovascular Medicine. 2006;**16**(6):209-215. DOI: 10.1016/j.tcm.2006.03.011

[48] Kali A, Shetty KS. Endocan: A novel circulating proteoglycan. Indian Journal of Pharmacology. 2014;**46**(6):579-583. DOI: 10.4103/0253-7613.144891

[49] Seidler DG, Dreier R. Decorin and its galactosaminoglycan chain: Extracellular regulator of cellular function? IUBMB Life. 2008;**60**(11):729-733. DOI: 10.1002/iub.115

[50] Nastase MV, Young MF, Schaefer L. Biglycan: A multivalent proteoglycan providing structure and signals. The Journal of Histochemistry and Cytochemistry. 2012;**60**(12):963-975. DOI: 10.1369/0022155412456380

[51] Newton JP, Hunter AP, Simmons DL, Buckley CD, Harvey DJ. CD31 (PECAM-1) exists as a dimer and is heavily N-glycosylated. Biochemical and Biophysical Research Communications. 1999;**261**(2):283-291. DOI: 10.1006/bbrc.1999.1018

[52] Lertkiatmongkol P, Paddock C, Newman DK, Zhu J, Thomas MJ, Newman PJ. The role of sialylated glycans in human platelet endothelial cell adhesion molecule 1 (PECAM-1)-mediated trans homophilic interactions and endothelial cell barrier function. The Journal of Biological Chemistry. 2016;**291**(50):26216-26225. DOI: 10.1074/jbc.M116.756502

[53] Påhlsson P, Strindhall J, Srinivas U, Lundblad A. Role of N-linked glycosylation in expression of E-selectin on human endothelial cells. European Journal of Immunology. 1995;**25**(9):2452-2459. DOI: 10.1002/eji.1830250907

[54] Yoshimura M, Ihara Y, Matsuzawa Y, Taniguchi N. Aberrant glycosylation of E-cadherin enhances cell-cell binding to suppress metastasis. The Journal of Biological Chemistry. 1996;**271**(23):13811-13815

[55] Sasaki N, Toyoda M. Glycoconjugates and related molecules in human vascular endothelial cells. International Journal of Vascular Medicine. 2013;**2013**:963596. DOI: 10.1155/2013/963596

[56] McCoy AJ, Pei XY, Skinner R, Abrahams JP, Carrell RW. Structure of beta-antithrombin and the effect of glycosylation on antithrombin's heparin affinity and activity. Journal of Molecular Biology. 2003;**326**(3):823-833

[57] Sperandio M, Gleissner CA, Ley K. Glycosylation in immune cell trafficking. Immunological Reviews. 2009;**230**(1):97-113. DOI: 10.1111/j.1600-065X.2009.00795

[58] Schnaar RL, Suzuki A, Stanley P. In: Varki A, Cummings RD, Esko JD, et al., editors. Essentials of Glycobiology. 2nd ed. Cold Spring Harbor (NY): Cold Spring Harbor Laboratory Press; 2009. Chapter 10 Glycosphingolipids

[59] Iwabuchi K. Involvement of glycosphingolipid-enriched lipid rafts in inflammatory responses. Frontiers in Bioscience. 2015;**20**:325-334

[60] Gillard BK, Jones MA, Marcus DM. Glycosphingolipids of human umbilical vein endothelial cells and smooth muscle cells. Archives of Biochemistry and Biophysics. 1987; **256**(2):435-445

[61] Nakayama H, Yoshizaki F, Prinetti A, Sonnino S, Mauri L, Takamori K, Ogawa H, Iwabuchi K. Lyn-coupled LacCer-enriched lipid rafts are required for CD11b/CD18-mediated neutrophil phagocytosis of nonopsonized microorganisms. Journal of Leukocyte Biology. 2008;**83**(3):728-741. DOI: 10.1189/jlb.0707478

[62] Iwabuchi K, Nagaoka I. Lactosylceramide-enriched glycosphingolipid signaling domain mediates superoxide generation from human neutrophils. Blood. 2002;**100**(4):1454-1464

[63] Iwabuchi K, Nakayama H, Oizumi A, Suga Y, Ogawa H, Takamori K. Role of ceramide from glycosphingolipids and its metabolites in immunological and inflammatory responses in humans. Mediators of Inflammation. 2015;**2015**:120748. DOI: 10.1155/2015/120748

[64] Zemunik T, Markotić A, Marusić A. Expression of neutral glycosphingolipids in cytokine-stimulated human endothelial cells. Biochemistry (Mosc). 2004;**69**(5):513-519

[65] van de Kar NC, Kooistra T, Vermeer M, Lesslauer W, Monnens LA, van Hinsbergh VW. Tumor necrosis factor alpha induces endothelial galactosyl transferase activity and verocytotoxin receptors. Role of specific tumor necrosis factor receptors and protein kinase C. Blood. 1995;**85**(3):734-743

[66] Schweppe CH, Bielaszewska M, Pohlentz G, Friedrich AW, Büntemeyer H, Schmidt MA, Kim KS, Peter-Katalinić J, Karch H, Müthing J. Glycosphingolipids in vascular endothelial cells: Relationship of heterogeneity in Gb3Cer/CD77 receptor expression with differential Shiga toxin 1 cytotoxicity. Glycoconjugate Journal. 2008;**25**(4):291-304. DOI: 10.1007/s10719-007-9091-7

[67] Müthing J, Duvar S, Heitmann D, Hanisch FG, Neumann U, Lochnit G, Geyer R, Peter-Katalinic J. Isolation and structural characterization of glycosphingolipids of in vitro propagated human umbilical vein endothelial cells. Glycobiology. 1999;**9**(5):459-468

[68] Cooling LW, Zhang DS, Koerner TAW. Lewis X and sialyl Lewis X glycosphingolipids. Trends in Glycoscience and Glycotechnology. 1997;**9**(46):191-209

[69] Zeng Y. Endothelial glycocalyx as a critical signalling platform integrating the extracellular haemodynamic forces and chemical signalling. Journal of Cellular and Molecular Medicine. 2017;**21**(8):1457-1462. DOI: 10.1111/jcmm.13081

[70] Weinbaum S, Zhang X, Han Y, Vink H, Cowin SC. Mechanotransduction and flow across the endothelial glycocalyx. Proceedings of the National Academy of Sciences. 2003;**100**(13):7988-7995. DOI: 10.1073/pnas.1332808100

[71] Secomb TW, Hsu R, Pries AR. Effect of the endothelial surface layer on transmission of fluid shear stress to endothelial cells. Biorheology. 2001;**38**(2-3):143-150

[72] Satchell S. The role of the glomerular endothelium in albumin handling. Nature Reviews. Nephrology. 2013;**9**(12):717-725. DOI: 10.1038/nrneph.2013.197

[73] Salmon AH, Satchell SC. Endothelial glycocalyx dysfunction in disease: Albuminuria and increased microvascular permeability. The Journal of Pathology. 2012;**226**(4):562-574. DOI: 10.1002/path.3964

[74] Salmon AH, Ferguson JK, Burford JL, Gevorgyan H, Nakano D, Harper SJ, Bates DO, Peti-Peterdi J. Loss of the endothelial glycocalyx links albuminuria and vascular dysfunction. Journal of the American Society of Nephrology. 2012;**23**(8):1339-1350. DOI: 10.1681/ASN.2012010017

[75] Padberg JS, Wiesinger A, di Marco GS, Reuter S, Grabner A, Kentrup D, Lukasz A, Oberleithner H, Pavenstädt H, Brand M, Kümpers P. Damage of the endothelial glycocalyx in chronic kidney disease. Atherosclerosis. 2014;**234**(2):335-343. DOI: 10.1016/j.atherosclerosis.2014.03.016

[76] Dane MJ, van den Berg BM, Avramut MC, Faas FG, van der Vlag J, Rops AL, Ravelli RB, Koster BJ, van Zonneveld AJ, Vink H, Rabelink TJ. Glomerular endothelial surface layer acts as a barrier against albumin filtration. The American Journal of Pathology. 2013;**182**(5):1532-1540. DOI: 10.1016/j.ajpath.2013.01.049

[77] Lennon FE, Singleton PA. Hyaluronan regulation of vascular integrity. American Journal of Cardiovascular Disease. 2011;**1**(3):200-213

[78] Curry FR, Adamson RH. Tonic regulation of vascular permeability. Acta Physiologica. 2013;**207**(4):628-649. DOI: 10.1111/apha.12076

[79] Lipowsky HH. The endothelial glycocalyx as a barrier to leukocyte adhesion and its mediation by extracellular proteases. Annals of Biomedical Engineering. 2012;**40**(4):840-848. DOI: 10.1007/s10439-011-0427-x

[80] Kolářová H, Ambrůzová B, Svihálková Šindlerová L, Klinke A, Kubala L. Modulation of endothelial glycocalyx structure under inflammatory conditions. Mediators of Inflammation. 2014;**2014**:694312. DOI: 10.1155/2014/694312

[81] Ushiyama A, Kataoka H, Iijima T. Glycocalyx and its involvement in clinical pathophysiologies. Journal of Intensive Care. 2016;**4**(1):59. DOI: 10.1186/s40560-016-0182-z

[82] McDonald KK, Cooper S, Danielzak L, Leask RL. Glycocalyx degradation induces a pro-inflammatory phenotype and increased leukocyte adhesion in cultured endothelial cells under flow. PLoS One. 2016;**11**(12):e0167576. DOI: 10.1371/journal.pone.0167576

[83] Henry CB, Duling BR. TNF-alpha increases entry of macromolecules into luminal endothelial cell glycocalyx. American Journal of Physiology. Heart and Circulatory Physiology. 2000;**279**(6):H2815-H2823

[84] Constantinescu AA, Vink H, Spaan JA. Elevated capillary tube hematocrit reflects degradation of endothelial cell glycocalyx by oxidized LDL. American Journal of Physiology. Heart and Circulatory Physiology. 2001;**280**(3):H1051-H1057

[85] Mulivor AW, Lipowsky HH. Inflammation- and ischemia-induced shedding of venular glycocalyx. American Journal of Physiology. Heart and Circulatory Physiology. 2004;**286**(5):H1672-H1680. DOI: 10.1152/ajpheart.00832.2003

[86] Lipowsky HH, Gao L, Lescanic A. Shedding of the endothelial glycocalyx in arterioles, capillaries, and venules and its effect on capillary hemodynamics during inflammation. American Journal of Physiology. Heart and Circulatory Physiology. 2011;**301**(6):H2235-H2245. DOI: 10.1152/ajpheart.00803.2011

[87] Rodrigues SF, Granger DN. Blood cells and endothelial barrier function. Tissue Barriers. 2015;**3**(1-2):e978720. DOI: 10.4161/21688370.2014.978720

[88] Termeer CC, Hennies J, Voith U, Ahrens T, Weiss JM, Prehm P, Simon JC. Oligosaccharides of hyaluronan are potent activators of dendritic cells. Journal of Immunology. 2000;**165**(4):1863-1870

[89] Wright RD, Cooper D. Glycobiology of leukocyte trafficking in inflammation. Glycobiology. 2014;**24**(12):1242-1251. DOI: 10.1093/glycob/cwu101

[90] Nieuwdorp M, Meuwese MC, Vink H, Hoekstra JB, Kastelein JJ, Stroes ES. The endothelial glycocalyx: A potential barrier between health and vascular disease. Current Opinion in Lipidology. 2005;**16**(5):507-511

[91] Vink H, Constantinescu AA, Spaan JA. Oxidized lipoproteins degrade the endothelial surface layer: Implications for platelet-endothelial cell adhesion. Circulation. 2000;**101**(13):1500-1502

[92] Romero R, Gotsch F, Pineles B, Kusanovic JP. Inflammation in pregnancy: Its roles in reproductive physiology, obstetrical complications, and fetal injury. Nutrition Reviews. 2007;**65**(12 Pt 2):S194-S202

[93] Challis JR, Lockwood CJ, Myatt L, Norman JE, Strauss JF 3rd, Petraglia F. Inflammation and pregnancy. Reproductive Sciences. 2009;**16**(2):206-215. DOI: 10.1177/1933719108329095

[94] Jabbour HN, Sales KJ, Catalano RD, Norman JE. Inflammatory pathways in female reproductive health and disease. Reproduction. 2009;**138**(6):903-919. DOI: 10.1530/REP-09-0247

[95] Germain SJ, Sacks GP, Sooranna SR, Sargent IL, Redman CW. Systemic inflammatory priming in normal pregnancy and preeclampsia: The role of circulating syncytiotrophoblast microparticles. Journal of Immunology. 2007;**178**(9):5949-5956

[96] Sacks G, Sargent I, Redman C. An innate view of human pregnancy. Immunology Today. 1999;**20**(3):114-118

[97] Redman CW, Sargent IL. Preeclampsia and the systemic inflammatory response. Seminars in Nephrology. 2004;**24**(6):565-570

[98] Eggleton P, Haigh R, Winyard PG. Consequence of neo-antigenicity of the 'altered self'. Rheumatology. 2008;**47**(5):567-571. DOI: 10.1093/rheumatology/ken014

[99] Keswani SC, Chauhan N. Antiphospholipid syndrome. Journal of the Royal Society of Medicine. 2002;**95**(7):336-342

[100] Lyall F, Greer IA. The vascular endothelium in normal pregnancy and pre-eclampsia. Reviews of Reproduction. 1996;**1**(2):107-116

[101] Chaiworapongsa T, Romero R, Yoshimatsu J, Espinoza J, Kim YM, Park K, Kalache K, Edwin S, Bujold E, Gomez R. Soluble adhesion molecule profile in normal pregnancy and pre-eclampsia. The Journal of Maternal-Fetal & Neonatal Medicine. 2002;**12**(1):19-27. DOI: 10.1080/jmf.12.1.19.27

[102] Golias C, Tsoutsi E, Matziridis A, Makridis P, Batistatou A, Charalabopoulos K. Leukocyte and endothelial cell adhesion molecules in inflammation focusing on inflammatory heart disease. In Vivo. 2007;**21**(5):757-769

[103] Hidalgo A, Peired AJ, Wild M, Vestweber D, Frenette PS. Complete identification of E-selectin ligands on neutrophils reveals distinct functions of PSGL-1, ESL-1, and CD44. Immunity. 2007;**26**(4):477-489. DOI: 10.1016/j.immuni.2007.03.011

[104] Schnaar RL, Suzuki A, Stanley P. In: Varki A, Cummings RD, Esko JD, et al., editors. Essentials of Glycobiology. 2nd ed. Cold Spring Harbor (NY): Cold Spring Harbor Laboratory Press; 2009. Chapter 31 G-type lectins

[105] Sriramarao P, Berger E, Chambers JD, Arfors KE, Gehlsen KR. High mannose type N-linked oligosaccharides on endothelial cells may influence beta 2 integrin mediated neutrophil adherence in vitro. Journal of Cellular Biochemistry. 1993;**51**(3):360-368. DOI: 10.1002/jcb.240510316

[106] Diamond MS, Staunton DE, Marlin SD, Springer TA. Binding of the integrin Mac-1 (CD11b/CD18) to the third immunoglobulin-like domain of ICAM-1 (CD54) and its regulation by glycosylation. Cell. 1991;**65**(6):961-971

[107] Feduska JM, Garcia PL, Brennan SB, Bu S, Council LN, Yoon KJ. N-glycosylation of ICAM-2 is required for ICAM-2-mediated complete suppression of metastatic potential of SK-N-AS neuroblastoma cells. BMC Cancer. 2013;**13**:261. DOI: 10.1186/1471-2407-13-261

[108] Willhauck-Fleckenstein M, Moehler TM, Merling A, Pusunc S, Goldschmidt H, Schwartz-Albiez R. Transcriptional regulation of the vascular endothelial glycome by angiogenic and inflammatory signalling. Angiogenesis. 2010;**13**(1):25-42. DOI: 10.1007/s10456-010-9162-4

[109] van Kooyk Y, Rabinovich GA. Protein-glycan interactions in the control of innate and adaptive immune responses. Nature Immunology 2008;**9**(6):593-601. DOI: 10.1038/ni.f.203

[110] van Kooyk Y. C-type lectins on dendritic cells: Key modulators for the induction of immune responses. Biochemical Society Transactions 2008;**36**(Pt 6):1478-1481. DOI: 10.1042/BST0361478

[111] Varki A. Since there are PAMPs and DAMPs, there must be SAMPs? Glycan "self-associated molecular patterns" dampen innate immunity, but pathogens can mimic them. Glycobiology. 2011;**21**(9):1121-1124

[112] Erlebacher A. Immunology of the maternal-fetal interface. Annual Review of Immunology. 2013;**31**:387-411. DOI: 10.1146/annurev-immunol-032712-100003

[113] Laderach DJ, Compagno D, Toscano MA, Croci DO, Dergan-Dylon S, Salatino M, Rabinovich GA. Dissecting the signal transduction pathways triggered by galectin-glycan interactions in physiological and pathological settings. IUBMB Life. 2010;**62**(1):1-13. DOI: 10.1002/iub.281

[114] Nobumoto A, Nagahara K, Oomizu S, Katoh S, Nishi N, Takeshita K, Niki T, Tominaga A, Yamauchi A, Hirashima M. Galectin-9 suppresses tumor metastasis by blocking adhesion to endothelium and extracellular matrices. Glycobiology. 2008;**18**(9):735-744. DOI: 10.1093/glycob/cwn062

[115] Norling LV, Perretti M, Cooper D. Endogenous galectins and the control of the host inflammatory response. The Journal of Endocrinology. 2009;**201**(2):169-184. DOI: 10.1677/JOE-08-0512

[116] Cedeno-Laurent F, Dimitroff CJ. Galectins and their ligands: Negative regulators of anti-tumor immunity. Glycoconjugate Journal. 2012;**29**(8-9):619-625. DOI: 10.1007/s10719-012-9379-0

[117] Macauley MS, Crocker PR, Paulson JC. Siglec-mediated regulation of immune cell function in disease. Nature Reviews. Immunology. 2014;**14**(10):653-666. DOI: 10.1038/nri3737

[118] O'Sullivan JA, Carroll DJ, Bochner BS. Glycobiology of eosinophilic inflammation: Contributions of siglecs, glycans, and other glycan-binding proteins. Frontiers in Medicine. 2017;**4**:116. DOI: 10.3389/fmed.2017.00116

[119] Pillai S, Netravali IA, Cariappa A, Mattoo H. Siglecs and immune regulation. Annual Review of Immunology. 2012;**30**:357-392. DOI: 10.1146/annurev-immunol-020711-075018

[120] Varki A, Gagneux P. Multifarious roles of sialic acids in immunity. Annals of the New York Academy of Sciences. 2012;**1253**:16-36. DOI: 10.1111/j.1749-6632.2012.06517.x

[121] Crocker PR, Varki A. Siglecs in the immune system. Immunology. 2001;**103**(2):137-145

[122] Dam TK, Brewer CF. Maintenance of cell surface glycan density by lectin-glycan interactions: A homeostatic and innate immune regulatory mechanism. Glycobiology. 2010; **20**(9):1061-1064. DOI: 10.1093/glycob/cwq084

[123] Görög P, Pearson JD. Sialic acid moieties on surface glycoproteins protect endothelial cells from proteolytic damage. The Journal of Pathology. 1985;**146**(3):205-212. DOI: 10.1002/path.1711460307

[124] Schauer R. Achievements and challenges of sialic acid research. Glycoconjugate Journal. 2000;**17**(7-9):485-499

[125] Kreisman LS, Cobb BA. Infection, inflammation and host carbohydrates: A glyco-evasion hypothesis. Glycobiology. 2012;**22**(8):1019-1030. DOI: 10.1093/glycob/cws070

[126] Dam TK, Brewer CF. Lectins as pattern recognition molecules: The effects of epitope density in innate immunity. Glycobiology. 2010;**20**(3):270-279. DOI: 10.1093/glycob/cwp186

[127] Rabinovich GA, van Kooyk Y, Cobb BA. Glycobiology of immune responses. Annals of the New York Academy of Sciences. 2012;**1253**:1-15. DOI: 10.1111/j.1749-6632.2012.06492.x

[128] Myatt L, Webster RP. Vascular biology of preeclampsia. Journal of Thrombosis and Haemostasis. 2009;**7**(3):375-384. DOI: 10.1111/j.1538-7836.2008.03259.x

[129] Aird WC. Spatial and temporal dynamics of the endothelium. Journal of Thrombosis and Haemostasis. 2005;**3**(7):1392-1406. DOI: 10.1111/j.1538-7836.2005.01328.x

[130] Bach FH, Robson SC, Ferran C, Winkler H, Millan MT, Stuhlmeier KM, Vanhove B, Blakely ML, van der Werf WJ, Hofer E. Endothelial cell activation and thromboregulation during xenograft rejection. Immunological Reviews. 1994;**141**:5-30

[131] Zhang J, Defelice AF, Hanig JP, Colatsky T. Biomarkers of endothelial cell activation serve as potential surrogate markers for drug-induced vascular injury. Toxicologic Pathology. 2010;**38**(6):856-871. DOI: 10.1177/0192623310378866

[132] Hunt BJ, Jurd KM. Endothelial cell activation. A central pathophysiological process. BMJ. 1998;**316**(7141):1328-1329

[133] Magee LA, Pels A, Helewa M, Rey E, von Dadelszen P. Canadian Hypertensive Disorders of Pregnancy (HDP) Working Group; The hypertensive disorders of pregnancy (29.3). Best Practice & Research. Clinical Obstetrics & Gynaecology. 2015;**29**(5):643-657. DOI: 10.1016/j.bpobgyn.2015.04.001

[134] Laresgoiti-Servitje E. A leading role for the immune system in the pathophysiology of preeclampsia. Journal of Leukocyte Biology. 2013;**94**(2):247-257. DOI: 10.1189/jlb.1112603

[135] Naljayan MV, Karumanchi SA. New developments in the pathogenesis of preeclampsia. Advances in Chronic Kidney Disease. 2013;**20**(3):265-270. DOI: 10.1053/j.ackd.2013.02.003

[136] Ahmed A. New insights into the etiology of preeclampsia: Identification of key elusive factors for the vascular complications. Thrombosis Research. 2011;**127**(Suppl 3):S72-S75. DOI: 10.1016/S0049-3848(11)70020-2

[137] Karumanchi SA, Lindheimer MD. Preeclampsia pathogenesis: "triple a rating"-autoantibodies and antiangiogenic factors. Hypertension. 2008;**51**(4):991-992. DOI: 10.1161/HYPERTENSIONAHA.107.100735

[138] Verlohren S, Muller DN, Luft FC, Dechend R. Immunology in hypertension, preeclampsia, and target-organ damage. Hypertension. 2009;**54**(3):439-443. DOI: 10.1161/HYPERTENSIONAHA.108.120253

[139] Tranquilli AL, Brown MA, Zeeman GG, Dekker G, Sibai BM. The definition of severe and early-onset preeclampsia. Statements from the International Society for the Study of Hypertension in Pregnancy (ISSHP). Pregnancy Hypertens. 2013;**3**(1):44-47. DOI: 10.1016/j.preghy.2012.11.001

[140] Ball E, Bulmer JN, Ayis S, Lyall F, Robson SC. Late sporadic miscarriage is associated with abnormalities in spiral artery transformation and trophoblast invasion. The Journal of Pathology. 2006;**208**(4):535-542. DOI: 10.1002/path.1927

[141] Gun BD, Numanoglu G, Ozdamar SO. The comparison of vessels in elective and spontaneous abortion decidua in first trimester pregnancies: Importance of vascular changes in early pregnancy losses. Acta Obstetricia et Gynecologica Scandinavica. 2006;**85**(4):402-406. DOI: 10.1080/00016340500501731

[142] Lyall F. Priming and remodeling of human placental bed spiral arteries during pregnancy—A review. Placenta. 2005;**26**(Suppl A):S31-S36. DOI: 10.1016/j.placenta.2005.02.010

[143] Espinoza J, Romero R, Mee Kim Y, Kusanovic JP, Hassan S, Erez O, Gotsch F, Than NG, Papp Z, Jai KC. Normal and abnormal transformation of the spiral arteries during pregnancy. Journal of Perinatal Medicine. 2006;**34**(6):447-458. DOI: 10.1515/JPM.2006.089

[144] Burton GJ, Woods AW, Jauniaux E, Kingdom JC. Rheological and physiological consequences of conversion of the maternal spiral arteries for uteroplacental blood flow during human pregnancy. Placenta. 2009;**30**(6):473-482. DOI: 10.1016/j.placenta.2009.02.009

[145] Phipps E, Prasanna D, Brima W, Jim B. Preeclampsia: Updates in pathogenesis, definitions, and guidelines. Clinical Journal of the American Society of Nephrology. 2016;**11**(6):1102-1113. DOI: 10.2215/CJN.12081115

[146] Raymond D, Peterson E. A critical review of early-onset and late-onset preeclampsia. Obstetrical & Gynecological Survey. 2011;**66**(8):497-506. DOI: 10.1097/OGX.0b013e3182331028

[147] Raghupathy R. Cytokines as key players in the pathophysiology of preeclampsia. Medical Principles and Practice. 2013;**22**(Suppl 1):8-19. DOI: 10.1159/000354200

[148] Warrington JP, George EM, Palei AC, Spradley FT, Granger JP. Recent advances in the understanding of the pathophysiology of preeclampsia. Hypertension. 2013;**62**(4):666-673. DOI: 10.1161/HYPERTENSIONAHA.113.00588

[149] Abumaree MH, Chamley LW, Badri M, El-Muzaini MF. Trophoblast debris modulates the expression of immune proteins in macrophages: A key to maternal tolerance of the fetal allograft? Journal of Reproductive Immunology. 2012;**94**(2):131e41. DOI: 10.1016/j.jri.2012.03.488

[150] Abumaree MH, Stone PR, Chamley LW. The effects of apoptotic, deported human placental trophoblast on macrophages: Possible consequences for pregnancy. Journal of Reproductive Immunology. 2006;**72**(1e2):33e45. DOI: 10.1016/j.jri.2006.03.001

[151] Chamley LW, Holland OJ, Chen Q, Viall CA, Stone PR, Abumaree M. Review: Where is the maternofetal interface? Placenta. 2014;**35**(Suppl):S74-S80. DOI: 10.1016/j.placenta.2013.10.014

[152] Shen F, Wei J, Snowise S, DeSousa J, Stone P, Viall C, Chen Q, Chamley L. Trophoblast debris extruded from preeclamptic placentae activates endothelial cells: A mechanism by which the placenta communicates with the maternal endothelium. Placenta. 2014;**35**(10):839-847. DOI: 10.1016/j.placenta.2014.07.009

[153] LaMarca BD, Ryan MJ, Gilbert JS, Murphy SR, Granger JP. Inflammatory cytokines in the pathophysiology of hypertension during preeclampsia. Current Hypertension Reports. 2007;**9**(6):480-485

[154] Saito S, Sakai M. Th1/Th2 balance in preeclampsia. Journal of Reproductive Immunology. 2003;**59**(2):161-173

[155] Daniel Y, Kupferminc MJ, Baram A, Jaffa AJ, Wolman I, Shenhav M, Lessing JB. Plasma soluble endothelial selectin is elevated in women with pre-eclampsia. Human Reproduction. 1998;**13**(12):3537-3541

[156] Fei X, Hongxiang Z, Qi C, Daozhen C. Maternal plasma levels of endothelial dysfunction mediators including AM, CGRP, sICAM-1 and tHcy in pre-eclampsia. Advances in Clinical and Experimental Medicine. 2012;**21**(5):573-579

[157] Farzadnia M, Ayatollahi H, Hasan-Zade M, Rahimi HR. A comparative study of serum level of Vascular Cell Adhesion Molecule-1 (sVCAM-1), Intercellular Adhesion Molecule-1 (ICAM-1) and High Sensitive C-REACTIVE protein (hs-CRP) in normal and pre-eclamptic pregnancies. Iranian Journal of Basic Medical Sciences. 2013;**16**(5):689-693

[158] Haller H, Ziegler EM, Homuth V, Drab M, Eichhorn J, Nagy Z, Busjahn A, Vetter K, Luft FC. Endothelial adhesion molecules and leukocyte integrins in preeclamptic patients. Hypertension. 1997;**29**(1 Pt 2):291-296

[159] Wang Y, Zhang Y, Lewis DF, Gu Y, Li H, Granger DN, Alexander JS. Protease chymotrypsin mediates the endothelial expression of P- and E-selectin, but not ICAM and VCAM, induced by placental trophoblasts from pre-eclamptic pregnancies. Placenta. 2003;**24**(8-9):851-861

[160] Ziganshina MM, Krechetova LV, Vanko LV, Kulterbayeva MA, Sokolyan AV, Sukhikh GT. Time course of changes in the soluble forms of cell adhesion molecules in preeclampsia. Akusherstvo i ginekologiya/Obstetrics and Gynecology (Rus). 2011;(2):42-48

[161] Krauss T, Emons G, Kuhn W, Augustin HG. Predictive value of routine circulating soluble endothelial cell adhesion molecule measurements during pregnancy. Clinical Chemistry. 2002;**48**(9):1418-1425

[162] Szarka A, Rigó J Jr, Lázár L, Beko G, Molvarec A. Circulating cytokines, chemokines and adhesion molecules in normal pregnancy and preeclampsia determined by multiplex suspension array. BMC Immunology. 2010;**11**:59. DOI: 10.1186/1471-2172-11-59

[163] Veas CJ, Aguilera VC, Muñoz IJ, Gallardo VI, Miguel PL, González MA, Lamperti LI, Escudero CA, Aguayo CR. Fetal endothelium dysfunction is associated with circulating maternal levels of sE-selectin, sVCAM1, and sFlt-1 during pre-eclampsia. The Journal of Maternal-Fetal & Neonatal Medicine. 2011;**24**(11):1371-1377. DOI: 10.3109/14767058.2011.556204

[164] Robajac D, Vanhooren V, Masnikosa R, Miković Ž, Mandić V, Libert C, Nedić O. Preeclampsia transforms membrane N-glycome in human placenta. Experimental and Molecular Pathology. 2016;**100**(1):26-30. DOI: 10.1016/j.yexmp.2015.11.029

[165] Sukhikh GT, Ziganshina MM, Nizyaeva NV, Kulikova GV, Volkova JS, Yarotskaya EL, Kan NE, Shchyogolev AI, Tyutyunnik VL. Differences of glycocalyx composition in the structural elements of placenta in preeclampsia. Placenta. 2016;**43**:69-76. DOI: 10.1016/j.placenta.2016.05.002

[166] Stern R, Asari AA, Sugahara KN. Hyaluronan fragments: An information-rich system. European Journal of Cell Biology. 2006;**85**(8):699-715. DOI: 10.1016/j.ejcb.2006.05.009

[167] Frey H, Schroeder N, Manon-Jensen T, Iozzo RV, Schaefer L. Biological interplay between proteoglycans and their innate immune receptors in inflammation. The FEBS Journal. 2013;**280**(10):2165-2179. DOI: 10.1111/febs.12145

[168] Marini M, Bonaccini L, Thyrion GD, Vichi D, Parretti E, Sgambati E. Distribution of sugar remains in human placentas from pregnancies complicated by hypertensive disorders. Acta histochemica. 2011;**113**:815-825. DOI: 10.1016/j.acthis.2010.12.001

[169] Berg S, Engman A, Holmgren S, Lundahl T, Laurent TC. Increased plasma hyaluronan in severe pre-eclampsia and eclampsia. Scandinavian Journal of Clinical and Laboratory Investigation. 2001;**61**(2):131-137

[170] Romão M, Weel IC, Lifshitz SJ, Peraçoli MT. Elevated hyaluronan and extracellular matrix metalloproteinase inducer levels in women with preeclampsia. Archives of Gynecology and Obstetrics. 2014;**289**(3):575-579. DOI: 10.1007/s00404-013-3021-7

[171] Hentschke MR, Lucas LS, Mistry HD, Pinheiro da Costa BE, Poli-de-Figueiredo CE. Endocan-1 concentrations in maternal and fetal plasma and placentae in pre-eclampsia in the third trimester of pregnancy. Cytokine. 2015;**74**(1):152-156. DOI: 10.1016/j.cyto.2015.04.013

[172] Cakmak M, Yilmaz H, Bağlar E, Darcin T, Inan O, Aktas A, Celik HT, Ozdemir O, Atalay CR, Akcay A. Serum levels of endocan correlate with the presence and severity

of pre-eclampsia. Clinical and Experimental Hypertension. 2016;**38**(2):137-142. DOI: 10.3109/10641963.2015.1060993

[173] Adekola H, Romero R, Chaemsaithong P, Korzeniewski SJ, Dong Z, Yeo L, Hassan SS, Chaiworapongsa T. Endocan, a putative endothelial cell marker, is elevated in preeclampsia, decreased in acute pyelonephritis, and unchanged in other obstetrical syndromes. The Journal of Maternal-Fetal & Neonatal Medicine. 2015;**28**(14):1621-1632. DOI: 10.3109/14767058.2014.964676

[174] Siddiqui MF, Nandi P, Girish GV, Nygard K, Eastabrook G, de Vrijer B, Han VK, Lala PK. Decorin over-expression by decidual cells in preeclampsia: A potential blood biomarker. American Journal of Obstetrics and Gynecology. 2016;**215**(3):361.e1-361.e15. DOI: 10.1016/j.ajog.2016.03.020

[175] Khedun SM, Naicker T, Moodley J, Gathiram P. Urinary heparin sulfate proteoglycan excretion in black African women with pre-eclampsia. Acta Obstetricia et Gynecologica Scandinavica. 2002;**81**(4):308-312

[176] Rabelink TJ, de Zeeuw D. The glycocalyx-linking albuminuria with renal and cardiovascular disease. Nature Reviews. Nephrology. 2015;**11**(11):667-676. DOI: 10.1038/nrneph.2015.162

[177] Kim YH, Nijst P, Kiefer K, Tang WH. Endothelial glycocalyx as biomarker for cardiovascular diseases: Mechanistic and clinical implications. Current Heart Failure Reports. 2017;**14**(2):117-126. DOI: 10.1007/s11897-017-0320-5

Chapter 7

Endothelial Cell von Willebrand Factor Secretion in Health and Cardiovascular Disease

Luiza Rusu and Richard D. Minshall

Additional information is available at the end of the chapter

http://dx.doi.org/10.5772/intechopen.74029

Abstract

The main function of von Willebrand factor (vWF) is to initiate platelet adhesion upon vascular injury. The hallmark of acute and chronical inflammation is the widespread activation of endothelial cells which provokes excessive vWF secretion from the endothelial cell storage pool. The level of vWF in blood not only reflects the state of endothelial activation early on in the pathogenesis, but also predicts disease outcome. Elevation in the blood level of vWF occurs either by pathologic increase in the rate of basal vWF secretion or by increased evoked vWF release from dysfunctional/activated endothelial cells (ECs). The increase in plasma vWF is predictive of prothrombotic complications and multi-organ system failure associated with reduced survival in the context of severe inflammatory response syndrome, type II diabetes mellitus, stroke and other inflammatory cardiovascular disease states. This chapter focuses on the role of high circulating vWF levels in thrombotic and inflammatory disease while paying attention to the emerging vWF-related drug development strategies.

Keywords: cardiovascular disease, endothelial activation, von Willebrand factor, hemostasis, thrombosis, inflammation, ADAMTS-13, vWF-related therapeutical strategies

1. Introduction

Endothelial dysfunction, often as a result of chronic activation, is a primary determinant of the severity of disease states. Apart from other cell-specific defects, activation of endothelial cells (ECs) increases platelet binding to von Willebrand factor (vWF), a multimeric blood protein primarily synthesized, stored and secreted by ECs [1–6]. Under physiological conditions, vWF is secreted from ECs via two pathways that enable hemostasis; a continuous or basal secretory pathway that maintains a baseline blood vWF level, [7] and the other, a regulated secretory pathway induced by agonists such as thrombin [8, 9]. Basal vWF secretion involves elements of regulated secretion, with vWF targeted to Weibel-Palade bodies (WPBs) after Golgi processing, but continuously secreted from the storage pool [7]. Release of WPB contents into the extracellular space upon thrombin stimulation of ECs, thought to be pathophysiologically relevant in inflammatory cardiovascular disease, occurs via several processes: (1) signaling via [Ca^{2+}]/$G\alpha q$ and $G\alpha 12$/α-soluble NSF attachment protein (α-SNAP) [10] that (2) promotes engagement and activation of vesicle (v) and target (t) membrane-associated v-SNARE and t-SNARE proteins (vesicle- and target-soluble NSF attachment protein receptors) [11, 12] and (3) energy-dependent fusion of WPB with plasma membrane that promotes the formation of a secretion pore through which the exocytosis of WPB contents occurs [13–15].

Once secreted from WPBs, vWF circulates in a globular conformation under resting conditions [16] and is a carrier for circulating coagulation factor VIII, thereby protecting it from degradation [17–19]. The blood vWF level in health and inflammatory disease is predominantly EC derived, while the contribution of platelets is rather minimal [20]. In response to high shear stress and inflammatory mediators [21], normally quiescent ECs secrete long vWF multimers in large quantities from the storage pool into systemic circulation. vWF multimers are then extracellularly cleaved by a metalloprotease ADAMTS-13 (A Disintegrin and Metalloproteinase with a thrombospondin type 1 motif, member 13), unfold in the circulation and self-associate into particularly linked concatemers to form ultra-large vWF strings [22]. Platelets spontaneously bind to activated vWF via glycoprotein Ibα (GpIbα) interaction with the exposed A1 domain, initiating the thrombogenic process [23–26]. In addition to its classical role in platelet binding, the vWF A1 domain also plays a role in vWF-dependent inflammatory responses [27–29]. In this chapter, we will discuss the most recent findings related to vWF secretion from ECs, the finely tuned balance of vWF level and activity in hemostasis and thrombosis, and the mechanisms by which vWF/ADAMTS-13 axis links inflammation and thrombosis. The potential of vWF as a target in antithrombotic therapies is also discussed.

2. Molecular mechanisms of vWF secretion

2.1. von Willebrand factor and Weibel-Palade bodies at a glance

WPBs are unique secretory granules in ECs, which were first discovered in the 1960s by transmission electron microscopy [30]. Later on, vWF was identified inside WPBs of cultured human ECs [4, 5, 31]. vWF synthesis and maturation trigger WPB biogenesis [32, 33]. vWF is the best example of a protein that drives its own organelle formation [5, 34, 35]. To date, the structure of vWF consists in domains arranged as follows: D1D2D′D3A1A2A3D4C1C2C3C4C5C6CK. Of these, D1D2 is the pro-peptide and, the rest, from D′-CK is the fully functional, mature vWF [36]. The high density of vWF in the secretory granules enables a bolus of fully functional vWF to be released at the site of vascular injury or inflammation, which will promote efficient platelet binding and hemostasis or lead to thrombosis [37]. The physiological importance of proper WPBs formation can be appreciated in the context of various disease states associated with the release of immature, defective or low levels of VWF due to altered Golgi multimerization or defective tubular packing in WPBs (i.e. type 2B von Willebrand disease (vWD)) [38, 39].

WPBs originate from clathrin and clathrin adaptor-protein1-coated vesicles, [35, 40] which, when loaded with vWF cargo, bud from the trans-Golgi network, continue to mature and vWF contained in them becomes densely pack and highly multimeric vWF [35]. Once the vesicles had formed, they lose the clathrin coat, and the interactions between WPBs and the actin cytoskeleton are thought to either tether WPBs to the perinuclear cytosolic compartment or to relocate WPBs in the proximity of the plasma membrane in preparation for fusion and exocytosis [41]. Upon secretion of its contents, WPBs dissociate from the membrane and are recycled and refilled [35].

Interestingly, vWF secretion is influenced by plasma sodium level [42]. In mice subjected to mild water restriction, elevated endothelial vWF protein levels correlated with increased number of micro thrombi in capillaries [42]. Hypernatremia causes up-regulation of vWF gene expression via nuclear factor of activated T-cells 5 (NFAT5) binding to the vWF promoter [42]. Another regulator of vWF was found to be autophagy [43]. Endothelial cell-specific ATG7 (critical factor in autophagy) deficient mice have prolonged bleeding times as compared to control, and decreased vWF secretion of immature vWF [43].

At least two different secretion mechanisms of WPB cargo have been reported so far: selective, time-dependent 'kiss-and-run' release [13] and differential release of the distinct components of these storage granules [8]. Apart from vWF, WPBs also contain other inflammatory and vasoactive mediators: P-selectin, Rab-27, coagulation factor XIIIa, tissue plasminogen activator, interleukin-8 (IL-8), eotaxin, endothelin-1, endothelin-converting enzyme, calcitonin-gene-related peptide, α1,3-fucosyltransferase VI and angiopoietin 2 [44]. vWF and the other components—stockpiled in and liberated as needed from WPBs—provide the ECs with the ability to react acutely to restore homeostasis; vWF plays a role in hemostasis and thrombosis, and also, in the regulation of inflammation [45], vascular permeability [27] and angiogenesis [46].

vWF is synthesized exclusively by ECs, megakaryocytes and platelets and stored in specialized secretory granules. EC WPBs and platelet α-granules share several characteristics, as both organelles contain vWF, P-selectin and CD63 [47, 48]. But, in platelets, vWF detection by immune-gold labeling is restricted to a subset of spherical α-granules [48]. In this vane, spherical secretory α-granules are quite distinct from WPBs. First, the vWF content of platelets is relatively low: 0.05–0.1 U per 3×10^8 platelets [49]. For comparison, plasma vWF concentration is 1–1.8 U/mL (10 μg/mL blood), of which only 15% of plasma vWF comes from platelets, while the majority 85% of the total vWF comes from ECs [4, 20, 34, 50]. Second, ECs combine basal and regulated vWF release, while platelets do not have a mechanism of basal secretion and, thus, substantial platelet activation would be needed for platelet vWF secretion to significantly contribute to the elevated blood vWF observed in different disease states. Finally, excessive secretion of EC-derived vWF in inflammation is attributed to the large capacity of ECs to make and store vWF in EC-specific storage pool, that is, in WPBs.

Thus, EC secretory granules supply the vasculature with circulating vWF to control hemostasis and thrombosis, while platelets play only a secondary role in this process [20, 49]. A balanced level of EC-derived vWF is critical to overcome the thrombotic complications in pathological settings, therefore it is important to understand the underlying endothelial constitutive and evoked exocytosis mechanisms which provide the bloodstream vWF in health and disease.

2.2. Basal versus regulated vWF secretion

Secretion of vWF occurs by one of the following three modes:

1. regulated secretion from WPBs, in response to a specific agonist (secretagogue) on-demand upon vascular injury [51, 52];
2. basal (constitutive-like or continuous) secretagogue-independent secretion of vWF from WPBs [7];
3. constitutive, secretagogue-independent release of vWF from non-WPB compartments [34, 40].

Over the years, there have been in the field opposite views about how much vWF is released through each of these three pathways and what determines the balance between basal (constitutive-like) and regulated vWF secretion is still under debate [34, 53, 54].

2.2.1. Basal vWF secretion

In resting ECs, secretion of vWF was thought to take place predominantly via conventional constitutive vWF secretion which is susceptible to protein synthesis inhibitor cycloheximide [34]. However, the importance of this pathway was exaggerated initially, as it could be drawn from the more recently published studies listed below. A vWF multimeric analysis in ECs challenged this view, indicating that highly multimeric vWF might be released solely from WPB storage pool [53]. Most recently, the issue was revisited when a study using metabolic labeling of vWF in human umbilical vein ECs (HUVECs) showed that most of the vWF secreted from unstimulated cells is not mediated by conventional constitutive secretion, but rather by basal release from the WPBs [7, 55]. Giblin and colleagues [7] recently brought more evidence to dismiss the belief that multimeric vWF passes uninterrupted from the Golgi to plasma membrane. They showed that freshly synthetized vWF is held for at least 24 h in WPBs before unstimulated release occurred, escaping cycloheximide-induced inhibition of protein synthesis, and, thus, consistent with release from the storage pool [7]. Similarly, Romani de Wit and coworkers [56] studied the dynamics of GFP-vWF-positive WPBs in resting HUVECs over time, and they were able to capture multiple image frames of WPBs traveling long distances toward the cell periphery. Intriguingly, resting ECs displayed membrane-apposed accumulation of GFP-vWF-containing vesicles [33, 56, 57]. It is worth mentioning here that only whenever a component of the cytoplasmic machinery is ablated the constitutive vWF secretion becomes predominant [40]. Taken together, these studies of WPBs behavior suggest that only the multimeric form of vWF is stored and that ECs secrete multimeric vWF via a continuous secretory pathway, which is a source of vWF in the bloodstream. If the WPB storage compartment is the source of the continuously secreted form of vWF that travels in the bloodstream, then the ability to regulate this constitutive vWF secretory route has significant clinical implications. Disruption of continuous vWF secretion may be implicated in the pathophysiology of type 2 vWD, which is due to both reduced vWF-dependent platelet function and reduced highly multimeric vWF in plasma.

http://dx.doi.org/10.5772/intechopen.74029

2.2.2. *Regulated vWF secretion*

The release of vWF from the regulated pathway occurs only following stimulation of ECs with an appropriate agonist, providing the endothelium with the means to react to its microenvironment by finely tuning the rate of release.

The notion that blood collected under stress clots faster was known for a while. In the 1970s, it was found that desmopressin (a synthetic analog of vassopresin) can elevate vWF level twofolds in healthy individuals [58] The follow-up studies showed that desmopressin activates vasopressin receptor 2 (V2R) on ECs and triggers cyclic adenosine monophosphate (cAMP)-mediated release of vWF from EC WPBs [58]. A multitude of agonists have been reported to induce vWF release via regulated secretion. These include thrombin [51], calcium ionophores [34], hypoxia [59], vasopressin [58], histamine [14], complement [60], platelet-activating factor [61] and interleukins [62]. Importantly, high shear stress is modulating regulated vWF release [63].

2.3. G protein signaling in hemostasis and thrombosis

In order to understand how to control WPB secretion for therapeutic purposes, the signaling mechanisms of vWF secretion need to be elucidated.

The exocyst is a cytoplasmic protein complex which targets secretory granules from the trans-Golgi network to the plasma membrane; it facilitates docking and priming of the secretory granule to the plasma membrane, prior to SNARE-mediated fusion [64]. When WPBs are trafficked to the plasma membrane, the vesicles are aligned such that v-SNAREs from the vesicles and t-SNAREs from target membrane can assemble as α-helix zippers which pull the membranes together. This SNARE zipper model was studied in detail in synapses [65]. Interestingly, all major players of these complexes identified in neurons are also present in the endothelium, including SNAP23, syntaxin 2, 3 and 4, and vesicle-associated membrane protein 3 (VAMP3) complex which are thought to regulate vWF exocytosis [11].

Release of WPBs contents into the extracellular space is thought to occur via GTPase-dependent processes [10]. It has been postulated that G proteins mediate cell type and signaling microdomain-specific functions. According to the classic G protein signaling model, heterotrimeric G proteins are located in the proximity of the plasma membrane where they can be activated by seven transmembrane spanning receptors, the canonical G protein-coupled receptors (GPCRs), to provoke downstream signaling events. G proteins are GTPases that typically function through GTP hydrolysis and cycling between nucleotide free GDP-bound and GTP-bound forms. GTPases also control the timing and specificity of vesicle trafficking and the exocyst partners recognition events, without GTP hydrolysis [66, 67]; the distinction between cycling and non-cycling GTPases might be more obvious when examining the effect of GTP hydrolysis-deficient mutant proteins that would be expected to cause gain-of-function on non-cycling GTPases and loss-of-function on cycling GTPases [66]. Furthermore, several studies indicate heterotrimeric G proteins can rapidly shuttle between the plasma membrane and intracellular membranes to exercise their function upon cell-specific organelles, along the secretory routes. Activation of GPCRs and G protein α and $\beta\gamma$ subunits of Gs, Gi, Gq/11 and G12/13 can stimulate secretory granule release [10, 68]. It has been shown, for example, by fluorescence polarization, that G protein i/o $\beta\gamma$ subunit competes with synaptotagmin for specific interaction sites on t-SNAREs, namely syntaxin 1 and SNAP25B (Synaptosomal-associated protein 25) [69]. G protein i/o binds to the SNARE at the plasma membrane, but in the presence of synaptotagmin and calcium, inhibits vesicle fusion with the plasma membrane, suggesting the G $\beta\gamma$-SNARE axis has an inhibitory role during synaptic exocytosis [69]. In the exocrine pancreas, G proteins have been shown to play a role in early transport events [68].

A role for G proteins Gαq/11 and Gα12/13 in hemostasis has been previously reported [70, 71]. Platelets from Gαq-deficient mice fail to respond to low doses of platelet-activating agonists and these mice have prolonged bleeding times and reduced thrombus formation after intravenous administration of adrenaline/collagen [71, 72]. Studies in megakaryocyte-restricted Gα12/13 double knockout mice reveal that these mice have prolonged bleeding time and reduced thrombus formation, suggesting that Gα13-dependent signaling in platelets is also relevant for hemostasis and thrombosis [70]. Interestingly, we found that, in addition to Gαs stimulatory-G protein [58, 73], Gα12 and Gαq/11 facilitate exocytosis of vWF from ECs [10]. Importantly, in Gα12 overexpression studies, Gα12 is able to localize to the plasma membrane because of its palmitoylation at cysteine 11 [74]. Palmitoylation targets Gα12 to lipid rafts fractions [75]. Both wild-type Gα12wt and Gα12QL (constitutive active) were observed in lipid rafts fractions, and therefore, the localization of Gα12 to discreet endothelial microdomains may be independent of Gα12 activation [76]. Other studies reported direct G protein-dependent regulation of the SNARE protein fusion machinery is required for secretory granule exocytosis [77], and Gα12 was shown by the yeast two-hybrid method to interact with a member of the exocytotic assembly, α-SNAP [66]. Using cultured human ECs and knockout mouse models, we showed that depletion of Gα12 or α-SNAP inhibited both basal and thrombin-induced vWF secretion and that Gα12$^{-/-}$ mice exhibit mildly reduced blood levels of vWF, but intact vWF multimeric pattern, and impaired thrombus formation [10]. Our studies suggest that Gα12 may interact directly with α-SNAP to promote the docking and fusion of WPBs [10]. Furthermore, Gα12 and Gαq subunits, which are known to regulate actin cytoskeleton rearrangements in ECs via activation of RhoA GTPase, promote WPB docking on the plasma membrane, providing both direct and indirect mechanisms linking GPCR activation and SNARE complex fusion [10].

2.4. Kinetics of WPB secretion

Secretion of vWF from ECs is mediated by fusion of WPBs with the plasma membrane in a manner dependent on the ATPase N-ethylmaleimide-sensitive-factor (NSF), soluble-NSF-attachment protein alpha (α-SNAP) and SNAREs [78]. NSF binds to SNARE complexes to facilitate the disassembly of the zippered bundles [79]. Because NSF lacks a direct binding domain for members of the SNARE family, it connects via an adaptor, α-SNAP [80]. Six NSF proteins assemble together at the plasma membrane, and each NSF hexamer requires three α-SNAPs to mediate binding to the SNAREs [78]. Once the NSF/α-SNAP/SNARE complex is formed, NSF hydrolyses ATP, providing the energy necessary for the disassembly of the

SNARE complex [81]. Therefore, the rate of exocytosis depends on α-SNAP and NSF activity [78]. Using PC12 cells as an α-SNAP-regulated exocytosis model, it was shown that α-SNAP, in absence of NSF activity, can actually block exocytosis and that this α-SNAP-dependent event occurs by direct binding of α-SNAP to free syntaxin, thus preventing SNARE complex assembly [82]. It is documented that α-SNAP is activated in the exocyst complex by phosphorylation [83], that α-SNAP binds and stimulates NSF ATPase activity, [84] that Gα12 interacts with α-SNAP, [66] and that S-nitrosylation of NSF inhibits WPB exocytosis [85]. α-SNAP regulates exocytosis of granules from different types of cells [86]. α-SNAP binding to the SNARE complex in the fused membrane mediates recruitment and activation of NSF resulting of exocytosis from ECs [10, 87]. The Gα12 binding site for α-SNAP was recently identified by using a library of substitution mutants within myc-tagged Gα12QL in which regions of the cDNA encoding consecutive six aminoacids were replaced with a sequence encoding the following six aminoacids: asparagine-alanine-alanine-isoleucine-arginine-serine (NAAIRS) by oligonucleotide-directed mutagenesis and expressed in a cell line as described previously [88], followed by evaluation of direct binding between Gα12 NAAIRS mutants and α-SNAP by glutathione S-transferase (GST) pulldown [10]. Based on the evidence generated by the GST pulldown assay, we constructed an α-*S*NAP *B*inding *D*omain peptide to which we added a myristoyl group and micellar nanoformulation for cellular entry, to further assess the role of Gα12 interaction with α-SNAP in vWF secretion [89, 90].

2.5. Spatial and temporal regulators of the exocyst complex

Secretion of vWF from ECs is mediated by small GTPases via both second messengers Ca^{2+} and cAMP-dependent signaling pathways [91–93]. Small GTPases are the effectors of the exocyst complex, involved in temporal coordination, spatial segregation and proof-reading of membrane trafficking events [94]. Rab and Ral GTPases are thought to be involved in vesicle tethering, whereas RhoGTPases are spatial regulators of the exocyst complex [95].

RalA was the first GTPase found to co-sediment with WPBs in density gradients [96]. Ral A is activated by its exchange factor, Ral guanine-nucleotide dissociation stimulator (RalGDS) [97], which is kept inactive by β-arrestin under static conditions [98]. Upon GPCR activation, Ral GDS uncouples from β-arrestin and functions in its GTP-bound state. RalGDS downregulation with siRNA in thrombin-stimulated HUVECs leads to accumulation of WPBs in the proximity of the plasma membrane, but exocytosis is incomplete, suggesting RalGDS/ β-arrestin complex is necessary to link thrombin receptors to WPBs exocytosis [98]. Ral A facilitates WPBs trafficking and delivery to the plasma membrane [91]. Ral A has been implicated in actin cytoskeleton dynamic rearrangements through its direct interactions with effectors filamin A and RalBP1/RLIP76 (a RAC/CDC42 guanine-nucleotide activating protein (GAP) [99]. RalBP1 links RhoGTPases and RalGTPases, and, of note, RalBP1 GAP has an ATP binding domain, although it is not clear whether this domain is a motor required for assembly of the exocyst [99]. Studies conducted in our laboratory suggest that human pulmonary artery ECs treated with filamin A siRNA attenuates constitutive and thrombin-induced vWF secretion [100]. It has been proposed that Ral A/Ca^{2+}-dependent signaling might be a prerequisite for the exocytotic machinery [101].

The second point of intervention for the Rab and Ral GTPases is anchoring and fusion of WPBs with the plasma membrane [8]. Ral A also promotes exocytosis by increasing phospholipase D1 (PLD1) activity and subsequent phosphatidic acid (PA) production, thereby facilitating plasma membrane fusion as described in more detail in Section 2.6 of this chapter. The Rabs are a family of over 60 members of small GTPases that control membrane identity and the actions of the intracellular vesicles; each type of secretory vesicle in the cells has a unique set of Rab family members, as reviewed in [102]; of these, six Rab proteins were found in association with WPBs:Rab3 isoform b [103], Rab3 isoform d [104], Rab27a [105], Rab3 isoform a, Rab15, Rab33a, Rab37 [106] and Rab35 [107]. Rab 27a is located on the cytosolic face of WPBs, is used as a marker of organelle identity, and has multifunctional capacities: it could either mildly inhibit the secretion of WPBs by associating with its effector MyRIP (myosin VIIa and Rab-interacting protein), thus anchoring WPBs to actin filaments and keeping them from attaching to the plasma membrane until the right timing, [57] or it could strongly activate the secretion of WPBs by associating with an alternate effector, synaptotagmin-like protein 4 (or granuphilin) (Slp4-a), [108] which links the secretory granules to the plasma membrane via syntaxin-binding protein 1 and syntaxin 2 and 3 [108, 109]. The ratio of Rab27a occupancy by Slp4-a or MyRIP dictates whether Rab27a is stimulatory or inhibitory with regards to WPB exocytosis [103]. Furthermore, Rab27 was shown to work synergistically with Rab15 to control exocytosis; Zografou et al. recently showed that simultaneous knockdown of the two Rabs using siRNA in HUVEC leads to a greater reduction in vWF secretion compared with knockdown of either Rab alone [106]. Their experiments further showed that Munc13-4, a known effector of Rab27a, co-localized with Rab15 on WPBs. The three proteins, Rab27a, Rab15 and Munc13-4, thus form a complex and work in tandem to help regulate exocytosis of vWF [106]. Rab 33b has an inhibitory effect on vWF secretion [106].

A recent genome-wide screen identified a completely new signaling pathway associated with WPB exocytosis. Rab 35, which is controlled by Rab GAP TBC1D10A, promotes ACAP2 (ArfGAP with coiled-coil, Ank repeat and pleckstrin homology domain-containing protein) activation, which inhibits histamine-induced Ca^{2+}-dependent vWF and P-selectin expression in human ECs. This study used constitutively active mutants of Rab35, downregulation with siRNA and a fluorescence activated cell sorting (FACS)-based vWF secretory assay to prove that Rab35 promotes histamine-induced vWF secretion in a TBC1D10A- and ACAP2-dependent manner [107]. Of note, ACAP2 GAP targets Arf 6 which is a positive regulator of vWF secretion from human ECs, as shown by total internal reflection fluorescence (TIRF) microscopy and FACS-based vWF secretory essay [107]. Arf 6 GTPase activity at the plasma membrane elevates phosphatidylinositol 4,5-bisphosphate (PI (4,5) P_2) levels via PI (4)P5-kinase activation, acting antagonistically to Rab35 through TBC1D10A Rab GAP [107]. Finally, among the Rabs found to be in association with WPBs, only Rab27 is known to be involved in basal secretion [57, 108].

2.6. Endothelial cell secretory microdomains

GTPase-mediated exocyst activity of the SNARE assembly occurs in specific regions of the plasma membrane with distinct lipid profiles [110]. Namely, we know there is an increase in

PA production in HUVECs upon stimulation with histamine, which is a known agonist to induce exocytosis of WPB contents [111]. The increase in PA production is mediated by recruitment and activation of PLD1, an enzyme that hydrolyses phosphatidylcholine to produce PA [111]. PLD1 downregulation using shRNA resulted in a reduced secretion of vWF upon histamine stimulation [111]. PLD1 is commonly thought of as a general promoter of membrane fusion because of its role in producing fusogenic conical lipids such as PA [112]. PLD1 requires activation by one or more factors specific to the cell type and activation pathway, including small GTPases such as those of the ADP-ribosylation factor/Rho families as well as RalA, RalGDS or protein kinase C [113]. Thus, RalA and RalGDS not only play a role in the exocytosis process itself, as discussed in Section 2.5, but are also directly associated with the cytosolic face of WPBs. Therefore, it has been suggested that RalA could serve as an upstream activator of PLD1, promoting PLD1 movement to the membrane and subsequent generation of PA-enriched membrane microdomains important for membrane fusion [97].

2.7. Zyxin and other proteins that regulate vWF release from endothelial cells

Data published by Han et al. show that zyxin, a focal adhesion LIM domain-containing protein, is involved in thrombin-mediated remodeling of the actin cytoskeleton [114]. The molecular structure of zyxin predicts its function in cytoskeletal dynamics [115]. Zyxin has proline-rich repeats at the N terminus followed by a leucine-rich nuclear export signal (NES) and three copies of a cysteine- and histidine-rich motif called the LIM domain at the C terminus [115]. Regulators of cytoskeletal dynamics, such as Enap/vasodilator-stimulated phosphoprotein (VASP) family members and α-actinin interact with the proline-rich region of zyxin. Zyxin can generate new actin structures in a VASP-dependent manner, independently of the Arp2/3 complex that cooperates with members of the Wiskott-Aldrich syndrome family of proteins (WASP) to nucleate actin filaments [114, 116]. Zyxin is a VASP-dependent actin polymerization machine in cells [117], and Han et al. showed zyxin binds to the C-terminal domain of protease-activated receptor 1 (PAR-1) [114]. Upon disruption of PAR-1-zyxin interaction, thrombin-induced formation of actin stress fibers was inhibited further supporting the hypothesis that zyxin functions as a signal transducer in PAR-1 signaling. In contrast, downregulation of zyxin did not affect thrombin-induced activation of RhoA or Gi, Gq and G12/13 heterotrimeric G proteins, implicating a novel signaling pathway regulated by PAR-1 that is not mediated by G proteins. Depletion of zyxin using siRNA inhibited thrombin-induced actin stress fiber formation and serum response element (SRE)-dependent gene transcription. In addition, depletion of zyxin resulted in delay of endothelial barrier restoration after thrombin treatment. In 2017, Han et al. reported that downregulation of zyxin in HUVECs with shRNA inhibits cAMP-dependent secretion of vWF [116]. In zyxin shRNA-expressing cells, formation of the actin framework around exocytic WPBs was scarce. Moreover, phosphorylation of zyxin at serines 142 and 143 (S142/S143) is critical for vWF secretion since the zyxin mutant could not rescue the defect in zyxin shRNA-treated cells [116]. They showed that a protein kinase A (PKA)-specific inhibitor blocked zyxin phosphorylation at S142/S143 and concluded that zyxin acts downstream of PKA [116]. Han et al. thus proposed a novel model for cytoskeleton reorganization around WPBs undergoing exocytosis. Upon epinephrine stimulation, pre-existing filaments are reorganized to form actin frameworks around exocytotic granules, limiting granule movement and promoting their localization in close proximity to the plasma membrane [116]. Then, actin monomers are recruited from the cytosol to form coat structures around granules within actin frameworks that promote fusion [116]. It was postulated that ECs use this synergistic strategy for effective and precise exocytosis. Under their experimental conditions, zyxin downregulation with shRNA had no effect on vWF release upon thrombin or histamine stimulation, whereas these mice exhibited impaired epinephrine-stimulated vWF release, prolonged bleeding time and thrombosis. Live cell super-resolution microscopy allowed visualization of zyxin-dependent reorganization of pre-existing actin filaments around WPBs before fusion. Using the total internal reflection fluorescence structured illumination microscopy (TIRF-SIM) technique, it was possible to achieve simultaneous visualization of the dynamics of fine cortical actin filaments and the behavior of the exocytotic granule in close proximity of the plasma membrane. Zyxin promotes the recruitment of the actin regulatory protein α-actinin; α-actinin is an actin crosslinking protein [114]. To prove the co-localization of zyxin with its interacting partners, they co-expressed zyxin construct tagged with mCherry for fluorescence microscopy detection (zyxin-mCherry) and Lifeact tagged with green fluorescence protein (GFP-Lifeact) (Life act is an actin binding peptide used in microscopy to monitor the behavior of actin filaments). Interestingly, the assembly of the pre-existing filaments started when WPBs were still tubular, so the formation of the actin framework appeared as a pre-fusion event by TIRF-SIM. Alexa Fluor 647-G actin incorporation assay indicated that pre-existing actin filaments reorganize to form the actin framework around the tubular WPBs, and G-actin was also recruited to form the actin coat structure in proximity to WPBs fused to the membrane and connected with the actin frameworks. Once WPBs became spherical and fluorescently-labeled, vWF was expulsed and fluorescence intensity declined in the expulsed area. The authors explain that the exocytotic events shown by variable-angle TIRF are mediated by the contraction of the actin coat which squeezes out WPB contents, followed by retraction of the depleted WPBs in the cytoplasm [116].

3. Dynamics of vWF reactivity in acute diseases

3.1. vWF as a surrogate marker of endothelial dysfunction

Association between vascular dysfunction and increased vWF levels is well established. The first study found a correlation between factor VIII antigen (another name for vWF) and kidney vascular damage in the context of glomerulonephritis in the 1970s [118]. Since this time, there have been many reports of inflammatory diseases associated with elevated vWF, that is, in acute systemic inflammation disorders such as sepsis, acute respiratory distress syndrome or systemic inflammatory response syndrome [73], T2DM [119] and TTP [120].

Upon activation of ECs, vWF acts as an acute phase reactant and correlates with serum C-reactive protein (CRP) level, another acute phase reactant [121, 122]. Other hemostatic proteins also behave in this way (i.e. factor VIII, fibrinogen and plasminogen inhibitor 1). Active vWF corresponds to the form of vWF required for platelet receptor GpIb binding [123–125].

http://dx.doi.org/10.5772/intechopen.74029

Detection of active vWF is now possible using an assay based on a nanobody AU/vWF a11 which allows investigators to distinguish between the active and latent conformations of the vWF A1 domain [123]. Several pathological conditions are associated with a disturbed balance in vWF activation and inactivation kinetics and thereby increased levels of active vWF and thrombotic complications [126]. The same active vWF assay revealed that levels of circulating active vWF increased approximately twofold in patients with acquired and congenital TTP [123, 126]. More and more evidence indicates that vWF is a biomarker of EC activation, but there are numerous discrepancies among the various clinical studies [127, 128]. In a more recent effort to advance the use of plasma vWF as a clinical marker of vascular inflammation, Hyseni et al. measured plasma concentrations of active vWF in a cohort of 275 patients with systemic inflammatory response syndrome [45]. They reported that patients with an elevated level of active vWF on admission had a twofold higher mortality rate [45]. In contrast, despite strongly elevated vWF levels, no predictions of mortality could be obtained based on total vWF [45]. Elevated active vWF is thus now regarded as an independent biomarker of poor outcome in patients with acute lung injury [129]. Mechanical ventilation is necessary to support the critical ill, but it also exacerbates injury through mechanical stress-activated signaling pathways, therefore it is expected to affect the disease outcome [130]. Consistent with these findings, an earlier 28-day study of 50 patients van der Heijden et al. reported that high vWF levels correlated with pulmonary compliance [Vt/(Pplat –PEEP)], where Vt = tidal volume, Pplat = plateau pressure, PEEP = positive end-expiratory pressure throughout the course of septic shock while patients were mechanically ventilated [131].

3.2. vWF/ADAMTS13 axis in vascular health and disease

In order to fulfill its functions, vWF remodels in a few distinct ways [16, 132–136]. In ECs, vWF forms tubular structures inside acidic WPBs secretory granules [137]. The switch that converts highly packed vWF tubules into ultra-large vWF strings in the blood stream is critically important but poorly understood. Recently, more insight has been gained into the mechanism of rapid transition from tightly packed vWF tubules into intraendothelial granules to vWF strings that function at physiological pH. It is likely that distal to the fused end of the WPB, alkalinisation induces a rapid conformational change in the structure of vWF, which propagates causing vWF to unfurl in a concerted manner at the site of secretion, resulting in the loss of the storage conformation [132].

The highly multimeric, elongated form of vWF is not present in healthy plasma, but it is found in various pathological settings. This observation can be explained by the fact that vWF senses shear forces and remodels accordingly [134]. Atomic force micrographs have demonstrated at the single molecule level that under static conditions, vWF assumes a globular conformation, whereas, under high shear flow, vWF turns into an extended chain format [16] that forms ultra-large strings to which platelets bind to initiate clot formation at sites of vascular damage [25] and, when shear stress is above 30.000 s^{-1}, factor VIII is released from its carrier protein to provide factor VIII to the coagulation cascade [138]. We now realize that, while ultra-large MW (molecular weight) vWF is essential for the normal hemostasis, this multimeric array should not become too large because it alters the thrombotic propensity [15, 16, 133, 134, 138–147].

The last biosynthetic step required for the formation of normal vWF is the limited proteolysis of the multimeric array by the circulating metalloprotease ADAMTS13 [126, 135]. ADAMTS-13 is produced mainly by the hepatic stellate cells [148]. Secondarily, the enzyme is synthesize in other cell type (ECs, podocytes, platelets and glial cells), but the physiological importance of these other sources was not yet established [149]. ADAMTS-13 plasma concentration is in the range of 0.7–1.4 μg/mL [150]. Interestingly, ADAMTS-13 is secreted into the circulation as an active enzyme and has a plasma half-life of approximately 2–4 days [151]. The mechanism of ADAMTS-13 clearance is not completely elucidated. It has been suggested that the hepatic asialoglycoprotein receptor could be involved in ADAMTS-13 clearance [152]. It is believed that newly released multimeric forms of vWF become tethered to the EC surface through the interaction with P-selectin [153, 154] and become partially unfolded [16], allowing for ADAMTS13 cleavage of the multimeric arrays [136]. The physiological proteolytic processing of vWF by ADAMTS13 occurs between Tyr1605-Met1606 in the central A2 domain of vWF, and is facilitated by partially unfolding vWF by flow conditions in the microcirculation [124, 126, 155–162].

Too little cleavage of the newly released vWF produces a tendency for microvascular thrombotic occlusion, as in TTP [120], and too much cleavage by ADAMTS13 results in type 2 like vWD and a bleeding phenotype [38]. Cleavage is dramatically increased during systemic inflammation [45] and other prothrombotic conditions, and there is an inverse relationship between plasma levels of vWF and ADAMTS-13; under high shear stress/inflammatory conditions, the circulating vWF can acquire autoimmune resistance to proteolysis by ADAMTS-13 or ADAMTS-13 is quickly exhausted as there is more vWF to cleave than available cleaving enzyme for consumption [45]. Additionally, a decrease in the vWF-inactivating protease ADAMTS13 is dependent on the severity of the disease and organ dysfunction [163].

In mice models, vWF-deficiency abrogates the ADAMTS13-deficient prothrombotic state [164] and endotoxemia-induced thrombosis in mice [165], consistent with the observation that vWF-deficient mice subjected to the polymicrobial model of sepsis exhibit increased survival [29]. It has been recently reported that neutrophil-derived small peptides or human neutrophil peptides (HNPs) also known as α-defensins can inhibit cleavage of vWF by ADAMTS13 [166]; these peptides [167] have sequence similarities with the ADAMTS-13 spacer domain RRY motif and can bind to the cleavage site for ADAMTS-13 on the vWF A2 domain. It was shown that HNPs levels are high in TTP patients [166]. Pro-inflammatory cytokine IL-6 limits ADAMTS-13 function [168, 169], while IL-8 and TNF-α stimulate further the release of vWF from WPBs [168].

In conclusion, excessive levels of the highly prothrombotic and multimeric form of vWF and/or ADAMTS13 deficiency constitute a unifying pathologic mechanism linking inflammation to thrombosis [170].

3.3. vWF role in ischemic stroke

Stroke remains a major health concern and a leading cause of death in the adult population. As a result of intracerebral thrombosis, cerebral ischemia/reperfusion injury causes brain tissue

http://dx.doi.org/10.5772/intechopen.74029

damage [171]. vWF promotes intracerebral thrombo-inflammatory response in the context of acute stroke [167, 172–175] and the vWF/ADAMTS13 axis was found to be involved in acute and chronic ischemic cerebrovascular events in patients [175]. vWF-deficient mice are protected from ischemic stroke [174]. It is well known that circulating vWF originates primarily from the endothelium, with a minor contribution from platelets [20]. Our current understanding of the role of different pools of vWF in the pathophysiology of acute stroke is based on mouse models [176]. EC-vWF mice are chimeric mice that express vWF only in ECs. Irradiated mice transplanted with bone marrow from vWF−/− mice to repopulate myeloid cells lack vWF in platelets but express vWF in ECs. Plt-mice are chimeric $vWF^{-/-}$ mice transplanted with normal bone marrow, and therefore have vWF in platelets [176]. The wild-type (WT), $vWF^{-/-}$, Plt-vWF and EC-vWF mice were subjected to 1 h ischemia followed by 23 h reperfusion and the outcome was compared [176]. The infarct volume and neurological outcome were comparable in WT and EC-vWF mice and decreased in $vWF^{-/-}$ mice. The stroke outcome in EC-vWF mice was documented using triphenyl-tetrazolium chloride-stained serial brain sections after 1 h transient middle cerebral artery occlusion. Also, it was observed in EC-VWF mice that there was a reduced local cerebral blood flow as assessed by Doppler flowmeter and a higher rate of thrombus formation in comparison to $vWF^{-/-}$ mice assessed by intravital microscopy. Stroke, infarction, vascular spasm and iatrogenic thrombotic events cause ischemia, which has a dramatic impact on vital organs. Post-ischemic reperfusion changes the pH, and extracellular alkalinization stimulates the physiological mechanisms that directly promote EC activation and can double vWF release in a $[Ca^{2+}]$-dependent manner [171]. Delaying the pH recovery with a Na^+/H^+ exchange subtype I pump inhibitor (applied in the perfusion media) [171] might prove to be a promising new way of inhibiting EC activation upon reperfusion injury. Taken together, EC-vWF seems to be the primary determinant of vWF-dependent ischemic stroke [171, 176], while platelet vWF plays a minor role [20, 176]. The ability to control vWF secretion from dysfunctional endothelium might be a valuable therapeutic target in stroke prone patients.

3.4. vWF role in sepsis

Apart from its primary role in hemostasis, vWF has a dual role in the pathophysiology of severe sepsis. On the one hand, vWF is involved in host-defense with a possible initial protective role in preventing complement activation [121]. In addition to its classical role in platelet binding, the vWF A1 domain also plays a role in vWF-dependent inflammatory responses. vWF and platelets promote leukocyte diapedesis, downstream of leukocyte tethering, rolling and adhesion in a mouse model of thioglycollate-induced peritonitis [177]. Polymorphonuclear leukocytes seem to directly interact with vWF via P-selectin glycoprotein ligand-1 and β2-integrins [178] As shown in mice in which inflammation was provoked by two different methods, [27] vWF-regulated leukocyte recruitment can be blocked by administration of a blocking anti-vWF llama nanobody, KB-VWF-006, which has picomolar affinity for the vWF A1 domain [27].

On the other hand, sepsis is not only a systemic inflammatory condition, it is also a state of dysfunctional endothelium and coagulation. One of the early on signs of systemic endothelial activation is sepsis-induced elevation of plasma vWF levels [121, 129, 163, 179]. Sepsis can promote DIC, which is common in critically ill patients. When unfolded, highly multimeric sepsis-induced vWF interacts with platelets [26] and generates small clots in the microvasculature [45, 124]. Microvascular thrombosis appears to be a major pathological mechanism in sepsis pathology resulting in multi-organ dysfunction syndrome (MODS) [124]. Hence, sepsis-induced vWF secretion in excess in DIC and MODS are inevitably linked. In addition, sepsis-induced ultra-large high molecular weight multimeric vWF permits complement activation, [121] leading to a positive feedback cycle of inflammation and thrombosis.

In murine model of sepsis, mice subjected to cecal ligation and puncture (CLP) have increased circulating levels of vWF that promote a procoagulant phenotype and poor outcome [29]. vWF-deficient mice subjected to the CLP model of sepsis exhibit increased survival [180]. For the purpose of testing whether Gα12 modulates vWF secretion in sepsis pathological setting, we subjected Gα12$^{-/-}$ mice and WT control mice to the CLP model of polymicrobial sepsis and monitored survival [181]. Our preliminary results indicate that 80% of the Gα12$^{-/-}$ mice survived, while all WT mice succumbed in the first 96 h [182]. To further determine whether decreased vWF was responsible for the protective effect of G12 deficiency, we restored circulating vWF level in Gα12$^{-/-}$ mice, by intravenous administration of purified vWF [10], to the level observed in WT mice. This procedure resulted in the loss of the protective effect of G12 deletion [182]. Furthermore, we employed a pharmacological G12 inhibition approach to prove G12 involvement in sepsis-induced vWF secretion [183]. We hypothesized that a synthetic peptide derived from Gα12 would inhibit α-SNAP-dependent WPB priming and fusion with the plasma membrane [89, 182], thereby inhibiting vWF secretion from activated ECs, and reducing the risk of thrombotic microangiopathy during sepsis [182].

3.5. vWF role in other inflammatory diseases

Transient elevations of plasma vWF level were also observed after epinephrine infusion [184], and chronic elevation of circulating vWF (2–3-fold) was reported in hyperthyroidism, which is thought to be due to β-adrenergic receptor stimulation. In contrast, hypothyroidism is associated with a 15% decrease in vWF level, although this is reversible with appropriate treatment [185].

vWF secretion from ECs might play a role in sickle cell disease pathogenesis [186, 187]. Erythrocytes bind specifically to vWF [186] and stasis, or the reduction of blood flow and shear, promotes binding of erythrocytes to vWF which form fibrin-rich regions in venous thrombi [186].

4. vWF-related antithrombotic treatment strategies

Despite recent major advances in the vascular biology of thrombosis, we face unmet treatment needs which warrant search for novel antithrombotic medication. Inhibition of vWF secretion constitutes an attractive therapeutic strategy to counteract thrombus initiation and propagation as the plasma concentration of vWF increases in high risk populations and predicts cardiovascular disease outcome. In this section, we review the drugs with the potential of vWF antagonism, illustrating how they might become an option to overcome current limitations of antithrombotic therapy.

Most of the studies involving anti-vWF antibodies were conducted in animal models. Monoclonal antibodies have been widely tested in murine, monkey and rabbit models of cardiovascular disease, including coronary thrombosis, stroke and in-stent stenosis: GPG-290, 6B4-Fab, AJW200, 82D6A6 and SZ-123 [188, 189]. These are all agents with antithrombotic and anti-inflammatory effects which do not prolong bleeding time and do not provoke thrombocytopenia. However, to date, none of these have made it into clinical trials. Hillgruber and colleagues recently published a study that found a massive accumulation of vWF in skin biopsies of patients suffering from leukocytoclastic vasculitis, an immune complex (IC)-mediated vasculitis (ICV) frequently encountered in dermatology that is caused by IC precipitation in the vessel wall followed by recruitment of neutrophils [28]. These results were confirmed in a murine model of vasculitis [28], and importantly, they identified ICs as possible vWF secretagogues. Of note, polyclonal anti-vWF blocking antibodies had an anti-inflammatory effect, reducing leukocyte recruitment and edema formation in a murine model of vascular inflammation [28]. Although the physiological implications of elevated vWF levels (increasing up to 400% of the normal level in various conditions [190, 191]) require additional investigation, it is currently believed that plasma vWF level is a surrogate marker of increased risk of vascular complications in septic patients and in those with vascular disease, which makes vWF antagonism a promising therapeutic target in thrombosis and inflammation.

Aptamers and nanobodies have been demonstrated to directly interfere with the vWF pathway, suggesting their powerful antithrombotic properties and acceptable level of safety may prove to be useful strategies. Aptamers are oligonucleotides that have similar characteristics with monoclonal antibodies and with small molecules. ARC1779 is an aptamer that binds to the A1 domain of vWF, blocking its interaction with GpIb and thereby inhibiting vWF-dependent platelet function. Clinical trials with ARC1779 were conducted and completed, but until truly meaningful clinical endpoints can be obtained that indicate effective inhibition of thrombosis without increasing bleeding, the utility of aptamers will remain unclear. Before the clinical trial was prematurely closed by the sponsor, the clinical and laboratory data after 14 days of dosing in nine patients with TTP aged 18–75 were very promising, and the authors optimistically proposed the study continuation (www.clinicaltrials.com; [192]) suggesting further development may be in order.

Nanobodies have the advantage of being highly specific therapeutic agents. Caplacizumab (ALX-0081) is an anti-vWF humanized nanobody that selectively targets vWF A1 domain, locking platelets launching on VWF A1 domain via interaction with their receptor GPIb. TITAN phase II trial concluded that caplacizumab administration in 75 patients with acquired TTP lead to a rapid resolution of the acute TTP episode, but it was adversely seconded by mild bleeding when compared to placebo group [193–195].

Unlike the vWF aptamer or antibodies, a pharmacological inhibitor of vWF secretion would have the advantage of acting from the inside of ECs, thereby limiting the amount of vWF available to support binding of platelets and thrombus formation. Studies thus far from our group suggest inhibition of Gα12-dependent activation of vWF secretion from WPBs may in fact be one such option [89, 90, 181, 182, 196]. Ongoing studies are demonstrating that inhibition of vWF secretion from ECs, using a novel peptide inhibitor to block Gα12/α-SNAP-dependent WPB exocytosis [89], reduces DIC and mortality in septic mice [89, 90, 182, 183, 196].

5. Conclusions

The development of antithrombotic drugs continues to be an active area of research. As there is not a straightforward relationship between therapeutic intervention and improvement of endothelial function, but rather a complicated interrelation between multiple subcellular "targets", research has focused on understanding the underlying mechanisms leading to vWF elevation in the circulation. Development of novel non-invasive diagnostic methods that facilitate early detection of endothelial damage and dysfunction and expand our knowledge of the etiology of cardiovascular disease are aggressively being pursued. In this overview, we present currently available literature concerning the contribution of endothelial cell activation/dysfunction to the increase in the level of plasma vWF in the context of inflammatory cardiovascular disease. While differential diagnosis of infectious and non-infectious organ damage associated with high vWF levels is not possible using vWF as a marker, elevated levels of vWF correlate very well with organ failure and poor survival and thus encourage further pursuit of this line of research toward novel drug therapy.

Author details

Luiza Rusu* and Richard D. Minshall

*Address all correspondence to: luizarusu123@gmail.com

Ohio State University, University of Illinois at Chicago, USA

References

[1] Vlot AJ, Koppelman SJ, Bouma BN, Sixma JJ. Factor VIII and von Willebrand factor. Thrombosis and Haemostasis. 1998;**79**(3):456-465

[2] Borchiellini A, Fijnvandraat K, ten Cate JW, Pajkrt D, van Deventer SJ, Pasterkamp G, et al. Quantitative analysis of von Willebrand factor propeptide release in vivo: Effect of experimental endotoxemia and administration of 1-deamino-8-D-arginine vasopressin in humans. Blood. 1996;**88**(8):2951-2958

[3] Blann AD. How a damaged blood vessel wall contibutes to thrombosis and hypertenasion. Pathophysiology of Haemostasis and Thrombosis. 2003;**33**(5–6):445-448

[4] Sadler JE, Shelton-Inloes BB, Sorace JM, Harlan JM, Titani K, Davie EW. Cloning and characterization of two cDNAs coding for human von Willebrand factor. Proceedings of the National Academy of Sciences of the United States of America. 1985;**82**(19): 6394-6398

[5] Wagner DD, Saffaripour S, Bonfanti R, Sadler JE, Cramer EM, Chapman B, et al. Induction of specific storage organelles by von Willebrand factor propolypeptide. Cell. 1991; **64**(2):403-413

[6] Nishio K, Anderson PJ, Zheng XL, Sadler JE. Binding of platelet glycoprotein Ibalpha to von Willebrand factor domain A1 stimulates the cleavage of the adjacent domain A2 by ADAMTS13. Proceedings of the National Academy of Sciences of the United States of America. 2004;**101**(29):10578-10583

[7] Giblin JP, Hewlett LJ, Hannah MJ. Basal secretion of von Willebrand factor from human endothelial cells. Blood. 2008;**112**(4):957-964

[8] Cleator JH, Zhu WQ, Vaughan DE, Hamm HE. Differential regulation of endothelial exocytosis of P-selectin and von Willebrand factor by protease-activated receptors and cAMP. Blood. 2006;**107**(7):2736-2744

[9] Borissoff JI, Spronk HM, Heeneman S, ten Cate H. Is thrombin a key player in the 'coagulation-atherogenesis' maze? Cardiovascular Research 2009;**82**(3):392-403

[10] Rusu L, Andreeva A, Visintine DJ, Kim K, Vogel SM, Stojanovic-Terpo A, et al. G protein-dependent basal and evoked endothelial cell vWF secretion. Blood. 2014;**123**(3): 442-450

[11] Pulido IR, Jahn R, Gerke V. VAMP3 is associated with endothelial weibel-palade bodies and participates in their Ca(2+)-dependent exocytosis. Biochimica et Biophysica Acta. 2011;**1813**(5):1038-1044

[12] Fu J, Naren AP, Gao X, Ahmmed GU, Malik AB. Protease-activated receptor-1 activation of endothelial cells induces protein kinase Calpha-dependent phosphorylation of syntaxin 4 and Munc18c: Role in signaling p-selectin expression. The Journal of Biological Chemistry. 2005;**280**(5):3178-3184

[13] Babich V, Meli A, Knipe L, Dempster JE, Skehel P, Hannah MJ, et al. Selective release of molecules from Weibel-Palade bodies during a lingering kiss. Blood. 2008;**111**(11):5282-5290

[14] Erent M, Meli A, Moisoi N, Babich V, Hannah MJ, Skehel P, et al. Rate, extent and concentration dependence of histamine-evoked Weibel-Palade body exocytosis determined from individual fusion events in human endothelial cells. The Journal of Physiology. 2007;**583**(Pt 1):195-212

[15] Goerge T, Niemeyer A, Rogge P, Ossig R, Oberleithner H, Schneider SW. Secretion pores in human endothelial cells during acute hypoxia. The Journal of Membrane Biology. 2002;**187**(3):203-211

[16] Seyfried BK, Friedbacher G, Rottensteiner H, Schwarz HP, Ehrlich H, Allmaier G, et al. Comparison of plasma-derived and recombinant von Willebrand factor by atomic force microscopy. Thrombosis and Haemostasis. 2010;**104**(3):523-530

[17] Gralnick HR, Coller BS. Studies of the human factor VIII/von Willebrand's factor protein. II. Identification and characterization of the von Willebrand protein. Blood. 1975; **46**(3):417-430

[18] Nogami K, Shima M, Nishiya K, Hosokawa K, Saenko EL, Sakurai Y, et al. A novel mechanism of factor VIII protection by von Willebrand factor from activated protein C-catalyzed inactivation. Blood. 2002;**99**(11):3993-3998

[19] Nachman RL, Jaffe EA. The platelet-endothelial cell–VIII axis. Thrombosis and Haemostasis. 1976;**35**(1):120-123

[20] Kanaji S, Fahs SA, Shi Q, Haberichter SL, Montgomery RR. Contribution of platelet vs. endothelial VWF to platelet adhesion and hemostasis. Journal of Thrombosis and Haemostasis. 2012;**10**(8):1646-1652

[21] Lazzari MA, Sanchez-Luceros A, Woods AI, Alberto MF, Meschengieser SS. Von Willebrand factor (VWF) as a risk factor for bleeding and thrombosis. Hematology. 2012;**17**(Suppl 1):S150-S152

[22] Chen J, Ling M, Fu X, Lopez JA, Chung DW. Simultaneous exposure of sites in von willebrand factor for glycoprotein Ib binding and ADAMTS13 cleavage: Studies with Ristocetin. Arteriosclerosis, Thrombosis, and Vascular Biology; **32**(11):2625-2630

[23] Andre P, Denis CV, Ware J, Saffaripour S, Hynes RO, Ruggeri ZM, et al. Platelets adhere to and translocate on von Willebrand factor presented by endothelium in stimulated veins. Blood. 2000;**96**(10):3322-3328

[24] Ruggeri ZM. Von Willebrand factor. Current Opinion in Hematology. 2003;**10**(2):142-149

[25] Ruggeri ZM. Von Willebrand factor, platelets and endothelial cell interactions. Journal of Thrombosis and Haemostasis. 2003;**1**(7):1335-1342

[26] Ruggeri ZM, De Marco L, Gatti L, Bader R, Montgomery RR. Platelets have more than one binding site for von Willebrand factor. The Journal of Clinical Investigation. 1983; **72**(1):1-12

[27] Ayme G, Adam F, Legendre P, Bazaa A, Proulle V, Denis CV, et al. A novel single-domain antibody against von Willebrand factor A1 domain resolves leukocyte recruitment and vascular leakage during inflammation-brief report. Arteriosclerosis, Thrombosis, and Vascular Biology. 2017;**37**(9):1736-1740

[28] Hillgruber C, Steingraber AK, Poppelmann B, Denis CV, Ware J, Vestweber D, et al. Blocking von Willebrand factor for treatment of cutaneous inflammation. The Journal of Investigative Dermatology. 2014;**134**(1):77-86

[29] Lerolle N, Dunois-Larde C, Badirou I, Motto DG, Hill G, Bruneval P, et al. Von Willebrand factor is a major determinant of ADAMTS-13 decrease during mouse sepsis induced by cecum ligation and puncture. Journal of Thrombosis and Haemostasis. 2009; **7**(5):843-850

[30] Weibel ER, Palade GE. New cytoplasmic components in arterial endothelia. The Journal of Cell Biology. 1964;**23**:101-112

[31] Zimmerman TS, Ratnoff OD, Powell AE. Immunologic differentiation of classic hemophilia (factor 8 deficiency) and von Willebrand's dissase, with observations on combined deficiencies of antihemophilic factor and proaccelerin (factor V) and on an acquired circulating anticoagulant against antihemophilic factor. The Journal of Clinical Investigation. 1971;**50**(1):244-254

[32] van Mourik JA, Romani de Wit T, Voorberg J. Biogenesis and exocytosis of Weibel-Palade bodies. Histochemistry and Cell Biology 2002;**117**(2):113-122

[33] Voorberg J, Fontijn R, Calafat J, Janssen H, van Mourik JA, Pannekoek H Biogenesis of von Willebrand factor-containing organelles in heterologous transfected CV-1 cells. The EMBO Journal 1993;**12**(2):749-758

[34] Sporn LA, Marder VJ, Wagner DD. Inducible secretion of large, biologically potent von Willebrand factor multimers. Cell. 1986;**46**(2):185-190

[35] Zenner HL, Collinson LM, Michaux G, Cutler DF. High-pressure freezing provides insights into Weibel-Palade body biogenesis. Journal of Cell Science. 2007;**120**(Pt 12):2117-2125

[36] Zhou YF, Eng ET, Zhu J, Lu C, Walz T, Springer TA. Sequence and structure relationships within von Willebrand factor. Blood. 2012;**120**(2):449-458

[37] Wagner DD, Marder VJ. Biosynthesis of von Willebrand protein by human endothelial cells: Processing steps and their intracellular localization. The Journal of Cell Biology. 1984;**99**(6):2123-2130

[38] Scaglione GL, Lancellotti S, Papi M, De Spirito M, Maiorana A, Baronciani L, et al. The type 2B p.R1306W natural mutation of von Willebrand factor dramatically enhances the multimer sensitivity to shear stress. Journal of Thrombosis and Haemostasis. 2013;**11**(9): 1688-1698

[39] Valentijn KM, Eikenboom J. Weibel-Palade bodies: A window to von Willebrand disease. Journal of Thrombosis and Haemostasis. 2013;**11**(4):581-592

[40] Lui-Roberts WW, Collinson LM, Hewlett LJ, Michaux G, Cutler DF. An AP-1/clathrin coat plays a novel and essential role in forming the Weibel-Palade bodies of endothelial cells. The Journal of Cell Biology. 2005;**170**(4):627-636

[41] Rondaij MG, Bierings R, Kragt A, Gijzen KA, Sellink E, van Mourik JA, et al. Dynein-dynactin complex mediates protein kinase A-dependent clustering of Weibel-Palade

bodies in endothelial cells. Arteriosclerosis, Thrombosis, and Vascular Biology. 2006; **26**(1):49-55

[42] Dmitrieva NI, Burg MB. Secretion of von Willebrand factor by endothelial cells links sodium to hypercoagulability and thrombosis. Proceedings of the National Academy of Sciences of the United States of America. 2014;**111**(17):6485-6490

[43] Torisu T, Torisu K, Lee IH, Liu J, Malide D, Combs CA, et al. Autophagy regulates endothelial cell processing, maturation and secretion of von Willebrand factor. Nature Medicine. 2013;**19**(10):1281-1287

[44] Rondaij MG, Bierings R, Kragt A, van Mourik JA, Voorberg J. Dynamics and plasticity of Weibel-Palade bodies in endothelial cells. Arteriosclerosis, Thrombosis, and Vascular Biology. 2006;**26**(5):1002-1007

[45] Hyseni A, Kemperman H, de Lange DW, Kesecioglu J, de Groot PG, Roest M. Active von Willebrand factor predicts 28-day mortality in patients with systemic inflammatory response syndrome. Blood. 2014

[46] Xiao J, Feng Y, Li X, Li W, Fan L, Liu J, et al. Expression of ADAMTS13 in normal and abnormal placentae and its potential role in angiogenesis and placenta development. Arteriosclerosis, Thrombosis, and Vascular Biology. 2017;**37**(9):1748-1756

[47] van Nispen tot Pannerden H, de Haas F, Geerts W, Posthuma G, van Dijk S, Heijnen HF. The platelet interior revisited: Electron tomography reveals tubular alpha-granule subtypes. Blood. 2010;**116**(7):1147-1156

[48] Sehgal S, Storrie B. Evidence that differential packaging of the major platelet granule proteins von Willebrand factor and fibrinogen can support their differential release. Journal of Thrombosis and Haemostasis. 2007;**5**(10):2009-2016

[49] Howard MA, Montgomery DC, Hardisty RM. Factor-VIII-related antigen in platelets. Thrombosis Research. 1974;**4**(5):617-624

[50] Nichols WL, Hultin MB, James AH, Manco-Johnson MJ, Montgomery RR, Ortel TL, et al. Von Willebrand disease (VWD): Evidence-based diagnosis and management guidelines, the National Heart, Lung, and Blood Institute (NHLBI) expert panel report (USA). Haemophilia. 2008;**14**(2):171-232

[51] Levine JD, Harlan JM, Harker LA, Joseph ML, Counts RB. Thrombin-mediated release of factor VIII antigen from human umbilical vein endothelial cells in culture. Blood. 1982; **60**(2):531-534

[52] Nightingale T, Cutler D. The secretion of von Willebrand factor from endothelial cells; an increasingly complicated story. Journal of Thrombosis and Haemostasis. 2013;**11**(Suppl 1): 192-201

[53] Tsai HM, Nagel RL, Hatcher VB, Seaton AC, Sussman II. The high molecular weight form of endothelial cell von Willebrand factor is released by the regulated pathway. British Journal of Haematology. 1991;**79**(2):239-245

[54] van den Biggelaar M, Hernandez-Fernaud JR, van den Eshof BL, Neilson LJ, Meijer AB, Mertens K, et al. Quantitative phosphoproteomics unveils temporal dynamics of thrombin signaling in human endothelial cells. Blood. 2014;**123**(12):e22-e36

[55] Johnsen J, Lopez JA. VWF secretion: What's in a name? Blood. 2008;**112**(4):926-927

[56] Romani de Wit T, Rondaij MG, Hordijk PL, Voorberg J, van Mourik JA. Real-time imaging of the dynamics and secretory behavior of Weibel-Palade bodies. Arteriosclerosis, Thrombosis, and Vascular Biology. 2003;**23**(5):755-761

[57] Nightingale TD, White IJ, Doyle EL, Turmaine M, Harrison-Lavoie KJ, Webb KF, et al. Actomyosin II contractility expels von Willebrand factor from Weibel-Palade bodies during exocytosis. The Journal of Cell Biology. 2011;**194**(4):613-629

[58] Kaufmann JE, Oksche A, Wollheim CB, Gunther G, Rosenthal W, Vischer UM. Vasopressin-induced von Willebrand factor secretion from endothelial cells involves V2 receptors and cAMP. The Journal of Clinical Investigation. 2000;**106**(1):107-116

[59] Pinsky DJ, Naka Y, Liao H, Oz MC, Wagner DD, Mayadas TN, et al. Hypoxia-induced exocytosis of endothelial cell Weibel-Palade bodies. A mechanism for rapid neutrophil recruitment after cardiac preservation. The Journal of Clinical Investigation. 1996;**97**(2):493-500

[60] Hattori R, Hamilton KK, McEver RP, Sims PJ. Complement proteins C5b-9 induce secretion of high molecular weight multimers of endothelial von Willebrand factor and translocation of granule membrane protein GMP-140 to the cell surface. The Journal of Biological Chemistry. 1989;**264**(15):9053-9060

[61] Hashemi S, Palmer DS, Aye MT, Ganz PR. Platelet-activating factor secreted by DDAVP-treated monocytes mediates von Willebrand factor release from endothelial cells. Journal of Cellular Physiology. 1993;**154**(3):496-505

[62] Denis CV, Kwack K, Saffaripour S, Maganti S, Andre P, Schaub RG, et al. Interleukin 11 significantly increases plasma von Willebrand factor and factor VIII in wild type and von Willebrand disease mouse models. Blood. 2001;**97**(2):465-472

[63] Galbusera M, Zoja C, Donadelli R, Paris S, Morigi M, Benigni A, et al. Fluid shear stress modulates von Willebrand factor release from human vascular endothelium. Blood. 1997;**90**(4):1558-1564

[64] Datta YH, Ewenstein BM. Regulated secretion in endothelial cells: Biology and clinical implications. Thrombosis and Haemostasis. 2001;**86**(5):1148-1155

[65] Jahn R, Fasshauer D. Molecular machines governing exocytosis of synaptic vesicles. Nature. 2012;**490**(7419):201-207

[66] Andreeva AV, Kutuzov MA, Vaiskunaite R, Profirovic J, Meigs TE, Predescu S, et al. G alpha12 interaction with alphaSNAP induces VE-cadherin localization at endothelial junctions and regulates barrier function. The Journal of Biological Chemistry. 2005;**280**(34):30376-30383

[67] Andreeva AV, Kutuzov MA, Voyno-Yasenetskaya TA. Scaffolding proteins in G-protein signaling. Journal of Molecular Signaling. 2007;**2**:13

[68] Sassmann A, Gier B, Grone HJ, Drews G, Offermanns S, Wettschureck N. The Gq/G11-mediated signaling pathway is critical for autocrine potentiation of insulin secretion in mice. The Journal of Clinical Investigation. 2010;**120**(6):2184-2193

[69] Zurawski Z, Page B, Chicka MC, Brindley RL, Wells CA, Preininger AM, et al. Gbetagamma directly modulates vesicle fusion by competing with synaptotagmin for binding to neuronal SNARE proteins embedded in membranes. The Journal of Biological Chemistry. 2017;**292**(29):12165-12177

[70] Moers A, Nieswandt B, Massberg S, Wettschureck N, Grüner S, Konrad I, et al. G13 is an essential mediator of platelet activation in hemostasis and thrombosis. Nature Medicine. 2003;**9**(11):1418-1422

[71] Offermanns S, Toombs CF, Hu YH, Simon MI. Defective platelet activation in G alpha (q)-deficient mice. Nature. 1997;**389**(6647):183-186

[72] Moers A, Wettschureck N, Gruner S, Nieswandt B, Offermanns S. Unresponsiveness of platelets lacking both Gaq and Ga13. The Journal of Biological Chemistry. 2004;**279**: 45354-45359

[73] Mannucci PM. Desmopressin (DDAVP) in the treatment of bleeding disorders: The first 20 years. Blood. 1997;**90**(7):2515-2521

[74] Ponimaskin E, Harteneck C, Schultz G, Schmidt MF. A cysteine-11 to serine mutant of G alpha12 impairs activation through the thrombin receptor. FEBS Letters. 1998;**429**(3):370-374

[75] Vaiskunaite R, Kozasa T, Voyno-Yasenetskaya TA. Interaction between the G alpha subunit of heterotrimeric G(12) protein and Hsp90 is required for G alpha(12) signaling. The Journal of Biological Chemistry. 2001;**276**(49):46088-46093

[76] Waheed AA, Jones TL. Hsp90 interactions and acylation target the G protein Galpha 12 but not Galpha 13 to lipid rafts. The Journal of Biological Chemistry. 2002;**277**(36):32409-32412

[77] Blackmer T, Larsen EC, Bartleson C, Kowalchyk JA, Yoon EJ, Preininger AM, et al. G protein betagamma directly regulates SNARE protein fusion machinery for secretory granule exocytosis. Nature Neuroscience. 2005;**8**(4):421-425

[78] Barnard RJ, Morgan A, Burgoyne RD. Stimulation of NSF ATPase activity by alpha-SNAP is required for SNARE complex disassembly and exocytosis. The Journal of Cell Biology. 1997;**139**(4):875-883

[79] Zhao C, Smith EC, Whiteheart SW. Requirements for the catalytic cycle of the N-ethylmaleimide-sensitive factor (NSF). Biochimica et Biophysica Acta. 2012;**1823**(1):159-171

[80] Clary DO, Griff IC, Rothman JE. SNAPs, a family of NSF attachment proteins involved in intracellular membrane fusion in animals and yeast. Cell. 1990;**61**(4):709-721

[81] Whiteheart SW, Rossnagel K, Buhrow SA, Brunner M, Jaenicke R, Rothman JE. N-ethylmaleimide-sensitive fusion protein: A trimeric ATPase whose hydrolysis of ATP is required for membrane fusion. The Journal of Cell Biology. 1994;**126**(4):945-954

[82] Barszczewski M, Chua JJ, Stein A, Winter U, Heintzmann R, Zilly FE, et al. A novel site of action for alpha-SNAP in the SNARE conformational cycle controlling membrane fusion. Molecular Biology of the Cell. 2008;**19**(3):776-784

[83] Hirling H, Scheller RH. Phosphorylation of synaptic vesicle proteins: Modulation of the alpha SNAP interaction with the core complex. Proceedings of the National Academy of Sciences of the United States of America. 1996;**93**(21):11945-11949

[84] Morgan A, Dimaline R, Burgoyne RD. The ATPase activity of N-ethylmaleimide-sensitive fusion protein (NSF) is regulated by soluble NSF attachment proteins. The Journal of Biological Chemistry. 1994;**269**(47):29347-29350

[85] Matsushita K, Morrell CN, Cambien B, Yang SX, Yamakuchi M, Bao C, et al. Nitric oxide regulates exocytosis by S-nitrosylation of N-ethylmaleimide-sensitive factor. Cell. 2003; **115**(2):139-150

[86] Rodríguez F, Bustos MA, Zanetti MN, Ruete MC, Mayorga LS, Tomes CN. α-SNAP prevents docking of the acrosome during sperm exocytosis because it sequesters monomeric syntaxin. PLoS One. 2011;**6**(7):e21925

[87] Niles WD, Malik AB. Endocytosis and exocytosis events regulate vesicle traffic in endothelial cells. The Journal of Membrane Biology. 1999;**167**(1):85-101

[88] Meigs TE, Juneja J, DeMarco CT, Stemmle LN, Kaplan DD, Casey PJ. Selective uncoupling of G alpha 12 from rho-mediated signaling. The Journal of Biological Chemistry. 2005; **280**(18):18049-18055

[89] Minshall RD, Rusu L. Compositions and method for treating thrombosis. Google Patents; 2014

[90] Rusu L, Schlapfer M, Offermanns S, Du X, Minshall RD. Abstract 659: Inhibition of vWF secretion with novel G alpha12 N-terminal alpha-SNAP binding domain peptide increases survival in septic rodents. Arteriosclerosis, Thrombosis, and Vascular Biology. 2015;**35**(Suppl 1):A659-A65A

[91] Rondaij MG, Sellink E, Gijzen KA, ten Klooster JP, Hordijk PL, van Mourik JA, et al. Small GTP-binding protein Ral is involved in cAMP-mediated release of von Willebrand factor from endothelial cells. Arteriosclerosis, Thrombosis, and Vascular Biology 2004;**24**(7): 1315-1320

[92] Birch KA, Ewenstein BM, Golan DE, Pober JS. Prolonged peak elevations in cytoplasmic free calcium ions, derived from intracellular stores, correlate with the extent of thrombin-stimulated exocytosis in single human umbilical vein endothelial cells. Journal of Cellular Physiology. 1994;**160**(3):545-554

[93] Klarenbach SW, Chipiuk A, Nelson RC, Hollenberg MD, Murray AG. Differential actions of PAR2 and PAR1 in stimulating human endothelial cell exocytosis and permeability: The role of rho-GTPases. Circulation Research. 2003;**92**(3):272-278

[94] Wu H, Rossi G, Brennwald P. The ghost in the machine: Small GTPases as spatial regulators of exocytosis. Trends in Cell Biology. 2008;**18**(9):397-404

[95] Roumanie O, Wu H, Molk JN, Rossi G, Bloom K, Brennwald P. Rho GTPase regulation of exocytosis in yeast is independent of GTP hydrolysis and polarization of the exocyst complex. The Journal of Cell Biology. 2005;**170**(4):583-594

[96] de Leeuw HP, Wijers-Koster PM, van Mourik JA, Voorberg J. Small GTP-binding protein RalA associates with Weibel-Palade bodies in endothelial cells. Thrombosis and Haemostasis. 1999;**82**(3):1177-1181

[97] Rondaij MG, Bierings R, van Agtmaal EL, Gijzen KA, Sellink E, Kragt A, et al. Guanine exchange factor RalGDS mediates exocytosis of Weibel-Palade bodies from endothelial cells. Blood. 2008;**112**(1):56-63

[98] Bhattacharya M, Anborgh PH, Babwah AV, Dale LB, Dobransky T, Benovic JL, et al. Beta-arrestins regulate a Ral-GDS Ral effector pathway that mediates cytoskeletal reorganization. Nature Cell Biology. 2002;**4**(8):547-555

[99] Mott HR, Owen D. RLIP76 (RalBP1): The first piece of the structural puzzle. Small GTPases. 2010;**1**(3):157-160

[100] Rusu L. Molecular Mechanisms of vWF Secretion [Doctoral]. Indigo: University of Illinois at Chicago; 2013

[101] Xie L, Kang Y, Liang T, Dolai S, Xie H, Parsaud L, et al. RalA GTPase tethers insulin granules to L- and R-type calcium channels through binding $\alpha 2$ δ-1 subunit. Traffic. 2013;**14**(4):428-439

[102] Stenmark H. Rab GTPases as coordinators of vesicle traffic. Nature Reviews. Molecular Cell Biology. 2009;**10**(8):513-525

[103] Bierings R, Hellen N, Kiskin N, Knipe L, Fonseca AV, Patel B, et al. The interplay between the Rab27A effectors Slp4-a and MyRIP controls hormone-evoked Weibel-Palade body exocytosis. Blood. 2012;**120**(13):2757-2767

[104] Knop M, Aareskjold E, Bode G, Gerke V. Rab3D and annexin A2 play a role in regulated secretion of vWF, but not tPA, from endothelial cells. The EMBO Journal. 2004;**23**(15): 2982-2992

[105] Hannah MJ, Hume AN, Arribas M, Williams R, Hewlett LJ, Seabra MC, et al. Weibel-Palade bodies recruit Rab27 by a content-driven, maturation-dependent mechanism that is independent of cell type. Journal of Cell Science. 2003;**116**(Pt 19):3939-3948

[106] Zografou S, Basagiannis D, Papafotika A, Shirakawa R, Horiuchi H, Auerbach D, et al. A complete Rab screening reveals novel insights in Weibel-Palade body exocytosis. Journal of Cell Science. 2012;**125**(Pt 20):4780-4790

[107] Biesemann A, Gorontzi A, Barr F, Gerke V. Rab35 protein regulates evoked exocytosis of endothelial Weibel-Palade bodies. The Journal of Biological Chemistry. 2017;**292**(28): 11631-11640

[108] Mizuno K, Fujita T, Gomi H, Izumi T. Granuphilin exclusively mediates functional granule docking to the plasma membrane. Scientific Reports. 2016;**6**:23909

[109] van Breevoort D, van Agtmaal EL, Dragt BS, Gebbinck JK, Dienava-Verdoold I, Kragt A, et al. Proteomic screen identifies IGFBP7 as a novel component of endothelial cell-specific Weibel-Palade bodies. Journal of Proteome Research. 2012;**11**(5):2925-2936

[110] Ammar M, Kassas N, Chasserot-Golaz S, Bader M-F, Vitale N. Lipids in regulated exocytosis: What are they doing? Frontiers in Endocrinology. 2013;**4**(125)

[111] Disse J, Vitale N, Bader MF, Gerke V. Phospholipase D1 is specifically required for regulated secretion of von Willebrand factor from endothelial cells. Blood. 2009;**113**(4):973-980

[112] Roth MG. Molecular mechanisms of PLD function in membrane traffic. Traffic. 2008;**9**(8): 1233-1239

[113] Jenkins GM, Frohman MA. Phospholipase D: A lipid centric review. Cellular and Molecular Life Sciences. 2005;**62**(19–20):2305-2316

[114] Han J, Liu G, Profirovic J, Niu J, Voyno-Yasenetskaya T. Zyxin is involved in thrombin signaling via interaction with PAR-1 receptor. The FASEB Journal. 2009;**23**(12):4193-4206

[115] Macalma T, Otte J, Hensler ME, Bockholt SM, Louis HA, Kalff-Suske M, et al. Molecular characterization of human zyxin. The Journal of Biological Chemistry. 1996;**271**(49): 31470-31478

[116] Han X, Li P, Yang Z, Huang X, Wei G, Sun Y, et al. Zyxin regulates endothelial von Willebrand factor secretion by reorganizing actin filaments around exocytic granules. Nature Communications. 2017;**8**:14639

[117] Fradelizi J, Noireaux V, Plastino J, Menichi B, Louvard D, Sykes C, et al. ActA and human zyxin harbour Arp2/3-independent actin-polymerization activity. Nature Cell Biology. 2001;**3**(8):699-707

[118] Boneu B, Abbal M, Plante J, Bierme R. Letter: Factor-VIII complex and endothelial damage. Lancet. 1975;**1**(7922):1430

[119] Berk KA, Oudshoorn TP, Verhoeven AJM, Mulder MT, Roks AJM, Dik WA, et al. Diet-induced weight loss and markers of endothelial dysfunction and inflammation in treated patients with type 2 diabetes. Clinical Nutrition ESPEN. 2016;**15**:101-106

[120] Bianchi V, Robles R, Alberio L, Furlan M, Lammle B. Von Willebrand factor-cleaving protease (ADAMTS13) in thrombocytopenic disorders: A severely deficient activity is specific for thrombotic thrombocytopenic purpura. Blood. 2002;**100**(2):710-713

[121] Feng S, Liang X, Kroll MH, Chung DW, Afshar-Kharghan V. Von Willebrand factor is a cofactor in complement regulation. Blood. 2015;**125**(6):1034-1037

[122] Pottinger BE, Read RC, Paleolog EM, Higgins PG, Pearson JD. Von Willebrand factor is an acute phase reactant in man. Thrombosis Research. 1989;**53**(4):387-394

[123] Groot E, de Groot PG, Fijnheer R, Lenting PJ. The presence of active von Willebrand factor under various pathological conditions. Current Opinion in Hematology. 2007; **14**(3):284-289

[124] De Filippis V, Lancellotti S, Maset F, Spolaore B, Pozzi N, Gambaro G, et al. Oxidation of Met1606 in von Willebrand factor is a risk factor for thrombotic and septic complications in chronic renal failure. The Biochemical Journal. 2012;**442**(2):423-432

[125] Lancellotti S, De Filippis V, Pozzi N, Oggianu L, Rutella S, Scaglione GL, et al. Oxidized von Willebrand factor is efficiently cleaved by serine proteases from primary granules of leukocytes: Divergence from ADAMTS-13. Journal of Thrombosis and Haemostasis. 2011;**9**(8):1620-1627

[126] Crawley JT, de Groot R, Xiang Y, Luken BM, Lane DA. Unraveling the scissile bond: How ADAMTS13 recognizes and cleaves von Willebrand factor. Blood. 2011;**118**(12): 3212-3221

[127] Paulus P, Jennewein C, Zacharowski K. Biomarkers of endothelial dysfunction: Can they help us deciphering systemic inflammation and sepsis? Biomarkers. 2011;**16**(Suppl 1): S11-S21

[128] Reinhart K, Bayer O, Brunkhorst F, Meisner M. Markers of endothelial damage in organ dysfunction and sepsis. Critical Care Medicine. 2002;**30**(Suppl 5):S302-S312

[129] Ware LB, Conner ER, Matthay MA. Von Willebrand factor antigen is an independent marker of poor outcome in patients with early acute lung injury. Critical Care Medicine. 2001;**29**(12):2325-2331

[130] Hepokoski M, Englert JA, Baron RM, Crotty-Alexander LE, Fuster MM, Beitler JR, et al. Ventilator-induced lung injury increases expression of endothelial inflammatory mediators in the kidney. American Journal of Physiology. Renal Physiology. 2017;**312**(4):F654-FF60

[131] van der Heijden M, Pickkers P, van Nieuw Amerongen GP, van Hinsbergh VW, Bouw MP, van der Hoeven JG, et al. Circulating angiopoietin-2 levels in the course of septic shock: Relation with fluid balance, pulmonary dysfunction and mortality. Intensive Care Medicine. 2009;**35**(9):1567-1574

[132] Zhou YF, Eng ET, Nishida N, Lu C, Walz T, Springer TA. A pH-regulated dimeric bouquet in the structure of von Willebrand factor. The EMBO Journal. 2011;**30**(19):4098-4111

[133] Muller JP, Lof A, Mielke S, Obser T, Bruetzel LK, Vanderlinden W, et al. pH-dependent interactions in dimers govern the mechanics and structure of von Willebrand factor. Biophysical Journal. 2016;**111**(2):312-322

[134] Muller JP, Mielke S, Lof A, Obser T, Beer C, Bruetzel LK, et al. Force sensing by the vascular protein von Willebrand factor is tuned by a strong intermonomer interaction. Proceedings of the National Academy of Sciences of the United States of America. 2016; **113**(5):1208-1213

[135] Furlan M, Robles R, Lammle B. Partial purification and characterization of a protease from human plasma cleaving von Willebrand factor to fragments produced by in vivo proteolysis. Blood. 1996;**87**(10):4223-4234

[136] Dong JF, Moake JL, Nolasco L, Bernardo A, Arceneaux W, Shrimpton CN, et al. ADAMTS-13 rapidly cleaves newly secreted ultralarge von Willebrand factor multimers on the endothelial surface under flowing conditions. Blood. 2002;**100**(12):4033-4039

[137] Michaux G, Abbitt KB, Collinson LM, Haberichter SL, Norman KE, Cutler DF. The physiological function of von Willebrand's factor depends on its tubular storage in endothelial Weibel-Palade bodies. Developmental Cell. 2006;**10**(2):223-232

[138] Bonazza K, Rottensteiner H, Schrenk G, Frank J, Allmaier G, Turecek PL, et al. Shear-dependent interactions of von Willebrand factor with factor VIII and protease ADAMTS 13 demonstrated at a single molecule level by atomic force microscopy. Analytical Chemistry. 2015;**87**(20):10299-10305

[139] Aponte-Santamaria C, Huck V, Posch S, Bronowska AK, Grassle S, Brehm MA, et al. Force-sensitive autoinhibition of the von Willebrand factor is mediated by interdomain interactions. Biophysical Journal. 2015;**108**(9):2312-2321

[140] Davydovskaya P, Janko M, Gaertner F, Ahmad Z, Simsek O, Massberg S, et al. Blood platelet adhesion to printed von Willebrand factor. Journal of Biomedical Materials Research. Part A. 2012;**100(**(2):335-341

[141] Lippok S, Kolsek K, Lof A, Eggert D, Vanderlinden W, Muller JP, et al. Von Willebrand factor is dimerized by protein disulfide isomerase. Blood. 2016;**127**(9):1183-1191

[142] Lof A, Muller JP, Benoit M, Brehm MA. Biophysical approaches promote advances in the understanding of von Willebrand factor processing and function. Advances in Biological Regulation. 2017;**63**:81-91

[143] Papi M, Maulucci G, De Spirito M, Missori M, Arcovito G, Lancellotti S, et al. Ristocetin-induced self-aggregation of von Willebrand factor. European Biophysics Journal. 2010; **39**(12):1597-1603

[144] Posch S, Aponte-Santamaria C, Schwarzl R, Karner A, Radtke M, Grater F, et al. Mutual a domain interactions in the force sensing protein von Willebrand factor. Journal of Structural Biology. 2017;**197**(1):57-64

[145] Siedlecki CA, Lestini BJ, Kottke-Marchant KK, Eppell SJ, Wilson DL, Marchant RE. Shear-dependent changes in the three-dimensional structure of human von Willebrand factor. Blood. 1996;**88**(8):2939-2950

[146] Tobimatsu H, Nishibuchi Y, Sudo R, Goto S, Tanishita K. Adhesive forces between A1 domain of von Willebrand factor and N-terminus domain of glycoprotein Ibalpha measured by atomic force microscopy. Journal of Atherosclerosis and Thrombosis. 2015; **22**(10):1091-1099

[147] Wu T, Lin J, Cruz MA, Dong JF, Zhu C. Force-induced cleavage of single VWFA1A2A3 tridomains by ADAMTS-13. Blood. 2010;**115**(2):370-378

[148] Zhou W, Inada M, Lee TP, Benten D, Lyubsky S, Bouhassira EE, et al. ADAMTS13 is expressed in hepatic stellate cells. Laboratory Investigation. 2005;**85**(6):780-788

[149] Plaimauer B, Fuhrmann J, Mohr G, Wernhart W, Bruno K, Ferrari S, et al. Modulation of ADAMTS13 secretion and specific activity by a combination of common amino acid polymorphisms and a missense mutation. Blood. 2006;**107**(1):118-125

[150] Rieger M, Ferrari S, Kremer Hovinga JA, Konetschny C, Herzog A, Koller L, et al. Relation between ADAMTS13 activity and ADAMTS13 antigen levels in healthy donors and patients with thrombotic microangiopathies (TMA). Thrombosis and Haemostasis. 2006;**95**(2):212-220

[151] Furlan M, Robles R, Morselli B, Sandoz P, Lammle B. Recovery and half-life of von Willebrand factor-cleaving protease after plasma therapy in patients with thrombotic thrombocytopenic purpura. Thrombosis and Haemostasis. 1999;**81**(1):8-13

[152] Barrett AJ, Rawlings ND, Woessner JF. Handbook of Proteolytic Enzymes. 2nd ed. Amsterdam, Boston: Elsvier Academic Press; 2004

[153] Padilla A, Moake JL, Bernardo A, Ball C, Wang Y, Arya M, et al. P-selectin anchors newly released ultralarge von Willebrand factor multimers to the endothelial cell surface. Blood. 2004;**103**(6):2150-2156

[154] Datta YH, Romano M, Jacobson BC, Golan DE, Serhan CN, Ewenstein BM. Peptido-leukotrienes are potent agonists of von Willebrand factor secretion and P-selectin surface expression in human umbilical vein endothelial cells. Circulation. 1995;**92**(11):3304-3311

[155] Lancellotti S, De Cristofaro R. Structure and proteolytic properties of ADAMTS13, a metalloprotease involved in the pathogenesis of thrombotic microangiopathies. Progress in Molecular Biology and Translational Science. 2011;**99**:105-144

[156] Lancellotti S, Dragani A, Ranalli P, Petrucci G, Basso M, Tartaglione R, et al. Qualitative and quantitative modifications of von Willebrand factor in patients with essential thrombocythemia and controlled platelet count. Journal of Thrombosis and Haemostasis. 2015;**13**(7):1226-1237

[157] Lynch CJ, Lane DA, Luken BM. Control of VWF A2 domain stability and ADAMTS13 access to the scissile bond of full-length VWF. Blood. 2014;**123**(16):2585-2592

[158] Xiang Y, de Groot R, Crawley JT, Lane DA. Mechanism of von Willebrand factor scissile bond cleavage by a disintegrin and metalloproteinase with a thrombospondin type 1 motif, member 13 (ADAMTS13). Proceedings of the National Academy of Sciences of the United States of America. 2011;**108**(28):11602-11607

[159] Xu AJ, Springer TA. Calcium stabilizes the von Willebrand factor A2 domain by promoting refolding. Proceedings of the National Academy of Sciences of the United States of America. 2012;**109**(10):3742-3747

[160] Zander CB, Cao W, Zheng XL. ADAMTS13 and von Willebrand factor interactions. Current Opinion in Hematology. 2015;**22**(5):452-459

[161] Zhang J, Ma Z, Dong N, Liu F, Su J, Zhao Y, et al. A conformation-sensitive monoclonal antibody against the A2 domain of von Willebrand factor reduces its proteolysis by ADAMTS13. PLoS One. 2011;**6**(7):e22157

[162] Zhou M, Dong X, Baldauf C, Chen H, Zhou Y, Springer TA, et al. A novel calcium-binding site of von Willebrand factor A2 domain regulates its cleavage by ADAMTS13. Blood. 2011;**117**(17):4623-4631

[163] Claus RA, Bockmeyer CL, Sossdorf M, Losche W. The balance between von-Willebrand factor and its cleaving protease ADAMTS13: Biomarker in systemic inflammation and development of organ failure? Current Molecular Medicine. 2010;**10**(2):236-248

[164] Chauhan AK, Walsh MT, Zhu G, Ginsburg D, Wagner DD, Motto DG. The combined roles of ADAMTS13 and VWF in murine models of TTP, endotoxemia, and thrombosis. Blood. 2008;**111**(7):3452-3457

[165] Patel KN, Soubra SH, Bellera RV, Dong JF, McMullen CA, Burns AR, et al. Differential role of von Willebrand factor and P-selectin on microvascular thrombosis in endotoxemia. Arteriosclerosis, Thrombosis, and Vascular Biology. 2008;**28**(12):2225-2230

[166] Pillai VG, Bao J, Zander CB, McDaniel JK, Chetty PS, Seeholzer SH, et al. Human neutrophil peptides inhibit cleavage of von Willebrand factor by ADAMTS13: A potential link of inflammation to TTP. Blood. 2016;**128**(1):110-119

[167] Kraft P, Drechsler C, Gunreben I, Nieswandt B, Stoll G, Heuschmann PU, et al. Von Willebrand factor regulation in patients with acute and chronic cerebrovascular disease: A pilot, case-control study. PLoS One. 2014;**9**(6):e99851

[168] Bernardo A, Ball C, Nolasco L, Moake JF, Dong JF. Effects of inflammatory cytokines on the release and cleavage of the endothelial cell-derived ultralarge von Willebrand factor multimers under flow. Blood. 2004;**104**(1):100-106

[169] Nguyen TC, Liu A, Liu L, Ball C, Choi H, May WS, et al. Acquired ADAMTS-13 deficiency in pediatric patients with severe sepsis. Haematologica. 2007;**92**(1):121-124

[170] Nguyen TC, Gushiken F, Correa JI, Dong JF, Dasgupta SK, Thiagarajan P, et al. A recombinant fragment of von Willebrand factor reduces fibrin-rich microthrombi formation in mice with endotoxemia. Thrombosis Research. 2015;**135**(5):1025-1030

[171] Huck V, Niemeyer A, Goerge T, Schnaeker EM, Ossig R, Rogge P, et al. Delay of acute intracellular pH recovery after acidosis decreases endothelial cell activation. Journal of Cellular Physiology. 2007;**211**(2):399-409

[172] Bongers TN, de Maat MP, van Goor ML, Bhagwanbali V, van Vliet HH, Gomez Garcia EB, et al. High von Willebrand factor levels increase the risk of first ischemic stroke: Influence of ADAMTS13, inflammation, and genetic variability. Stroke. 2006;**37**(11):2672-2677

[173] Khan MM, Motto DG, Lentz SR, Chauhan AK. ADAMTS13 reduces VWF-mediated acute inflammation following focal cerebral ischemia in mice. Journal of Thrombosis and Haemostasis. 2012;**10**(8):1665-1671

[174] Kleinschnitz C, De Meyer SF, Schwarz T, Austinat M, Vanhoorelbeke K, Nieswandt B, et al. Deficiency of von Willebrand factor protects mice from ischemic stroke. Blood. 2009;**113**(15):3600-3603

[175] Denorme F, Kraft P, Pareyn I, Drechsler C, Deckmyn H, Vanhoorelbeke K, et al. Reduced ADAMTS13 levels in patients with acute and chronic cerebrovascular disease. PLoS One. 2017;**12**(6):e0179258

[176] Dhanesha N, Prakash P, Doddapattar P, Khanna I, Pollpeter MJ, Nayak MK, et al. Endothelial cell-derived von willebrand factor is the major determinant that mediates von Willebrand factor-dependent acute ischemic stroke by promoting postischemic thrombo-inflammation. Arteriosclerosis, Thrombosis, and Vascular Biology. 2016;**36**(9):1829-1837

[177] Petri B, Broermann A, Li H, Khandoga AG, Zarbock A, Krombach F, et al. Von Willebrand factor promotes leukocyte extravasation. Blood. 2010;**116**(22):4712-4719

[178] Pendu R, Terraube V, Christophe OD, Gahmberg CG, de Groot PG, Lenting PJ, et al. P-selectin glycoprotein ligand 1 and beta2-integrins cooperate in the adhesion of leukocytes to von Willebrand factor. Blood. 2006;**108**(12):3746-3752

[179] Bockmeyer CL, Reuken PA, Simon TP, Budde U, Lösche W, Bauer M, et al. ADAMTS13 activity is decreased in a septic porcine model. Significance for glomerular thrombus deposition. Thrombosis and Haemostasis. 2011;**105**(1):145-153

[180] Kasuda S, Matsui H, Ono S, Matsunari Y, Nishio K, Shima M, et al. Relevant role of von Willebrand factor in neutrophil recruitment in a mouse sepsis model involving cecal ligation and puncture. Haematologica. 2016;**101**(2):e52-e54

[181] Rusu L, Bae M, Castellon M, Stojanovic-Terpo A, Christman JW, Du X, et al., editors. Novel G alpha12 N-terminal alpha-SNAP Binding Domain Peptide Inhibits vWF secretion, Prevents Microvascular Thrombosis, and Increases Survival in Septic Mice. AHA Scientific Sessions; 2016 November 2016; New Orleans

[182] Rusu L, Bae M, Castellon M, Stojanovic-Terpo A, Christman JW, Du X, et al. Abstract 20799: Novel G alpha 12 N-terminal alpha-SNAP binding domain peptide inhibits vWF secretion, prevents microvascular thrombosis and increases survival in septic mice. Circulation. 2016;**134**(Suppl 1):A20799-A

[183] Rusu L, Christman JW, Du X, Minshall RD. Inhibition of vWF Secretion with Novel Gα12 N-terminal α-SNAP Binding Domain Peptide Increases Survival in Septic Mice. Experimental Biology 2016 Meeting; April 2016; San Diego: The FASEB Journal; 2016. p. S943.8

[184] Vischer UM, Wollheim CB. Epinephrine induces von Willebrand factor release from cultured endothelial cells: Involvement of cyclic AMP-dependent signalling in exocytosis. Thrombosis and Haemostasis. 1997;**77**(6):1182-1188

[185] Liu L, Wang X, Lin Z, Wu H. Elevated plasma levels of VWF:Ag in hyperthyroidism are mediated through beta-adrenergic receptors. Endocrine Research. 1993;**19**(2–3):123-133

[186] Smeets MWJ, Mourik MJ, Niessen HWM, Hordijk PL. Stasis promotes erythrocyte adhesion to von Willebrand factor. Arteriosclerosis, Thrombosis, and Vascular Biology. 2017;**37**(9):1618-1627

[187] Sparkenbaugh E, Pawlinski R. Interplay between coagulation and vascular inflammation in sickle cell diseas. British Journal of Haematology. 2013;**162**(1):3-14

[188] Ji S, Jiang M, Yan B, Shen F, He Y, Wan A, et al. The chimeric monoclonal antibody MHCSZ-123 against human von Willebrand factor A3 domain inhibits high-shear arterial thrombosis in a rhesus monkey model. Journal of Hematology & Oncology. 2017; **10**(1):111

[189] Zhao YM, Jiang M, Ji SD, He Y, Shen F, Li XM, et al. Anti-human VWF monoclonal antibody SZ-123 prevents arterial thrombus formation by inhibiting VWF-collagen and VWF-platelet interactions in rhesus monkeys. Biochemical Pharmacology. 2013;**85**(7): 945-953

[190] Clark P, Brennand J, Conkie JA, McCall F, Greer IA, Walker ID. Activated protein C sensitivity, protein C, protein S and coagulation in normal pregnancy. Thrombosis and Haemostasis. 1998;**79**(6):1166-1170

[191] Bender M. High VWF, low ADAMTS13 puts women at risk. Blood. 2012;**119**(6):1329-1330

[192] Cataland SR, Scully MA, Paskavitz J, Maruff P, Witkoff L, Jin M, et al. Evidence of persistent neurologic injury following thrombotic thrombocytopenic purpura. American Journal of Hematology. 2011;**86**(1):87-89

[193] Peyvandi F, Callewaert F. Caplacizumab for acquired thrombotic thrombocytopenic Purpura. The New England Journal of Medicine. 2016;**374**(25):2497-2498

[194] Peyvandi F, Scully M, Kremer Hovinga JA, Cataland S, Knobl P, Wu H, et al. Caplacizumab for acquired thrombotic thrombocytopenic Purpura. The New England Journal of Medicine. 2016;**374**(6):511-522

[195] Peyvandi F, Scully M, Kremer Hovinga JA, Knobl P, Cataland S, De Beuf K, et al. Caplacizumab reduces the frequency of major thromboembolic events, exacerbations and death in patients with acquired thrombotic thrombocytopenic purpura. Journal of Thrombosis and Haemostasis. 2017;**15**(7):1448-1452

[196] Rusu L, Schlapfer M, Atkinson J, Du X, Minshall RD. Abstract 20277: Inhibition of vWF secretion prevents microvascular thrombosis in CLP rodent models of sepsis. Circulation. 2014;**130**(Suppl 2):A20277-A

Chapter 8

Hyperglycemia-Induced Endothelial Dysfunction

Domokos Gero

Additional information is available at the end of the chapter

http://dx.doi.org/10.5772/intechopen.71433

Abstract

Glucose-induced endothelial dysfunction plays a fundamental role in the development of diabetic vascular complications and glycemic control (the foundation of diabetes care) provides limited protection against the cardiovascular complications. Therefore, identification of novel drug targets and treatment approaches for diabetes complications represent a key direction of current pharmaceutical research. The "unifying theory" of hyperglycemia-induced endothelial cell injury organizes the events of cellular dysfunction in a linear cascade and identifies mitochondrial superoxide generation as the triggering event of the injury. Exposure to high glucose concentration for long periods or repeated glycemic swings may induce changes in metabolic substrate availability and lead to mitochondrial hyperpolarization. Changes in the mitochondrial membrane potential induce superoxide production by the electron transport chain and result in oxidative stress. Mitochondrial superoxide is also responsible for the induction of other sources of reactive oxygen species (ROS) within the cells, including advanced glycation end products (AGEs) and the NADPH oxidase. Mitochondria also show morphological changes and impaired assembly of the respiratory complexes occurs, which results in cellular energy failure, cell senescence and vascular dysfunction. Current intervention strategies aim to inhibit the mitochondrial ROS production and novel therapeutic approaches are expected to provide valuable tools in diabetes therapy in the upcoming years.

Keywords: hyperglycemia, diabetes, endothelial cells, oxidative stress, mitochondria, electron transport chain, superoxide, bioenergetics

1. Introduction

The significance of hyperglycemia-induced endothelial damage is underlined by its pathogenic role in diabetes complications and the associated costs of diabetes management. The global prevalence of diabetes among adults over 18 years of age has risen from 4.7% in 1980 to 8.5% in 2014 with a steep increase over the age of 50, reaching the peak prevalence of

25% above 80 years of age [1, 2]. The (direct and indirect) medical costs for patients with diabetes are double the amount compared to expenses for nondiabetic individuals and three times higher in case of cardiovascular diseases such as myocardial infarction or stroke [3]. Currently, diabetes-related healthcare expenditure accounts for 10% of the total healthcare costs and it is estimated to increase by 70% over the next 25 years leading to a serious societal and economic burden [4]. Diabetes complications are responsible for the majority of the associated costs and excess costs gradually increase with the duration of the disease leading to substantially higher expenses after 8–10 years [3, 5]. Hyperglycemia-induced endothelial dysfunction is the major contributor to the development of vascular disease in diabetes mellitus [6]. While insulin resistance may be present in patients with no increase in plasma glucose level and it may contribute to endothelial dysfunction, the major pathway that is responsible for endothelial damage is glucose-induced oxidative stress in diabetes [6, 7].

2. Characteristics of the damage

2.1. Glucose and oxidative stress in diabetic vascular damage

Endothelial dysfunction is a pathological state of the endothelium and can be defined as an aberration of the normal endothelial function of vascular relaxation, blood clotting and immune function. In general, it means impaired endothelium-dependent vasodilation as a result of imbalance between vasodilating and vasoconstricting substances produced by (or acting on) the endothelium. Endothelial dysfunction can be a significant predictor of coronary artery disease and atherosclerosis and it increases the risk of stroke and heart attack [8]. In basic science and in clinical research, endothelial function is commonly assessed by the use of the acetylcholine-mediated vasodilatation test or by flow-mediated vasodilation, and this methodology is considered the 'gold standard' at this moment [8, 9]. Endothelial dysfunction is primarily responsible for the impaired vasorelaxation in diabetes but it is closely followed by the development of vascular smooth muscle cell dysfunction [10, 11]. Impaired relaxation may be caused by diminished production or increased destruction of vasodilating factors or impaired response to them in diabetes. Oxidative stress is considered as one of the major underlying mechanisms, which leads to endothelial dysfunction in hyperglycemia, since the therapeutic supplementation of antioxidants or antioxidant enzymes can restore the endothelium-dependent vasodilation in experimental models of diabetes [10].

Glucose-induced damage is apparently controversial: glucose is a major source of energy and a small increase in blood glucose, which has no obvious ill effect on the short term, can cause serious long-term complications in diabetes. Glucose uptake is noninsulin dependent in endothelial cells and it occurs via GLUT1 (glucose transporter 1), thus high blood glucose level results in similarly high intracellular glucose concentration in endothelial cells [12, 13]. Endothelial cells have few mitochondria and primarily use glycolysis to produce ATP molecules, which suggests low oxygen consumption and relatively low level of oxidant production [14]. Furthermore, higher glucose concentration would allow even higher rate of anaerobic metabolism to produce the necessary amount of ATP and limit aerobic metabolism, oxygen consumption and reactive oxygen species (ROS) production in the cells. Still, hyperglycemia is associated with the activation of various ROS-producing pathways and increased oxidant production in endothelial cells [15, 16]. Oxidants play a significant role in the destruction of nitric oxide and other signaling molecules and result in impaired vasoreactivity [10, 17, 18]. Inflammatory pathways may be implicated in the early stages of the injury and they are typically involved in the later stages of the disease and contribute to oxidant production and inflammatory cytokine secretion, which can also change the vascular function [19]. Oxidative stress also induces DNA damage that triggers endothelial cell senescence that might have an impact on vascular function in the later stages of the injury [20]. There are approximately 2–10 trillion (2–10 × 10^{12}) endothelial cells in the human body and they form the endothelial surface of 500 m^2 of blood vessels and require constant renewal [21–23]. Mostly, the resident stem cells (located in the vessel wall) take part in the repair processes but also circulating progenitor cells that arise from the bone marrow are involved in the process [22]. In diabetes, endothelial cell turnover is impaired and it might be a consequence of accelerated aging or reduced renewal of cells [24, 25]. While ROS-mediated injury dominates in the earlier stages of hyperglycemia-induced damage, cell senescence and impairment of endothelial cell turnover may play the leading part in the later stages.

2.2. Target cells of hyperglycemia

Hyperglycemia induces damage in a select cell population in the body, including mainly the mesangial cells in the kidney, neurons and Schwann cells in peripheral nerves and a subset of endothelial cells: only the microvascular and the arterial endothelial cells show impairment [26]. Interestingly, this dichotomy in the vulnerability is often preserved in *in vitro* experiments: microvascular endothelial cells are more susceptible to glucose-induced injury, whereas venous endothelial cells show reduced oxidant production and damage. This suggests that differences in the pressure, blood flow or vessel function in various parts of the circulation may not be accounted for the susceptibility. It is rather an inherent difference between the cells that explain the vulnerability of the microvasculature [27]. There are differences in the protein and RNA expression patterns, including the miRNA expression profiles, and the different responses of microvascular and macrovascular endothelial cells to various metabolic stimuli may be attributed to this difference [28].

Differences in glucose uptake may be partially responsible for the susceptibility: most cells tightly regulate the glucose transport rate and prevent the unrestricted uptake, but endothelial and mesangial cells are unable to decrease the transport rate [29, 30]. Glucose overload induces a gradual increase in the mitochondrial membrane potential and the elevated protonic potential increases the superoxide generation by the respiratory chain [31]. The mitochondrial membrane potential is regulated by uncoupling proteins in the cells: these channels release excess protons from the intermembrane space to the matrix and protect against mitochondrial hyperpolarization. Endothelial cells express uncoupling protein 2 (UCP2) and its transport capacity is controlled by oxidative stress: high levels of oxidants open the channel, whereas the absence of oxidants closes the channel [32, 33]. In venous endothelial cells, hyperglycemia upregulates the expression of UCP2 and it effectively protects against mitochondrial hyperpolarization and ROS production [34, 35]. This process does not work in microvascular endothelial cells: there is no change in UCP2 expression in response to elevated glucose concentration resulting in mitochondrial hyperpolarization with a simultaneous rise in mitochondrial superoxide generation [35]. In many cases, endothelial cells were found to produce excess levels of mitochondrial oxidants in response to hyperglycemia only in the presence of pro-inflammatory cytokines, suggesting further mechanisms to be involved in the hyperglycemia-induced cell-damaging processes but the potential implication of inflammatory pathways has not been clarified [36].

2.3. Time course of hyperglycemic injury

At cellular level, hyperglycemic damage occurs within a few days and induces compensatory and repair mechanisms that may have consequences in the cell population. Vascular endothelium covers a huge surface in the body and possesses a huge capacity to compensate for any damage that occurs over longer periods, thus changes in vascular function may occur with a delay.

In experimental models, glucose levels are often above 20–30 mmol/L and vascular dysfunction develops over weeks or within a few months [37]. The development of hyperglycemia-induced endothelial cell damage is neither instantaneous *in vitro*, it usually takes a few days of exposure to high glucose levels to induce a significant increase in the mitochondrial membrane potential and oxidant production [35, 38]. Hyperglycemia-induced ROS production induces RNA and DNA damage that may be responsible for the reduced proliferation rate observed in endothelial cells [39]. Reduced proliferation and senescence occur after more than 10 doublings of endothelial cells exposed to 25 mmol/L glucose *in vitro* [25].

On the other hand, diabetic vascular complications occur after years of hyperglycemic exposure and poor glycemic control accelerates the development of the disease [40, 41]. Although complications usually first appear some years after clinical diagnosis, retinopathy and nephropathy were often present (in 10–37% of patients) at the time of clinical diagnosis or within the first year after diagnosis [42]. Glucose levels that induce endothelial damage are moderately elevated in most patients due to improved diabetes care and diabetes self-management education and support (DSME/S) [43, 44].

Endothelial cell senescence and reduced proliferation are the dominant features in diabetes, still pathological proliferation of blood vessels occurs in diabetic retinopathy [45]. This controversy is explained by the fact that progressive retinal angiogenesis is preceded by a series of events that is characterized by reduced cell proliferation and stimulates neovascularization in the retina [45]. Proliferative diabetic retinopathy is not the primary pathogenic response to hyperglycemia but a compensatory response to retinal hypoxia. Diabetic retinopathy starts with the loss of two cell types of the retinal capillaries: the endothelial cells and the vessel supporting pericytes and the earliest pathologic signs are acellular, nonperfused capillary segments in the retina [45]. Pericyte loss may precede the endothelial damage in the retina and it is caused by angiotensin II overexpression induced by oxidative stress in diabetes. However, the increased number of migrating pericytes and loss of pericytes from the straight

http://dx.doi.org/10.5772/intechopen.71433

parts of capillaries may also occur as a result of hypoxia, and thus might be a consequence of prior endothelial damage. On the other hand, the loss of pericytes results in reduced proliferation of stalk endothelial cells leading to fewer phalanx cells and promotes hypoxia in the retina. Hypoxia is the main stimulus of uncontrolled proliferation in diabetic vessels and both angiotensin II and vascular endothelial growth factor (VEGF) are involved in the neovascularization. In the pathological angiogenesis, not only the retinal endothelial cells take part but also the bone marrow-derived progenitor cells that may explain how enhanced proliferation capacity replaces the cell loss at the later stage.

3. Triggers of endothelial dysfunction and damage

3.1. Hyperglycemia and 'glucose memory'

Glucose-induced endothelial damage is not only caused by constantly high glucose concentration but also by transiently elevated glucose levels. In experimental models, damage induced by intermittent high glucose is comparable or more severe than the injury induced by constantly high glucose concentration. Glucose levels studied in most experimental models are often much higher than the values that cause irreversible damage in humans on the long term and result in accelerated progression of diabetic complications.

Diagnostic criteria for diabetes are based on the relationship between plasma glucose values and the risk of diabetes-specific microvascular complications: blood glucose concentration that causes diabetic vascular damage has been empirically determined and diagnostic criteria were established. The World Health Organization (WHO) introduced new diagnostic criteria in 1980, which were globally accepted, but had to lower the cut-off values for diabetes in 1999 since growing body of evidence supported the development of complications at lower blood glucose levels [46, 47]. The updated threshold values has raised considerable dispute and are often criticized for not preventing complications but further lowering has not been achieved because of the risk of hypoglycemia. The definition of hyperglycemia is challenging, since blood glucose values show a physiological increase after a meal and this calls for separate normal values for fasting, postprandial and random blood glucose levels. Still, it is evident that "high" glucose levels that induce damage in endothelial cells in the long term are very close to the normal blood glucose values, less than a twofold increase in the blood glucose level triggers injury in the cells. In the past, osmotic damage was presumed to play a pathogenic role in glucose-induced cellular injury but the minor changes in osmolality rule out this possibility. In healthy human subjects, the rise in blood glucose levels after a meal typically reaches or goes beyond these values, making the definition of hyperglycemia rather confusing [48]. From the pathogenic viewpoint of hyperglycemia, absolute cut-off values cannot be established to separate normoglycemic and hyperglycemic concentration ranges.

While earlier studies confirmed that the risk of cardiovascular complications corresponds to the average increase in glucose level (measured as glycated hemoglobin, HbA1c), more recent studies also found independent associations with the postprandial peaks [49]. These results highly suggest the action of secondary mediators that are rather induced by the fluctuations in blood glucose (glycemic variability) than by an absolute increase. Experimental models confirmed that glycemic swings caused at least as severe tissue damage as constant hyperglycemia, and persistence of high-glucose memory was postulated in cells and animals that were exposed to normoglycemic conditions following a hyperglycemic exposure [50–52]. Endothelial cells when returned to normal glucose concentration after exposure to high glucose showed increased ROS production and activation of poly(ADP-ribose) polymerase (PARP) even a week following the normalization of the glucose level and in this respect they showed similar characteristics to cells maintained at high glucose [52]. The persistence of oxidative stress in endothelial cells *in vitro* confirms that 'glucose memory' is an inherent feature of these cells. It also means that once hyperglycemia activates the various ROS-producing pathways they continue to produce oxidants for multiple days or weeks in endothelial cells even if the glucose level is fully normalized. Oxidative stress is the key feature of the changes induced by hyperglycemia, and 'metabolic memory' is another term used that refers to the characteristic metabolic changes [51]. The length of high glucose memory is unknown in humans but it is suspected to last longer than *in vitro* because (1) inflammatory pathways are also involved and (2) the response is not limited by the life cycle of single cells but it is possibly carried over to multiple cell generations.

Blockade of the early changes has been confirmed to prevent or slow down the progression of complications but the reversal at a later phase may not be achieved by glycemic control [53]. Benefits of intensive glucose control can be detected after 3 years of treatment if no retinopathy or mild disease is present at the start of the treatment strategy in type 1 diabetes [54]. The importance of blocking the glucose-induced damage early on in type 2 diabetes has been confirmed by the results of the United Kingdom Prospective Diabetes Study (UKPDS) [41]. On the other hand, there is little benefit of strict glucose control if established cardiovascular disease is already present at the start of the treatment regimen [53]. Similarly, in diabetic rats, a 6-month long period of good glycemic control following 2 months of poor glycemic control results in significantly reduced progression, whereas no benefit is observed on retinopathy if good glycemic control was started after 6 months of poor glycemic control: both nitrosative stress and tissue damage were similarly advanced as with 12 months of poor glycemic control [55, 56]. These suggest that the processes started by hyperglycemia may be partially reversed if normoglycemia follows a shorter period of high glucose exposure. It is still unclear whether the detrimental effects of transient hyperglycemia is buffered within the individual cells or it is the entire population of endothelial cells that compensate for the changes and the reason why progressive damage occurs following an extended hyperglycemic period is the loss of the renewal capacity of the cells.

3.2. Downstream molecules responsible for the damage

The mechanism of high glucose memory is still obscure and little is known about the pathways involved. Hyperglycemia modifies the metabolism of the cells and is suspected to induce various downstream pathways or molecules that are responsible for maintaining the tissue damaging actions. Oxidative stress pathways act as executors of tissue damage but the linkage between hyperglycemia and the sustained activation of oxidative pathways still remains rather elusive.

Alterations in the metabolome in diabetes are suspected to maintain the metabolic changes for extended periods even if there is little change in the expression profile of proteins [57]. Excess glucose load induces changes in a series of metabolite levels and the normalization of these levels may not occur as rapidly as glucose lowering. Apart from glucose, the concentrations of glucose-1-phosphate, lactate, glucosamine, mannose, mannosamine, hydroxybutyrate and glyoxalate also elevate in the plasma in diabetes [58]. All of the above intermediates and the increased fatty acids increase the tricarboxylic acid (TCA) cycle flux in the cells. Perturbation of the TCA cycle flux is also supported by other metabolomics studies in diabetes [59]. Associations between diabetes risk and the plasma levels of branched chain (BCAA, isoleucine, leucine and valine) and aromatic (phenylalanine, tyrosine) amino acids have been found suggesting that the changes not only involve the carbohydrate and lipid metabolism but also the catabolism of proteins and amino acids [60]. Catabolism of BCAAs provides intermediates for the TCA cycle and potentially drives the TCA flux. Apart from the systemic changes that affect the milieu of the cells, specific changes of amino acid levels have been observed in endothelial cells: hyperglycemia increases the concentration of alanine, proline, glycine, serine and glutamine within the cells and induces elevation of the aminoadipate, cystathionine and hypotaurine levels [61]. Whether these changes are only markers of hyperglycemia or they play a pathogenic role in oxidative stress induction is still undetermined.

4. Mechanisms of ROS production in hyperglycemia

4.1. Glucose-induced oxidative stress pathways

Changes in glucose metabolism are presumed to be directly responsible for provoking oxidant production in endothelial cells. Endothelial cells predominantly use glucose as energy source and rely on glycolysis to generate ATP molecules [14]. Glycolytic flux exceeds the rate of oxidative phosphorylation (OXPHOS) by two orders of magnitude in endothelial cells *in vitro* and similar ratio is suspected *in vivo* [62, 63]. The contribution of fatty acid oxidation to energy production is thought to be negligible in capillary endothelial cells, though endothelial cells take up fatty acids and transport them to the neighboring cells, thus play important role in transendothelial fatty acid delivery [64]. Since the function of capillary endothelial cells is to deliver oxygen and fuel sources to other cells in tissues, they do not consume much oxygen or store energy but preserve them to other perivascular cells. Thus, excess glucose is not converted to glycogen for storage in endothelial cells, but is pushed toward glycolysis [65]. Glutamine is a further energy source in endothelial cells via glutaminolysis that directly produces one GTP molecule (that can be converted to ATP) and further five ATP molecules from $NADH^+$ and $FADH_2$ via OXPHOS. Glutamine is the most abundant amino acid in the plasma, and glutaminolysis is a valuable energy source if glycolytic output is low since it feeds alpha-ketoglutarate to the TCA cycle and similarly produces lactate (or pyruvate). However, all the energy producing steps in glutaminolysis occur in the mitochondria via the TCA cycle and OXPHOS and mitochondrial impairment may affect the energy efficacy of glutaminolysis [66].

The metabolic balance between glycolysis and OXPHOS is controlled by nutrients (the ATP and NADH output) via Sirtuin 1 (SIRT1) and AMP-activated protein kinase (AMPK) in the cells. SIRT1 is a NAD^+-dependent histone deacetylase enzyme that regulates energy homeostasis via gene expression changes induced by deacetylating a variety of histone proteins, transcription factors and coregulators [67]. The activity of SIRT1 is primarily controlled by NAD^+ abundance and NAD^+/NADH ratio. AMPK is a master sensor of the energy level in the cells: it detects the cellular ATP concentration and is activated by a decrease in the ATP level. There is a complex interplay between AMPK and SIRT1: the two enzymes indirectly activate each other. Activated SIRT1 deacetylates LKB1 (tumor suppressor liver kinase B1) that phosphorylates and activates AMPK [68, 69], whereas AMPK activates SIRT1 by increasing the NAD^+/NADH ratio either by inducing the NAD^+ biosynthesis enzyme NamPRT (nicotinamide phosphoribosyltransferase) or by a NamPRT-independent mechanism [70]. Thus, caloric restriction activates both AMPK and SIRT1, whereas both enzymes are suppressed if energy sources are abundant like in hyperglycemia [71, 72]. In caloric restriction, SIRT1 deacetylates and activates peroxisome proliferation activating receptor-γ (PPAR-γ) coactivator 1-α (PGC-1) and forkhead box O1 protein 1 (FOXO1) and leads to glucose sparing: suppressed glycolysis and increased mitochondrial activity and they also activate gluconeogenesis [73, 74]. On the other hand, in hyperglycemia, the activity of AMPK and SIRT1 is suppressed and it results in enhanced glycolysis, inhibition of gluconeogenesis and decreased mitochondrial biogenesis and OXPHOS [73].

Overload of glycolysis and the pentose phosphate pathway are the initial steps that trigger alternate pathways of glucose metabolism (**Figure 1**). Prior perturbation of mitochondrial metabolism (TCA cycle overload and impaired OXPHOS) is highly possible since inhibition of mitochondrial superoxide generation prevents the activation of the above pathways but the exact mechanism that initiates these events is unknown [26]. The high glycolytic input and low OXPHOS capacity may gradually block the main metabolic steps and shunt the metabolism to alternative pathways. These include the methylglyoxal, hexosamine and polyol pathways: dihydroxyacetone phosphate (DHAP) is diverted to the methylglyoxal pathway and leads to protein kinase C (PKC) activation, and fructose-6-phosphate (F6P) increases the flux through the hexosamine pathway and excess glucose enters the polyol pathway when converted to sorbitol [66, 75]. Suppressed expression of the gluconeogenetic enzyme glucose-6-phosphate dehydrogenase (G6PDH) prevents shunting of glucose to the pentose phosphate pathway that further increases the glycolytic load [76, 77]. All these processes lead to ROS production and the generation of advanced glycation end products (AGEs), the products of nonenzymatic glycation and oxidation of proteins and lipids that accumulate in diabetes. AGEs signal through the receptor of AGE (RAGE), a cell surface receptor that is also activated by the damage-associated molecular patterns (DAMP) HMGB1 (high-mobility group box 1) and S100 proteins [78]. RAGE activates nuclear factor kappa B (NF-κB) and controls several inflammatory genes, thus links hyperglycemia to inflammation. Since RAGE itself is upregulated by NF-κB, inflammation is maintained by positive feedback in hyperglycemia as AGEs, the ligands are continuously produced.

http://dx.doi.org/10.5772/intechopen.71433

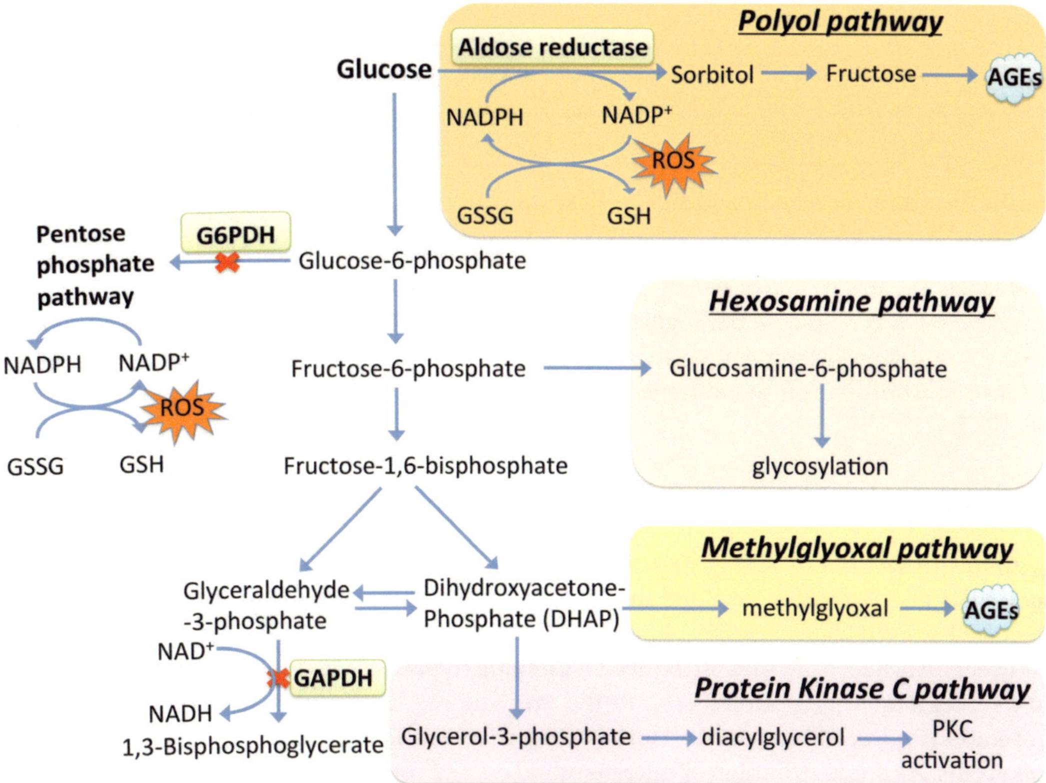

Figure 1. Hyperglycemia-induced ROS-producing pathways in the cytoplasm. AGEs: advanced glycation end-products; G6PDH: glucose-6-phosphate dehydrogenase; GAPDH: glyceraldehyde-3-phosphate dehydrogenase; GSH/GSSG: reduced/oxidized glutathione; NAD^+/NADH: nicotinamide adenine dinucleotide; NADP+/NADPH: nicotinamide adenine dinucleotide phosphate and ROS: reactive oxygen species.

Interestingly, hyperglycemia induces a long-lasting suppression in SIRT1 and AMPK activity in endothelial cells: the activity of both enzymes remains low weeks after the normalization of glucose level following a week long hyperglycemia [68]. Thus, SIRT1 and AMPK have been implicated in glucose memory since restoration of their activity reduces the ROS production and PARP activity in the cells.

One further molecule that possibly takes part in the maintenance of oxidative stress in hyperglycemic endothelial cells is p66SHC (66-kDa Src homology 2 domain-containing protein) [79]. p66SHC is induced by hyperglycemia and it contributes to oxidative stress and endothelial damage. Genetic ablation of p66SHC reduces the oxidative stress in diabetic animals, protects against vascular dysfunction and blocks the progression of nephropathy [79, 80]. p66SHC is a redox enzyme that associates with 70 kDa heat shock protein (Hsp70) and localizes within the intermembrane space in the mitochondria. Upon oxidative stress, p66SHC is released from the complex and transfers electrons from the electron transfer chain (from cytochrome c specifically) to oxygen and produces hydrogen peroxide (H_2O_2) [81]. Under basal conditions, p66SHC is also present as an inactive enzyme in the cytoplasm where it becomes activated via phosphorylation in response to cellular stress and translocates to the mitochondria. The active p66SHC diverts a fraction of the mitochondrial electron flow between complexes III and IV to produce ROS instead of water and is involved in the opening of the permeability transition pore during apoptosis. In hyperglycemia, p66SHC may function as a shunt pathway if complex IV activity is impaired. The activity of p66SHC is also regulated by acetylation: it is a direct target of SIRT1 and diminished SIRT1 activity increases the acetylation and activity of p66SHC in hyperglycemia [82]. Furthermore, acetylation of p66SHC promotes the phosphorylation-mediated activation of the protein, and since the acetylation-resistant p66SHC isoform partially protects against the vascular impairment, it may play a pathogenic role in diabetic vascular dysfunction. The linkage to SIRT1 and the protection associated with the loss of p66SHC suggest that p66SHC make a substantial contribution to oxidative stress in diabetes and it may represent the key target of SIRT1.

4.2. Unifying hypothesis: the role of mitochondrial oxidants

With the growth of our knowledge about glucose-induced cellular damage and the various molecules and pathways involved in the process, the pathomechanism of glucose-induced damage has become inexplicable. In an effort to explain the puzzling complexity of the cellular events, Michael Brownlee introduced a unifying hypothesis in which he placed the events in an integrating linear model [26]. In the unifying mechanism, mitochondrial superoxide generation is placed in center stage followed by all other ROS-producing pathways as secondary events. As the contribution of mitochondrial energy production seems negligible in endothelial cells, this proposition was a striking novelty at first, but it renders the series of events logically based on a wealth of scientific results. First of all, the unifying framework assumes that the main ROS-producing mechanisms implicated in hyperglycemic cellular damage are interrelated and a common pathway is responsible for their activation [75]. Secondly, the overload of glycolysis rather occurs as a single downstream perturbation of metabolism that leaves behind glycolytic intermediates than by multiple blockades of glycolytic enzymes in response to excess glucose input. Thus, inhibition of a downstream step of glucose catabolism in the mitochondria might be responsible for the activation of the ROS-producing shunt pathways in the cytoplasm. The observation that prevention of mitochondrial superoxide generation inhibits the cytoplasmic ROS production pathways (PKC activation, sorbitol accumulation and AGE production) also supported the assumption that mitochondrial damage precedes the glycolytic impairment [83].

The exact nature of hyperglycemic perturbation of mitochondrial metabolism remains enigmatic, and it is still debatable whether superoxide itself or the steps leading to its increased production is the triggering event of glucose-induced damage. High TCA flux and elevated glycolytic pyruvate input were detected in hyperglycemia and these may serve as inducers of mitochondrial ROS production but might also be the consequences of dysfunctional OXPHOS [83]. Various pharmacological interventions that reduce the mitochondrial ROS production effectively inhibit the hyperglycemic damage [26, 38, 75]. Higher flux through the electron transport chain is expected to reduce the accumulation of glycolytic intermediates and prevent the activation of oxidative stress pathways but only some of the interventions increased the electron transport (e.g. uncoupling agents and proteins), whereas others (e.g. antioxidants) did not change it or severely reduced it (complex II inhibition). Also, the increased electron flow may induce a proportional rise in superoxide generation by the electron transport chain if electron leakage is unaffected. Furthermore, endothelial cells, in which the mitochondrial DNA is selectively depleted (rho zero cells) and lacks a functional electron transport chain, fail to activate PKC, the polyol and hexosamine pathways and they do not produce AGEs, though their mitochondrial metabolism is impaired and they are expected to accumulate glycolytic intermediates [26]. These observations led to the proposition that mitochondrial superoxide generated by the electron transport chain is responsible for the initiation of hyperglycemic endothelial damage [26, 83, 84].

4.3. The mechanism of glucose-induced mitochondrial superoxide generation

Mitochondria produce superoxide nonenzymatically via multiple respiratory complexes in the electron transport chain and enzymatically via the mitochondrial xanthine oxidase [85–87]. The nonenzymatic production of superoxide occurs when a single electron is directly transferred to oxygen by prosthetic groups of the respiratory complexes or by reduced coenzymes that act as soluble electron carriers. The electron transport chain may leak electrons to oxygen and it is the main source of superoxide in hyperglycemia. Mitochondrial monoamine oxidase (MAO) and p66SHC also produce H_2O_2 within the mitochondria that may contribute to oxidative stress in hyperglycemia [88].

Molecular oxygen is biradical; it has two unpaired electrons in the outer orbitals, which makes it chemically reactive. In the ground state, the unpaired electrons are arranged in the triplet state, and as a result of spin restrictions, molecular oxygen is not highly reactive: it can only react with one electron at a time. If one of the unpaired electrons is excited and changes its spin (oxygen goes from the triplet state to the short-lived singlet state), it will become a powerful oxidant that is highly reactive [86]. The reduction of oxygen by one electron at a time produces superoxide ($O_2^{\bullet-}$) anion that might be converted to hydrogen peroxide (either spontaneously or through a reaction catalyzed by superoxide dismutase), which may be fully reduced to water or partially reduced to hydroxyl radical ($OH^{\bullet}$). In addition, superoxide may react with other radicals including nitric oxide ($NO^{\bullet}$) and form peroxynitrite ($ONOO^{\bullet-}$), another very powerful oxidant. The respiratory components are thermodynamically capable of transferring one electron to oxygen and form superoxide in the highly reducing environment of the mitochondria, since the standard reduction potential of oxygen to superoxide is −0.160 V and the respiratory chain incorporates components with standard reduction potentials between −0.32 V (NAD(P)H) and +0.39 V (cytochrome a_3 in Complex IV) [86].

In the respiratory chain, electrons move along the electron transport chain going from donor to acceptor molecules until they are transferred to molecular oxygen (the standard reduction potential of oxygen/H_2O couple is +0.82 V), while the generated free energy is used to synthesize ATP from ADP and inorganic phosphate. Respiratory Complex I transfers electrons from NADH and Complex II from $FADH_2$ to coenzyme Q (CoQ, ubiquinone), which is the substrate of Complex III. Complex III transfers electrons from reduced CoQ to cytochrome C, which is used by Complex IV to reduce oxygen into water. The step-by-step transfer of electrons allows the free energy to be released in small increments. The energy released as electrons flow through the respiratory chain is converted into a H^+ gradient through the inner mitochondrial membrane: protons are transported from the mitochondrial matrix to the intermembrane space (by Complexes I, III and IV) and a proton concentration gradient forms across the inner mitochondrial membrane [89]. Since the mitochondrial outer membrane is freely permeable to protons, the pH of the mitochondrial matrix is higher (the proton concentration is lower) than that of the intermembrane space and the cytosol. An electric potential (mitochondrial membrane potential) of 140–160 mV is formed across the inner membrane by pumping of positively charged protons outward from the matrix, which becomes negatively charged [90]. Thus, free energy released during the oxidation of NADH or $FADH_2$ is converted to an electric potential and a proton concentration gradient—collectively, the proton-motive force—and this energy is used by ATP synthase (Complex V) for ATP generation via the chemiosmotic coupling [91]. While the majority of oxygen molecules are used for water formation during the above processes, superoxide is generated at an estimated rate of 0.1–2% of oxygen consumption under normal respiration (State 3) and physiological operation of the respiratory chain [85, 88].

The electron transport chain may produce superoxide by multiple mechanisms but electron leakage before Complex III is suspected to represent the main source of superoxide in hyperglycemic endothelial cells [26, 83]. Complexes I and III are the respiratory complexes that are capable to produce large amounts of superoxide under certain conditions (**Figure 2**). Complex I may produce superoxide by two mechanisms: (1) the reduced flavin mononucleotide (FMN) center can transfer electrons to oxygen instead of CoQ when the $NADH/NAD^+$ ratio is high (and the CoQ binding site is blocked or the CoQ pool is mostly reduced) and (2) by reverse electron transfer (RET) from the CoQ binding site if there is high electron supply from Complex II and the electrons are forced back to Complex I instead of proceeding to Complex III (by a reduced CoQ pool and high proton-motive force) [85, 92]. In Complex III, superoxide is produced from the semiquinone anionic state of CoQ (semiubiquinone) by directly reacting with oxygen instead of completing the Q-cycle [85, 93]. Reduced CoQ diffuses through the bilipid layer of the membrane to its binding site in Complex III and transfers the electrons to the iron-sulfur protein (Rieske protein) in two steps that produce a semiquinone intermediate state of CoQ after the first electron transfer, which is the source of superoxide. In the presence of respiratory inhibitors, Complex I may produce the highest amount of superoxide, especially through RET, but the contribution of Complexes I and III to superoxide production is unknown in healthy mitochondria [86]. Superoxide is also produced in the matrix by other enzymes that interact with the NADH pool and by enzymes connected to the inner membrane CoQ pool. These include α-ketoglutarate dehydrogenase that may produce superoxide if its substrate (α-ketoglutarate) concentration and the $NADH/NAD^+$ ratio increase in the matrix. In the membrane, α-glycerophosphate dehydrogenase may produce superoxide partly via RET and Complex II, which transfer electrons from succinate to CoQ, is also suspected to generate some superoxide [85].

http://dx.doi.org/10.5772/intechopen.71433

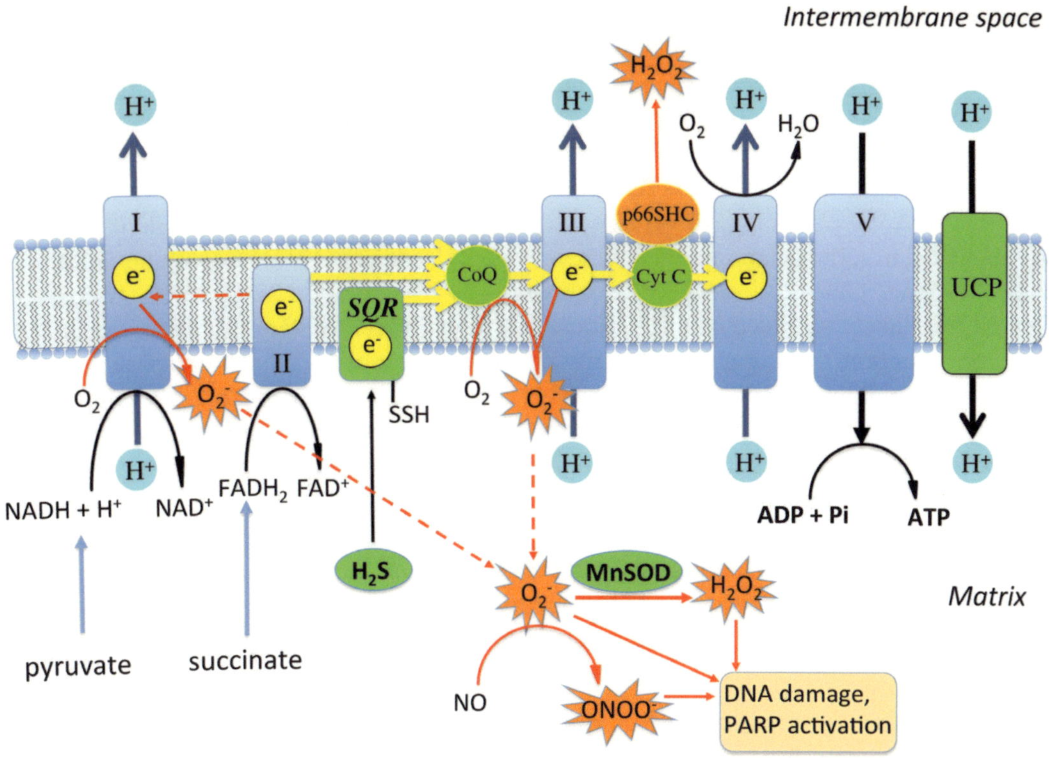

Figure 2. Oxidant production by the mitochondrial electron transport chain. CoQ: coenzyme Q, ubiquinone; Cyt C: cytochrome C; FAD+/$FADH_2$: flavin adenine dinucleotide; H_2O_2: hydrogen peroxide; MnSOD: manganese-dependent superoxide dismutase; $NO^\bullet$: nitric oxide; $O_2^{\bullet-}$: superoxide, $ONOO^{\bullet-}$: peroxynitrite; PARP: poly(ADP-ribose) polymerase; p66SHC: 66-kDa Src homology 2 domain-containing protein; SQR: sulfide:quinone oxidoreductase and UCP: uncoupling protein.

In hyperglycemic endothelial cells, the increased production of superoxide originates from the reduced CoQ pool before Complex III [75, 83]. The high electron donor input from glycolysis and the TCA cycle may increase the membrane potential and inhibit the electron transfer at Complex III, thus increase the concentration of reduced and free radical intermediates of CoQ. Superoxide generation may occur as direct 'leakage' of electrons to oxygen, as a result of the longer half-life of CoQ intermediates in the lipid bilayer and bound to Complex III or via RET through Complex I. Superoxide generation is also promoted by the increased membrane potential and proton concentration gradient through the inner membrane [31, 35, 83, 94]. Superoxide production was found to increase exponentially above 140 mV with the increase of the mitochondrial membrane potential [95]. Since with the generation of each superoxide molecule one electron is lost compared to the number of protons, superoxide production per se may increase the membrane potential and the proton gradient or might be responsible for the maintenance of the elevated membrane potential. Furthermore, the proton and charge transfer of Complexes III and IV are disproportional since Complex III picks up two protons from the matrix side of the inner membrane (the negatively charged N-face) and releases four protons to the intermembrane space side (positively charged P-face), whereas Complex IV abstracts four protons from the matrix and releases two protons to the intermembrane space per transfer of two electrons. Thus, Complex III transfers four protons but only two positive charges, whereas Complex IV transfers two protons and four positive charges [89, 96], which may lead to an increase in the membrane potential if there is a mismatch between the activity of the two complexes. Also, while it is possible to generate considerably higher membrane potential than the physiological value, since the proton-motive force is sufficient to generate about 240 mV, the proton permeability of biological membranes increases above 130 mV; thus, the higher values are associated with energy loss [95]. To optimize the energy efficiency, OXPHOS is tightly regulated by the ATP concentration (or ATP/ADP ratio) in the matrix: high ATP concentration in the matrix allosterically inhibits Complex IV of the respiratory chain and decreases the mitochondrial membrane potential [97]. Complex IV has a low reserve capacity and it may represent the major controlling site of respiration and mitochondrial ATP synthesis [95]. This immediate regulation is supplemented by the phosphorylation-mediated regulation of respiratory complexes, which transmit the extramitochondrial and extracellular stimuli to adapt OXPHOS to stress conditions [95]. Phosphorylation sites were detected in all respiratory complexes and there is a growing list of stress factors that may induce phosphorylation of the complexes or mitochondrial hyperpolarization that might be associated with the adaptive process. This is how inflammatory cytokines may affect superoxide generation in diabetes.

Hyperglycemia-induced mitochondrial superoxide production is a functional change of the respiratory chain; no difference is detectable in the assembly or the relative amounts of the respiratory complexes in the early phases of the injury [26, 35]. At later stages, changes in the expression or assembly of some components of the respiratory chain may occur and these are typically associated with impaired functionality [98, 99]. The glucose-induced changes in the mitochondrial superoxide production are reversible: normalization of the membrane potential suppresses the ROS production in endothelial cells [26, 35, 83, 94, 100]. While elevated mitochondrial membrane potential is detectable in endothelial cells exposed to high glucose concentration, the overexpression of either uncoupling protein 1 (UCP1) or uncoupling protein 2 (UCP2) normalizes the membrane potential and reduces the ROS production [26, 35, 83]. The function of UCP2 is regulated by ROS itself: the proton conductance of the protein is controlled by glutathionylation, and if ROS is present, it increases the proton leakage, whereas in the absence of ROS, the channel closes, thus this feedback may control the mitochondrial potential and the ROS production simultaneously [32, 33]. Furthermore, hydrogen sulfide donors that normalize the mitochondrial potential by electron supplementation via sulfide:quinone oxidoreductase (SQR) also inhibit the superoxide generation induced by hyperglycemia [94, 100].

The mitochondrial matrix possesses antioxidant enzymes to defend against oxidative damage. Manganese-dependent superoxide dismutase (MnSOD, also known as superoxide dismutase 2 (SOD2)) is the mitochondrial enzyme that neutralizes superoxide produced by the respiratory chain and converts it to H_2O_2. Since functional mitochondria constantly produce ROS, it is necessary to scavenge oxygen radicals. The importance of MnSOD is underlined by the fact that MnSOD-deficient mice exhibit extensive mitochondrial injury and only survive for less than 3 weeks [101]. Mutations associated with reduced activity of MnSOD accelerate diabetic nephropathy and neuropathy [102–104]. On the other hand, overexpression of MnSOD prevents hyperglycemic injury in endothelial cells, suggesting that the respiratory chain is the source of oxidants in hyperglycemia [26, 83]. The amount of superoxide produced by the respiratory chain may not be excessively higher in hyperglycemia, since the overexpression of the MnSOD can efficiently scavenge the oxidants or low amounts of mitochondria-targeted antioxidants are able to neutralize ROS in hyperglycemia [26, 38, 83].

5. Mechanism of damage: cell damaging responses to ROS production in hyperglycemia

In cells exposed to hyperglycemia, mitochondrial ROS production activates various mechanisms to reduce the oxidant production. This includes immediate responses that may control the mitochondrial potential in the short term and also longer term responses that may protect against the increase of the mitochondrial potential, but these mostly reduce the energy efficiency of OXPHOS. Hyperglycemia and ROS production activate the uncoupling proteins in the mitochondrial inner membrane that allow higher proton transfer from the intermembrane space to the matrix without coupled ATP production [32, 33]. This activity not only reduces the mitochondrial membrane potential but also decreases the amount of ATP generated in the mitochondria.

Hyperglycemia also increases the consumption of hydrogen sulfide, an inorganic substrate of the mitochondria that can act as an endogenous electron donor [105–107]. Since H_2S oxidation may provide electrons to CoQ without the additional protons, it can reduce the mitochondrial potential and promote ATP synthesis; thus, H_2S may represent an alternative energy source that is used in small quantities or function as a buffer to control the mitochondrial potential. Hyperglycemia reduces the mitochondrial H_2S pool and the plasma concentration of H_2S, and it may deplete the buffering capacity of H_2S in the mitochondria [94, 108, 109].

These immediate reactions are supplemented with the morphological changes of mitochondria. Mitochondria are dynamically changing organelles in the cells: they may form long tubes that cross the whole length of the cell or short rods that are as long as wide or any length in between. Mitochondria continuously change their shape by fusion (elongation) and fission (fragmentation) and they move along microtubular tracks within the cells. This process is believed to help maintain functional mitochondria; it allows rapid redistribution of mitochondrial proteins and may help the elimination of dysfunctional parts or proteins. Hyperglycemia stimulates the fission of mitochondria that can reduce the mitochondrial membrane potential but also helps dissociate the respiratory complexes and decrease the chance of assembly of various proteins within a complex [110–114]. Altogether, it results in partly assembled respiratory complexes and higher superoxide production that will reduce the energy efficiency of mitochondria [98, 99]. Mitochondrial fission is a later process induced by high glucose exposure, and it occurs only after the superoxide production is induced.

Mitochondrial ROS production plays an active role in the initiation of fragmentation, since administration of a mitochondrial scavenger prevents the hyperglycemia-induced fission of mitochondria [113]. Blocking of mitochondrial fission will also restore the acetylcholine-mediated eNOS (endothelial nitric oxide synthase) phosphorylation and cGMP response in hyperglycemic endothelial cells, suggesting that the vascular impairment is partly caused by mitochondrial fission itself [114].

Mitochondrial ROS production results in DNA damage in the mitochondria that activates the mitochondrial DNA repair enzymes [115]. Oxidative DNA damage activates poly(ADP-ribose) polymerase 1 (PARP1) in the mitochondria similar to the situation in the nucleus [116]. PARP1 adds ADP-ribose polymers (PARs) to the mitochondrial base excision repair (BER) enzymes, exo/endonuclease G (EXOG) and DNA polymerase gamma (Polγ) and affects the mitochondrial DNA repair [116]. Activation of mitochondrial PARP1, as opposed to nuclear PARP1, may decrease the DNA repair and slow down the mitochondrial biogenesis. Integrity of the mitochondrial DNA (mtDNA) also relies on mitochondrial transcription factor A (TFAM), a protein that may act as a physical shield of the mitochondrial DNA, since it forms histone-like structures with mtDNA and is present in large amounts in mitochondria (~900 molecules for each mtDNA). Apart from protecting the DNA from damaging agents, it tightly binds to heavily damaged DNA parts, blocks the transcription and may promote the repair of affected sites [115]. TFAM is also implicated in mitochondrial biogenesis and the maintenance of stable mtDNA copy number. In diabetic retinas, the level of TFAM is reduced, and it decreases the mitochondrial biogenesis that can lead to fewer mitochondria and less efficient OXPHOS [117].

Oxidant production will also induce several changes in the function of proteins that may be associated with cellular injury and result in altered cell metabolism, senescence and vascular dysfunction. Oxidative stress leads to oxidative DNA damage and DNA strand breaks that activates the predominantly nuclear PARP1 and may lead to ATP depletion and necrosis or apoptosis [118]. However, the level of PARP activation is mostly lower than to induce cell death; it results in higher NAD^+ consumption and changes in the PARylation pattern of proteins [50]. The higher NAD^+ utilization and decreased mitochondrial output may decrease the nuclear and cytoplasmic NAD^+ concentrations and by reducing the amount of substrate for SIRT1 (another NAD^+-dependent enzyme), it will block the deacetylation of proteins [67, 68, 82]. A third posttranslational modification that changes in hyperglycemia is protein S-sulfhydration (or persulfidation), a reaction between H_2S and reactive cysteine residues [119]. Protein S-sulfhydration is a highly prevalent modification that typically increases the activity of target proteins. The antioxidant master regulator Nrf2 (nuclear factor E2-related factor 2) transcription factor is also activated by H_2S via sulfhydration of its key controller, Kelch-like erythroid cell-derived protein with Cap 'n' collar (CNC) homology (ECH)-associated protein 1 (Keap1) [120, 121]. A further target is ATP synthase in the respiratory chain: H_2S increases cellular bioenergetics via S-sulfhydration of Complex V [122]. Since hyperglycemia reduces the H_2S level in the cells and plasma, it will also decrease the protein S-sulfhydration and results in lower Nrf2 activity and OXPHOS efficiency [108, 109]. All these changes contribute to the dysfunction of proteins in hyperglycemia and promote cellular dysfunction.

There are further changes in the cellular metabolism that reduce the ATP output, which include diminished glucose uptake, blockage of anaerobic metabolism and inappropriate assembly of mitochondrial respiratory complexes. High extracellular glucose immediately stimulates glucose uptake, but decreases the glucose transport over longer term in endothelial cells [123, 124]. Downregulation of GLUT1 glucose transporter is responsible for the diminished glucose uptake, and it may contribute to the low ATP output. Hyperglycemia reduces the activity of the glycolytic enzyme glyceraldehyde-3-phosphate dehydrogenase (GAPDH) via PARylation and reduces the anaerobic glucose metabolism [125]. Aerobic metabolism is also decreased by mitochondrial fragmentation and disassembly of mitochondrial respiratory complexes that develop over longer exposure to hyperglycemia [93, 99, 113]. Altogether these changes reduce the ATP generation in the cells and block the anaerobic compensation for the diminished mitochondrial activity.

Oxidative stress will induce DNA strand breaks in the mitochondria and promote mutations and senescence of endothelial cells. Accelerated aging of endothelial cells and the lack of endothelial progenitor cells decrease the functional endothelial cell pool in hyperglycemia [126]. The number of bone marrow-derived progenitor cells is lower in the circulation in diabetes and the progenitor cells possess diminished proliferation capacity [24, 127]. It will reduce the resupply of endothelial cells and may place extra workload on the pre-existing vascular endothelium extending the exposure to glucose, inflammatory mediators and oxidants.

Vascular dysfunction is characterized by inappropriate relaxation in response to acetylcholine, which is mediated by endothelial nitric oxide (NO) [128–131]. NO is synthesized from the guanidinium group of L-arginine by eNOS via a NADPH-dependent reaction. Mitochondrial superoxide may interact with NO, which leads to a loss of bioavailable NO, and form peroxynitrite ($ONOO^-$), a very reactive radical that activates PARP1 [132–134]. Furthermore, tetrahydrobiopterin (the pteridine cofactor of eNOS) is an essential regulator of the enzyme: when tetrahydrobiopterin availability is inadequate, it becomes 'uncoupled' and produces superoxide, using molecular oxygen as substrate, instead of NO [135]. Tetrahydrobiopterin levels are lower in animal models of diabetes and tetrahydrobiopterin supplementation restores the vascular relaxation in these models suggesting a pathogenic role in diabetes [136, 137]. Another key element of vascular dysfunction is the reduced H_2S bioavailability in diabetes. H_2S and NO interact at multiple levels: H_2S stimulates eNOS expression and activity, promotes the action of NO by maintaining a reduced soluble guanylate cyclase (sGC) and by inhibition of the vascular cGMP phosphodiesterase (PDE5) and prolongs the half-life of cGMP [138–140]. Increased mitochondrial H_2S consumption and its diminished concentration in hyperglycemic endothelial cells inhibit the NO-dependent vasodilation and contribute to vascular damage in diabetes.

6. Potential therapeutic approaches

6.1. Therapeutic approaches targeting the mitochondria

Glycemic control has been the main therapeutic modality for prevention and treatment of hyperglycemic injury and diabetes complications. However, recent studies confirmed that glycemic control provides limited protection against the cardiovascular events, and adjunct therapy is necessary to reduce the risk of complications. Previous efforts found aldose reductase (a key enzyme of the polyol pathway) to serve as potential drug target and found that inhibition of aldose reductase may prevent the pathological changes that occur in response to high sorbitol levels [141]. The results of the clinical trials were less impressive than expected from preclinical studies, still the first aldose reductase inhibitor has been marketed in Asia for the treatment of diabetes complications [142].

Following the discovery that mitochondrial superoxide is responsible for the induction of all ROS-producing pathways in hyperglycemic endothelial cells, an intense search began for mitochondrial drug targets and inhibitors of mitochondrial superoxide generation [26, 83, 84]. Mitochondria-specific targeting moieties have been developed and linked to antioxidants or superoxide dismutase (SOD) mimetics [143, 144]. The majority of these molecules use the triphenylphosphonium (TPP) targeting group and attain 100- to 500-fold accumulation in the mitochondria [145, 146]. Both the mitochondria-targeted ubiquinol (MitoQ) and piperidine nitroxide TEMPO (mitoTEMPO) proved beneficial in diabetes models [147–149]. Overexpression of MnSOD was found to protect against diabetic retinopathy in a transgenic model, but long-term delivery of MnSOD is unresolved in humans [150].

While no protein target has been identified, various phenotypic screens were performed, which allowed the target-agnostic discovery of potential drug candidates [38, 151]. In cell-based models, paroxetine emerged as a mitochondrial free radical scavenger and glucocorticoid steroids as UCP2 inducers in hyperglycemic endothelial cells [35, 38]. In another screen, which also used multiple assay variables as output and examined the OXPHOS-associated gene expression, the antihelmintic drug mebendazole and the Chinese herbal medicine deoxysappanone B emerged as inhibitors of mitochondrial ROS production [151]. The protective effect of all of these drugs might be a direct consequence of the normalization of the mitochondrial membrane potential or free radical scavenging.

The mitochondrial antioxidant effect of select microtubular drugs, which was independently confirmed by the previous two studies, might be related to their mitochondrial fusion promoting effect, since excessive mitochondrial fission and fragmentation occur in hyperglycemia [38, 151]. To identify compounds that promote mitochondrial fusion, a separate phenotypic screening program was conducted [152]. This study identified hydrazone M1, a small molecule that restore the mitochondrial network in cells but its efficacy has not been tested in diabetes [152, 153]. Also, compounds that block the mitochondrial fission are expected to improve the mitochondrial function and reduce the mitochondrial ROS production in hyperglycemia, but these inhibitors (mitochondrial division inhibitor-1 (mdivi-1), dynasore, P110 and 15-oxospiramilactone) have not been tested in diabetes [154, 155].

In another effort to identify compounds that reduce the mitochondrial ROS production but do not interfere with energy production, isolated mitochondria were used for high throughput screening and hit compounds were selected based on a dual output of ROS production and respiration rate [156, 157]. CN-POBS (N-cyclohexyl-4-(4-nitrophenoxy)benzenesulfonamide) was identified as a selective inhibitor of ROS production by the ubiquinone-binding site of complex I, and S3QELs ("sequels," selective suppressors of site III_{OQ} electron leak) were found to act as inhibitors of the outer ubiquinone-binding site similar to terpestacin [156–158]. Unfortunately, there are no data about their action against hyperglycemia-induced ROS production. Statins also block the mitochondrial ROS production but they simultaneously reduce the mitochondrial respiration and may cause toxicity [38, 151]. A further inhibitor of mitochondrial respiration is H_2S, a known inhibitor of complex IV, that turns out to act as stimulator of mitochondrial metabolism at low concentrations via electron donation [106]. H_2S supplementation either using sodium sulfide or mitochondria-targeted donor molecules inhibits the hyperglycemia-induced ROS production and endothelial dysfunction at low concentrations [35, 94]. Long-term administration of H_2S is effective against diabetic nephropathy and retinopathy in animal models [159, 160].

Finally, many of the currently used anti-diabetic medications also possess mitochondrial targets and they might be partly responsible for their beneficial effects on endothelial cells and the vasculature. The biguanide metformin apart from activating AMPK also acts as a mild and transient inhibitor of respiratory complex I [161]. The sulfonylurea glibenclamide inhibits the mitochondrial ATP-sensitive potassium channel (mitoK_{ATP}), decreases the mitochondrial membrane potential and ROS production and increases the respiration rate [162, 163]. Thiazolidinediones (TZDs) also possess a specific mitochondrial target (mTOT, mitochondrial target of TZDs), which comprise a recently identified protein complex. TZDs bind to a pyruvate carrier complex in the mitochondria and modulate the pyruvate entry into the mitochondria that may explain their antioxidant effect [164]. The discovery of these novel mitochondrial targets is expected to promote target-based drug discovery efforts and may provide new compounds in the upcoming years.

6.2. Therapeutic approaches to replace the injured endothelial cells

Endothelial cells exposed to oxidative stress and the proinflammatory environment undergo accelerated aging in hyperglycemia, thus stimulation of cell replacement with fresh endothelial cells may help restore the vascular function [126]. While it is difficult to estimate the exact number of endothelial cells, a reduction of progenitor cell count and functionality was detected in diabetes, and it is expected to result in a decreased number of functional endothelial cells in the vasculature [24, 127]. Even in the retina, where neovascularization (proliferative diabetic retinopathy) is the characteristic event, progenitor cell therapy is expected to cause improvement and treat the ischemic vascular abnormalities [165]. Currently, it is difficult to predict which treatment strategy will prove effective in diabetes, but probably the drug-induced enhancement of progenitor cell potency has the highest translational potential in diabetes [166, 167]. Drugs that were suggested for progenitor cell enhancement include statins, losartan (angiotensin II receptor antagonist), aliskiren (direct renin inhibitor), hydrogen sulfide, thymosin β4 and the CXCR4 (C-X-C chemokine receptor type 4) antagonist plerixafor (AMD3100, 1,1-[1,4-Phenylenebis(methylene)]bis-1,4,8,11-tetraazacyclotetradecane) [167]. As some of these drugs are in use in diabetic patients, an evaluation of the effect of these compounds on diabetic progenitor cells might be available in the near future [168]. If mobilization and enhancement of endothelial progenitor cells are achieved, it could help the endothelial recovery in the vasculature in diabetic patients, which may lead to an extension of indication of these drugs.

7. Conclusion

Reversible changes occur in the early phase of hyperglycemic injury that might be pharmacologically targetable. Blocking the high glucose-induced mitochondrial superoxide production represents the major goal in endothelial cells, but it does not provide a drug target that can be directly assessed [169, 170]. The involvement of mitochondria in the pathogenesis of various diseases intensified the interest in druggable targets and promoted selective delivery of compounds to the mitochondria [146]. Normalization of the mitochondrial membrane potential or administration of mitochondria-specific free radical scavengers reverses the adverse effects of hyperglycemia and may present experimental therapeutic approaches in diabetes [16, 38, 100]. Early administration of mitochondrial antioxidants or drugs that restore the mitochondrial metabolism is expected to prevent the later changes that occur in diabetes.

The later stages of hyperglycemic injury also include morphological changes and impaired assembly of the respiratory complexes that necessitate different treatment strategies. Mitochondrial fusion promoting drugs might represent promising approaches in this phase of diabetes complications but their efficacy has not been tested in diabetes [152, 153]. Alternatively, stimulation of the endothelial progenitor cells to help replace the senescent endothelial cells may prove beneficial in diabetes [126].

Altogether, advancement in our understanding of glucose-induced cellular and mitochondrial damage and identification of new drug targets are expected to provide novel strategies in diabetes treatment.

Acknowledgements

D.G. received funding from the People Programme (Marie Curie Actions) of the European Union's Seventh Framework Programme under the grant agreement number 628100.

Author details

Domokos Gero[1,2]*

*Address all correspondence to: gerodomokos@yahoo.com

1 Institute of Pathophysiology, Semmelweis University Medical School, Budapest, Hungary

2 University of Exeter Medical School, Exeter, UK

References

[1] Roglic G, World Health Organization, Global report on diabetes. Geneva, Switzerland: World Health Organization; 2016. 86 p

[2] Tamayo T et al. The prevalence and incidence of diabetes in Germany. Deutsches Ärzteblatt International. 2016;**113**(11):177-182

[3] Ulrich S et al. Cost burden of type 2 diabetes in Germany: Results from the population-based KORA studies. BMJ Open. 2016;**6**(11):e012527

[4] Hex N et al. Estimating the current and future costs of Type 1 and Type 2 diabetes in the UK, including direct health costs and indirect societal and productivity costs. Diabetic Medicine. 2012;**29**(7):855-862

[5] Brown JB et al. Type 2 diabetes: Incremental medical care costs during the first 8 years after diagnosis. Diabetes Care. 1999;**22**(7):1116-1124

[6] Hadi HA, Suwaidi JA. Endothelial dysfunction in diabetes mellitus. Vascular Health and Risk Management. 2007;**3**(6):853-876

[7] Georgescu A. Vascular dysfunction in diabetes: The endothelial progenitor cells as new therapeutic strategy. World Journal of Diabetes. 2011;**2**(6):92-97

[8] Esper RJ et al. Endothelial dysfunction: A comprehensive appraisal. Cardiovascular Diabetology. 2006;**5**:4

[9] Raitakari OT, Celermajer DS. Flow-mediated dilatation. British Journal of Clinical Pharmacology. 2000;**50**(5):397-404

[10] De Vriese AS et al. Endothelial dysfunction in diabetes. British Journal of Pharmacology. 2000;**130**(5):963-974

[11] Montero D et al. Vascular smooth muscle function in type 2 diabetes mellitus: A systematic review and meta-analysis. Diabetologia. 2013;**56**(10):2122-2133

[12] Bakker W et al. Endothelial dysfunction and diabetes: Roles of hyperglycemia, impaired insulin signaling and obesity. Cell and Tissue Research. 2009;**335**(1):165-189

[13] Artwohl M et al. Insulin does not regulate glucose transport and metabolism in human endothelium. European Journal of Clinical Investigation. 2007;**37**(8):643-650

[14] Eelen G et al. Endothelial cell metabolism in normal and diseased vasculature. Circulation Research. 2015;**116**(7):1231-1244

[15] Giacco F, Brownlee M. Oxidative stress and diabetic complications. Circulation Research. 2010;**107**(9):1058-1070

[16] Quijano C et al. Enhanced mitochondrial superoxide in hyperglycemic endothelial cells: Direct measurements and formation of hydrogen peroxide and peroxynitrite. American Journal of Physiology. Heart and Circulatory Physiology. 2007;**293**(6):H3404-H3414

[17] Coppey LJ et al. Effect of antioxidant treatment of streptozotocin-induced diabetic rats on endoneurial blood flow, motor nerve conduction velocity, and vascular reactivity of epineurial arterioles of the sciatic nerve. Diabetes. 2001;**50**(8):1927-1937

[18] Haj-Yehia AI et al. Effects of the superoxide dismutase-mimic compound TEMPOL on oxidant stress-mediated endothelial dysfunction. Antioxidants & Redox Signaling. 1999;**1**(2):221-232

[19] Ceriello A. Diabetic complications: From oxidative stress to inflammatory cardiovascular disorders. Medicographia. 2011;**33**(1):29-34

[20] Maeda M et al. Intermittent high glucose implements stress-induced senescence in human vascular endothelial cells: Role of superoxide production by NADPH oxidase. PLoS One. 2015;**10**(4):e0123169

[21] Galley HF, Webster NR. Physiology of the endothelium. British Journal of Anaesthesia. 2004;**93**(1):105-113

[22] Patrick V, Lepore J. Blood vessels and the endothelium. In: Warrell DA, Cox TM, Firth JD, editors. Oxford Textbook of Medicine. Oxford, UK: Oxford University Press; 2010

[23] Bianconi E et al. An estimation of the number of cells in the human body. Annals of Human Biology. 2013;**40**(6):463-471

[24] Loomans CJ et al. Endothelial progenitor cell dysfunction: A novel concept in the pathogenesis of vascular complications of type 1 diabetes. Diabetes. 2004;**53**(1):195-199

[25] Rogers SC et al. Exposure to high or low glucose levels accelerates the appearance of markers of endothelial cell senescence and induces dysregulation of nitric oxide synthase. The Journals of Gerontology. Series A, Biological Sciences and Medical Sciences. 2013;**68**(12):1469-1481

[26] Brownlee M. The pathobiology of diabetic complications: A unifying mechanism. Diabetes. 2005;**54**(6):1615-1625

[27] Calcutt NA et al. Therapies for hyperglycaemia-induced diabetic complications: From animal models to clinical trials. Nature Reviews. Drug Discovery. 2009;**8**(5):417-429

[28] McCall MN et al. MicroRNA profiling of diverse endothelial cell types. BMC Medical Genomics. 2011;**4**:78

[29] Heilig CW et al. Overexpression of glucose transporters in rat mesangial cells cultured in a normal glucose milieu mimics the diabetic phenotype. The Journal of Clinical Investigation. 1995;**96**(4):1802-1814

[30] Kaiser N et al. Differential regulation of glucose transport and transporters by glucose in vascular endothelial and smooth muscle cells. Diabetes. 1993;**42**(1):80-89

[31] Korshunov SS, Skulachev VP, Starkov AA. High protonic potential actuates a mechanism of production of reactive oxygen species in mitochondria. FEBS Letters. 1997;**416**(1):15-18

[32] Mailloux RJ, Harper ME. Uncoupling proteins and the control of mitochondrial reactive oxygen species production. Free Radical Biology & Medicine. 2011;**51**(6):1106-1115

[33] Mailloux RJ, Harper ME. Mitochondrial proticity and ROS signaling: Lessons from the uncoupling proteins. Trends in Endocrinology and Metabolism. 2012;**23**(9):451-458

[34] Koziel A et al. The influence of high glucose on the aerobic metabolism of endothelial EA.hy926 cells. Pflügers Archiv. 2012;**464**(6):657-669

[35] Gero D, Szabo C. Glucocorticoids suppress mitochondrial oxidant production via upregulation of uncoupling protein 2 in hyperglycemic endothelial cells. PLoS One. 2016;**11**(4):e0154813

[36] Busik JV, Mohr S, Grant MB. Hyperglycemia-induced reactive oxygen species toxicity to endothelial cells is dependent on paracrine mediators. Diabetes. 2008;**57**(7): 1952-1965

[37] Engerman R, Bloodworth JM Jr, Nelson S. Relationship of microvascular disease in diabetes to metabolic control. Diabetes. 1977;**26**(8):760-769

[38] Gero D et al. Cell-based screening identifies paroxetine as an inhibitor of diabetic endothelial dysfunction. Diabetes. 2013;**62**(3):953-964

[39] Davidson SM, Yellon DM. Does hyperglycemia reduce proliferation or increase apoptosis? Am J Physiol Heart Circ Physiol. 2006;**291**(3):H1486 author reply H1487

[40] Cheng AY, Leiter LA. Glucose lowering and cardiovascular disease: What do we know and what should we do? European Journal of Cardiovascular Prevention and Rehabilitation. 2010;**17**(Suppl 1):S25-S31

[41] UK Prospective Diabetes Study (UKPDS) Group. Intensive blood-glucose control with sulphonylureas or insulin compared with conventional treatment and risk of complications in patients with type 2 diabetes (UKPDS 33). Lancet. 1998;**352**(9131):837-853

[42] Harris MI. Classification, Diagnostic Criteria, and Screening for Diabetes. In: Harris MI et al., editors. Diabetes in America. Chapter 2, pages 15-36, NIH publication 95-168 (Published by NIH/NIDDK, Bethesda, MD). 1995

[43] Powers MA et al. Diabetes Self-management education and support in Type 2 diabetes: A joint position statement of the American Diabetes Association, the American Association of Diabetes Educators, and the Academy of Nutrition and Dietetics. Diabetes Care. 2015;**38**(7):1372-1382

[44] Si D et al. Comparison of diabetes management in five countries for general and indigenous populations: An internet-based review. BMC Health Services Research. 2010;**10**:169

[45] Hammes HP et al. Diabetic retinopathy: Targeting vasoregression. Diabetes. 2011;**60**(1):9-16

[46] WHO Expert Committee on Diabetes Mellitus: Second report. World Health Organization Technical Report Series. 1980;**646**:1-80

[47] Alberti KG, Zimmet PZ. Definition, diagnosis and classification of diabetes mellitus and its complications. Part 1: Diagnosis and classification of diabetes mellitus provisional report of a WHO consultation. Diabetic Medicine. 1998;**15**(7):539-553

[48] Felig P, Wahren J, Hendler R. Influence of oral glucose ingestion on splanchnic glucose and gluconeogenic substrate metabolism in man. Diabetes. 1975;**24**(5):468-475

[49] Bonora E, Muggeo M. Postprandial blood glucose as a risk factor for cardiovascular disease in Type II diabetes: The epidemiological evidence. Diabetologia. 2001;**44**(12):2107-2114

[50] Horvath EM et al. Rapid 'glycaemic swings' induce nitrosative stress, activate poly(ADP-ribose) polymerase and impair endothelial function in a rat model of diabetes mellitus. Diabetologia. 2009;**52**(5):952-961

[51] Ihnat MA, Thorpe JE, Ceriello A. Hypothesis: The 'metabolic memory', the new challenge of diabetes. Diabetic Medicine. 2007;**24**(6):582-586

[52] Ihnat MA et al. Reactive oxygen species mediate a cellular 'memory' of high glucose stress signalling. Diabetologia. 2007;**50**(7):1523-1531

[53] Skyler JS et al. Intensive glycemic control and the prevention of cardiovascular events: Implications of the ACCORD, ADVANCE, and VA diabetes trials: A position statement of the American Diabetes Association and a scientific statement of the American College of Cardiology Foundation and the American Heart Association. Circulation. 2009;**119**(2):351-357

[54] Diabetes Control Complications Trial Research Group, et al. The effect of intensive treatment of diabetes on the development and progression of long-term complications in insulin-dependent diabetes mellitus. The New England Journal of Medicine. 1993;**329**(14):977-986

[55] Kowluru RA, Kanwar M, Kennedy A. Metabolic memory phenomenon and accumulation of peroxynitrite in retinal capillaries. Experimental Diabetes Research. 2007;**2007**:21976

[56] Kowluru RA. Effect of reinstitution of good glycemic control on retinal oxidative stress and nitrative stress in diabetic rats. Diabetes. 2003;**52**(3):818-823

[57] Galderisi A et al. Metabolomics reveals new metabolic perturbations in children with type 1 diabetes. Pediatric Diabetes. 2017. DOI: 10.111/pedi.12524

[58] Padberg I et al. A new metabolomic signature in type-2 diabetes mellitus and its pathophysiology. PLoS One. 2014;**9**(1):e85082

[59] Li M et al. GC/TOFMS analysis of metabolites in serum and urine reveals metabolic perturbation of TCA cycle in db/db mice involved in diabetic nephropathy. American Journal of Physiology. Renal Physiology. 2013;**304**(11):F1317-F1324

[60] Sas KM et al. Metabolomics and diabetes: Analytical and computational approaches. Diabetes. 2015;**64**(3):718-732

[61] Yuan W et al. Amine metabolomics of hyperglycemic endothelial cells using capillary LC-MS with isobaric tagging. Journal of Proteome Research. 2011;**10**(11):5242-5250

[62] Krutzfeldt A et al. Metabolism of exogenous substrates by coronary endothelial cells in culture. Journal of Molecular and Cellular Cardiology. 1990;**22**(12):1393-1404

[63] Harjes U, Bensaad K, Harris AL. Endothelial cell metabolism and implications for cancer therapy. British Journal of Cancer. 2012;**107**(8):1207-1212

[64] Dagher Z et al. Acute regulation of fatty acid oxidation and amp-activated protein kinase in human umbilical vein endothelial cells. Circulation Research. 2001;**88**(12):1276-1282

[65] Noyman I et al. Hyperglycemia reduces nitric oxide synthase and glycogen synthase activity in endothelial cells. Nitric Oxide. 2002;**7**(3):187-193

[66] Goveia J, Stapor P, Carmeliet P. Principles of targeting endothelial cell metabolism to treat angiogenesis and endothelial cell dysfunction in disease. EMBO Molecular Medicine. 2014;**6**(9):1105-1120

[67] Yu J, Auwerx J. Protein deacetylation by SIRT1: An emerging key post-translational modification in metabolic regulation. Pharmacological Research. 2010;**62**(1):35-41

[68] Zheng Z et al. Sirtuin 1-mediated cellular metabolic memory of high glucose via the LKB1/AMPK/ROS pathway and therapeutic effects of metformin. Diabetes. 2012;**61**(1):217-228

[69] Ruderman NB et al. AMPK and SIRT1: A long-standing partnership? American Journal of Physiology. Endocrinology and Metabolism. 2010;**298**(4):E751-E760

[70] Canto C, Auwerx J. Targeting sirtuin 1 to improve metabolism: All you need is NAD(+)? Pharmacological Reviews. 2012;**64**(1):166-187

[71] Saha AK et al. Insulin resistance due to nutrient excess: Is it a consequence of AMPK downregulation? Cell Cycle. 2011;**10**(20):3447-3451

[72] Saha AK et al. Downregulation of AMPK accompanies leucine- and glucose-induced increases in protein synthesis and insulin resistance in rat skeletal muscle. Diabetes. 2010;**59**(10):2426-2434

[73] Houtkooper RH, Pirinen E, Auwerx J. Sirtuins as regulators of metabolism and healthspan. Nature Reviews. Molecular Cell Biology. 2012;**13**(4):225-238

[74] Rodgers JT et al. Nutrient control of glucose homeostasis through a complex of PGC-1alpha and SIRT1. Nature. 2005;**434**(7029):113-118

[75] Brownlee M. Biochemistry and molecular cell biology of diabetic complications. Nature. 2001;**414**(6865):813-820

[76] Leopold JA et al. Glucose-6-phosphate dehydrogenase overexpression decreases endothelial cell oxidant stress and increases bioavailable nitric oxide. Arteriosclerosis, Thrombosis, and Vascular Biology. 2003;**23**(3):411-417

[77] Zhang Z et al. Increasing glucose 6-phosphate dehydrogenase activity restores redox balance in vascular endothelial cells exposed to high glucose. PLoS One. 2012;**7**(11):e49128

[78] Ramasamy R, Yan SF, Schmidt AM. Receptor for AGE (RAGE): Signaling mechanisms in the pathogenesis of diabetes and its complications. Annals of the New York Academy of Sciences. 2011;**1243**:88-102

[79] Menini S et al. Deletion of p66Shc longevity gene protects against experimental diabetic glomerulopathy by preventing diabetes-induced oxidative stress. Diabetes. 2006; **55**(6):1642-1650

[80] Camici GG et al. Genetic deletion of p66(Shc) adaptor protein prevents hyperglycemia-induced endothelial dysfunction and oxidative stress. Proceedings of the National Academy of Sciences of the United States of America. 2007;**104**(12):5217-5222

[81] Giorgio M et al. Electron transfer between cytochrome c and p66Shc generates reactive oxygen species that trigger mitochondrial apoptosis. Cell. 2005;**122**(2):221-233

[82] Kumar S et al. Sirtuin1-regulated lysine acetylation of p66Shc governs diabetes-induced vascular oxidative stress and endothelial dysfunction. Proceedings of the National Academy of Sciences of the United States of America. 2017;**114**(7):1714-1719

[83] Nishikawa T et al. Normalizing mitochondrial superoxide production blocks three pathways of hyperglycaemic damage. Nature. 2000;**404**(6779):787-790

[84] Nishikawa T, Edelstein D, Brownlee M. The missing link: A single unifying mechanism for diabetic complications. Kidney International. Supplement. 2000;**77**:S26-S30

[85] Murphy MP. How mitochondria produce reactive oxygen species. The Biochemical Journal. 2009;**417**(1):1-13

[86] Turrens JF. Mitochondrial formation of reactive oxygen species. The Journal of Physiology. 2003;**552**(Pt 2):335-344

[87] Rus DA et al. Induction of mitochondrial xanthine oxidase activity during apoptosis in the rat mammary gland. Frontiers in Bioscience. 2007;**12**:1184-1189

[88] Kluge MA, Fetterman JL, Vita JA. Mitochondria and endothelial function. Circulation Research. 2013;**112**(8):1171-1188

[89] Dzbek J, Korzeniewski B. Control over the contribution of the mitochondrial membrane potential (DeltaPsi) and proton gradient (DeltapH) to the protonmotive force (Deltap). In silico studies. The Journal of Biological Chemistry. 2008;**283**(48):33232-33239

[90] Kunz W et al. Kinetic limitations in the overall reaction of mitochondrial oxidative phosphorylation accounting for flux-dependent changes in the apparent delta GexP/delta mu H+ ratio. FEBS Letters. 1988;**233**(1):17-21

[91] Mitchell P. Coupling of phosphorylation to electron and hydrogen transfer by a chemi-osmotic type of mechanism. Nature. 1961;**191**:144-148

[92] Treberg JR, Quinlan CL, Brand MD. Evidence for two sites of superoxide production by mitochondrial NADH-ubiquinone oxidoreductase (complex I). The Journal of Biological Chemistry. 2011;**286**(31):27103-27110

[93] Bleier L, Drose S. Superoxide generation by complex III: From mechanistic rationales to functional consequences. Biochimica et Biophysica Acta. 2013;**1827**(11-12): 1320-1331

[94] Suzuki K et al. Hydrogen sulfide replacement therapy protects the vascular endothelium in hyperglycemia by preserving mitochondrial function. Proceedings of the National Academy of Sciences of the United States of America. 2011;**108**(33):13829-13834

[95] Kadenbach B et al. New extension of the Mitchell Theory for oxidative phosphorylation in mitochondria of living organisms. Biochimica et Biophysica Acta. 2010;**1800**(3):205-212

[96] Nicholls DG, Ferguson SJ. Bioenergetics 3. 3rd ed. San Diego, CA: Academic Press. xviii; 2002. p. 297

[97] Ramzan R et al. Mitochondrial respiration and membrane potential are regulated by the allosteric ATP-inhibition of cytochrome c oxidase. Biochimica et Biophysica Acta. 2010;**1797**(9):1672-1680

[98] Ferreira FM et al. Diabetes and mitochondrial bioenergetics: Alterations with age. Journal of Biochemical and Molecular Toxicology. 2003;**17**(4):214-222

[99] Munusamy S et al. Alteration of renal respiratory Complex-III during experimental type-1 diabetes. BMC Endocrine Disorders. 2009;**9**:2

[100] Gero D et al. The novel mitochondria-targeted hydrogen sulfide (H2S) donors AP123 and AP39 protect against hyperglycemic injury in microvascular endothelial cells in vitro. Pharmacological Research. 2016;**113**(Pt A):186-198

[101] Lebovitz RM et al. Neurodegeneration, myocardial injury, and perinatal death in mitochondrial superoxide dismutase-deficient mice. Proceedings of the National Academy of Sciences of the United States of America. 1996;**93**(18):9782-9787

[102] Nishi H et al. DNA typing of HLA class II genes in Japanese patients with dilated cardiomyopathy. Journal of Molecular and Cellular Cardiology. 1995;**27**(10):2385-2392

[103] Nomiyama T et al. The polymorphism of manganese superoxide dismutase is associated with diabetic nephropathy in Japanese type 2 diabetic patients. Journal of Human Genetics. 2003;**48**(3):138-141

[104] Vincent AM et al. SOD2 protects neurons from injury in cell culture and animal models of diabetic neuropathy. Experimental Neurology. 2007;**208**(2):216-227

[105] Hildebrandt TM, Grieshaber MK. Three enzymatic activities catalyze the oxidation of sulfide to thiosulfate in mammalian and invertebrate mitochondria. The FEBS Journal. 2008;**275**(13):3352-3361

[106] Modis K et al. Intramitochondrial hydrogen sulfide production by 3-mercaptopyruvate sulfurtransferase maintains mitochondrial electron flow and supports cellular bioenergetics. The FASEB Journal. 2013;**27**(2):601-611

[107] Szabo C et al. Poly(ADP-ribose) polymerase inhibitors ameliorate nephropathy of type 2 diabetic Leprdb/db mice. Diabetes. 2006;**55**(11):3004-3012

[108] Jain SK et al. Low levels of hydrogen sulfide in the blood of diabetes patients and streptozotocin-treated rats causes vascular inflammation? Antioxidants & Redox Signaling. 2010;**12**(11):1333-1337

[109] Suzuki K et al. Clinical implication of plasma hydrogen sulfide levels in Japanese patients with Type 2 diabetes. Internal Medicine. 2017;**56**(1):17-21

[110] Wang W et al. Mitochondrial fission triggered by hyperglycemia is mediated by ROCK1 activation in podocytes and endothelial cells. Cell Metabolism. 2012;**15**(2):186-200

[111] Yu T, Jhun BS, Yoon Y. High-glucose stimulation increases reactive oxygen species production through the calcium and mitogen-activated protein kinase-mediated activation of mitochondrial fission. Antioxidants & Redox Signaling. 2011;**14**(3):425-437

[112] Yu T, Robotham JL, Yoon Y. Increased production of reactive oxygen species in hyperglycemic conditions requires dynamic change of mitochondrial morphology. Proceedings of the National Academy of Sciences of the United States of America. 2006;**103**(8): 2653-2658

[113] Makino A, Scott BT, Dillmann WH. Mitochondrial fragmentation and superoxide anion production in coronary endothelial cells from a mouse model of type 1 diabetes. Diabetologia. 2010;**53**(8):1783-1794

[114] Shenouda SM et al. Altered mitochondrial dynamics contributes to endothelial dysfunction in diabetes mellitus. Circulation. 2011;**124**(4):444-453

[115] Larsen NB, Rasmussen M, Rasmussen LJ. Nuclear and mitochondrial DNA repair: Similar pathways? Mitochondrion. 2005;**5**(2):89-108

[116] Szczesny B et al. Opposing roles of mitochondrial and nuclear PARP1 in the regulation of mitochondrial and nuclear DNA integrity: Implications for the regulation of mitochondrial function. Nucleic Acids Research. 2014;**42**(21):13161-13173

[117] Santos JM et al. Mitochondrial biogenesis and the development of diabetic retinopathy. Free Radical Biology & Medicine. 2011;**51**(10):1849-1860

[118] Gero D, Szabo C. Poly(ADP-ribose) polymerase: A new therapeutic target? Current Opinion in Anaesthesiology. 2008;**21**(2):111-121

[119] Paul BD, Snyder SH. H(2)S signalling through protein sulfhydration and beyond. Nature Reviews. Molecular Cell Biology. 2012;**13**(8):499-507

[120] Xie L et al. Hydrogen sulfide induces Keap1 S-sulfhydration and suppresses diabetes-accelerated atherosclerosis via Nrf2 activation. Diabetes. 2016;**65**(10):3171-3184

[121] Nguyen T, Nioi P, Pickett CB. The Nrf2-antioxidant response element signaling pathway and its activation by oxidative stress. The Journal of Biological Chemistry. 2009; **284**(20):13291-13295

[122] Modis K et al. S-Sulfhydration of ATP synthase by hydrogen sulfide stimulates mitochondrial bioenergetics. Pharmacological Research. 2016;**113**(Pt A):116-124

[123] Alpert E et al. Delayed autoregulation of glucose transport in vascular endothelial cells. Diabetologia. 2005;**48**(4):752-755

[124] Cohen G et al. The roles of hyperglycaemia and oxidative stress in the rise and collapse of the natural protective mechanism against vascular endothelial cell dysfunction in diabetes. Archives of Physiology and Biochemistry. 2007;**113**(4-5):259-267

[125] Du X et al. Inhibition of GAPDH activity by poly(ADP-ribose) polymerase activates three major pathways of hyperglycemic damage in endothelial cells. The Journal of Clinical Investigation. 2003;**112**(7):1049-1057

[126] Jarajapu YP, Grant MB. The promise of cell-based therapies for diabetic complications: Challenges and solutions. Circulation Research. 2010;**106**(5):854-869

[127] Tepper OM et al. Human endothelial progenitor cells from type II diabetics exhibit impaired proliferation, adhesion, and incorporation into vascular structures. Circulation. 2002;**106**(22):2781-2786

[128] Ignarro LJ et al. Endothelium-derived relaxing factor produced and released from artery and vein is nitric oxide. Proceedings of the National Academy of Sciences of the United States of America. 1987;**84**(24):9265-9269

[129] Ignarro LJ et al. Endothelium-derived relaxing factor from pulmonary artery and vein possesses pharmacologic and chemical properties identical to those of nitric oxide radical. Circulation Research. 1987;**61**(6):866-879

[130] Furchgott RF, Martin W. Interactions of endothelial cells and smooth muscle cells of arteries. Chest. 1985;**88**(4 Suppl):210S-213S

[131] Furchgott RF, Vanhoutte PM. Endothelium-derived relaxing and contracting factors. The FASEB Journal. 1989;**3**(9):2007-2018

[132] Beller CJ et al. Activation of the peroxynitrite-poly(adenosine diphosphate-ribose) polymerase pathway during neointima proliferation: A new target to prevent restenosis after endarterectomy. Journal of Vascular Surgery. 2006;**43**(4):824-830

[133] Gero D, Szabo C. Role of the peroxynitrite-poly (ADP-ribose) polymerase pathway in the pathogenesis of liver injury. Current Pharmaceutical Design. 2006;**12**(23): 2903-2910

[134] Radovits T et al. The peroxynitrite decomposition catalyst FP15 improves ageing-associated cardiac and vascular dysfunction. Mechanisms of Ageing and Development. 2007;**128**(2):173-181

[135] Alp NJ, Channon KM. Regulation of endothelial nitric oxide synthase by tetrahydrobiopterin in vascular disease. Arteriosclerosis, Thrombosis, and Vascular Biology. 2004; **24**(3):413-420

[136] Pannirselvam M et al. Cellular basis of endothelial dysfunction in small mesenteric arteries from spontaneously diabetic (db/db −/−) mice: Role of decreased tetrahydrobiopterin bioavailability. British Journal of Pharmacology. 2002;**136**(2):255-263

[137] Pieper GM. Acute amelioration of diabetic endothelial dysfunction with a derivative of the nitric oxide synthase cofactor, tetrahydrobiopterin. Journal of Cardiovascular Pharmacology. 1997;**29**(1):8-15

[138] Szabo C. Hydrogen sulfide, an enhancer of vascular nitric oxide signaling: Mechanisms and implications. American Journal of Physiology. Cell Physiology. 2017;**312**(1):C3-C15

[139] Hosoki R, Matsuki N, Kimura H. The possible role of hydrogen sulfide as an endogenous smooth muscle relaxant in synergy with nitric oxide. Biochemical and Biophysical Research Communications. 1997;**237**(3):527-531

[140] Coletta C et al. Hydrogen sulfide and nitric oxide are mutually dependent in the regulation of angiogenesis and endothelium-dependent vasorelaxation. Proceedings of the National Academy of Sciences of the United States of America. 2012;**109**(23): 9161-9166

[141] Tang WH, Martin KA, Hwa J. Aldose reductase, oxidative stress, and diabetic mellitus. Frontiers in Pharmacology. 2012;**3**:87

[142] Grewal AS et al. Updates on aldose reductase inhibitors for management of diabetic complications and non-diabetic diseases. Mini Reviews in Medicinal Chemistry. 2016;**16**(2):120-162

[143] Kagan VE et al. Mitochondrial targeting of electron scavenging antioxidants: Regulation of selective oxidation vs random chain reactions. Advanced Drug Delivery Reviews. 2009;**61**(14):1375-1385

[144] Apostolova N et al. Mitochondria-targeted antioxidants as a therapeutic strategy for protecting endothelium in cardiovascular diseases. Current Medicinal Chemistry. 2014;**21**(25):2989-3006

[145] Murphy MP. Targeting lipophilic cations to mitochondria. Biochimica et Biophysica Acta. 2008;**1777**(7-8):1028-1031

[146] Frantz MC, Wipf P. Mitochondria as a target in treatment. Environmental and Molecular Mutagenesis. 2010;**51**(5):462-475

[147] Chacko BK et al. Prevention of diabetic nephropathy in Ins2(+/)(−)(AkitaJ) mice by the mitochondria-targeted therapy MitoQ. The Biochemical Journal. 2010;**432**(1):9-19

[148] Shahzad K et al. Nlrp3-inflammasome activation in non-myeloid-derived cells aggravates diabetic nephropathy. Kidney International. 2015;**87**(1):74-84

[149] Qi H et al. Glomerular endothelial mitochondrial dysfunction is essential and characteristic of diabetic kidney disease susceptibility. Diabetes. 2017;**66**(3):763-778

[150] Kanwar M et al. Oxidative damage in the retinal mitochondria of diabetic mice: Possible protection by superoxide dismutase. Investigative Ophthalmology & Visual Science. 2007;**48**(8):3805-3811

[151] Wagner BK et al. Large-scale chemical dissection of mitochondrial function. Nature Biotechnology. 2008;**26**(3):343-351

[152] Wang D et al. A small molecule promotes mitochondrial fusion in mammalian cells. Angewandte Chemie (International Ed. in English). 2012;**51**(37):9302-9305

[153] Andreux PA, Houtkooper RH, Auwerx J. Pharmacological approaches to restore mitochondrial function. Nature Reviews. Drug Discovery. 2013;**12**(6):465-483

[154] Rovira-Llopis S et al. Mitochondrial dynamics in type 2 diabetes: Pathophysiological implications. Redox Biology. 2017;**11**:637-645

[155] Reddy PH. Inhibitors of mitochondrial fission as a therapeutic strategy for diseases with oxidative stress and mitochondrial dysfunction. Journal of Alzheimer's Disease. 2014;**40**(2):245-256

[156] Orr AL et al. Suppressors of superoxide production from mitochondrial complex III. Nature Chemical Biology. 2015;**11**(11):834-836

[157] Orr AL et al. Inhibitors of ROS production by the ubiquinone-binding site of mitochondrial complex I identified by chemical screening. Free Radical Biology & Medicine. 2013;**65**:1047-1059

[158] Jung HJ et al. Terpestacin inhibits tumor angiogenesis by targeting UQCRB of mitochondrial complex III and suppressing hypoxia-induced reactive oxygen species production and cellular oxygen sensing. The Journal of Biological Chemistry. 2010;**285**(15):11584-11595

[159] Safar MM, Abdelsalam RM. H2S donors attenuate diabetic nephropathy in rats: Modulation of oxidant status and polyol pathway. Pharmacological Reports. 2015;**67**(1):17-23

[160] Si YF et al. Treatment with hydrogen sulfide alleviates streptozotocin-induced diabetic retinopathy in rats. British Journal of Pharmacology. 2013;**169**(3):619-631

[161] Viollet B et al. Cellular and molecular mechanisms of metformin: An overview. Clinical Science (London, England). 2012;**122**(6):253-270

[162] Doughan AK, Harrison DG, Dikalov SI. Molecular mechanisms of angiotensin II-mediated mitochondrial dysfunction: Linking mitochondrial oxidative damage and vascular endothelial dysfunction. Circulation Research. 2008;**102**(4):488-496

[163] Skalska J et al. Antidiabetic sulphonylureas activate mitochondrial permeability transition in rat skeletal muscle. British Journal of Pharmacology. 2005;**145**(6):785-791

[164] Colca JR et al. Identification of a mitochondrial target of thiazolidinedione insulin sensitizers (mTOT)—Relationship to newly identified mitochondrial pyruvate carrier proteins. PLoS One. 2013;**8**(5):e61551

[165] Lois N et al. Endothelial progenitor cells in diabetic retinopathy. Frontiers in Endocrinology (Lausanne). 2014;**5**:44

[166] Sukmawati D, Tanaka R. Introduction to next generation of endothelial progenitor cell therapy: A promise in vascular medicine. American Journal of Translational Research. 2015;**7**(3):411-421

[167] Ye L, Poh KK. Enhancing endothelial progenitor cell for clinical use. World Journal of Stem Cells. 2015;**7**(6):894-898

[168] Cappellari R et al. Plerixafor improves the endothelial health balance. The effect of diabetes analysed by polychromatic flow cytometry. Atherosclerosis. 2016;**251**:373-380

[169] Santos R et al. A comprehensive map of molecular drug targets. Nature Reviews. Drug Discovery. 2017;**16**(1):19-34

[170] Hopkins AL, Groom CR. The druggable genome. Nature Reviews. Drug Discovery. 2002;**1**(9):727-730

Chapter 9

Impact of Advanced Glycation End Products on Endothelial Function and Their Potential Link to Atherosclerosis

Ezequiel Alvarez, Beatriz Paradela-Dobarro, Mercedes González-Peteiro and José Ramón González-Juanatey

Additional information is available at the end of the chapter

http://dx.doi.org/10.5772/intechopen.73025

Abstract

The role of advanced glycation end products (AGEs) in cardiovascular diseases is a matter of interest in the last years and the strong association between the action of AGEs on their receptor (RAGE) and atherosclerosis has attracted increased attention. The aim of this chapter is to review the results of our laboratory and others on the molecular mechanisms triggered by AGEs in the endothelium that could participate in the atherosclerotic process. These mechanisms and molecular pathways could be the source of new therapeutic targets against atherosclerosis or vascular disease. Oxidative stress in endothelium induced by AGEs triggers molecular signaling pathways that produce an inflammatory response or even endothelial dysfunction. Adhesion molecules expression at the membranes of endothelial cells as a consequence of this response or induced by other mechanisms involving AGEs mediates the adhesion of leukocytes to endothelium. This adhesion is a key step in the atherogenesis process and the possible involvement of AGE-RAGE axis in this process should be considered as a potential therapeutic target. Finally, potential pharmacological modulation of AGE-RAGE axis activity at the endothelium is suggested, but the specific pharmacological tools available nowadays are missing; respectively, drugs used for the treatment of cardiovascular and metabolic diseases could be helpful for AGE-RAGE axis modulation, thus also affecting endothelial (dys)function.

Keywords: advanced glycation end products, atherosclerosis, endothelial dysfunction, oxidative stress, receptor for advanced glycation end products, vascular adhesion molecules, vascular inflammation

IntechOpen

1. Introduction

Cardiovascular diseases resulting from atherosclerosis have become the most important cause of mortality and morbidity in the general population [1]. Although atherosclerosis develops as a consequence of multiple risk factors such as hypertension, dyslipidemia, diabetes, aging and smoking, the common pathway for its development is endothelial dysfunction and vascular inflammation [2]. In the last two decades, the role of advanced glycation end products (AGEs) in the development of endothelial dysfunction has gained increasing interest [3–5], initially as a possible molecular mechanism of diabetic cardiovascular complications [3], and, in the last years, as an independent risk factor of vascular injury [6].

AGEs are products of non-enzymatic molecular modifications of proteins and lipids that affect the structure and function of the target molecule. They are produced endogenously by spontaneous reactions, but pathophysiological conditions may accelerate their formation and they also contribute to disease by different mechanisms.

AGEs comprise a heterogeneous group: the most studied are pentosidine and Nε-carboxymethyl-lysine (CML) and quantitatively, the most important in the tissues are the hydroimidazolones like CML [7]. AGEs are formed by a combination of glycation, oxidation, and/or carbonylation reactions both in the extra- and in the intracellular space. Other processes involving lipid peroxidations in the cell membranes lead to the formation of advanced lipid end products, as for example, malondialdehyde [8]. The classical mechanism of AGE formation is the slow Maillard reaction between glucose or reducing sugars and proteins [9]. The interaction between the carbonyl groups of reducing sugars and amino groups of proteins results in the formation of a Schiff base within a few hours. Intramolecular rearrangement of the Schiff base results in more stable Amadori products [9]. An example of these types of products is glycated hemoglobin or glycated albumin, the former is widely used in clinical practice for diagnosis and follow-up of diabetes mellitus and the last could be regarded as a smart alternative to modified hemoglobin for the same purposes, with less dependence on hematological diseases and intracellular conditions. Finally, the process of oxidation of the Amadori products leads to reactive carbonyl compounds and subsequently to the formation of AGEs within weeks to months. AGEs can also be formed intracellularly. Glucose is altered into reactive carbonyl compounds during glycolysis pathway, of which the best-known is methylglyoxal. The chemical reaction between these carbonyl compounds and proteins can result in AGEs [10].

Absorption of exogenous AGEs also contributes to their accumulation in tissues. Tobacco smoke contains highly reactive glycation products which rapidly form AGEs *in vitro* and *in vivo* and therefore, increase the serum AGEs levels in smokers compared to non-smokers [11]. The content of AGEs in food depends on the temperature at which food products are prepared, with oven frying being the most severe inducer [12]. Approximately 10% of the ingested AGEs are absorbed from the gastrointestinal tract into the blood [13]. The final level of AGEs accumulation depends on their clearance and the metabolic mechanisms by the kidney and liver, respectively. Increased level of AGEs can be found in patients with either renal [13] or liver failure [14].

The role of AGEs in cardiovascular diseases is a matter of interest in the last years [15], and the strong association between the axis of action of AGEs and their receptor (RAGE) and atherosclerosis or cardiovascular ischemic disease [3, 16, 17] has attracted increased attention.

The aim of this chapter is to review the results of our laboratory and others on the molecular mechanisms triggered by AGEs in the endothelium that could participate in the atherosclerotic process. These mechanisms and molecular pathways could help in the development of new therapeutic targets against atherosclerosis or vascular disease.

2. Molecular mechanisms triggered by AGEs in the endothelium

It is generally accepted that AGEs target cells by three main mechanisms. First, proteins modified by AGEs have altered biological function, either enzymatic activity, binding properties or structural conformation. Second, extracellular matrix components modified by AGEs interact abnormally with other matrix components and with matrix receptors, such as integrins. This includes also the formation of new links or the alteration of those previously existing, between proteins, which may alter the physical properties of extracellular matrix and cell environment. Third, plasma proteins modified by AGEs bind to cell surface receptors, of which the receptor for AGEs (RAGE) is acknowledged to be the most important, activating intracellular signaling pathways and various cellular responses.

Binding of AGEs to RAGE is responsible for the generation of reactive oxygen species (ROS) and the activation of transcription factors such as nuclear factor-κB (NF-κB), with subsequent changes in the expression of many genes involved in vascular inflammation and endothelial dysfunction [18–20]. Besides from the involvement of AGEs-RAGE axis, the precursors of AGEs, like Amadori products or early glycated products also have a role in the global response of non-enzymatic glycation of proteins, so we will also discuss their effects on endothelial cells.

2.1. AGEs-induced ROS production in the endothelium

One of the first and best studied actions of AGEs on endothelial cells is the induction of ROS. The suggested mechanisms for this action are several and range from the activation of ROS-producing enzymes to the reduction of ROS-neutralizing enzymes. In the first group of enzymes or enzyme complexes are nicotinamide adenine dinucleotide phosphate (NADPH) oxidase [21] and mitochondria [22], whereas in the second, there are endothelial nitric oxide (NO) synthase (eNOS) [23], superoxide dismutase (SOD) and glutathione peroxidase [24, 25]. The molecular mechanisms of these actions have been related to the activation of NF-κB via RAGE [26, 27].

ROS production in endothelial cells has important consequences on endothelial activation. In brain microvascular endothelial cells, AGEs-induced ROS production enhances vascular endothelial growth factor (VEGF) expression, which mediates an increase in cell permeability [28], and platelet tissue factor up-regulation [29]. Other mechanisms of AGEs on endothelial cells promoting endothelial activation or dysfunction are the generation of asymmetric dimethylarginine (ADMA, a metabolic by-product of natural protein modification processes in the cytoplasm of cells, that acts as a competitive inhibitor of NOS) [30], or impaired calcium signaling [31].

It is important to note that the effects of AGEs' precursors (i.e. Amadori products or glycated proteins) on endothelial cells, differ from the effects of AGEs themselves. Several works have focused on this issue (see, for a review, [32]). Amadori products modify eNOS activity and gene expression, promoting apoptosis of endothelial cells [33, 34]. A recent study performed by our group has highlighted the important molecular and functional differences between early glycated human serum albumin (gHSA) and advanced glycated albumin (AGE-HSA), obtained commercially or by glucose incubation during 4 weeks at 37°C in aseptic conditions, respectively [35]. The respective control molecules of these treatments were unmodified commercial HSA and HSA incubated for the same time than AGE-HSA, but without glucose (Ct-HSA). Molecular characterization of the early and advanced glycation products formed on each modified albumin (gHSA and AGE-HSA) were studied by matrix assisted laser desorption/ionization—time of flight (MALDI-TOF)-mass spectrometry. Once characterized, the effects on ROS production of human umbilical vein endothelial cells (HUVECs) under the stimuli of gHSA or AGE-HSA were compared [35]. Low concentrations of gHSA enhanced long-lasting ROS production in HUVECs, whereas AGE-HSA induced extracellular ROS production after short time of incubation and at lower concentrations than gHSA. Extracellular ROS production of HUVEC was measured by the cytochrome C reduction method, whereas intracellular ROS production of HUVEC was measured by 5(6)-carboxy-2′,7′-dichlorofluorescein diacetate (cDCF-DA; Sigma-Aldrich), an intracellular dye for that purpose [36].

Treatment of HUVECs with gHSA (25–100 μg/mL) for different times (4–12 h) induced significant increments of extracellular ROS production with respect to treatment with the same concentration of un-modified albumin (HSA, used as control) [36]. The maximal response (i.e. the quantity of ROS) was obtained with 25 μg/mL gHSA after 4 h of treatment (**Figure 1a**). The effects of AGE-HSA were studied under the same conditions. AGE-HSA increased the extracellular ROS production at lower concentrations (12 μg/mL) and after shorter time of exposure than gHSA (2 h). Another important difference is that, at long incubation periods, the ROS-inducing effects of gHSA were maintained, whereas no significant increases on ROS production were observed with AGE-HSA at 4–8 h (**Figure 1b**).

Similar experiments were designed to measure the intracellular ROS production by using cDCF-DA after 4 h of treatment the HUVECs with gHSA or AGE-HSA (12–50 μg/mL).

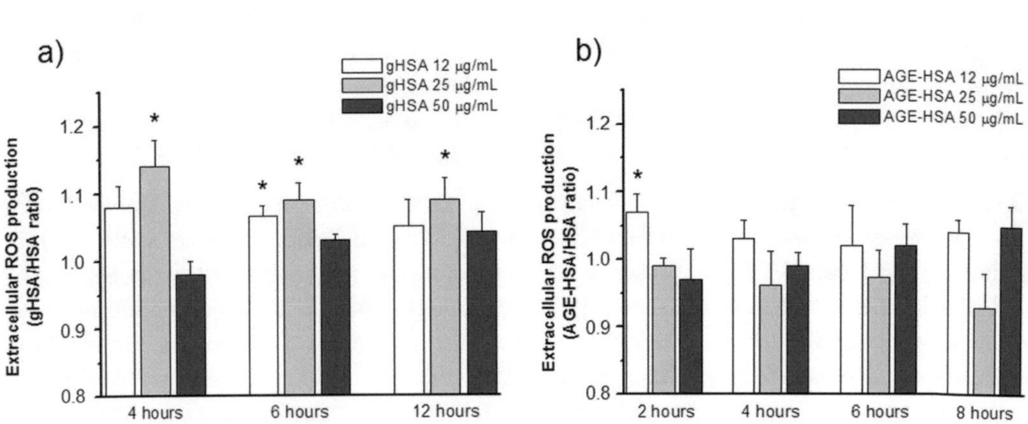

Figure 1. Extracellular ROS production in HUVECs after treatment with different concentrations of (a) gHSA (12–50 mg/mL) or (b) AGE-HSA (12–50 mg/mL), for periods of time indicated on each graph. Columns represent the ratio of ROS produced by treatment/HSA and are expressed as mean ± S.E.M. (vertical bars) of at least three independent experiments. *$p < 0.05$ with respect to the control values (Student's t test).

Interestingly, at 25 μg/mL, gHSA significantly enhanced the intracellular ROS production, whereas AGE-HSA only showed a trend to slightly increase it (**Figure 2**).

Therefore, differences in the induction of ROS production were observed between gHSA (a low glycated product) and AGE-HSA (a high glycated product). Although the effects of AGE-HSA are accepted to be mediated by RAGE, the receptor that mediates the effects of gHSA has not been revealed yet [37], since, the effects of gHSA are not mediated by RAGE [38].

2.2. Expression of adhesion molecules mediating leukocyte adhesion to endothelium

RAGE-ligands interaction induces a series of signal transduction cascades and lead to the activation of transcription factor NF-κB as well as increased expression of cytokines, chemokines, and adhesion molecules [39]. Expression of inducible adhesion molecules is a final common pathway in the development of vascular inflammation and pathology, rendering the vasculature a selective target for circulating peripheral blood cells [27, 40].

A number of studies have demonstrated induction of vascular cell adhesion molecule-1 (VCAM-1) expression in a RAGE-dependent manner when endothelial cells are exposed to AGEs [18]. Moreover, engagement of RAGE by AGEs results in enhanced expression of other adhesion molecules, such as E-selectin and intercellular cell adhesion molecule-1 (ICAM-1) [40–42]. High expression of adhesion molecules in endothelial cells may promote adhesive interactions of circulating monocytes with the endothelial surface, resulting, eventually, in transendothelial migration [43].

We confirmed that AGE-HSA up-regulated ICAM-1 and VCAM-1 expression more than gHSA, in terms of mRNA quantitative changes, measured by total messenger RNA retrotranscription and quantitative real-time polymerase chain reaction (qPCR) [35]. Even while

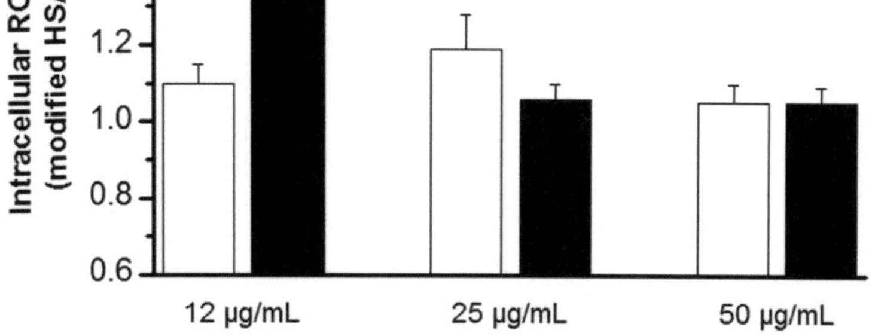

Figure 2. Intracellular ROS production in HUVECs after 4 h of treatment with different concentrations of gHSA (white columns) and AGE-HSA (black columns), as indicated in the x-axis. Results are shown as the ratio modified HSA/control HSA, expressed as mean, in columns, ± S.E.M. (vertical bars) of at least four independent experiments. Comparisons were made between each ratio level and the unit (*$p < 0.05$; Student's *t* test).

the effects of gHSA seemed to be limited to 4 h- treatment, AGE-HSA up-regulated VCAM-1 and ICAM-1 expression for longer periods of time (from 2 to 6 h). Differences on the active concentrations of both glycation products were also observed: whereas gHSA was only active at 25 μg/mL, AGE-HSA was also effective at 12 and 100 μg/mL (**Figure 3**).

To further confirm the increase in the expression of these adhesion molecules, protein levels of VCAM-1 and ICAM-1 were analyzed by western blot analysis after the treatment of HUVECs with two relevant concentrations of gHSA and AGE-HSA: 25 and 100 μg/mL, in comparison with the same concentrations of unmodified HSA and Ct-HSA, respectively. There was a significant elevation of VCAM-1 and ICAM-1 levels caused by the effect of both AGE-HSA concentrations tested. On the other hand, only the concentration of 25 μg/mL gHSA (but not 100 μg/mL) enhanced the ICAM-1 protein levels (**Figure 4**).

The functional translation of VCAM-1 and ICAM-1 up-regulation was analyzed by the adhesion of peripheral blood mononuclear cells (PBMCs) to HUVEC monolayers after treatment with both types of modified albumins for 4 h (**Figure 5**). After these treatments, the adhesion of calcein-AM-stained PBMCs to HUVEC monolayers after 1 h of incubation and washing of non-adhered

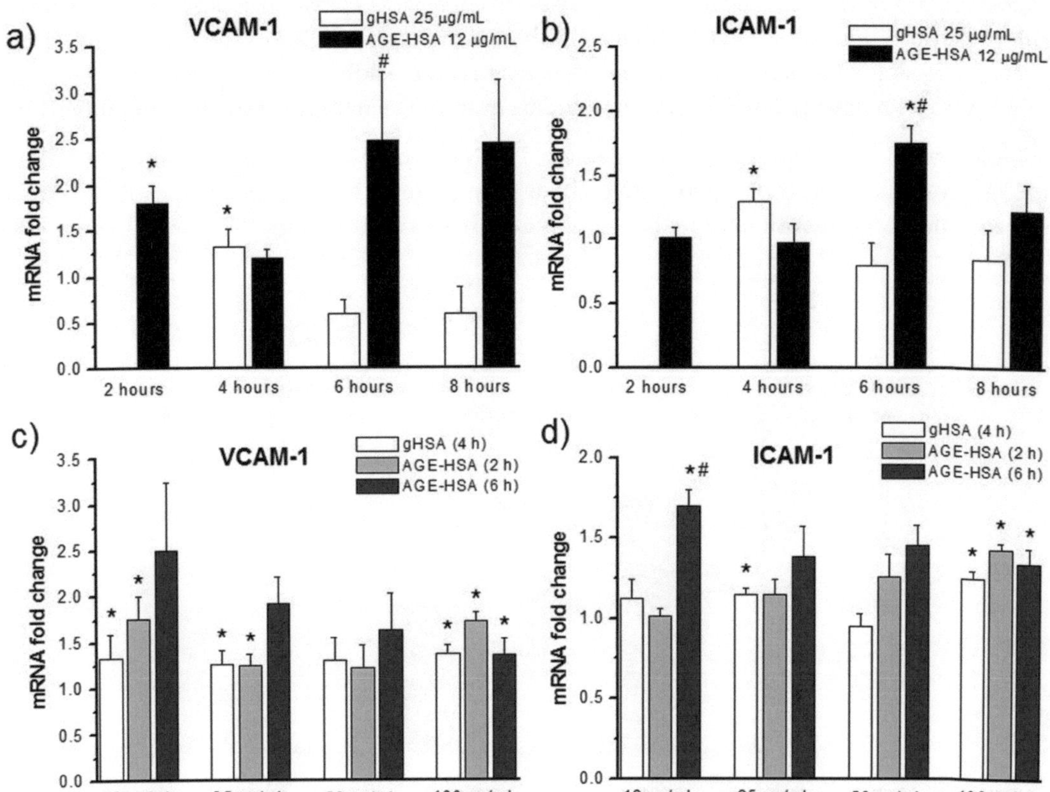

Figure 3. The expression levels of mRNA of VCAM-1 (a and c) and ICAM-1 (b and d) after treatment with gHSA or AGE-HSA at the concentrations and times indicated on HUVEC cultures. Results are shown as the ratio treatment/respective control, expressed as mean (columns) ± S.E.M. (vertical bars) of at least four independent experiments. Comparisons were made between each ratio level and the unit (*$p < 0.05$; Student's *t* test) and between AGE-HSA and gHSA treated experiments ate the same time of incubation (a and b) or concentration (c and d; #$p < 0.05$; Student's *t* test).

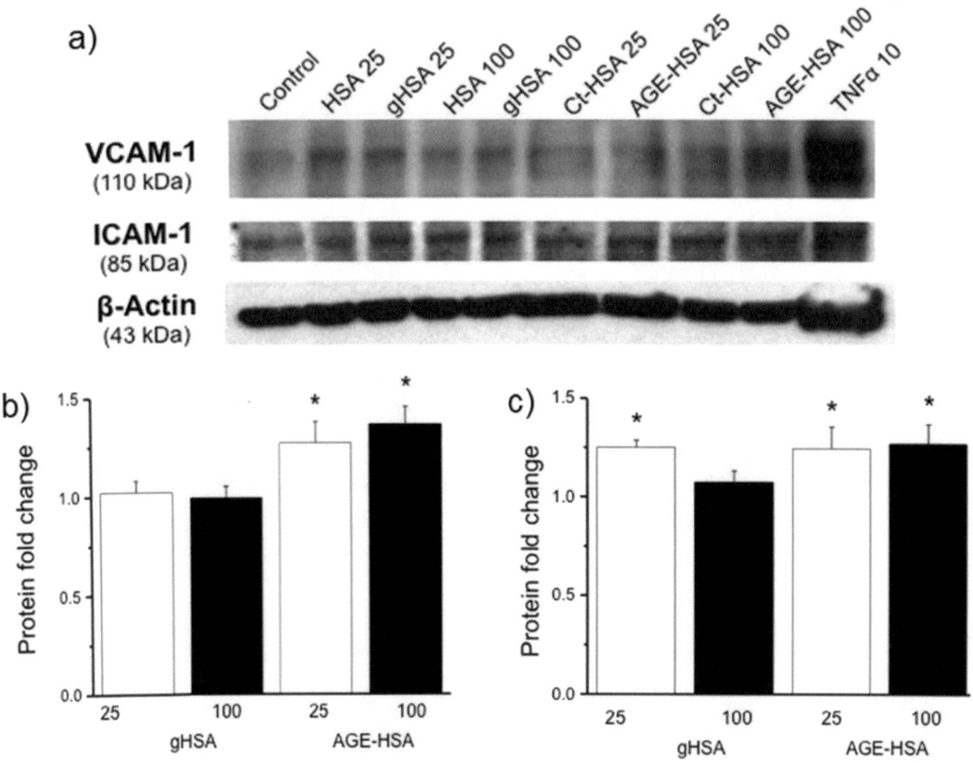

Figure 4. The expression levels of VCAM-1 and ICAM-1 measured by western blot in HUVEC protein extracts obtained after 4 h of treatment with gHSA or AGE-HSA (25 or 100 μg/mL, as indicated). TNF-α (10 ng/mL) was used as a positive inducer control. (a) Representative blots for VCAM-1, ICAM-1 and β-actin. Columns represent the fold change of protein expression for (b) VCAM-1 and (c) ICAM-1 calculated by optical densitometry with respect to β-actin and expressed as mean values (columns) ± S.E.M. (vertical bars) of at least three independent experiments. *$p < 0.05$ with respect to unmodified HSA or Ct-HSA for gHSA and AGE-HSA, respectively (Student's *t* test).

PBMCs was quantified by fluorescence. In these conditions, gHSA (25 μg/mL) induced no significant effect in PBMCs adhesion in comparison with the control HSA. However, AGE-HSA (25 μg/mL) induced a significant increase in the adhesion of PBMC to HUVEC monolayers.

The effects of gHSA and AGE-HSA on PBMCs transmigration through HUVEC monolayers were studied in comparison to the ICAM-1 and VCAM-1 changes of expression. For these experiments HUVEC with transfected green fluorescent protein were grown until confluence onto transwells with 5 μm of pore size (Millipore). After treatment with AGE-HSA (25 and 100 μg/mL) for 4 h PBMCs were layered over the HUVECs and incubated at 37°C. TNF-α (10 ng/mL) was used as a positive control because it induces endothelial cell activation and promotes PBMCs transmigration through the endothelial monolayer. The number of transmigrated PBMCs were estimated by quantification of nuclei acids content with CyQUANT® GR dye (Molecular probes, Invitrogen) at the end of the experiment. Unless for the case of TNF-α, no changes were observed for any of the stimuli after 3 h of treatment. However, after 24 h of HUVEC incubation with 25 μg/mL AGE-HSA, a significant increase in the migration of PBMCs was observed as compared to control (**Figure 6**). On the contrary, higher concentration of AGE-HSA (100 μg/mL), showed no effect in the transmigration of PBMCs. The positive control with TNF-α increased the migration of PBMCs even more than after 3 h (**Figure 6**).

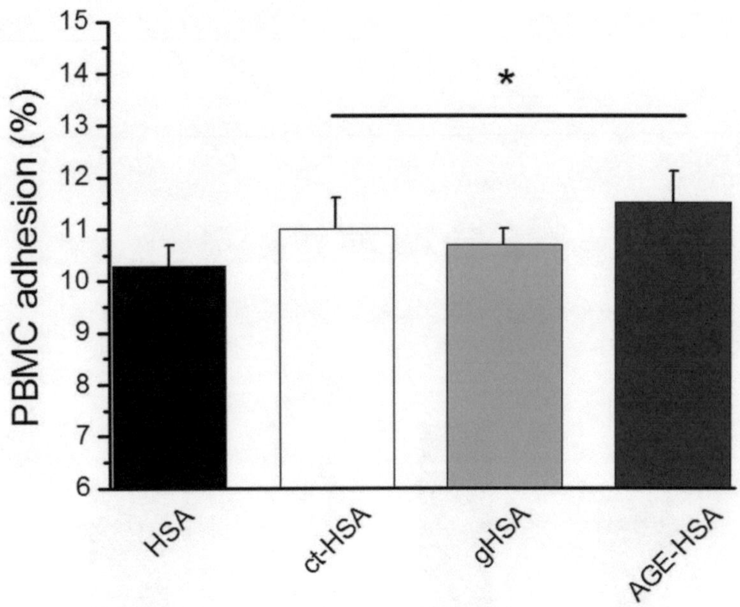

Figure 5. Quantification of the adhesion of PBMCs to a HUVEC monolayer, after treatment of HUVECs during 4 h with gHSA (25 µg/mL) or AGE-HSA (25 µg/mL), compared with HSA (25 µg/mL) or ct-HSA (25 µg/mL), respectively. The graph represents the mean percentage of adhesion (columns) ± S.E.M. (vertical bars) of at least three independent experiments. *$p < 0.05$ between the columns indicated (ANOVA followed by Tukey's test).

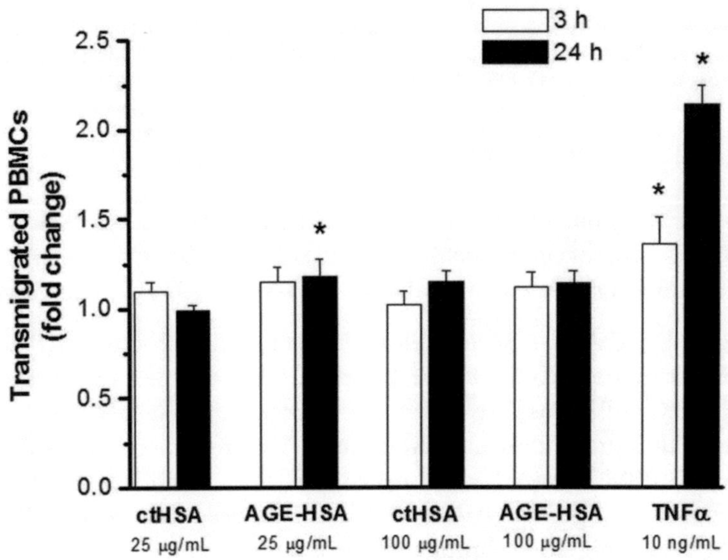

Figure 6. Transmigration of PBMCs through HUVEC monolayers after 3 h (white columns) or 24 h (black columns). Columns represent the mean (columns) ± S.E.M. (in vertical bars) of the increase of PBMCs transmigration after treatment compared to untreated control. *$p < 0.05$ with respect to untreated control (Student's *t* test).

Given the results obtained in the adhesion molecules expression in HUVECs, another approach was performed repeating the study with *in vivo* glycated albumin obtained from healthy volunteers and from cardiovascular patients, which donated their blood after signing informed consent.

http://dx.doi.org/10.5772/intechopen.73025

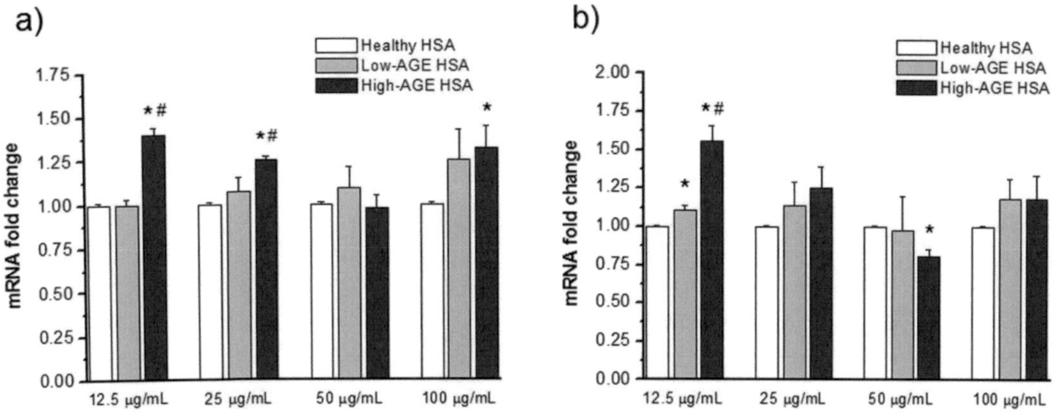

Figure 7. The expression of mRNA for ICAM-1 (a) and VCAM-1 (b) after the treatment of HUVECs with HSA isolated from healthy volunteers (healthy HSA) or with low-AGE HSA and high-AGE HSA from cardiovascular patients for 4 h. Columns represent the fold increase of mRNA expression for each gene and are expressed as mean values (columns) ± S.E.M. (vertical bars) of at least three independent experiments. $^{*}p < 0.05$ with respect to healthy HSA. $\#p < 0.05$ with respect to low-AGE HSA (Student's t test).

The whole study and protocols were approved by the Ethics Committee for Human Studies at Galicia (Spanish region) in accordance to the 1975 Declaration of Helsinki. Particularly, we analyzed the effect of HSAs categorized in healthy or nonglycated (from healthy volunteers), low-AGE or high-AGE (from cardiovascular patients), according to their content in AGE adducts. Glycation level was estimated by the molecular weight increment of isolated HSAs, due to the incorporation of different glycation products to the molecule. This was measured by mass spectrometry with a 4800 MALDI-TOF/TOF analyzer (Applied Biosystems). On this basis, attending to the increase of HSA molecular weight with respect to non-modified HSA, three stocks of HSA were prepared and categorized as healthy-nonglycated HSA, low-, and high-AGE HSA (molecular weights of 66,481, 66,665 and 66,778 Da for healthy, low-, and high-AGE HSA, respectively). HUVECs were incubated with a range of concentrations of these types of HSAs (12–200 μg/mL) for 4 h. In these conditions, the treatment with high-AGE HSA significantly increased the mRNA expression of ICAM-1 at concentrations of 12.5 and 25 μg/mL with respect to healthy-nonglycated HSA (**Figure 7a**; $p < 0.001$). An increase was also observed at 100 μg/mL concentration with respect to healthy HSA ($p = 0.046$). Moreover, high-AGE HSA was able to induce a significant increase with respect to low-AGE HSA at 12.5 and 25 μg/mL (**Figure 7a**; $p < 0.05$).

In the case of VCAM-1 expression, high-AGE HSA only induced an increase in the mRNA expression at 12.5 μg/mL with respect to healthy HSA and low-AGE HSA (**Figure 7b**; $p < 0.05$). At this concentration, low-AGE HSA also induced an increase in the expression of VCAM-1 with respect to healthy HSA (**Figure 7b**; $p < 0.05$). Finally, at a concentration of 50 μg/mL, high-AGE HAS induced a reduction in the expression of VCAM-1 with respect to healthy HSA ($p < 0.05$). This reduction in the expression of VCAM-1 was only transient as the mRNA levels recovered again at higher concentrations. Altogether, these results suggest that *in vivo* glycation of albumin could have a pro-inflammatory effect in endothelial cells, which would trigger chronic endothelial dysfunction.

PBMCs adhesion to HUVECs was also studied with *in vivo* glycated albumins at 12.5, 25 and 100 μg/mL. HUVECs were treated with these concentrations for 24 h. After that, HUVECs

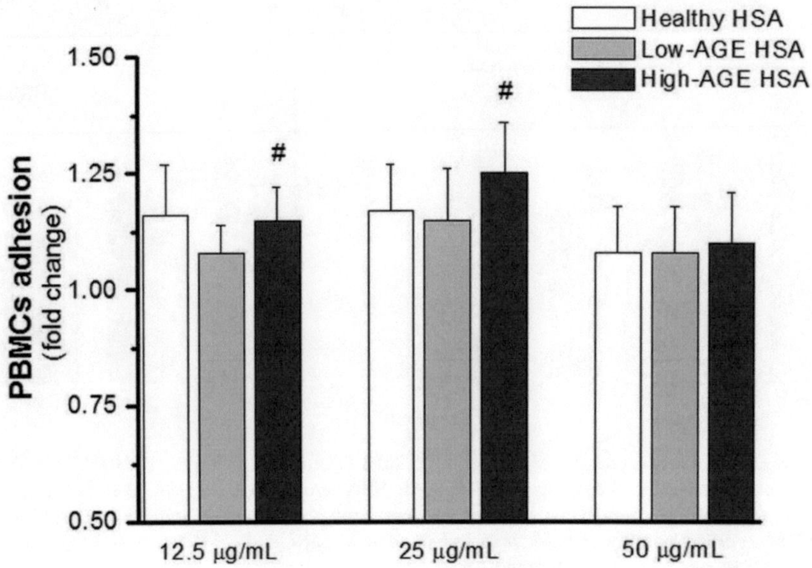

Figure 8. PBMCs adhesion to HUVEC monolayers treated with albumin from healthy volunteers (healthy HSA) or low-AGE HSA and high-AGE HSA from cardiovascular patients for 24 h. Columns represent the fold change of percentage of PBMCs adhered with respect to commercial HSA, expressed as mean values (columns) ± S.E.M. (vertical bars) of at least three independent experiments. #$p < 0.05$ with respect to low-AGE HSA (Student's *t* test).

were incubated with PBMCs for 1 h. A slight but significant increase in PBMCs adhesion (measured as explained above) was observed with high-AGE HSA with respect to low-AGE HSA at 12.5 µg/mL ($p < 0.05$), but not with respect to healthy HSA (**Figure 8**; $p < 0.05$). A trend toward an increase in PBMCs adhesion was also observed after treatment with high-AGE HSA with respect to low-AGE HSA at 25 µg/mL ($p = 0.06$). This suggests that *in vivo* glycated albumin needs more time to induce PBMCs adhesion than highly *in vitro* glycated albumin (AGE-HSA).

3. Potential implications for pharmacological modulation of AGE-RAGE axis activity

In an attempt to counteract the inflammatory effects of AGE-HSA, we selected three RAGE inhibitors: a soluble form of RAGE (sRAGE; R&D systems), used at 0.25, 0.5 and 1 ng/mL; a monoclonal antibody against RAGE (anti-RAGE; R&D systems), used at 5, 10 and 20 µg/mL; and the RAGE antagonist FPS-ZM1 (Calbiochem, Merck Millipore), used at 125, 250, 500 and 1000 nM. HUVECs were pre-treated with different concentrations of these inhibitors and 50 min later treated with 25 µg/mL AGE-HSA. The inhibitory effect of these agents on the expression of VCAM-1 and ICAM-1 in HUVECs was studied.

However, contrary to what we expected, blockade of RAGE by using sRAGE, anti-RAGE antibody and FPS-ZM1 was not sufficient to counteract the AGE-induced VCAM-1 and ICAM-1 up-regulation at any of the concentrations tested under our experimental conditions. Our results may suggest that on endothelium, other RAGE-independent mechanisms may also

http://dx.doi.org/10.5772/intechopen.73025

be acting to increase adhesion molecule expression and induce inflammation. Other possible explanation for these results is that the pharmacological tools actually available to block RAGE activity are not able to block the effects of AGEs at the endothelial level. However, the results obtained on *in vivo* models of disease are promising, as we comment below.

To investigate the effects of RAGE blockade in pathological conditions, many studies have used soluble forms of RAGE or anti-RAGE antibodies, which can antagonize RAGE-ligand interaction to competitively inhibit the activation of RAGE signaling [39, 44, 45]. Evidence from these studies has shown that RAGE blockade protected against various disease challenges. Soluble RAGE, which competes with cellular RAGE for ligand binding, has been able to reduce inflammatory responses in several models tested. Streptozotocin-induced diabetic apoE−/− mice treated with once daily injections of murine sRAGE showed suppressed acceleration of atherosclerotic lesions in a dose-dependent manner [46]. In parallel with decreased atherosclerotic lesion area and the complexity of the atheroma plaque composition, the levels of tissue factor, VCAM-1, AGEs, and nuclear translocation of NF-kB were decreased in the aortas of sRAGE-treated mice [42, 46]. In other work, sRAGE-treated mice displayed significant stabilization of the lesion area at the aortic root. Compared with diabetic mice receiving albumin (placebo), those receiving sRAGE had significantly diminished activity of monocyte chemoattractant protein-1 (MCP-1), cyclooxygenase-2 (COX-2), VCAM-1 and matrix metalloprotease 9 (MMP-9) within aortic tissue [47]. Similarly, administration of sRAGE resulted in a highly significant decrease in atherosclerotic lesion area in parallel with decreased vascular expression of pro-inflammatory RAGE ligand S100/calgranulins and VCAM-1 and MMPs [48]. Moreover, sRAGE-treated non-diabetic mice displayed significantly decreased atherosclerosis and vascular inflammation [47, 48].

Further studies using anti-RAGE IgG fragments to block ligand binding to RAGE have confirmed these results, especially at the highest dose (up to 10 μg/mL) tested [49]. Exposure of HUVECs to AGE-bovine serum albumin induced expression of VCAM-1 and increased adhesiveness of the monolayer for T lymphoblast of the Molt-4 cell line, which was inhibited by addition of anti-RAGE IgG or sRAGE [40]. Activation of signaling pathway on endothelial cells by advanced oxidation products resulted in overexpression of VCAM-1 and ICAM-1 at both, gene and protein levels, something that was prevented by blocking RAGE with either anti-RAGE IgG or excess sRAGE [27]. Administration of anti-RAGE IgG or sRAGE strongly blocked the increase in vascular permeability in diabetic rats injected with human diabetic red blood cells [50]. Mice treated with sRAGE or anti-RAGE F(ab')2 fragments displayed significantly lower intima/media ratio (a marker of negative vascular remodeling after injury) compared to vehicle-treated animal models of femoral artery injury [51]. However, despite the fact that both, sRAGE and anti-RAGE IgG were able to reduce inflammatory responses in all models tested so far [42, 46, 50, 52], no significant decrease in ICAM-1 and VCAM-1 expression was observed after pre-treatment with soluble RAGE or anti-RAGE antibody, under our experimental conditions.

A recently developed high-affinity RAGE-specific inhibitor: FPS-ZM1 (N-benzyl-4-chloro-N-cyclohexylbenzamide; Calbiochem, Merck Millipore) [53] was also studied. This inhibitor was developed to interact with the ligand-binding domain of the receptor and block RAGE signaling. In our *in vitro* experimental conditions this approach was also unable to inhibit AGE-induced VCAM-1 and ICAM-1 up-regulation.

It is worth mentioning that, most of the above-mentioned works did not elucidate the precise AGE(s) that trigger signal transduction mechanisms upon interacting with RAGE. Kislinger et al. [54] studied the effect of CML-adducts and showed that CML-mediated VCAM-1 expression on HUVECs was also suppressed in the presence of excess sRAGE or anti-RAGE IgG. Nevertheless, they suggest that the findings presented in their work do not rule out other specific AGE products of glycation or oxidation, such as pentosidine, pyralline, methylglyoxal, and imidazolone [55–57], which are present in our modified albumins. Additionally, they also specified that their findings do not rule out either the presence of other receptors or cellular interaction sites for CML adducts, being possible that other receptors for AGE [58–60] may also engage CML- and AGE-modified adducts. These situations might explain why no reduction in the up-regulation of adhesion molecules is observed after pre-treatment with sRAGE and anti-RAGE antibody under our experimental conditions.

Additionally, Amadori-modified albumin stimulates adhesion of monocytes to endothelial cells through enhanced transcription of the cell surface adhesion molecules E-selectin, VCAM-1 and ICAM-1 [61], implicating an initial endothelial cell activation occurring at atherosclerosis-prone vascular sites [62, 63]. However, Amadori products do not compete with AGE-albumin for binding to AGE receptors such as RAGE [64]. Aortic endothelial cells express specific receptors for Amadori-modified albumin [37, 65]. Although less information is available for the receptor for Amadori products and signaling through Amadori-modified albumin receptors remains obscure, calnexin [66] and nucleophosmin [67, 68] have been reported to be the fructosyl-lysine specific binding proteins [66–68]. Binding of Amadori-modified albumin to calnexin-like receptors may participate in degradation and/or activation of signal transduction processes involved in mediating the biologic activities of Amadori-modified albumin [66]. The E-selectin expression induced by Amadori-modified albumin was 10 or 20 times higher than that induced with three types of AGEs-HSAs and was not suppressed by anti-RAGE antibody [69]. This would explain why RAGE antagonism would not counteract the increase in adhesion molecules expression.

In agreement with this hypothesis, Esposito et al. [70] found that anti-RAGE antibody completely prevented leukocyte adhesion to endothelial cells grown for 8 weeks in high-glucose-containing media, but it did not reduce the adhesion at 24 h. These results demonstrate that AGEs are important mediators of high-glucose-induced endothelial dysfunction after long-term exposure, whereas the same changes in acute exposure occur with the action of mediators other than AGEs. As the formation of Amadori products is highly probable after 24 h incubation in high glucose medium, but not the formation of AGEs, the effects on the inflammation parameters observed by Esposito et al. [70], and not prevented by anti-RAGE antibodies, might be due to the effect of the early glycated products, and not AGEs.

Besides from directly blocking RAGE, alternative pharmacological approaches might turn out to be more promising. Namely, it has been shown that both RAGE and sRAGE can be regulated by currently available pharmacological agents [71]. Other drugs currently in use for diabetic complications have been shown to have an effect on AGE accumulation. These include the antihypertensive angiotensin-converting enzyme inhibitor (ACEI) ramipril [72] and the glucose-lowering drug metformin [73], which both reduce AGE. Forbes et al. [74] demonstrated that compared with placebo, the ACEI perindopril increased human plasma sRAGE levels and reduced plasma AGE concentrations, suggesting an additional mechanistic effect of ACE inhibition in the treatment and prevention of vascular disease. The inhibition of ACE in

http://dx.doi.org/10.5772/intechopen.73025

rats increased the renal expression of sRAGE and decreased the expression of renal full-length RAGE protein [74]. These investigators also showed that plasma sRAGE levels were significantly increased by inhibition of ACE in both diabetic rats and human subjects with type 1 diabetes [74]. Olmesartan, an angiotensin II type 1 receptor blocker, inhibited the AGE-evoked ROS generation and reduced the expression levels of monocyte chemoattractant protein 1 and ICAM-1 in endothelial cells, subsequently blocking T-cell adhesion to endothelial cells [75].

Other potential agents that may affect circulating sRAGE include the thiazolidinediones [76, 77] and statins [78–80], both of which are known to modulate AGE-RAGE axis. Marx et al. [76] investigated the effects of the two thiazolidinediones available, rosiglitazone and pioglitazone, on RAGE expression in HUVECs. Exposure of HUVECs to thiazolidinedione resulted in a similar reduction in RAGE mRNA expression, via inhibition of NF-κB activation, and in RAGE cell surface expression, demonstrating how these drugs may influence RAGE expression and its deleterious inflammatory activity in subjects with DM [76]. Blockade of the interaction of S100A12 (an endogenous ligand of RAGE) with RAGE by statins at an early stage may prevent inflammation in atherosclerosis and counteract the harmful effects mediated by C reactive protein [81].

Finally, recent results testing new potential drugs have been reported. Curcumin, a polyphenolic natural compound is able to trap methylglyoxal, an important precursor of AGEs [82]. Added on endothelial cell cultures curcumin reduced the intracellular ROS levels and improved cell viability compared with the treatment of methylglyoxal alone. There was also a significant reduction in the expression levels of ICAM-1 [82]. Liquiritin, the 4′-O-glucoside of the flavanone liquiritigenin, reduced AGEs-induced apoptosis and ROS generation in HUVECs and also significantly increased AGEs-reduced SOD activity [83]. It even down-regulated the RAGE protein expression and significantly blocked NF-κB activation [83].

4. Conclusions

Oxidative stress induction by AGEs at endothelium triggers molecular signaling pathways that produce an inflammatory response or even endothelial dysfunction. Adhesion molecules expression at the membrane surface of endothelial cells as a consequence of this response or induced by AGEs by other mechanisms mediates the adhesion of leukocytes to endothelium. This adhesion is a key step in the atherogenesis process and the possible involvement of AGE-RAGE axis in it should be considered as potential therapeutic target. Finally, possible pharmacological modulation of AGE-RAGE axis activity at the endothelium is suggested, but specific pharmacological tools available nowadays are not efficient enough; momentarily, drugs used for cardiovascular and metabolic problems could be helpful in modulating the AGE-RAGE axis.

Acknowledgements

This study was supported by the *Plan Estatal de Investigación Científica y Técnica y de Innovación 2013–2016* and the *Instituto de Salud Carlos III* (grant number PI14/01140), co-financed by European Regional Development Fund. *Axudas para a consolidación e estructuración de unidades de investigación competitivas, Xunta de Galicia* (grant number ED431B 2016/022). The work of Beatriz Paradela-Dobarro was supported by *Instituto de Salud Carlos III* (grant number FI11/00325).

Author details

Ezequiel Alvarez[1,2*], Beatriz Paradela-Dobarro[1,2], Mercedes González-Peteiro[3] and José Ramón González-Juanatey[2,4]

*Address all correspondence to: ezequiel.alvarez.castro@gmail.com

1 Instituto de Investigación Sanitaria de Santiago de Compostela (IDIS), Santiago de Compostela, A Coruña, Spain

2 CIBER de Enfermedades Cardiovasculares (CIBERCV), Madrid, Spain

3 Departamento de Enfermería, Universidad de Santiago de Compostela, Santiago de Compostela, Spain

4 Instituto de Investigación Sanitaria de Santiago de Compostela (IDIS), Servicio de Cardiología y Unidad de Hemodinámica, Complexo Hospitalario Universitario de Santiago de Compostela (CHUS), SERGAS, Santiago de Compostela, A Coruña, Spain

References

[1] Global, regional, and national life expectancy, all-cause mortality, and cause-specific mortality for 249 causes of death, 1980-2015: A systematic analysis for the Global Burden of Disease Study 2015. Lancet. 2016;**388**(10053):1459-1544

[2] Cahill PA, Redmond EM. Vascular endothelium—Gatekeeper of vessel health. Atherosclerosis. 2016;**248**:97-109

[3] Basta G, Schmidt AM, De Caterina R. Advanced glycation end products and vascular inflammation: Implications for accelerated atherosclerosis in diabetes. Cardiovascular Research. 2004;**63**(4):582-592

[4] Sena CM, Pereira AM, Seica R. Endothelial dysfunction—A major mediator of diabetic vascular disease. Biochimica et Biophysica Acta. 2013;**1832**(12):2216-2231

[5] Wautier JL, Schmidt AM. Protein glycation: A firm link to endothelial cell dysfunction. Circulation Research. 2004;**95**(3):233-238

[6] de Vos LC et al. Advanced glycation end products: An emerging biomarker for adverse outcome in patients with peripheral artery disease. Atherosclerosis. 2016;**254**:291-299

[7] Thornalley PJ et al. Quantitative screening of advanced glycation endproducts in cellular and extracellular proteins by tandem mass spectrometry. The Biochemical Journal. 2003;**375**(Pt 3):581-592

[8] Jaisson S, Gillery P. Evaluation of nonenzymatic posttranslational modification-derived products as biomarkers of molecular aging of proteins. Clinical Chemistry. 2010;**56**(9): 1401-1412

[9] Ott C et al. Role of advanced glycation end products in cellular signaling. Redox Biology. 2014;**2**:411-429

[10] Degenhardt TP, Thorpe SR, Baynes JW. Chemical modification of proteins by methylglyoxal. Cellular and Molecular Biology (Noisy-le-Grand, France). 1998;**44**(7):1139-1145

[11] Cerami C et al. Tobacco smoke is a source of toxic reactive glycation products. Proceedings of the National Academy of Sciences of the United States of America. 1997;**94**(25): 13915-13920

[12] Goldberg T et al. Advanced glycoxidation end products in commonly consumed foods. Journal of the American Dietetic Association. 2004;**104**(8):1287-1291

[13] Koschinsky T et al. Orally absorbed reactive glycation products (glycotoxins): An environmental risk factor in diabetic nephropathy. Proceedings of the National Academy of Sciences of the United States of America. 1997;**94**(12):6474-6479

[14] Yagmur E et al. Elevation of nepsilon-(carboxymethyl)lysine-modified advanced glycation end products in chronic liver disease is an indicator of liver cirrhosis. Clinical Biochemistry. 2006;**39**(1):39-45

[15] Prasad A, Bekker P, Tsimikas S. Advanced glycation end products and diabetic cardiovascular disease. Cardiology in Review. 2012;**20**(4):177-183

[16] Fukami K, Yamagishi S, Okuda S. Role of AGEs-RAGE system in cardiovascular disease. Current Pharmaceutical Design. 2014;**20**(14):2395-2402

[17] Chiang KH et al. Plasma levels of soluble receptor for advanced glycation end products are associated with endothelial function and predict cardiovascular events in nondiabetic patients. Coronary Artery Disease. 2009;**20**(4):267-273

[18] Basta G et al. Advanced glycation end products activate endothelium through signal-transduction receptor RAGE: A mechanism for amplification of inflammatory responses. Circulation. 2002;**105**(7):816-822

[19] Wautier MP et al. Activation of NADPH oxidase by AGE links oxidant stress to altered gene expression via RAGE. American Journal of Physiology. Endocrinology and Metabolism. 2001;**280**(5):E685-E694

[20] Yan SF, Ramasamy R, Schmidt AM. The RAGE Axis: A fundamental mechanism signaling danger to the vulnerable vasculature. Circulation Research. 2010;**106**(5):842-853

[21] Lubrano V, Balzan S. Roles of LOX-1 in microvascular dysfunction. Microvascular Research. 2016;**105**:132-140

[22] Shen GX. Mitochondrial dysfunction, oxidative stress and diabetic cardiovascular disorders. Cardiovascular & Hematological Disorders Drug Targets. 2012;**12**(2):106-112

[23] Ren X et al. Advanced glycation end-products decreases expression of endothelial nitric oxide synthase through oxidative stress in human coronary artery endothelial cells. Cardiovascular Diabetology. 2017;**16**(1):52

[24] Liu GD et al. The augmentation of O-GlcNAcylation reduces glyoxal-induced cell injury by attenuating oxidative stress in human retinal microvascular endothelial cells. International Journal of Molecular Medicine. 2015;**36**(4):1019-1027

[25] Chen J et al. C-reactive protein upregulates receptor for advanced glycation end products expression and alters antioxidant defenses in rat endothelial progenitor cells. Journal of Cardiovascular Pharmacology. 2009;**53**(5):359-367

[26] Morita M et al. Advanced glycation end products-induced reactive oxygen species generation is partly through NF-kappa B activation in human aortic endothelial cells. Journal of Diabetes and its Complications. 2013;**27**(1):11-15

[27] Guo ZJ et al. Advanced oxidation protein products activate vascular endothelial cells via a RAGE-mediated signaling pathway. Antioxidants & Redox Signaling. 2008;**10**(10): 1699-1712

[28] Niiya Y et al. Advanced glycation end products increase permeability of brain microvascular endothelial cells through reactive oxygen species-induced vascular endothelial growth factor expression. Journal of Stroke and Cerebrovascular Diseases. 2012;**21**(4):293-298

[29] Niiya Y et al. Susceptibility of brain microvascular endothelial cells to advanced glycation end products-induced tissue factor upregulation is associated with intracellular reactive oxygen species. Brain Research. 2006;**1108**(1):179-187

[30] Ando R et al. Involvement of advanced glycation end product-induced asymmetric dimethylarginine generation in endothelial dysfunction. Diabetes & Vascular Disease Research. 2013;**10**(5):436-441

[31] Naser N et al. Advanced glycation end products acutely impair Ca(2+) signaling in bovine aortic endothelial cells. Frontiers in Physiology. 2013;**4**:38

[32] Schalkwijk CG, Miyata T. Early- and advanced non-enzymatic glycation in diabetic vascular complications: The search for therapeutics. Amino Acids. 2012;**42**(4):1193-1204

[33] Amore A et al. Amadori-configurated albumin induces nitric oxide-dependent apoptosis of endothelial cells: A possible mechanism of diabetic vasculopathy. Nephrology, Dialysis, Transplantation. 2004;**19**(1):53-60

[34] Amore A et al. Nonenzymatically glycated albumin (Amadori adducts) enhances nitric oxide synthase activity and gene expression in endothelial cells. Kidney International. 1997;**51**(1):27-35

[35] Paradela-Dobarro B et al. Key structural and functional differences between early and advanced glycation products. Journal of Molecular Endocrinology. 2016;**56**(1):23-37

[36] Rodino-Janeiro BK et al. Glycated albumin, a precursor of advanced glycation end-products, up-regulates NADPH oxidase and enhances oxidative stress in human endothelial

cells: Molecular correlate of diabetic vasculopathy. Diabetes/Metabolism Research and Reviews. 2010;**26**(7):550-558

[37] Wu VY, Cohen MP. Identification of aortic endothelial cell binding proteins for Amadori adducts in glycated albumin. Biochemical and Biophysical Research Communications. 1993;**193**(3):1131-1136

[38] Zhang M et al. Glycated proteins stimulate reactive oxygen species production in cardiac myocytes: Involvement of Nox2 (gp91phox)-containing NADPH oxidase. Circulation. 2006;**113**(9):1235-1243

[39] Chuah YK et al. Receptor for advanced glycation end products and its involvement in inflammatory diseases. International Journal of Inflammation. 2013;**2013**:403460

[40] Schmidt AM et al. Advanced glycation endproducts interacting with their endothelial receptor induce expression of vascular cell adhesion molecule-1 (VCAM-1) in cultured human endothelial cells and in mice. A potential mechanism for the accelerated vasculopathy of diabetes. The Journal of Clinical Investigation. 1995;**96**(3):1395-1403

[41] Boulanger E et al. AGEs bind to mesothelial cells via RAGE and stimulate VCAM-1 expression. Kidney International. 2002;**61**(1):148-156

[42] Kislinger T et al. Receptor for advanced glycation end products mediates inflammation and enhanced expression of tissue factor in vasculature of diabetic apolipoprotein E-null mice. Arteriosclerosis, Thrombosis, and Vascular Biology. 2001;**21**(6):905-910

[43] Aronson D, Rayfield EJ. How hyperglycemia promotes atherosclerosis: Molecular mechanisms. Cardiovascular Diabetology. 2002;**1**:1

[44] Chen Y et al. Blockade of late stages of autoimmune diabetes by inhibition of the receptor for advanced glycation end products. Journal of Immunology. 2004;**173**(2):1399-1405

[45] Zeng S et al. Blockade of receptor for advanced glycation end product (RAGE) attenuates ischemia and reperfusion injury to the liver in mice. Hepatology. 2004;**39**(2):422-432

[46] Park L et al. Suppression of accelerated diabetic atherosclerosis by the soluble receptor for advanced glycation endproducts. Nature Medicine. 1998;**4**(9):1025-1031

[47] Bucciarelli LG et al. RAGE blockade stabilizes established atherosclerosis in diabetic apolipoprotein E-null mice. Circulation. 2002;**106**(22):2827-2835

[48] Wendt T et al. Receptor for advanced glycation endproducts (RAGE) and vascular inflammation: Insights into the pathogenesis of macrovascular complications in diabetes. Current Atherosclerosis Reports. 2002;**4**(3):228-237

[49] Liliensiek B et al. Receptor for advanced glycation end products (RAGE) regulates sepsis but not the adaptive immune response. The Journal of Clinical Investigation. 2004;**113**(11): 1641-1650

[50] Wautier JL et al. Receptor-mediated endothelial cell dysfunction in diabetic vasculopathy. Soluble receptor for advanced glycation end products blocks hyperpermeability in diabetic rats. The Journal of Clinical Investigation. 1996;**97**(1):238-243

[51] Sakaguchi T et al. Central role of RAGE-dependent neointimal expansion in arterial restenosis. The Journal of Clinical Investigation. 2003;**111**(7):959-972

[52] Goova MT et al. Blockade of receptor for advanced glycation end-products restores effective wound healing in diabetic mice. The American Journal of Pathology. 2001; **159**(2):513-525

[53] Deane R et al. A multimodal RAGE-specific inhibitor reduces amyloid beta-mediated brain disorder in a mouse model of Alzheimer disease. The Journal of Clinical Investigation. 2012;**122**(4):1377-1392

[54] Kislinger T et al. N(epsilon)-(carboxymethyl)lysine adducts of proteins are ligands for receptor for advanced glycation end products that activate cell signaling pathways and modulate gene expression. The Journal of Biological Chemistry. 1999;**274**(44):31740-31749

[55] Sell DR, Monnier VM. Structure elucidation of a senescence cross-link from human extracellular matrix. Implication of pentoses in the aging process. The Journal of Biological Chemistry. 1989;**264**(36):21597-21602

[56] Njoroge FG, Sayre LM, Monnier VM. Detection of D-glucose-derived pyrrole compounds during Maillard reaction under physiological conditions. Carbohydrate Research. 1987;**167**: 211-220

[57] Westwood ME, Thornalley PJ. Molecular characteristics of methylglyoxal-modified bovine and human serum albumins. Comparison with glucose-derived advanced glycation end-product-modified serum albumins. Journal of Protein Chemistry. 1995;**14**(5):359-372

[58] Vlassara H, Bucala R. Recent progress in advanced glycation and diabetic vascular disease: Role of advanced glycation end product receptors. Diabetes. 1996;**45**(Suppl 3):S65-S66

[59] Araki N et al. Macrophage scavenger receptor mediates the endocytic uptake and degradation of advanced glycation end products of the Maillard reaction. European Journal of Biochemistry. 1995;**230**(2):408-415

[60] el Khoury J et al. Macrophages adhere to glucose-modified basement membrane collagen IV via their scavenger receptors. The Journal of Biological Chemistry. 1994;**269**(14): 10197-10200

[61] Desfaits AC, Serri O, Renier G. Gliclazide reduces the induction of human monocyte adhesion to endothelial cells by glycated albumin. Diabetes, Obesity & Metabolism. 1999;**1**(2): 113-120

[62] Dai G et al. Distinct endothelial phenotypes evoked by arterial waveforms derived from atherosclerosis-susceptible and -resistant regions of human vasculature. Proceedings of the National Academy of Sciences of the United States of America. 2004;**101**(41):14871-14876

[63] Nakashima Y et al. Upregulation of VCAM-1 and ICAM-1 at atherosclerosis-prone sites on the endothelium in the ApoE-deficient mouse. Arteriosclerosis, Thrombosis, and Vascular Biology. 1998;**18**(5):842-851

[64] Schmidt AM et al. Isolation and characterization of two binding proteins for advanced glycosylation end products from bovine lung which are present on the endothelial cell surface. The Journal of Biological Chemistry. 1992;**267**(21):14987-14997

[65] Wu VY, Cohen MP. Receptors specific for Amadori-modified glycated albumin on murine endothelial cells. Biochemical and Biophysical Research Communications. 1994;**198**(2): 734-739

[66] Wu VY, Shearman CW, Cohen MP. Identification of calnexin as a binding protein for Amadori-modified glycated albumin. Biochemical and Biophysical Research Communications. 2001;**284**(3):602-606

[67] Krantz S et al. Purification and partial amino acid sequencing of a fructosyllysine-specific binding protein from cell membranes of the monocyte-like cell line U937. Biochimica et Biophysica Acta. 1995;**1266**(1):109-112

[68] Brandt R et al. Nucleophosmin is a component of the fructoselysine-specific receptor in cell membranes of Mono Mac 6 and U937 monocyte-like cells. Biochimica et Biophysica Acta. 2004;**1670**(2):132-136

[69] Higai K, Shimamura A, Matsumoto K. Amadori-modified glycated albumin predominantly induces E-selectin expression on human umbilical vein endothelial cells through NADPH oxidase activation. Clinica Chimica Acta. 2006;**367**(1-2):137-143

[70] Esposito C et al. Long-term exposure to high glucose up-regulates VCAM-induced endothelial cell adhesiveness to PBMC. Kidney International. 2001;**59**(5):1842-1849

[71] Koyama H, Yamamoto H, Nishizawa Y. RAGE and soluble RAGE: Potential therapeutic targets for cardiovascular diseases. Molecular Medicine. 2007;**13**(11-12):625-635

[72] Forbes JM et al. Reduction of the accumulation of advanced glycation end products by ACE inhibition in experimental diabetic nephropathy. Diabetes. 2002;**51**(11):3274-3282

[73] Sena CM et al. Metformin restores endothelial function in aorta of diabetic rats. British Journal of Pharmacology. 2011;**163**(2):424-437

[74] Forbes JM et al. Modulation of soluble receptor for advanced glycation end products by angiotensin-converting enzyme-1 inhibition in diabetic nephropathy. Journal of the American Society of Nephrology. 2005;**16**(8):2363-2372

[75] Yamagishi S et al. Olmesartan blocks inflammatory reactions in endothelial cells evoked by advanced glycation end products by suppressing generation of reactive oxygen species. Ophthalmic Research. 2008;**40**(1):10-15

[76] Marx N et al. Thiazolidinediones reduce endothelial expression of receptors for advanced glycation end products. Diabetes. 2004;**53**(10):2662-2668

[77] Tan KC et al. Thiazolidinedione increases serum soluble receptor for advanced glycation end-products in type 2 diabetes. Diabetologia. 2007;**50**(9):1819-1825

[78] Paradela-Dobarro B et al. Statins modulate feedback regulation mechanisms between advanced glycation end-products and C-reactive protein: Evidence in patients with acute myocardial infarction. European Journal of Pharmaceutical Sciences. 2013;**49**(4):512-518

[79] Okamoto T et al. Angiogenesis induced by advanced glycation end products and its prevention by cerivastatin. The FASEB Journal. 2002;**16**(14):1928-1930

[80] Cuccurullo C et al. Suppression of RAGE as a basis of simvastatin-dependent plaque stabilization in type 2 diabetes. Arteriosclerosis, Thrombosis, and Vascular Biology. 2006; **26**(12):2716-2723

[81] Mahajan N, Bahl A, Dhawan V. C-reactive protein (CRP) up-regulates expression of receptor for advanced glycation end products (RAGE) and its inflammatory ligand EN-RAGE in THP-1 cells: Inhibitory effects of atorvastatin. International Journal of Cardiology. 2010;**142**(3):273-278

[82] Sun YP et al. Curcumin inhibits advanced glycation end product-induced oxidative stress and inflammatory responses in endothelial cell damage via trapping methylglyoxal. Molecular Medicine Reports. 2016;**13**(2):1475-1486

[83] Zhang X et al. Liquiritin attenuates advanced glycation end products-induced endothelial dysfunction via RAGE/NF-kappaB pathway in human umbilical vein endothelial cells. Molecular and Cellular Biochemistry. 2013;**374**(1-2):191-201

Chapter 10

Endothelial Dysfunction in Type 2 Diabetes: Targeting Inflammation

Cristina M. Sena, Fernanda Carrilho and
Raquel M. Seiça

Additional information is available at the end of the chapter

http://dx.doi.org/10.5772/intechopen.76994

Abstract

Several experimental and clinical studies have indicated a prominent role of vascular inflammation in the development of endothelial dysfunction. In endothelial dysfunction, the endothelium loses its physiological features, decrements nitric oxide bioavailability, and shifts towards a vasoconstrictor, pro-thrombotic and pro-inflammatory state. Within arterial wall, the interplay between the pro-inflammatory and pro-oxidant milieus promotes vascular dysfunction, and perivascular adipose tissue seems to play an important role. Inflammation is now considered a key event in vascular dysfunction and the development of vascular disease associated with obesity and type 2 diabetes. This concept is supported by the fact that anti-inflammatory adipokines such as adiponectin protect endothelial function, and interventions resulting in reduced inflammation such as the administration of salicylates prevent vascular dysfunction and cardiovascular events. Thus, the aim of this review is to address the role of inflammation and its mechanisms in endothelial dysfunction associated with diabetes, describing the impact of these conditions on vascular function.

Keywords: type 2 diabetes, endothelial dysfunction, oxidative stress, inflammation, adipokines

1. Introduction

Endothelial dysfunction is one of the major causes for vascular complications, accompanied by oxidative stress and inflammation. In diabetic and obesity/insulin resistance states, the endothelial dysfunction is incremented promoting the development and progression of vascular diseases [1].

Endothelial dysfunction involves reduced endothelium-dependent vasodilatation and a prothrombotic, pro-inflammatory and oxidant milieu [2]. The endothelial nitric oxide (NO) synthase (eNOS), renin-angiotensin-aldosterone and kallikrein-kinin response systems all fail to maintain normal vascular homeostasis in conditions of hyperglycemia, reactive oxidative species (ROS), free fatty acid (FFA) stress, and pro-inflammatory signaling [3, 4].

The aim of this review is to address the role of inflammation and its mechanisms in endothelial dysfunction associated with diabetes, describing the impact of these conditions on vascular function. We searched PubMed and Google Scholar primarily for original research articles published up to 2017 that were focused on the pathophysiology of endothelial dysfunction associated with type 2 diabetes. The main search terms used were "type 2 diabetes," "inflammation and endothelial dysfunction," "insulin resistance," and "therapies". We identified primarily full-text manuscripts written in English. We also searched Clinicaltrials.gov for information on ongoing clinical trials in endothelial dysfunction associated with type 2 diabetes.

2. Endothelial cell function

Vascular endothelium is crucial for the regulation of vascular homeostasis. It is metabolically active through the secretion of vasodilators and vasoconstrictors and acts as an active signal transducer for circulating factors that modify the vessel wall phenotype. The normal paracrine and autocrine functions of endothelial cells include the synthesis of a series of substances that moderate vascular tone, decrease leucocyte migration, control permeability, regulate proliferation and migration of smooth muscle cells, and regulate platelet adhesion and aggregation (**Figure 1**). Endothelium also regulates cellular adhesion, vessel wall inflammation, and angiogenesis.

The mechanisms implicated in the genesis of endothelial dysfunction are of extreme importance in developing adequate strategies to prevent or retard the clinical manifestations of cardiovascular diseases.

2.1. Endothelial dysfunction in diabetes

Dysfunction of vascular endothelium is considered not only as an important factor in the initiation of vascular complications, but also in its progression and clinical sequelae [5]. Endothelial dysfunction is the loss of endothelium physiological properties with a shift toward a vasoconstrictor, prothrombotic, and pro-inflammatory state [2].

The mechanisms underlying the development of endothelial dysfunction in type 2 diabetes are complex and include oxidative stress, inflammation, and chronic alterations in the hemodynamic balance. Several contributors to endothelial activation and dysregulation have been described: decreased tetrahydrobiopterin (BH_4) bioavailability and eNOS uncoupling, increased arginase, increased ROS production, decreased NO bioavailability, increased asymmetric dimethyl arginine, increased glycation and expression of receptor for advanced glycation end products (RAGE), nuclear factor κB (NFκB) activation, suppression of Kruppel-like Factor 2 [6], and phenotypic changes in perivascular adipose tissue leading to low grade inflammation and reduced adiponectin secretion [7, 8].

2.2. Inflammation

A state of subclinical systemic inflammation is characteristically present in obesity/insulin resistance and type 2 diabetes. The inflammation can be monitored by inflammatory markers such as high sensitivity C-reactive protein (hsCRP) and the inflammatory score derived from the pro-inflammatory plasma cytokines, interleukin (IL)-6, tumor necrosis factor α (TNFα), osteopontin, fractalkine, chemokine (C-C motif) ligand 2 (CCL2) and anti-inflammatory adiponectin, that inversely relate to insulin sensitivity (**Table 1**). The inflammatory score independently predicted fasting plasma glucose and insulin resistance in type 2 diabetic patients with high sensibility and specificity [9–12]. Moreover, other inflammatory biomarkers [i.e., growth differentiation factor-15 (GDF15), myeloid-related protein 8/14, pentraxin 3, lectin-like oxidized low-density lipoprotein receptor-1 (LOX-1)] have been considered surrogate markers of cardiovascular disease and atherosclerosis in type 2 diabetes patients [13–16].

GDF15 is a member of the transforming growth factor beta family, secreted from cells such as adipocytes and myocytes in response to cellular ischemia and oxidative stress both present in diabetes. GDF15 is a marker of oxidative stress and inflammation and provides independent prognostic information on cardiovascular events [17].

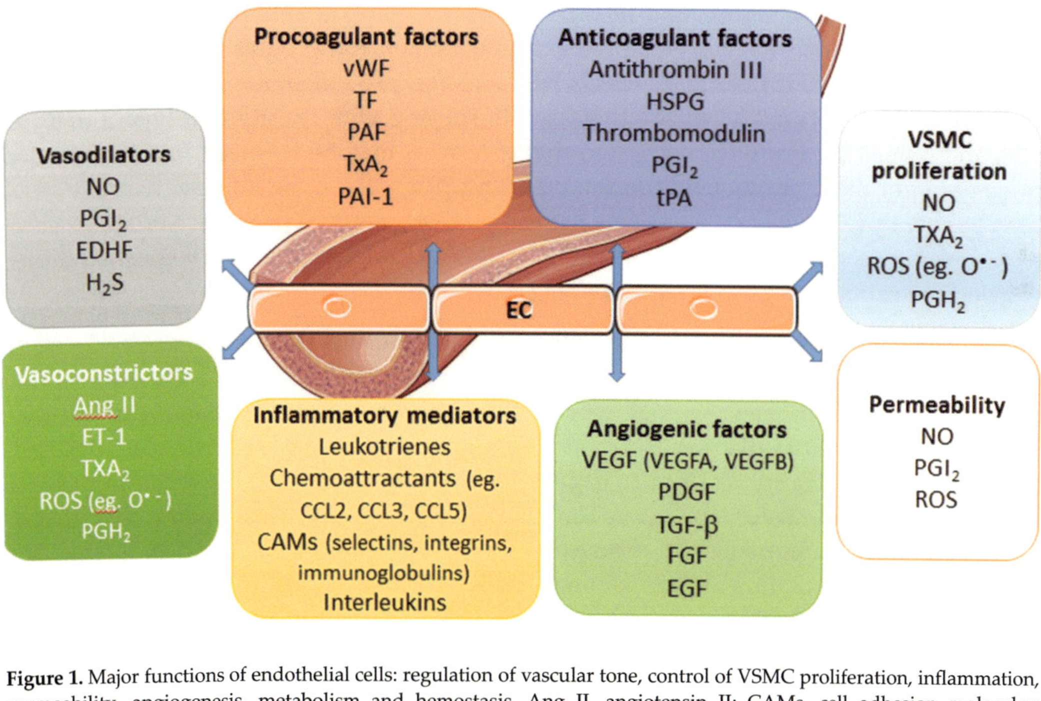

Figure 1. Major functions of endothelial cells: regulation of vascular tone, control of VSMC proliferation, inflammation, permeability, angiogenesis, metabolism and hemostasis. Ang II, angiotensin II; CAMs, cell adhesion molecules; CCL; chemokine (C-C motif) ligand; EC, endothelial cell; EDHF, endothelium derived hyperbolizing factor; EGF, epidermal growth factor; ET1, endothelin-1; FGF, fibroblast growth factor; H_2S; hydrogen sulfide; HSPG, heparan sulfate proteoglycans; ICAM, intercellular adhesion molecule; NO, nitric oxide; PAF, platelet-activating factor; PAI-1, Plasminogen activator inhibitor-1; PDGF, platelet-derived growth factor; PGH_2, prostaglandin H_2; PGI_2, prostacyclin; ROS, reactive oxygen species; TF, tissue factor; TFPI, tissue factor pathway inhibitor; TGF-β, transforming growth factor-β; t-PA, tissue plasminogen activator; TXA_2; thromboxane A_2; VCAM, vascular cell adhesion molecule; VEGF, vascular endothelial growth factor; VSMC, vascular smooth muscle cells; vWF, von Willebrand factor.

Myeloid-related protein 8/14 is a heterodimer consisting of two proteins that bind calcium and calgranulin A and B, which play an important role in the signaling pathways of calcium and in the interaction between the cytoskeleton and the membrane [18]. Myeloid-related protein 8/14 is synthesized by activated monocytes and neutrophils and is a pro-inflammatory protein expressed in atherosclerotic plaques associated with atherosclerosis in diabetic patients [19].

Pentraxin 3 is an acute-phase reactant produced by the peripheral tissues at sites of local inflammation and reflects impaired vascular endothelial function [20].

LOX-1 is a *lectin-like receptor* for *oxidized low-density* lipoproteins (ox-LDL), mainly expressed in endothelial cells, macrophages, smooth muscle cells, and monocytes. This receptor is upregulated by ox-LDL itself and by angiotensin II, endothelin, cytokines, and shear stress. The LOX-1 expressed on the cell surface can be proteolytically cleaved and released in a soluble form (sLOX-1) in the circulation under pathological conditions such as hyperlipidemia and type 2 diabetes [21, 22].

Additionally, galectin-3 might also be an independent marker of vascular remodeling and endothelial dysfunction accompanied by inflammation, proliferation, and atherosclerosis in both normal and diabetic individuals [23, 24]. Galectin-3 is a multifunctional protein that belongs to a family of β-galactoside binding proteins and widely distributes in the heart, brain, visceral **adipose tissue,** and blood vessels. Galectin-3 is able to bind the advanced glycation end products (AGEs) and advanced lipoxidation end products that accumulate in target organs and exert their toxic effects by triggering pro-inflammatory and pro-oxidant pathways [25]. Galectin-3 levels are increased in subjects with obesity and type 2 diabetes [26], and animal studies have suggested that galectin-3 may be involved in the onset and progression of these metabolic disorders by acting primarily at the adipose tissue level. A recent study by Olefsky and co-workers has shown that galectin-3 provides a crucial mechanistic link between inflammation and insulin resistance and that pharmacological inhibition of galectin-3 can increase insulin sensitivity [27].

Inflammation plays a crucial role in the etiology of vascular disease in diabetic states (**Figure 2**). The causes that trigger inflammation are pleiotropic and include most of the features that characterize type 2 diabetes. Arterial hypertension is also a low-grade inflammatory disease [28, 29] often present in diabetes along with hyperinsulinemia, insulin resistance, dyslipidemia, and obesity (**Figure 2**). Chronic exposure to glucotoxicity and lipotoxicity in diabetes induces a pro-inflammatory phenotype in macrophages residing or invading the adipose tissue and the vasculature [30, 31]. The dysfunctional endothelium may enhance leukocyte adhesion and the recruitment of inflammatory cells to the arterial wall, primarily through CCL2, a chemokine that promotes the attraction of immune cells to the sites of inflammation, thereby promoting lipid deposition and facilitating the atherosclerotic plaque formation [28, 32]. In addition, it is well known that the pro-inflammatory transcription factors NFκB and activator protein-1 and kinases such as c-Jun N-terminal kinase, p38 mitogen-activated protein kinase (MAPK) and extracellular signal-regulated kinase (ERK) are regulated by the cellular redox state [33, 34]. Proatherogenic factors in obesity and diabetes such as oxidized

Pro-inflammatory cytokines
TNF-α; Interleukins IL-1, IL-6, IL-8, IL-22
Local inflammation
iNOS
Cyclooxygenases—COX
Transcription factors as NFκB
Adhesion molecules
Intercellular adhesion molecule-1—ICAM-1
Vascular cellular adhesion molecule-1—VCAM-1
E-selectin
Chemokines
CCL2 (MCP-1)
CX3CL1 (fractalkine)
CCL5 (RANTES)
Toll-like receptors
Toll like receptor—TLR2
Toll like receptor—TLR4
Pro-fibrotic factors
Transforming growth factor—TGFβ
Connective tissue growth factor—CTGF

CCL2, chemokine (C-C motif) ligand 2; CCL5, chemokine (C-C motif) ligand 5; COX, cyclooxygenases; CTGF, connective tissue growth factor; CX3CL1, fractalkine; IL- Interleukin; iNOS, inducible nitric oxide synthase; ICAM-1, intercellular adhesion molecule-1; NFκB, nuclear factor κB; TGFβ, *transforming growth factor* β; TLR, toll like receptor; TNF-α; tumor necrosis factor α; VCAM-1, vascular cellular adhesion molecule-1.

Table 1. Inflammatory components of diabetic complications.

lipids, angiotensin II, and hyperglycemia increase the activity of NF-κB and MAPKs in endothelial cells and promote the activation of pro-inflammatory cytokines (e.g., IL-6), chemokines (e.g., CCL2, IL-8) [35], the expression of adhesion molecules [intercellular adhesion molecule-1 (ICAM-1), vascular cell adhesion molecule-1 (VCAM-1)] [36] and activation of inducible nitric oxide synthase (iNOS) [37], growth factors, and enzymes [38–40]. The subsequent increment in intracellular ROS production and the activation of the pro-inflammatory signaling complexes—the inflammasomes (including nucleotide binding and oligomerization domain-like receptor family pyrin domain containing 3 (NLRP3) inflammasome) is responsible for the activation of interleukins such as IL-1β and IL-18, triggering inflammation [41]. The NLRP3 inflammasomes of the innate immune system induce a microinflammatory state stimulating various pro-inflammatory cytokines involved in the pathogenesis of diabetes and its complications.

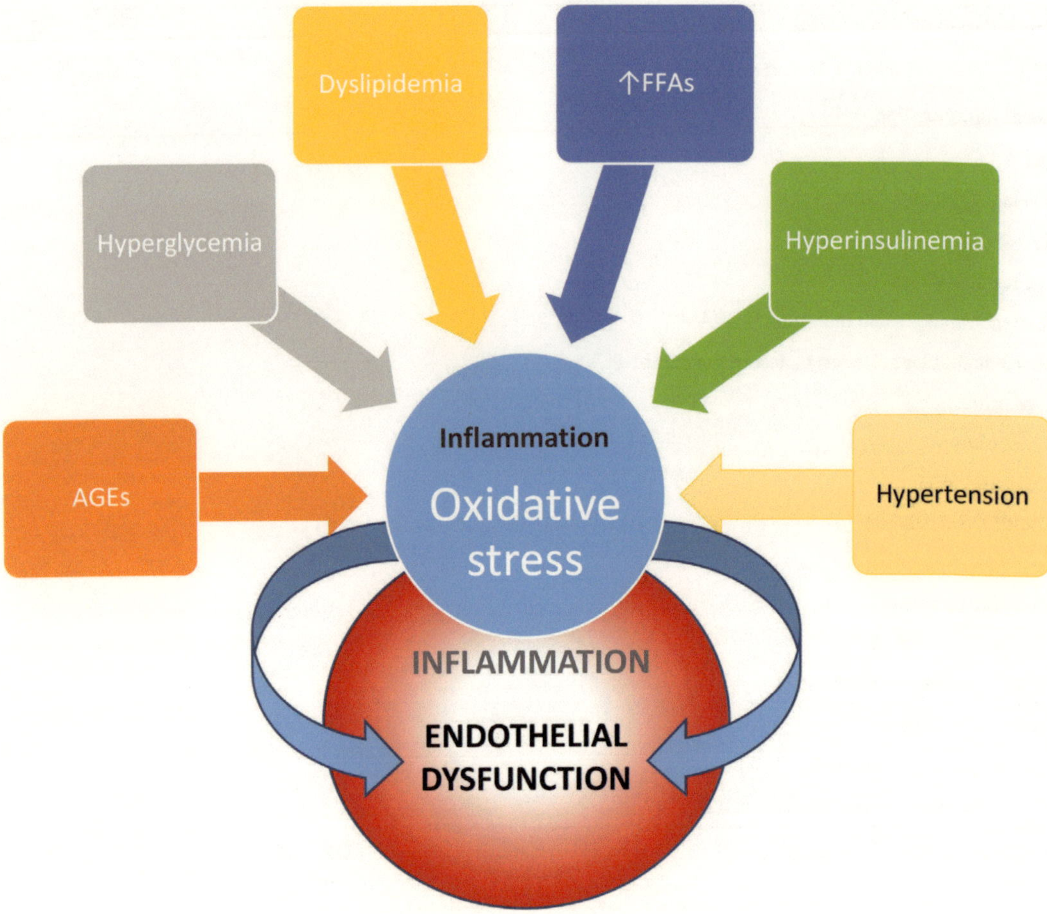

Figure 2. Risk factors for endothelial dysfunction associated with type 2 diabetes. Major role for oxidative stress and inflammation. AGEs, advanced glycation end products; FFAs, free fatty acids.

2.2.1. *Hyperglycemia-induced inflammation*

In diabetes, hyperglycemia can induce inflammation via different mechanisms [42]. The metabolic defects underlying diabetes cause mitochondrial superoxide overproduction in endothelial cells of blood vessels. This increased superoxide production leads to the activation of five major pathways involved in the pathogenesis of complications: polyol pathway flux, increased formation of advanced glycation end products (AGEs), increased expression of the receptor for AGEs and its activating ligands, activation of protein kinase C (PKC) isoforms and overactivity of the hexosamine pathway [43].

Hyperglycemia leads to increased reduction of glucose to sorbitol by aldose reductase with nicotinamide adenine dinucleotide phosphate (NADPH) consumption [44]. The cellular antioxidant capacity relies on the energy provided by NADPH to the glutathione and thioredoxin antioxidant systems. Thus, NADPH decrement will result in reduced antioxidant capacity and increased oxidative stress [44].

In endothelial cells, vascular smooth muscle cells, monocytes and macrophages, the intracellular synthesis of diacylglycerol is increased in hyperglycemia, leading to the activation of the PKC pathway [45, 46]. In monocytes, there is a subsequent release of the integrins CD11b, CD11c, and CD14 [47, 48]. CD11b or CD11c receptor occupation on the surface of human monocytes stimulates cell-specific pro-inflammatory pathways such as secretion of IL-8, macrophage inflammatory protein (MIP)1α and MIP1β [49]. CD14 + CD16+ monocytes are also linked with pro-inflammatory conditions [50].

Hyperglycemia also upregulates toll-like receptor (TLR) activity through an increment in ROS augmenting inflammation. In human monocytes, Dasu and colleagues [51] reported that high glucose induces TLR2 and TLR4 expression through PKC activation, by stimulating NADPH oxidase (NOX). Several other studies have demonstrated that under hyperglycemic conditions, reducing ROS and specifically NOX activity reduced TLR expression and activity [52, 53].

AGEs are generated in vivo as a normal consequence of metabolism, but their formation is accelerated under conditions of hyperglycemia, hyperlipidemia, and increased oxidative stress [54–57]. AGEs are highly reactive and can trigger inflammation by generating particularly TNF-α and IL-6 [58]. In addition, AGEs activate their receptors/binding sites (RAGE and lactoferrin-like polypeptide complex) in endothelial cells, monocytes, and macrophages leading to the activation of MAPK and NF-κB. AGEs also enhance the formation of oxidized low-density lipoprotein (oxLDL) and during hyperglycemia the expression of LOX-1 on monocytes and macrophages increases. These processes further facilitate the uptake of oxLDL by macrophages, thus increasing inflammation [59, 60].

Another important mechanism to cause hyperglycemia-induced endothelial dysfunction is the redox-dependent activation of endothelial NLRP3 inflammasomes [61]. Endothelial tight junction disruption in diabetes requires NLRP3 inflammasomes. High glucose activates NLRP3 inflammasome in endothelial cells via ROS production. Reducing ROS production abolished high glucose-induced inflammasome activation, tight junction disruption, and endothelial hyperpermeability in endothelial cells. The clinical potential of targeting inflammasome signaling axis for prevention of the early onset of diabetic vasculopathy is evident [61].

2.2.2. *Lipids-induced inflammation*

Lipids also induce a state of inflammation. In diabetes, lipids increment the inflammatory process by promoting oxidative stress and leukocyte activation and ultimately foster endothelial dysfunction and atherosclerosis progression. The ingestion of high fat diets results in increased leukocyte activation, which is reflected by an increase of surface expression of CD11b, CD11c and CD14 on monocytes and CD11b, CD66b and CD62L on neutrophils [47, 62, 63]. These results suggest a pro-inflammatory effect of dietary lipids on circulating inflammatory cells with detrimental effects on the vessel wall. After a meal, the remnants of triglyceride-rich lipoproteins and *oxLDL* are taken up by circulating leukocytes, macrophages, endothelial cells, and smooth muscle cells, activating the PKC pathway and resulting in *NF-κB* activation [64–66]. NF-κB promotes the transcription of various inflammatory genes, including genes encoding for cytokines, chemokines, and adhesion molecules [59]. In addition, FFA and cholesterol induce inflammation by activating TLR pathways and, subsequently,

NF-κB-mediated release of a broad range of cytokines and chemokines in different tissues [30, 31]. Cytokines released are involved in initiating and promoting a pro-inflammatory status, contributing to insulin resistance [67].

However, the use of anti-inflammatory therapies to treat these conditions is still controversial and often the results are inferior to the expected. On the other hand, indirect approaches regulating adipokines secretion or signaling seem to be promising [68].

2.2.3. *Macrophage polarization*

Macrophages are essential factors that contribute to the expression of inflammatory mediators and altered metabolism playing a critical role during the pathogenesis of atherosclerosis [69]. Polarized macrophages toward M1 phenotype aggravate atherosclerosis. The polarized macrophages not only exhibit increased inflammatory profile as observed in the expression of CCL2 and CCL5 but also change cholesterol homeostasis. The scavenger receptor class B type I (SR-B1) plays an important role in mediating the uptake of high-density lipoproteins (HDL)-derived cholesterol and cholesteryl ester in the liver and steroidogenic tissues, and its expression is reduced by M1 macrophages [70]. In addition, HDL prevents the induction of human macrophages into an M1 phenotype by preventing the accumulation of caveolin-1 to the cell membrane [71].

Adipokines play an important role particularly in the context of obesity and diabetes. Some have a direct vascular effect such as leptin and adiponectin [8, 72]. Increasing attention has been paid to the direct vascular effects of adipokines, especially adiponectin. Adiponectin is the most abundant adipokine secreted by adipose cells, which may couple the regulation of insulin sensitivity with energy metabolism as well as regulation of vascular function [8]. We have recently shown that adiponectin normalized endothelial cell function by a mechanism that involved increased eNOS phosphorylation and decreased perivascular adipose tissue inflammation [8]. In addition, hypoadiponectinemia-induced NLRP3 inflammasome was recently suggested as a novel mechanism of diabetic vascular endothelial dysfunction [73].

Some adipokines mediate the polarization of pro-inflammatory M1 and anti-inflammatory M2 macrophages and the influence of inflammation in the diabetic milieu. For instance, adiponectin and secreted frizzled-related protein 5 are both adipokines that have anti-inflammatory properties and that can stimulate M2 polarization [74, 75]. Both M1 and M2 macrophage phenotypes interchange dynamically depending on the environment. Depending on the stimulus, macrophages become polarized, which allows macrophages to critically contribute to tissue homeostasis, as they promote initiation and resolution of inflammatory responses. As a consequence, deregulation of the tissue macrophage polarization balance is an etiological agent of chronic inflammation present in obesity and insulin resistance [76].

In addition, it was previously reported that vitamin D promotes an antiatherogenic monocyte/macrophage phenotype in patients with diabetes [77]. Higher serum 25(OH)D levels correlated positively with a beneficial M2/M1 ratio, suggesting antiatherogenic properties [78]. Moreover, reversibility of the proatherogenic macrophage phenotype by vitamin D supplementation highlights vitamin D sufficiency as a potential therapeutic target to reduce inflammation and diabetic complications [77].

2.3. Therapeutic approaches

Human and animal studies have shown a correlation between inflammatory conditions and endothelial dysfunction [79, 80]. In clinical situations, none of the approaches to specifically and directly treat inflammation to prevent cardiovascular events or reduce atherosclerosis in human individuals were successful, although high-sensitivity C-reactive protein is shown to have a strong relationship with recurrent events of cardiovascular diseases in several clinical trials. Randomized placebo-controlled clinical trials evaluating anti-inflammatory agents are being conducted to clarify whether targeting the inflammation itself will reduce cardiovascular events and risks [81].

Diet-induced weight loss reduced the levels of biomarkers of endothelial dysfunction and inflammation in overweight and obese patients with type 2 diabetes independent of medication use and duration [82]. In addition, anti-inflammatory drugs, such as salicylates, have been shown to reverse insulin resistance and other related conditions that result from circulating cytokines which cause and maintain insulin resistance [83–87]. Fibrates seem to inhibit NFκB [88]. In two randomized, placebo-controlled trials, fenofibrate treatment reduced the postprandial production of TNF-α, IL-1β, IL-6, CCL2, and macrophage inflammatory protein-1α [88, 89]. Larger and longer trials are necessary to understand the effects of fibrates. In addition, expression of paraoxonase genes (PON 1, 2, 3) negatively correlates with a number of inflammatory diseases including atherosclerosis [90]. In contrast to PON1, mainly in the circulation, PON2 and PON3 are predominantly localized to intracellular compartments (although small amounts of hPON3 is also associated with HDL) and modulate cellular oxidative stress generated both by intracellular mechanisms and in response to extracellular stimuli [91]. PON1 protects LDL against oxidation and preserves function of HDL [91]. Recent evidence suggests that paraoxonase-1 may exert its anti-inflammatory, anti-oxidative functions leading to HDL-mediated eNOS activation in endothelial cells via inhibition of myeloperoxidase activity of inflammatory HDL [92]. There are several studies suggesting that paraoxonases have been and continue to be target/candidates for developing therapeutic interventions for inflammatory diseases [93].

Emerging anti-inflammatory approaches to vascular protection could be for instance: 5-lipoxygenase inhibitors, 5-lipoxygenase activating protein inhibitors, anti-cell adhesion molecules, SIRT activators, CCR2 and CCR5 antagonists [94], antibodies against TNF-α, and low doses of methotrexate [81].

Large-scale clinical trials are underway to investigate whether anti-inflammatory treatment improves cardiovascular outcomes, for example, methotrexate therapy (TETHYS trial and CIRT trial) [95, 96] and blockade of the cytokine IL-1β with canakinumab for the management of cardiovascular disease (CANTOS trial) [97, 98]. Additionally, randomized, placebo-controlled, double-masked clinical trials of salsalate [99, 100], IL1Ra [101, 102] and anti-TNF-α [103] are being used to determine whether these anti-inflammatory approaches modify disease risk in type 2 diabetes and atherosclerotic cardiovascular disease.

Another novel anti-inflammatory therapy could be based on the normalization of the glycocalyx function [104–106]. The endothelial glycocalyx is now recognized to be a gatekeeper of the vascular wall regulating many aspects of endothelial function including its permeability and integrity. A disturbed glycocalyx is associated with higher susceptibility to triggers of atherosclerosis and leukocyte/platelet adhesion [105–107].

In addition, it was recently described that inhibition of NLRP3 inflammasome with MCC950 has potential benefits reducing infarct size and preserving cardiac function in a pig model of myocardial infarction [108].

Understanding mediators of the resolution of inflammation deserves further development in order to reduce the progression of vascular complications associated with diabetes [32].

3. Conclusions

Inflammation is suggested to play a crucial role in the interaction between metabolic abnormalities and vascular dysfunction, which occur in diabetes. Indeed, elevated levels of circulating inflammatory markers are observed in patients with diabetes and obesity, promoting endothelial dysfunction. In the diabetic milieu, hyperglycemia and hyperlipidemia promote various intracellular and extracellular events and affect different cells in the vascular wall, leading to endothelial dysfunction. Obesity and type 2 diabetes also promote alterations in several pro-inflammatory cytokines, chemokines, and adipokines that will have an impact on vascular function. Knowing these mechanisms in detail will enable us to find new therapeutic targets for preventing or ameliorating the inflammation and subsequent vascular complications in diabetes.

Acknowledgements

The present work was supported by PTDC/BIM-MET/4447/2014; COMPETE: POCI-01-0145-FEDER-016784; PEst FCT: UID/NEU/04539/2013; COMPETE: POCI-01-0145-FEDER-007440.

Conflict of interest

No conflict of interest.

Author details

Cristina M. Sena[1]*, Fernanda Carrilho[2] and Raquel M. Seiça[1]

*Address all correspondence to: csena@ci.uc.pt

1 Physiology, IBILI, Faculty of Medicine, University of Coimbra, Portugal

2 Santarém Hospital, Portugal

References

[1] Muniyappa R, Sowers JR. Role of insulin resistance in endothelial dysfunction. Reviews in Endocrine & Metabolic Disorders. 2013;**14**:5-12

[2] Sena CM, Pereira AM, Seiça R. Endothelial dysfunction—A major mediator of diabetic vascular disease. Biochimica et Biophysica Acta. 2013;**1832**:2216-2231

[3] Roberts AC, Porter KE. Cellular and molecular mechanisms of endothelial dysfunction in diabetes. Diabetes & Vascular Disease Research. 2013;**10**:472-482

[4] Brady EM, Webb DR, Morris DH, Khunti K, Talbot DS, Sattar N, Davies MJ. Investigating endothelial activation and oxidative stress in relation to glycaemic control in a multiethnic population. Experimental Diabetes Research. 2012;**2012**:386041

[5] Cines DB, Pollak ES, Buck CA, Loscalzo J, Zimmerman GA, McEver RP, Pober JS, Wick TM, Konkle BA, Schwartz BS, Barnathan ES, McCrae KR, Hug BA, Schmidt AM, Stern DM. Endothelial cells in physiology and in the pathophysiology of vascular disorders. Blood. 1998;**91**:3527-3561

[6] Lee HY, Youn SW, Cho HJ, Kwon YW, Lee SW, Kim SJ, Park YB, Oh BH, Kim HS. FOXO1 impairs whereas statin protects endothelial function in diabetes through reciprocal regulation of Kruppel-like factor 2. Cardiovascular Research. 2013;**97**:143-152

[7] Omar A, Chatterjee TK, Tang Y, Hui DY, Weintraub NL. Proinflammatory phenotype of perivascular adipocytes. Arteriosclerosis, Thrombosis, and Vascular Biology. 2014;**34**:1631-1636

[8] Sena CM, Pereira A, Fernandes R, Letra L, Seiça RM. Adiponectin improves endothelial function in mesenteric arteries of rats fed a high-fat diet: Role of perivascular adipose tissue. British Journal of Pharmacology. 2017;**174**:3514-3526

[9] Daniele G, Guardado Mendoza R, Winnier D, Fiorentino TV, Pengou Z, Cornell J, Andreozzi F, Jenkinson C, Cersosimo E, Federici M, Tripathy D, Folli F. The inflammatory status score including IL-6, TNF-α, osteopontin, fractalkine, MCP-1 and adiponectin underlies whole-body insulin resistance and hyperglycemia in type 2 diabetes mellitus. Acta Diabetologica. 2014;**51**:123-131

[10] Kaptoge S, Seshasai SR, Gao P, Freitag DF, Butterworth AS, Borglykke A, Di Angelantonio E, Gudnason V, Rumley A, Lowe GD, Jørgensen T, Danesh J. Inflammatory cytokines and risk of coronary heart disease: New prospective study and updated meta-analysis. European Heart Journal. 2014;**35**:578-589

[11] Lubrano V, Balzan S. Consolidated and emerging inflammatory markers in coronary artery disease. World Journal of Experimental Medicine. 2015;**5**:21-32

[12] Pepys MB, Hirschfield GM. C-reactive protein: A critical update. The Journal of Clinical Investigation. 2003;**111**:1805-1812

[13] Puri R, Nissen SE, Shao M, Elshazly MB, Kataoka Y, Kapadia SR, Tuzcu EM, Nicholls SJ. Non-HDL cholesterol and triglycerides: Implications for coronary atheroma progression and clinical events. Arteriosclerosis, Thrombosis, and Vascular Biology. 2016;**36**:2220-2228

[14] Krintus M, Kozinski M, Kubica J, Sypniewska G. Critical appraisal of inflammatory markers in cardiovascular risk stratification. Critical Reviews in Clinical Laboratory Sciences. 2014;**51**:263-279

[15] Danesh J, Wheeler JG, Hirschfield GM, Eda S, Eiriksdottir G, Rumley A, Lowe GD, Pepys MB, Gudnason V. C-reactive protein and other circulating markers of inflammation in the prediction of coronary heart disease. The New England Journal of Medicine. 2004;**350**:1387-1397

[16] Myers GL, Christenson RH, Cushman M, Ballantyne CM, Cooper GR, Pfeiffer CM, Grundy SM, Labarthe DR, Levy D, Rifai N, Wilson PW. National academy of clinical biochemistry laboratory medicine practice guidelines: Emerging biomarkers for primary prevention of cardiovascular disease. Clinical Chemistry. 2009;**55**:378-384

[17] Wallentin L, Hijazi Z, Andersson U, Alexander JH, De Caterina R, Hanna M, Horowitz JD, Hylek EM, Lopes RD, Asberg S, Granger CB, Siegbahn A, ARISTOTLE Investigators. Growth differentiation factor 15, a marker of oxidative stress and inflammation, for risk assessment in patients with atrial fibrillation: Insights from the apixaban for reduction in stroke and other thromboembolic events in atrial fibrillation (ARISTOTLE) trial. Circulation. 2014;**130**:1847-1858

[18] Ionita MG, Vink A, Dijke IE, Laman JD, Peeters W, van der Kraak PH, Moll FL, de Vries JP, Pasterkamp G, de Kleijn DP. High levels of myeloid-related protein 14 in human atherosclerotic plaques correlate with the characteristics of rupture-prone lesions. Arteriosclerosis, Thrombosis, and Vascular Biology. 2009;**29**:1220-1227

[19] Peng WH, Jian WX, Li HL, Hou L, Wei YD, Li WM, Xu YW. Increased serum myeloid-related protein 8/14 level is associated with atherosclerosis in type 2 diabetic patients. Cardiovascular Diabetology. 2011;**10**:41

[20] Yang HS, Woo JE, Lee SJ, Park SH, Woo JM. Elevated plasma pentraxin 3 levels are associated with development and progression of diabetic retinopathy in Korean patients with type 2 diabetes mellitus. Investigative Ophthalmology & Visual Science. 2014;**55**:5989-5897

[21] Chen M, Nagase M, Fujita T, Narumiya S, Masaki T, Sawamura T. Diabetes enhances lectin-like oxidized LDL receptor-1 (LOX-1) expression in the vascular endothelium: possible role of LOX-1 ligand and AGE. Biochemical and Biophysical Research Communications. 2001;**287**:962-968

[22] Tan KC, Shiu SW, Wong Y, Leng L, Bucala R. Soluble lectin-like oxidized low density lipoprotein receptor-1 in type 2 diabetes mellitus. Journal of Lipid Research. 2008;**49**:1438-1444

[23] Papapanagiotou A, Siasos G, Kassi E, Gargalionis AN, Papavassiliou AG. Novel inflammatory markers in hyperlipidemia: Clinical implications. Current Medicinal Chemistry. 2015;**22**:2727-2743

[24] Ozturk D, Celik O, Satilmis S, Aslan S, Erturk M, Cakmak HA, Kalkan AK, Ozyilmaz S, Diker V, Gul M. Association between serum galectin-3 levels and coronary atherosclerosis and plaque burden/structure in patients with type 2 diabetes mellitus. Coronary Artery Disease. 2015;**26**:396-401

[25] Pugliese G, Iacobini C, Ricci C, Blasetti Fantauzzi C, Menini S. Galectin-3 in diabetic patients. Clinical Chemistry and Laboratory Medicine. 2014;**52**:1413-1423

[26] Weigert J, Neumeier M, Wanninger J, Bauer S, Farkas S, Scherer MN, Schnitzbauer A, Schäffler A, Aslanidis C, Schölmerich J, Buechler C. Serum galectin-3 is elevated in obesity and negatively correlates with glycosylated hemoglobin in type 2 diabetes. The Journal of Clinical Endocrinology and Metabolism. 2010;**95**:1404-1411

[27] Li P, Liu S, Lu M, Bandyopadhyay G, Oh D, Imamura T, Johnson AMF, Sears D, Shen Z, Cui B, Kong L, Hou S, Liang X, Iovino S, Watkins SM, Ying W, Osborn O, Wollam J, Brenner M, Olefsky JM. Hematopoietic-derived galectin-3 causes cellular and systemic insulin resistance. Cell. 2016;**167**:973-984

[28] Libby P. Inflammation in atherosclerosis. Nature. 2002;**420**:868-874

[29] Wenzel P, Knorr M, Kossmann S, Stratmann J, Hausding M, Schuhmacher S, Karbach SH, Schwenk M, Yogev N, Schulz E, Oelze M, Grabbe S, Jonuleit H, Becker C, Daiber A, Waisman A, Münzel T. Lysozyme M-positive monocytes mediate angiotensin II-induced arterial hypertension and vascular dysfunction. Circulation. 2011;**124**:1370-1381

[30] Nguyen MT, Favelyukis S, Nguyen AK, Reichart D, Scott PA, Jenn A, Liu-Bryan R, Glass CK, Neels JG, Olefsky JM. A subpopulation of macrophages infiltrates hypertrophic adipose tissue and is activated by free fatty acids via toll-like receptors 2 and 4 and JNK-dependent pathways. The Journal of Biological Chemistry. 2007;**282**:35279-35292

[31] Vandanmagsar B, Youm YH, Ravussin A, Galgani JE, Stadler K, Mynatt RL, Ravussin E, Stephens JM, Dixit VD. The NLRP3 inflammasome instigates obesity-induced inflammation and insulin resistance. Nature Medicine. 2011;**17**:179-188

[32] Libby P, Tabas I, Fredman G, Fisher EA. Inflammation and its resolution as determinants of acute coronary syndromes. Circulation Research. 2014;**114**:1867-1879

[33] Oliveira-Marques V, Marinho HS, Cyrne L, Antunes F. Role of hydrogen peroxide in NF-kappaB activation: From inducer to modulator. Antioxidants & Redox Signaling. 2009;**11**:2223-2243

[34] Son Y, Kim S, Chung HT, Pae HO. Reactive oxygen species in the activation of MAP kinases. Methods in Enzymology. 2013;**528**:27-48

[35] Janssen-Heininger YMW, Poynter ME, Baeuerle PA. Recent advances towards understanding redox mechanisms in the activation of nuclear factor κB. Free Radical Biology and Medicine. 2000;**28**:1317-1327

[36] Matsumoto K, Sera Y, Nakamura H, Ueki Y, Miyake S. Serum concentrations of soluble adhesion molecules are related to degree of hyperglycemia and insulin resistance in patients with type 2 diabetes mellitus. Diabetes Research and Clinical Practice. 2002;**55**:131-138

[37] Soskić SS, Dobutović BD, Sudar EM, Obradović MM, Nikolić DM, Djordjevic JD, Radak DJ, Mikhailidis DP, Isenović ER. Regulation of inducible nitric oxide synthase (iNOS) and its potential role in insulin resistance, diabetes and heart failure. Open Cardiovascular Medicine Journal. 2011;**5**:153-163

[38] Montezano AC, Burger D, Paravicini TM, Chignalia AZ, Yusuf H, Almasri M, He Y, Callera GE, He G, Krause KH, Lambeth D, Quinn MT, Touyz RM. Nicotinamide adenine dinucleotide phosphate reduced oxidase 5 (Nox5) regulation by angiotensin II and endothelin-1 is mediated via calcium/calmodulin-dependent, rac-1-independent pathways in human endothelial cells. Circulation Research. 2010;**106**:1363-1373

[39] Ning RB, Zhu J, Chai DJ, Xu CS, Xie H, Lin XY, Zeng JZ, Lin JX. RXR agonists inhibit high glucose-induced upregulation of inflammation by suppressing activation of the NADPH oxidase-nuclear factor-kappaB pathway in human endothelial cells. Genetics and Molecular Research. 2013;**12**:6692-6707

[40] Xia F, Wang C, Jin Y, Liu Q, Meng Q, Liu K, Sun H. Luteolin protects HUVECs from TNF-alpha-induced oxidative stress and inflammation via its effects on the Nox4/ROS-NF- kappaB and MAPK pathways. Journal of Atherosclerosis and Thrombosis. 2014;**21**:768-783

[41] Rathinam VAK, Fitzgerald KA. Inflammasome complexes: Emerging mechanisms and effector functions. Cell. 2016;**165**:792-800

[42] Hansen NW, Hansen AJ, Sams A. The endothelial border to health: Mechanistic evidence of the hyperglycemic culprit of inflammatory disease acceleration. IUBMB Life. 2017;**69**:148-161

[43] Giacco F, Brownlee M. Oxidative stress and diabetic complications. Circulation Research. 2010;**107**:1058-1070

[44] Brownlee M. Biochemistry and molecular cell biology of diabetic complications. Nature. 2001;**414**:813-820

[45] Araki E, Nishikawa T. Oxidative stress: A cause and therapeutic target of diabetic complications. Journal of Diabetes Investigation. 2010;**1**:90-96

[46] Geraldes P, King GL. Activation of protein kinase C isoforms and its impact on diabetic complications. Circulation Research. 2010;**106**:1319-1331

[47] Gower RM, Wu H, Foster GA, Devaraj S, Jialal I, Ballantyne CM, Knowlton AA, Simon SI. CD11c/CD18 expression is upregulated on blood monocytes during hypertriglyceridemia and enhances adhesion to vascular cell adhesion molecule-1. Arteriosclerosis, Thrombosis, and Vascular Biology. 2011;**31**:160-166

[48] Kizub IV, Klymenko KI, Soloviev AI. Protein kinase C in enhanced vascular tone in diabetes mellitus. International Journal of Cardiology. 2014;**174**:230-242

[49] Rezzonico R, Imbert V, Chicheportiche R, Dayer JM. Ligation of CD11b and CD11c β2 integrins by antibodies or soluble CD23 induces macrophage inflammatory protein 1α (MIP-1α) and MIP-1β production in primary human monocytes through a pathway dependent on nuclear factor-κB. Blood. 2001;**97**:2932-2940

[50] Geng S, Chen K, Yuan R, Peng L, Maitra U, Diao N, Chen C, Zhang Y, Hu Y, Qi CF, Pierce S, Ling W, Xiong H, Li L. The persistence of low-grade inflammatory monocytes contributes to aggravated atherosclerosis. Nature Communications. 2016;**7**:13436

[51] Dasu MR, Devaraj S, Zhao L, Hwang DH, Jialal I. High glucose induces toll-like receptor expression in human monocytes: Mechanism of activation. Diabetes. 2008;**57**:3090-3098

[52] Thallas-Bonke V, Thorpe SR, Coughlan MT, Fukami K, Yap FY, Sourris KC, Penfold SA, Bach LA, Cooper ME, Forbes JM. Inhibition of NADPH oxidase prevents advanced glycation end product-mediated damage in diabetic nephropathy through a protein kinase C-α-dependent pathway. Diabetes. 2008;**57**:460-469

[53] Chen JX, Stinnett A. Critical role of the NADPH oxidase subunit p47phox on vascular TLR expression and neointimal lesion formation in high-fat diet-induced obesity. Laboratory Investigation. 2008;**88**:1316-1328

[54] Sena CM, Matafome P, Louro T, Nunes E, Fernandes R, Seiça RM. Metformin restores endothelial function in aorta of diabetic rats. British Journal of Pharmacology. 2011;**163**:424-437

[55] Thallas-Bonke V, Coughlan MT, Tan AL, Harcourt BE, Morgan PE, Davies MJ, Bach LA, Cooper ME, Forbes JM. Targeting the AGE-RAGE axis improves renal function in the context of a healthy diet low in advanced glycation end-product content. Nephrology. 2013;**18**:47-56

[56] Kellow NJ, Savige GS. Dietary advanced glycation end-product restriction for the attenuation of insulin resistance, oxidative stress and endothelial dysfunction: a systematic review. European Journal of Clinical Nutrition. 2013;**67**:239-248

[57] Pereira AM, Fernandes R, Crisóstomo J, Seiça RM, Sena CM. The Sulforaphane and pyridoxamine supplementation normalize endothelial dysfunction associated with type 2 diabetes. Scientific Reports. 2017;**7**:14357

[58] Tomino Y, Hagiwara S, Gohda T. AGE-RAGE interaction and oxidative stress in obesity-related renal dysfunction. Kidney International. 2011;**80**:133-135

[59] De Vries MA, Klop B, Janssen HW, Njo TL, Westerman EM, Cabezas MC. Postprandial inflammation: Targeting glucose and lipids. Advances in Experimental Medicine and Biology. 2014;**824**:161-170

[60] Ott C, Jacobs K, Haucke E, Navarrete Santos A, Grune T, Simm A. Role of advanced glycation end products in cellular signaling. Redox Biology. 2014;**2**:411-429

[61] Chen Y, Wang L, Pitzer AL, Li X, Li PL, Zhang Y. Contribution of redox-dependent activation of endothelial NLRP3 inflammasomes to hyperglycemia-induced endothelial dysfunction. Journal of Molecular Medicine (Berlin). 2016;**94**:1335-1347

[62] Hiramatsu K, Arimori S. Increased superoxide production by mononuclear cells of patients with hypertriglyceridemia and diabetes. Diabetes. 1988;**37**:832-837

[63] Van Oostrom AJ, Rabelink TJ, Verseyden C, Sijmonsma TP, Plokker HW, De Jaegere PP, Cabezas MC. Activation of leukocytes by postprandial lipemia in healthy volunteers. Atherosclerosis. 2004;**177**:175-182

[64] Bentley C, Hathaway N, Widdows J, Bejta F, De Pascale C, Avella M, Wheeler-Jones CP, Botham KM, Lawson C. Influence of chylomicron remnants on human monocyte activation in vitro. Nutrition, Metabolism, and Cardiovascular Diseases. 2011;**21**:871-878

[65] Pirillo A, Norata GD, Catapano AL. LOX-1, OxLDL, and atherosclerosis. Mediators of Inflammation. 2013:152786

[66] Shi Y, Cosentino F, Camici GG, Akhmedov A, Vanhoutte PM, Tanner FC, Lüscher TF. Oxidized low- density lipoprotein activates p66Shc via lectin-like oxidized low-density lipoprotein receptor-1, protein kinase C-beta, and c-Jun N-terminal kinase kinase in human endothelial cells. Arteriosclerosis, Thrombosis, and Vascular Biology. 2011;**31**: 2090-2097

[67] Timar R, Timar B, Degeratu D, Serafinceanu C, Oancea C. Metabolic syndrome, adiponectin and proinflammatory status in patients with type1 diabetes mellitus. The Journal of International Medical Research. 2014;**42**:1131-1138

[68] Freitas Lima LC, Braga VA, do Socorro de França Silva M, Cruz JC, Sousa Santos SH, de Oliveira Monteiro MM, Balarini CM. Adipokines, diabetes and atherosclerosis: An inflammatory association. Frontiers in Physiology. 2015;**6**:304

[69] Moore KJ, Sheedy FJ, Fisher EA. Macrophages in atherosclerosis: A dynamic balance. Nature Reviews Immunology. 2013;**13**:709-721

[70] Valacchi G, Sticozzi C, Lim Y, Pecorelli A. Scavenger receptor class B type I: A multifunctional receptor. Annals of the New York Academy of Sciences. 2011;**1229**:E1-E7

[71] Lee MK, Moore XL, Fu Y, Al-Sharea A, Dragoljevic D, Fernandez-Rojo MA, Parton R, Sviridov D, Murphy AJ, Chin-Dusting JP. High-density lipoprotein inhibits human M1 macrophage polarization through redistribution of caveolin-1. British Journal of Pharmacology. 2016;**173**:741-751

[72] Koh KK, Park SM, Quon MJ. Leptin and cardiovascular disease: response to therapeutic interventions. Circulation. 2008;**117**:3238-3249

[73] Zhang J, Xia L, Zhang F, Zhu D, Xin C, Wang H, Zhang F, Guo X, Lee Y, Zhang L, Wang S, Guo X, Huang C, Gao F, Liu Y, Tao L. A novel mechanism of diabetic vascular endothelial dysfunction: Hypoadiponectinemia-induced NLRP3 inflammasome activation. Biochimica et Biophysica Acta. 2017;**1863**:1556-1567

[74] Ohashi K, Parker JL, Ouchi N, Higuchi A, Vita JA, Gokce N, Pedersen AA, Kalthoff C, Tullin S, Sams A, Summer R, Walsh K. Adiponectin promotes macrophage polarization toward an anti-inflammatory phenotype. The Journal of Biological Chemistry. 2010;**285**:6153-6160

[75] Ouchi N, Higuchi A, Ohashi K, Oshima Y, Gokce N, Shibata R, Akasaki Y, Shimono A, Walsh K. Sfrp5 is an anti-inflammatory adipokine that modulates metabolic dysfunction in obesity. Science. 2010;**329**:454-457

[76] Gregor MF, Hotamisligil GS. Inflammatory mechanisms in obesity. Annual Review of Immunology. 2011;**29**:415-445

[77] Riek AE, Oh J, Sprague JE, Timpson A, de las Fuentes L, Bernal-Mizrachi L, Schechtman KB, Bernal-Mizrachi C. Vitamin D suppression of endoplasmic reticulum stress promotes an antiatherogenic monocyte/macrophage phenotype in type 2 diabetic patients. The Journal of Biological Chemistry 2012;**287**:38482-38494

[78] Anandabaskar N, Selvarajan S, Dkhar SA, Kamalanathan SK, Tamilarasu K, Bobby Z. Effect of vitamin D supplementation on vascular functions and oxidative stress in type 2 diabetic patients with vitamin D deficiency. Indian Journal of Endocrinology and Metabolism. 2017;**21**:555-563

[79] Karbach S, Wenzel P, Waisman A, Munzel T, Daiber A. eNOS uncoupling in cardiovascular diseases-the role of oxidative stress and inflammation. Current Pharmaceutical Design. 2014;**20**:3579-3594

[80] Steven S, Munzel T, Daiber A. Exploiting the pleiotropic antioxidant effects of established drugs in cardiovascular disease. International Journal of Molecular Sciences. 2015;**16**:18185-18223

[81] Goldfine AB, Shoelson SE. Therapeutic approaches targeting inflammation for diabetes and associated cardiovascular risk. The Journal of Clinical Investigation. 2017;**127**:83-93

[82] Berk KA, Oudshoorn TP, Verhoeven AJM, Mulder MT, Roks AJM, Dik WA, Timman R, Sijbrands EJG. Diet-induced weight loss and markers of endothelial dysfunction and inflammation in treated patients with type 2 diabetes. Clinical Nutrition ESPEN. 2016;**15**:101-106

[83] Paul A, Calleja L, Camps J, Osada J, Vilella E, Ferré N, Mayayo E, Joven J. The continuous administration of aspirin attenuates atherosclerosis in apolipoprotein E-deficient mice. Life Sciences. 2000;**68**:457-465

[84] Rius B, López-Vicario C, González-Périz A, Morán-Salvador E, García-Alonso V, Clária J, Titos E. Resolution of inflammation in obesity-induced liver disease. Frontiers in Immunology. 2012;**3**:257

[85] Rogge MM. The role of impaired mitochondrial lipid oxidation in obesity. Biological Research for Nursing. 2009;**10**:356-373

[86] Mirza MS. Obesity, visceral fat and NAFLD: Querying the role of adipokines in the progression of nonalcoholic fatty liver disease. ISRN Gastroenterology. 2011;**11**:592404

[87] Tous M, Ferré N, Rull A, Marsillach J, Coll B, Alonso-Villaverde C, Camps J, Joven J. Dietary cholesterol and differential monocyte chemoattractant protein-1 gene expression in aorta and liver of apo E-deficient mice. Biochemical and Biophysical Research Communications. 2006;**340**:1078-1084

[88] Rosenson RS, Huskin AL, Wolff DA, Helenowski IB, Rademaker AW. Fenofibrate reduces fasting and postprandial inflammatory responses among hypertriglyceridemia patients with the metabolic syndrome. Atherosclerosis. 2008;**198**:381-388

[89] Okopién B, Krysiak R, Herman ZS. Effects of short-term fenofibrate treatment on circulating markers of inflammation and hemostasis in patients with impaired glucose tolerance. The Journal of Clinical Endocrinology and Metabolism. 2006;**91**:1770-1778

[90] Camps J, Marsillach J, Joven J. The paraoxonases: Role in human diseases and methodological difficulties in measurement. Critical Reviews in Clinical Laboratory Sciences. 2009;**46**:83-106

[91] Reddy ST, Devarajan A, Bourquard N, Shih D, Fogelman AM. Is it just paraoxonase 1 or are other members of the paraoxonase gene family implicated in atherosclerosis? Current Opinion in Lipidology. 2008;**19**:405-408

[92] Kratzer A, Giral H, Landmesser U. High-density lipoproteins as modulators of endothelial cell functions: Alterations in patients with coronary artery disease. Cardiovascular Research. 2014;**103**:350-361

[93] Chistiakov DA, Melnichenko AA, Orekhov AN, Bobryshev YV. Paraoxonase and atherosclerosis-related cardiovascular diseases. Biochimie. 2017;**132**:19-27

[94] Zhao Q. Dual targeting of CCR2 and CCR5: therapeutic potential for immunologic and cardiovascular diseases. Journal of Leukocyte Biology. 2010;**88**:41-55

[95] Everett BM, Pradhan AD, Solomon DH, Paynter N, MacFadyen J, Zaharris E, Gupta M, Clearfield M, Libby P, Hasan AAK, Glynn RJ, Ridker PM. Rationale and design of the cardiovascular inflammation reduction trial: A test of the inflammatory hypothesis of atherothrombosis. American Heart Journal. 2013;**166**:199-207

[96] Moreira DM, Lueneberg ME, da Silva RL, Fattah T, Mascia Gottschall CA. Rationale and design of the TETHYS trial: The effects of methotrexate therapy on myocardial infarction with ST-segment elevation. Cardiology. 2013;**126**:167-170

[97] Rissanen A, Howard CP, Botha J, Thuren T, Global Investigators. Effect of anti-IL-1β antibody (canakinumab) on insulin secretion rates in impaired glucose tolerance or type 2 diabetes: Results of a randomized, placebo-controlled trial. Diabetes, Obesity & Metabolism. 2012;**14**:1088-1096

[98] Ridker PM, Howard CP, Walter V, Everett B, Libby P, Hensen J, Thuren T, CANTOS Pilot Investigative Group. Effects of interleukin-1β inhibition with canakinumab on hemoglobin A1c, lipids, C-reactive protein, interleukin-6, and fibrinogen: A phase IIb randomized, placebo-controlled trial. Circulation. 2012;**126**:2739-2748

[99] Goldfine AB, Jablonski KA, Shoelson SE, Creager M. Targeting inflammation using salsalate in patients with type 2 diabetes: Effects on flow-mediated dilation (TINSAL-FMD). Diabetes Care. 2013;**36**:4132-4139

[100] Nohria A, Kinlay S, Buck JS, Redline W, Copeland-Halperin R, Kim S, Beckman JA. The effect of salsalate therapy on endothelial function in a broad range of subjects. Journal of the American Heart Association. 2014;**3**:e000609

[101] Larsen CM, Faulenbach M, Vaag A, Ehses JA, Donath MY, Mandrup-Poulsen T. Sustained effects of interleukin-1 receptor antagonist treatment in type 2 diabetes. Diabetes Care. 2009;**32**:1663-1668

[102] van Asseldonk EJ, Stienstra R, Koenen TB, Joosten LA, Netea MG, Tack CJ. Treatment with Anakinra improves disposition index but not insulin sensitivity in nondiabetic subjects with the metabolic syndrome: A randomized, double-blind, placebo-controlled study. The Journal of Clinical Endocrinology and Metabolism. 2011;**96**:2119-2126

[103] Timper K, Hruz P, Beglinger C, Donath MY. Infliximab in the treatment of Crohn disease and type 1 diabetes. Diabetes Care. 2013;**36**:e90-e91

[104] Meuwese MC, Mooij HL, Nieuwdorp M, van Lith B, Marck R, Vink H, Kastelein JJ, Stroes ES. Partial recovery of the endothelial glycocalyx upon rosuvastatin therapy in patients with heterozygous familial hypercholesterolemia. Journal of Lipid Research. 2009;**50**:148-153

[105] Drake-Holland AJ, Noble MI. Update on the important new drug target in cardiovascular medicine—The vascular glycocalyx. Cardiovascular & Hematological Disorders Drug Targets. 2012;**12**:76-81

[106] Tarbell JM, Cancel LM. The glycocalyx and its significance in human medicine. Journal of Internal Medicine. 2016;**280**:97-113

[107] Van Teeffelen JW, Brands J, Stroes ES, Vink H. Endothelial glycocalyx: Sweet shield of blood vessels. Trends in Cardiovascular Medicine. 2007;**17**:101-105

[108] Van Hout GP, Bosch L, Ellenbroek GH, de Haan JJ, Van Solinge WW, Cooper MA, Arslan F, de Jager SC, Robertson AA, Pasterkamp G, Hoefer IE. The selective NLRP3-inflammasome inhibitor MCC950 reduces infarct size and preserves cardiac function in a pig model of myocardial infarction. European Heart Journal. 2017;**38**:828-836

Chapter 11

Angiogenesis in Adipose Tissue: How can Moderate Caloric Restriction Affects Obesity-Related Endothelial Dysfunction?

Katarzyna Korybalska

Additional information is available at the end of the chapter

http://dx.doi.org/10.5772/intechopen.72624

Abstract

The plasticity of adipose tissue (AT) is related to its angiogenic ability. Angiogenesis is a multistep process which involves endothelial cell (EC) proliferation, migration, invasion and finally tube formation. AT as a secretory organ produces adipokines, which contributes to the development of subclinical inflammation. The inflammation-related adipokines deteriorate EC function and in consequence change the production of endothelial mediators responsible for vascular homeostasis and angiogenesis, leading to cardiovascular diseases (CVD) in obese patients. Additionally, the recent observation suggests that AT is poorly oxygenated in obesity. Hypoxia limits the healthy expansion of AT and stimulates a molecular response, enhancing nuclear factor kappa-B (NF-kB) and hypoxia-inducible factor (HIF-1) expression. HIF-1α induction does not start a normal angiogenic process but rather induces inflammatory response and fibrosis that is strongly associated with insulin resistance (IR). It is believed that EC dysfunction in obesity can be reduced by caloric restriction (CR). Moderate CR reflects a real-life situation and could be optimal to achieve an EC improvement. It reduces adiposity leading to pro-angiogenic, anti-inflammatory and—to a lesser extent—anti-oxidative cellular effects, which not only preserves the healthy EC phenotype but also leads to an improvement of AT remodeling and prevent systemic IR.

Keywords: obesity, angiogenesis, endothelial dysfunction, adipokines, caloric restriction

1. Introduction

Obesity (adiposity) is a serious health problem, especially in well-developed countries. The regional distribution of fat determines our health. Excessive accumulation of fat in the upper body's region (central obesity) is a stronger predictor of morbidity than excess fat in the lower body [1]. Central obesity is associated with insulin resistance (IR) and this condition predisposes to cardiovascular disease (CVD) [2]. Adipose tissue (AT) is not only an energy storage organ but also produces adipokines, which contribute to the development of subclinical inflammation [3]. The compounds released from AT are capable of affecting endothelial cell (EC) functions [4]. The mechanism of obesity-induced endothelial dysfunction is multifactorial mainly due to the omnidirectional impact of various adipokines, leading to the following abnormalities such as elevated blood pressure, formation of atherosclerotic plaques, oxidative stress, prothrombotic state and alterations in glucose and lipid metabolism [5]. AT remodeling is pathologically accelerated in an obese state due to local hypoxia. Reduced angiogenesis is a severe immune cell infiltration with subsequent pro-inflammatory responses which additionally deteriorates EC functions [6]. Therefore, one of the main goals of therapeutic interventions in obesity is to correct abnormalities in EC function and to protect endothelial integrity.

It is believed that EC dysfunction in obesity can be reduced by caloric restriction (CR), but it is unclear whether this benefit requires significant or moderate weight loss. In recent studies conducted on overweight humans, short- and long-lasting CR (6–52 weeks) have shown to improve a number of health outcomes [7–9]. The important issue is that most individuals have difficulty sustaining prolonged CR and the improvement of EC function may be problematic to achieve. Our cooperation with physicians, dieticians and psychologists allows us to claim that it is usually optimal for obese patients if CR is not so burdensome and yet, at the same time, effective. Therefore, we propose a mild CR as a way to lose body weight in obese individuals. Such a type of CR reflects a real-life situation and seems to be optimal to achieve an improvement of EC.

2. Adipose tissue

AT was earlier characterized as a connective tissue which stores triglycerides. An increase in global obesity and diabetes has attracted great interest to the function of this tissue. Nowadays, AT is considered an important regulator of energy balance, which plays a major role in nutrient homeostasis after feeding and releases free fatty acids (FFAs) during fasting. As such, it is regarded as an endocrine organ producing adipokines, which affect many organs and thus the homeostasis in the body (**Figure 1**).

AT is mainly found in subcutaneous and visceral depots. In obesity, AT is accumulated in different organs, including heart, liver, kidneys, bone marrow, lungs and the adventitia of major blood vessels, where secreted adipokines affect their function. Excess visceral adiposity is strongly correlated with IR, hypertension and dyslipidemia, which contribute to high rates of mortality and morbidity [3, 10]. Most adipokines, which stimulate inflammatory responses, are dysregulated in obesity and promote obesity-induced metabolic dysfunction, leading to CVD. The production of pro-inflammatory cytokines by AT is upregulated in an obese state (**Table 1**) while the secretion of anti-inflammatory factors is reduced (**Table 2**).

Adipocytes are divided into two types: white adipocytes and brown adipocytes. Brown adipocyte tissue (BAT) converts nutrients into chemical energy in the form of heat. Brown fat cells

http://dx.doi.org/10.5772/intechopen.72624

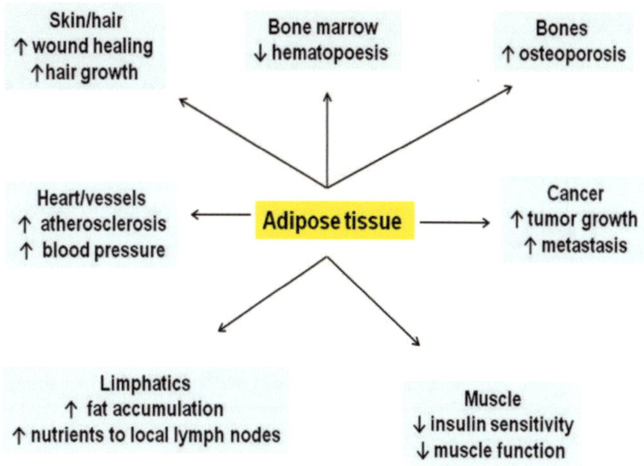

Figure 1. The impact of adipose tissue on multiple organs mediated by various factors released from adipocytes [3].

Pro-inflammatory adipokines

Adipokine	Function
Leptin	Appetite control though the central nervous system
Resistin	Induces insulin resistance by stimulating the Il-6 and TNF-α production in macrophages
Retinol-binding protein 4 (RBP4)	Induces insulin resistance by influencing glucose homeostasis
Lipocalin 2 (neutrophil gelatinase-associated lipocalin)	Promotes insulin resistance through TNF-α secretion from adipocytes
Angiopoietin-like protein 2 (ANGPTL-2)	Activates inflammatory response in endothelium and promotes insulin resistance
Tumor necrosis factor-α (TNF-α)	Attenuates insulin signaling in muscles and adipose tissue (IR)
Interleukin 6 (Il-6)	Involved in insulin resistance. It has various function in different organs
Interleukin 18 (IL-18)	Inflammation, involved in plaque instability and endothelial activation
Monocyte chemoattractant protein 1 (MCP-1/CCL-2)	Inflammation, involved in monocyte chemotaxis
CXC-chemokine ligand 5 (CXCL5)	Secreted from macrophages in AT. Responsible for IR
Chemerin	Inflammation, involved in monocyte chemotaxis and stimulates lipolysis
Nicotinamide phosphor ribosyltransferase (NAmPT, Visfatin)	Modulator of B cell differentiation, correlates with visceral adiposity, monocyte chemoattractant

Table 1. Pro-inflammatory adipokines and their functions [11, 12].

express a unique thermogenic and mitochondrial genetic program that promotes mitochondrial biogenesis, energy uncoupling and energy dissipation, in turn providing essential heat to the organism. Energy dissipation is possible in the presence of large amounts of mitochondria

Anti-inflammatory adipokines	
Adipokine	**Main function**
Adiponectin	Negatively correlates with inflammation and visceral fat accumulation, protects against metabolic dysfunction and IR
Secreted frizzled-related protein 5 (SFRP 5)	Anti-inflammatory, important for insulin sensitivity
Visceral adipose tissue-derived serine protease inhibitor (Vaspin)	Positively correlates with BMI and insulin sensitivity, increases glucose tolerance
Omentin-1	Expressed in visceral fat, protects against IR. Its level is reduced in obesity
Apelin	It plays different functions in various organs. Its production is enhanced by insulin. Has angiogenic and hypotensive properties

Table 2. Anti-inflammatory adipokines and their functions [11, 12].

with the uncoupling protein-1 (UCP-1). This provides heat rather than adenosine triphosphate (ATP) production [13].

White adipose tissue (WAT) stores triglycerides during energy consumption and releases fatty acids during starvation. WAT is also an active endocrine organ that secretes a large number of adipokines. Adipokines act centrally to regulate appetite and energy expenditure. They peripherally affect insulin sensitivity, promote subclinical inflammation and lipid uptake and accommodate the conversion of steroid hormones. Fats can be classified as subcutaneous or visceral. WAT has a specific morphology. Histologically, subcutaneous fat contains mature large adipocytes, whereas visceral fat consists of small adipocytes. Subcutaneous and visceral depots contribute to metabolism in different ways. An increased subcutaneous fat deposition in the form of "pear-shaped" or female pattern of distribution might protect against certain aspects of metabolic dysfunction, especially against IR [14, 15]. However, visceral depots, in an "apple" or male pattern of distribution, are thought to be associated with metabolic complications and appear to increase the risk of diabetes, hyperlipidemia and CVD [16]. It has become popular to term subcutaneous adipose as 'good fat' and visceral as 'bad fat'.

3. AT remodeling in obesity

3.1. Infiltration of immune cells into AT

AT is mainly comprised of adipocytes, although other cell types contribute to its growth and function. These include pre-adipocytes, lymphocytes, macrophages, fibroblasts and vascular cells (**Figure 2**). AT can respond rapidly and dynamically to nutrient deprivation and also to its excess. One of the unique attributes of AT is its incredible capacity to change its dimensions. This effect can be accomplished by increasing the size of adipose cells (hypertrophy) or by recruiting new adipocytes from the resident pool of progenitors (hyperplasia).

AT expands first by hypertrophy until a critical threshold is reached, upon which signals are released for the induction of preadipocyte proliferation and differentiation (hyperplasia) [17].

http://dx.doi.org/10.5772/intechopen.72624

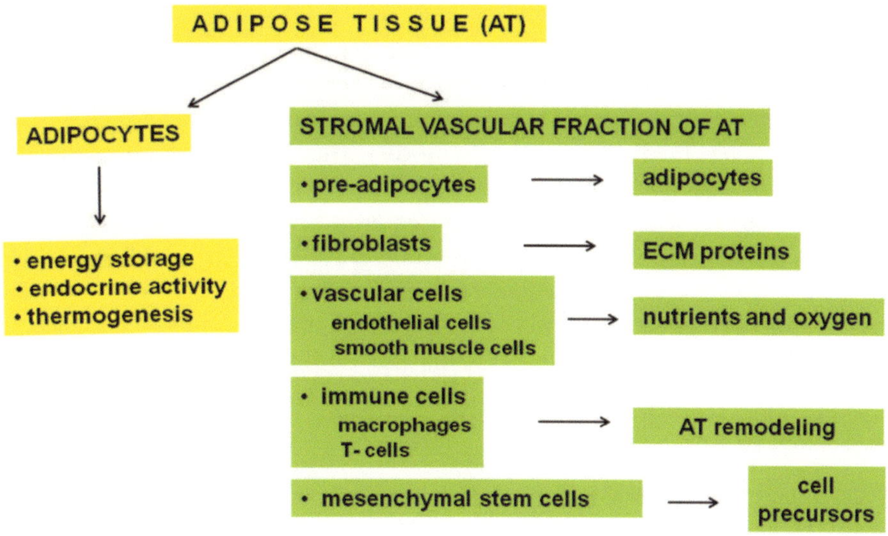

Figure 2. Components of adipose tissue [3, 12]. *Abbreviations*: AT, adipose tissue; ECM, extracellular matrix.

AT remodeling is pathologically accelerated in an obese state with reduced angiogenesis, extracellular matrix (ECM) overproduction and severe immune cell infiltration with subsequent pro-inflammatory responses. The large infiltration of macrophages in AT is linked to a systemic inflammation and IR. Moreover, the accumulation of macrophages is proportional to adiposity, and a sustained weight loss results in the lowering of inflammation, which suggests that this infiltration is reversible. Macrophages are also more abundant in the visceral than subcutaneous AT [6, 12]. Resident adipose macrophages display remarkable heterogeneity in their activities and functions. Hypertrophic adipocytes produce chemotactic factors, which promote monocyte accumulation in AT.

Macrophages can be classified into two broad groups: M1 and M2, based on the expression of particular antigens. Lumeng et al. proposed a model which emphasized that obesity is accompanied by a transformation of M2 anti-inflammatory macrophages (that are primarily accumulated during a negative energy balance) to more pro-inflammatory M1 macrophages [18]. The subsets of T cells presented in AT have been seen to be implicated in the macrophage activation. T helper cells ($CD4^+$) are present in a large numbers in the AT of lean persons and have a protective effect by impeding M1 macrophages, resulting in increased insulin sensitivity. T cytotoxic cell ($CD8^+$) can start the mobilization and activation of M1 macrophages and in this way it promotes an inflammation associated with IR. The M1 population positively correlates with IR and is characterized by overnutrition, where FFAs stimulate its pro-inflammatory responses [18]. In a lean state, resident macrophages are polarized toward the M2 state, which expresses a combination of anti-inflammatory factors that may help to preserve the normal adipocyte function by promoting AT repair and angiogenesis. Conversely, M1 macrophages induced by pro-inflammatory mediators express a repertoire of pro-inflammatory factors, which include tumor necrosis factor alpha (TNF-α), interleukin 6 (Il-6), inducible nitric oxidase synthase (iNOS) and produce reactive oxygen species (ROS) [3, 6]. The key function of macrophages is to remove apoptotic cells in an immunologically silent manner to prevent the release of harmful substances. The presence of apoptotic adipocytes surrounded by M1 macrophages (forming the so-called crown-like structures) is a characteristic feature in the obese with a full metabolic dysfunction. This pro-inflammatory state in AT is due to an impairment of the macrophage-mediated phagocytic process. The fibroblasts from metabolically dysfunctional AT produce excess ECM components that may contribute to metabolic dysregulation. The intercellular communication within AT is required for normal metabolic function. The obesity-associated changes in the cellular composition of AT lead to a modification of adipokine secretion [18, 19]. Consequently, obese patients can be categorized into those that have a fully dysfunctional metabolic phenotype and those that have a mildly dysfunctional metabolic phenotype (**Figure 3**) [19].

3.2. Angiogenesis in AT

Angiogenesis plays a central role in various physiological processes in a human body, not only during fetal development. Angiogenesis can be a hallmark of wound healing, menstrual cycle, cancer and various ischemic and inflammatory diseases. The pivotal process of angiogenesis can be simply described in multiple steps. First, angiogenic stimuli cause an increase in EC permeability and proliferation. Second, the proteolysis of the basement membrane components is a necessary process to promote the invasion of EC into the stroma of the neighboring

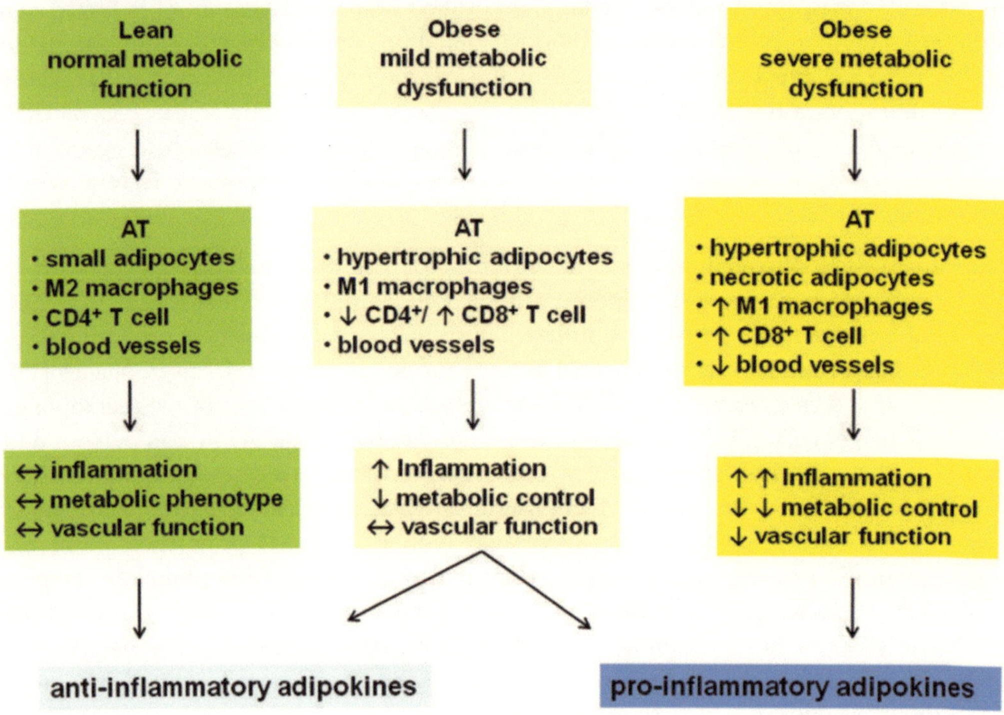

Figure 3. Adiposity-related metabolic dysfunction [3, 12]. *Abbreviations*: AT, adipose tissue; $CD4^+$, T helper cell; $CD8^+$, T cytotoxic cell; ↔, without changes.

tissue, in which the supportive activity of the tissue plasminogen activator system (t-PA and uPA—urokinase-type plasminogen activator) and matrix metalloproteinases (MMPs) are required. Third, the migrated ECs trigger lumen formation as the sprout forms a multicellular structure. Finally, the capillary is stabilized through the construction of a basement membrane, an adherent junction and ECs [20, 21].

AT possesses a relatively dense network of blood capillaries, ensuring an adequate exposure to nutrients and oxygen. The AT vasculature serves to transport systemic lipids to their storage depot in adipocytes, and transfers factors (e.g. adipokines) and nutrients (e.g. FFAs) from these cells in times of metabolic need. The microvasculature of AT is necessary for the expansion of adipose mass not only to prevent hypoxia, but also as a potential source of adipocyte progenitors in WAT. The blood capillary network also contributes to immunity and inflammation. AT macrophages serve multiple functions: (i) removal of necrotic adipocytes, (ii) production of pro-inflammatory and (iii) pro-angiogenic mediators [3, 22]. Obesity reduces the density of capillaries in AT, leading to localized hypoxia. The effect of hypoxia in obesity is complex and could be explained by: (i) the proportion of the cardiac output and blood flow that goes to WAT is not increased in the obese despite the expansion of the tissue mass, (ii) obese subjects do not exhibit the postprandial increase in the blood flow to AT that occurs in lean subjects and (iii) hypertrophied adipocytes are larger than normal, which impedes oxygen delivery to fat cells. Tissue hypoxia drives many cellular and molecular mechanisms. The first cellular mechanism responsible for local inflammation is macrophages recruitment. The necrosis of adipocytes, driven by hypoxia, is a prominent phagocytic stimulus that regulates macrophages infiltration. The second mechanism responsible for adipose inflammation is lipotoxicity. FFAs released from hypertrophic adipocytes could be transported to the liver and stored in lipid droplets. They could also be re-esterified to triglycerides in adipocytes. Those which escape re-esterification play a critical role as a primary energy source in several organs during prolonged fasting. FFAs are also ligands for TLR 4 (Toll-like receptor) presented in macrophages. FFAs binding with TLR 4 activate the inflammatory signaling cascade (NF-κB—nuclear factor kappa-B). The third mechanism is directly associated with oxygen deprivation (**Figure 4**) [22–24].

Hypoxia in AT has been investigated in human and animal models. Many adipokines related to inflammation (leptin, TNF-α and Il-6), MMPs, growth factors (VEGF—vascular growth factor and bFGF—basic fibroblast growth factor) are elevated in hypoxia [26]. The master regulator of hypoxia is hypoxia-inducible factor (HIF-1). It is a heterodimer composed of an oxygen-sensitive HIF-1α subunit and a constitutively expressed HIF-1β, which is not directly regulated by oxygen. A substantial number of genes are recognized to be hypoxia sensitive. The target genes include those involved in angiogenesis, cell proliferation, survival, apoptosis, vascular tone, glucose and energy metabolism. The genes, which regulate leptin, VEGF and MMPs expression, are controlled by HIF-1 and become elevated in response to low oxygen partial pressure (pO_2) in adipocytes. At the same time, the adiponectin gene is downregulated [27]. Glucose uptake by human adipocytes is strongly stimulated by hypoxia, presumably as a consequence of an increased amount of glucose transporters (GLUT). This may results in changes in insulin sensitivity. An experimental model of intermittent hypoxia has been shown to induce IR [28]. The effect of hypoxia on the WAT function has been discussed in terms of adipocytes, reflecting the fact that these are the cells that are characteristic of AT. Adipocytes

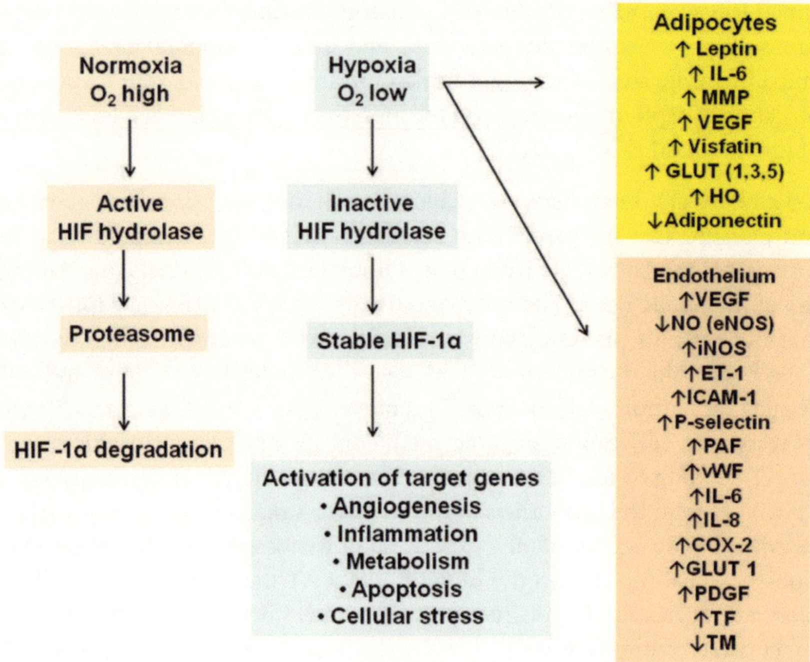

Figure 4. The response of adipocytes and endothelium to hypoxia [25, 26]. *Abbreviations*: HIF, hypoxia-inducible factor; Il-6, interleukin 6; MMP, matrix metalloproteinase; VEGF, vascular endothelial growth factor; GLUT, glucose transporter; HO, heme oxygenase; NO, nitric oxide; iNOS, inducible nitric oxide synthase; ET-1, endothelin 1; ICAM-1, intercellular cell adhesion molecule-1, PAF, platelet-activating factor; vWF, von Wilebrand factor; Il-8, interleukin 8; COX-2, cyclooxygenase 2; PDGF, platelet-derived growth factor; TF, tissue factor; TM, thrombomodulin.

generally account for no more than 50% of the total cell content of WAT (**Figure 2**). The other non-adipocyte cells such as immune cells, vascular cells and pre-adipocytes are also affected by hypoxia, producing inflammatory mediators. There are several transcription factors which are implicated in molecular response to hypoxia, including NF-κB, which modulates the transcription of target pro-inflammatory genes. However, the pivotal role in response to hypoxia is played by HIF-1, which leads to proper angiogenesis. Hypoxia promotes angiogenesis by stimulating VEGF production in ECs, which plays a central role in angiogenesis and neovascularization. It is a potent mitogen for vascular ECs. It also releases other mitogenic molecules (PDGF—platelet-derived growth factor, bFGF, ET-1—endothelin-1) for smooth muscle cells and many pro-inflammatory mediators (Il-6, Il-1α—interleukin 1α, Il-8—interleukin 8, MCP-1 —monocyte chemoattractant protein, iNOS) modulating the angiogenesis process [29].

Hypoxia can also act adversely by inhibiting the angiogenic response and by promoting EC death and apoptosis [30, 31]. The two major responses of ECs have been observed depending on the degree and duration of oxygen deficiency. Firstly, acute hypoxia rapidly activates the ECs to release chemoattractants (Il-8, PAF—platelet activating factor and MCP-1). This is a direct process which does not need gene induction. These inflammatory mediators are able to recruit and promote the adherence of leukocyte and platelets to endothelium, leading to a local inflammatory reaction in ischemic tissue. Secondly, longer periods of hypoxia increase the expression of specific genes encoding cytokines, growth factors and pro-coagulation molecules by HIF-1 activation [25]. Hypoxia in EC also induces NF-κB activation. This promotes the synthesis of pro-inflammatory cytokines, prostaglandins and adhesion molecules, which supports the further transmigration of leucocytes to AT. The adverse effect of NF-κB expression in hypoxia is EC death and apoptosis (**Figure 4**) [31].

EC proliferation and migration, crucial for angiogenesis, could also be affected by hypoxia. The expression of VEGF and its receptor Flt-1 are upregulated by hypoxic endothelium. Both VEGF and its receptor Flt-1 are responsible for the strong mitogenic response in a hypoxic condition. In spite of VEGF overexpression, hypoxia can also paradoxically inhibit the angiogenic response, which could be blocked by a soluble form of VEGFR1 (Flt-1) [29, 30].

Hypoxia can also affect vascular tone, favorable for vasoconstriction. The basal and stimulated nitric oxide (NO) release by endothelium is quickly inhibited by hypoxia. This seems to be due to a decrease in the constitutive endothelial NO synthase (eNOS) expression and the concomitant increase in ET-1 release. In conclusion, the increased production of different mitogens combined with the suppression of endothelial NO would be expected during vascular remodeling [32]. Additionally, hypoxia increases the procoagulant activity, which correlates with a marked decrease of thrombomodulin (TM) and an increase in the tissue factor (TF) expression (**Figure 4**) [25].

Angiogenesis plays a critical role in healthy AT expansion. To better understand this issue, the overexpressed HIF-1α in adipocytes in a transgenic mouse model was analyzed during hypoxia [33]. It was observed that there was no expression of the classical HIF-1α target genes such as VEGF, or any components of angiogenic or anaerobic glucose pathway was registered. Surprisingly, scientists observed fibrosis, which was induced by the upregulation of lysyl oxidase (LOX), elastin, collagens (I, III) and the tissue inhibitor of MMP-1 (TIMP-1). They proposed a hypothesis that the accumulation of ECM in WAT during hypoxia causes local fibrosis with a subsequent inflammatory response and IR [33]. Briefly, a healthy AT expansion consists of adequate angiogenic response and appropriate remodeling of the ECM. In contrast, a pathological AT expansion consists of a massive enlargement of existing adipocytes, reduced angiogenesis and consequent hypoxia [33, 34] (**Figure 5**). It has been reported that obese mice receiving anti-angiogenic reagents have a reduced body weight while their adipose mass shows increased metabolic rates [35]. This is due to the fact that there is a close interplay between adipogenesis and angiogenesis in obesity [36].

In the end of this section, it is worth to mention about some important angiogenic and angiostatic factors crucial for appropriate angiogenesis. Obesity is known to modify these mediators [37]. Below it is shortly discussed the essence of action of pro-angiogenic factors such as bFGF, IGF-1 (insulin growth factor-1) and Ang-1 (angiopoetin-1) and angiostatic factors such as TSP-1 (thrombospondin), endostatin, Ang-2 (angiopoetin-2), IP-10 (interferon-induced protein) and IFN-γ (interferon-γ).

bFGF is another essential pro-angiogenic factor besides VEGF. It changes ECs morphology, increases proliferation, migration and production of metalloproteinases which facilitates the

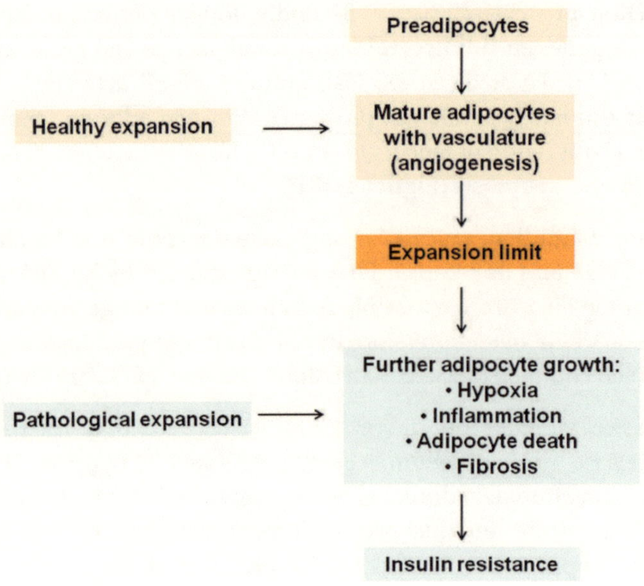

Figure 5. Healthy and unhealthy adipose tissue expansion [6, 26].

degradation of ECM. The autocrine secretion of bFGF by ECs is crucial for their migration and invasiveness [38]. Tsuboi et al. found correlations between bFGF and metalloproteinases in endothelial culture medium and suggested that expression of metalloproteinases is critical for migration and invasiveness of ECs and finally in the tube formations [39]. The clinical data analyzing the correlation between bFGF and abdominal obesity are still inconclusive [40, 41].

IGF-1 also called somatomedin C, has similar structure to insulin and possesses the affinity to insulin receptor. It is produced in the liver in response to growth hormone stimulation. As a mitogenic and anabolic factor, its effect is particularly important for the muscle, neural, hepatic, renal, lung and hematopoietic cells [42]. Additionally, the reduction of IGF-1 in rodents but not in humans is one of the most important effects of CR, which explains the maintenance of animal lifespan [43].

The key angiogenesis processes such as proliferation and migration are regulated by anti-angiogenic TSP-1. Bagavandoss and Wilks documented the anti-angiogenic effects of TSP-1 in various types of ECs, emphasize that its anti-angiogenic effect is mainly due to the inhibitory effect of endothelial proliferation [44]. Nowadays, TSP-1 is also classified as adipokine secreted by visceral fat, predisposing to IR and subclinical inflammation [45].

Endostatin is an endogenous inhibitor of angiogenesis, altering the action of VEGF and bFGF. The N-terminal sequence of this inhibitor is identical with a C-terminal fragment of XVIII collagen, presented in the basal membrane and extracellular matrix. Endostatin inhibits the proliferation, migration, adhesion and ability to tube formation. It blocks multiple signaling pathways, such TNF-α and NF-κB pathways, adhesion and also clotting process [46, 47]. Endostatin administration may reduce adipose tissue growth in animal model [35].

Maturation and stabilization of the blood vessels in the final stages of angiogenesis are controlled by a pair of opposing proteins—Ang-1 and Ang-2 [42]. Both proteins bind to the same Tie-2 (angiopoetin tyrosin kinase receptor) receptor on the surface of ECs resulting in opposite effects: Ang-1 acts as agonist and Ang-2 acts as antagonist. Ang-1 is secreted by adipocytes and Ang-2 by ECs [48]. Ang-1 concentration correlates with the percentage of adipose tissue in the body [49].

IP-10 is a chemotactic factor for T lymphocytes, produced by various cells such as monocytes, endothelium and fibroblasts in response to IFN-γ stimulation [50]. IP-10 overexpression occurs in subcutaneous fat tissue in obese patients [51], but no differences between obese patients with or without diabetes were reported [52].

Infiltrating macrophages and lymphocytes are an important cause of inflammation and IR in AT [3, 18, 19]. IFN-γ produced by lymphocytes changes the phenotype of macrophages to more pro-inflammatory—M1 [53]. Central obesity especially predisposes to high IFN-γ level [54] which is not modified by hypoglycemic treatment [55].

3.3. Crosstalk between adipocytes and endothelial cells

Vascular ECs play a major role in maintaining cardiovascular homeostasis. In addition to providing a physical barrier between the vessel wall and blood lumen, endothelium secretes a number of mediators that regulate vascular tone, coagulation, fibrinolysis and blood cells trafficking. Endothelium can extend its repertoire of functions by adaptation to various stimuli, including mechanical stress, oxidative and metabolic stress, inflammation, hypoxia and many others [32].

Obesity is a component of a metabolic syndrome, a constellation of metabolic risk factors that consist of (i) dyslipidemia, (ii) hypertension, (iii) glucose intolerance, (iv) IR, (v) prothrombotic and (vi) a pro-inflammatory state. Hyperglycemia, dyslipidemia, hyperinsulinemia and adipokines derived from AT play a more dominant role in microvascular complications. In addition to the endothelial pro-inflammatory activation and the decrease in NO production, endothelial barrier increases its permeability due to increased VEGF synthesis in response to hypoxia (HIF-1 activation) and the presence of FFAs released from adipose tissue as an effect of insulin resistance (**Figure 6**) [56]. The strong interaction between AT pro-inflammatory adipokines and endothelium makes obese patients much more prone to CVD [2]. Hanzu et al. exposed endothelium on the medium supplemented with extracts obtained from the visceral fat taken from obese and lean subjects. The adipokines secreted from the visceral fat taken from the obese adversely affected endothelium by increasing the expression of adhesion molecules and von Willebrand factor (vWF). That, in turn, intensified the endothelial cell proliferation and changed EC morphology. Researchers concluded that the observed effects are a result of the activation of NF-κB transcription factor signaling pathways [57].

Endothelial dysfunction in obesity is a multifactorial process and has different molecular aspects. Obesity is characterized by an increased generation of ROS. Because of endoplasmic reticulum stress and mitochondrial dysfunction, ROS are generated in the vascular wall and hypertrophied adipocytes. The effect of ROS on vascular function critically depends on their

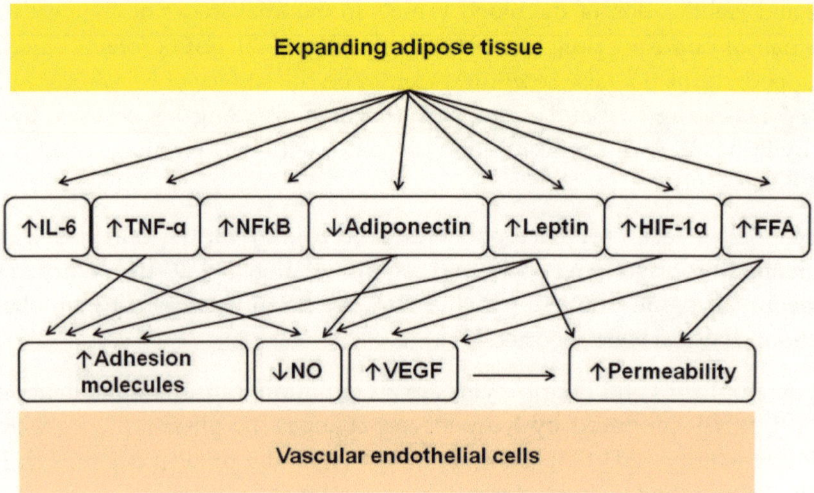

Figure 6. Crosstalk between adipocytes and endothelial cells [3, 4, 58]. *Abbreviations*: Il-6, interleukin 6; TNF-alpha, tumor necrosis factor-alpha; NF-κB, transcriptional factor; HIF-1α, transcriptional factor; FFA, free fatty acid; NO, nitric oxide; VEGF, vascular endothelial growth factor.

quantity. When formed in low amounts, they can act as intracellular secondary messengers, modulating the growth response of vascular smooth muscle cells and fibroblasts. A higher amount of ROS can cause widespread cellular toxicity. Many enzymes of the mitochondrial electron transport chain, such as COX (cyclooxygenase), LOX (lipooxygenase), xantin oxidase, myeloperoxidase, NADPH oxidase, uncoupling eNOS and leptin are the major contributors of ROS production in obesity, leading to a decrease in NO production and an increased production of vasoconstrictor ET-1. NO bioavailability is lowered as a result of peroxynitrite formation ($ONOO^-$). Peroxinitrite is also created as a result of the iNOS activity which is stimulated by an exaggerated production of TNF-α. The enzyme produces NO in a large amount and when combined with the superoxide (O_2^-), anion creates cytotoxic peroxinitrite. Finally, NO production can also be inhibited by an endogenous inhibitor—asymmetric dimethylarginine (ADMA), which competitively inhibits eNOS. The ADMA level is elevated in obese patients and could serve as another mechanism which alters the NO level [4, 32].

ROS accumulation and pro-inflammatory adipokines are implicated in the activation of NF-κB, which is involved in the immune response, apoptosis and inflammation regulating the expression of growth factors, pro-inflammatory cytokines and adhesion molecules [31]. Many products of the genes regulated by NF-κB also, in turn, activate NF-κB (e.g. TNF-α). Pro-inflammatory mediators created by NF-κB signaling, and derived from AT are implicated in EC activation with an increased expression of adhesion molecules (ICAM-1—intercellular cell adhesion molecule-1, VCAM-1—vascular cell adhesion molecule and selectins), and an increased production of chemotactic factors (MCP-1 and Il-8). This promotes the adhesion and migration of circulating leukocytes, initiating atherosclerotic lesion [32, 56].

ECs use glucose and FFAs as nutrients. Non-esterified FFAs are liberated from triglyceride-rich lipoproteins by the endothelial lipoprotein lipase. The endothelial glucose uptake is insulin independent. Physiologically, glucose uptake in endothelium occurs via the glucose transporter GLUT-1. The insulin receptor is presented on the EC surface. Insulin can dilate arteries by the PI3K-Akt-eNOS signaling pathway that stimulates NO release and is also able to rapidly release ET-1 (via MEK-ERK1/2-ET-1 pathway). Both effects occur via the insulin receptor [56]. Central obesity is associated with an increased FFAs level. Elevated FFAs may impair endothelial function as measured by flow-mediated dilatation (FMD) and might affect insulin-mediated vasodilatation [56]. FFAs alter some important intracellular pathways: they could affect ion transport (Na^+, K^+ and Ca^{2+}), vascular reactivity (PKC—protein kinase C) cell growth and ROS generation (NADPH oxidase). This action may have potentially relevant implications for obese patients, leading to a decrease in NO bioavailability. Another possible mechanism, induced by elevated FFAs, that could impair vasodilatation in obese patients, is the reduction of prostacyclin (PGI_2) production [32, 56].

The most essential adipokines implicated in EC dysfunction are leptin and adiponectin (**Tables 1** and **2**). Their specific properties affecting endothelium and angiogenesis processes are described below.

Leptin is secreted from WAT in proportion to the size of AT. It exerts a pressor effect by activating the central nervous system, which inhibits appetite. Its adverse multidirectional effects exerted on ECs include: (i) promoting oxidative stress, (ii) promoting thrombosis by inhibiting thrombomodulin level and increasing tissue factor, (iii) stimulating angiogenesis by promoting ECs proliferation and expression of adhesion molecules, MMPs and VEGF and (iv) stimulating pro-inflammatory cytokines such as TNF-α, Il-6 and MCP-1 [4, 59]. This stimulating effect of pro-inflammatory cytokines is responsible for ECs activation, and may cause hypertension. However, it has been recently shown that leptin may also have a vasodilatory effect. This heterogeneous effect relates to the predominant role of the endothelium-derived hyperpolarizing factor (EDHF) mechanism and is induced by a direct effect of NO release from ECs and an indirect effect of NO release from adipocytes, which triggered leptin, activates eNOS [60].

Adiponectin is the most abundantly secreted adipokine (plasma concentration: 2–20 μg/ml). Globular adiponectin (gAD) and full-length adiponectin (fAD) exert their effect by two receptors (Adipo R1 and Adipo R2). Both receptors are presented on ECs. Generally, adiponectin is responsible for insulin sensitivity by improving carbohydrate and lipid metabolism. Adiponectin exerts its insulin-sensitizing effect by increasing β-oxidation of FFAs, reducing serum triglyceride and FFAs. It also has antiatherogenic and anti-inflammatory properties. The production of adiponectin by adipocytes is inhibited by pro-inflammatory factors such as TNF-α and Il-6 as well as hypoxia and oxidative stress. Its antiatherogenic and anti-inflammatory properties within the vascular wall are mediated via: (i) increased phosphorylation of insulin receptor, (ii) modulation of NF-κB pathway (inhibiting adhesion molecules), (iii) inhibition of foam cell formation, (iv) decreased proliferation and migration of smooth muscle cells and (v) stimulation of NO production in ECs. The plasma adiponectin level highly correlates with the vasodilatory response. Conversely, hypoadiponectinemia is associated with a blunted endothelial function and coronary artery disease [3, 12]. Adiponectin can also induce angiogenesis by promoting signaling cross talk (AMPK-Akt-eNOS) in endothelium. Interestingly, a potent inhibition of endothelial angiogenic properties like proliferation and migration was also observed [61, 62].

The major risk factors for coronary artery disease, present in obese patients, impair the endothelium response to acetylcholine (ACh), which induces a paradoxical vasoconstriction rather than vasodilatation [32]. The endothelial damage can also be assessed by measuring some endothelial-derived markers. Hemostatic factors such as procoagulant von Wilebrant factor and anticoagulant TM are elevated in obesity. They are not only the markers of EC activation but also the markers of EC membrane injury. The factors responsible for EC activation, which mediate the interaction between leukocytes, platelets and the endothelium, are also elevated in obese patients (E-selectin, VCAM-1 and ICAM-1). These factors provide potentially relevant information about the EC condition and the tendency to vasoconstriction, coagulation, platelet aggregation and future cardiovascular morbidity and mortality [4, 32].

4. Caloric restriction

Caloric restriction (CR) is the most effective and reproducible dietary intervention known to affect aging process and increase the healthy lifespan in various model organisms from unicellular yeast to rodents and primates. There is no agreement on how severe a CR must be in order to confer benefits in different organs and systems. However, CR which in most cases involves a 20–40% reduction of dietary requirement relative to normal intake is a severe intervention that results in both beneficial and detrimental effects [63, 64]. Studies show that CR does not need to be prolonged for a long time to be effective, with the advantage that short-term CR is easier to include in clinical practice. In this context, a genomic analysis revealed that the results obtained from short- and long-term CR were similar [65]. It is one of the most common and cost-effective interventions used to induce body weight reduction and control CVD risk factors. It is important to note that the induction of negative energy balance is mandatory for achieving the metabolic benefits of weight loss. Benefits on CV risk factors by reducing the daily caloric intake have been widely described in obese subjects [7, 65–67]. CR reduces body weight, waist circumferences (visceral fat), serum lipids, insulin level and improves insulin sensitivity. The decrease in adiposity leads to a reduction of pro-inflammatory adipokines (e.g. leptin, Il-6, TNF-α, etc.), oxidative stress as well as to an increase in the anti-inflammatory adipokines (e.g. adiponectin, omentin, etc.) [7, 66–68]. Weight loss enhances FMD, which significantly improves endothelial function *in vitro* [8].

The molecular mechanism of CR is complex. It involves downregulation of insulin (also IGF-1 pathway) and insulin-like signaling, the signaling of mTOR (mammalian target of rapamycin) kinase pathway, a rise in the energy balance modulator sirtuins (particularly sirtuin 1) as well as a decrease in pro-inflammatory mediators, growth factors and ROS production [63]. Especially sirtuins are responsible for some beneficial and longevity-promoting effects of CR in many species of animals—from fruit flies to mammals. They are implicated in many physiological effects as control of circadian clock, mitochondrial biogenesis, aging, apoptosis and inflammation [69].

Large observational data support a detrimental effect of obesity on the risk of several cancers, including breast and colon cancer, two of the most common cancers in North America and Europe [63]. The most important causes predisposing to cancer development in obese people are elevated

http://dx.doi.org/10.5772/intechopen.72624

female sex hormones, hyperinsulinemia and a high level of pro-angiogenic and pro-inflammatory factors. Relatively little data exist on the effects of weight gain or weight loss on the risk of cancers [63]. The lack of data on weight loss is likely a function of the small number of individuals able to achieve a sustained weight loss. It is relatively often emphasized that the risk of colorectal cancer is reduced due to weight loss [70]. The best evidence that weight loss can reduce the risk of cancer comes from recent studies in bariatric surgery patients [71]. Tumors become malignant when they attract new blood vessels. Angiogenic switch could be slowed down when special drugs which can stop a key angiogenic mediator—VEGF are used. This concept of angiogenesis was first described by the pediatric surgeon Folkma [72]. The balance between pro- and anti-angiogenic factors allows neoangiogenesis to occur. Angiogenesis could be inhibited through an action on VEGF, bFGF and MMPs. Additionally, high level of mitogenic insulin resistance (IR) correlates with some angiogenic factors [73]. It is well documented that pro-inflammatory cytokines in obesity are mitogenic and pro-angiogenic. CR can decrease (i) insulin signaling, (ii) angiogenic mediators, (iii) inflammation lowering pro-inflammatory adipokines, NF-κB signaling and COX-2 expression, (iv) pro-angiogenic leptin and (v) increase anti-angiogenic adiponectin [74–76]. This anti-inflammatory effect of CR contributes significantly to crucial endothelial function in regulating angiogenesis, hemostasis, vascular tone and vascular wall integrity. This modified effect of CR exerted on endothelium is not only caused by decreased inflammation and angiogenic factors, but also by regulating fibrinolysis, the integrity of the basement membrane and extracellular matrix proteins [20]. Plasminogen activator inhibitor-1 (PAI-1), t-PA, u-PA and also MMPs are involved in angiogenesis. The circulating levels of PAI-1 and MMPs are consistently decreased in response to CR [4]. Rats fed a diet reduced by 40% showed improved vascular EC function, reduced free radical production, expression of NF-κB and a decreased expression of pro-inflammatory genes such as IL-6, TNF-α, sICAM-1 or iNOS [77]. Furthermore, the positive effect of a reduced caloric intake leads to an increased expression of eNOS and transcriptional factor Nrf2 (nuclear factor erythroid 2-related factor), which produces anti-oxidative stress proteins, and activates the VEGF-dependent metabolic pathways [64, 74, 77].

5. Effects of moderate caloric restriction on obese patients—personal observations

In the next section, we would like to present the data of our studies where we investigated the effect of moderate CR on: (i) endothelial cell function especially involved in angiogenesis, (ii) production of adipokines, angiogenic and angiostatic factor and (iii) oxidative stress. Based on our previous studies that have already been published [78] and the data from the literature, we hypothesized that moderate CR, because it is not so burdensome and reflect a real-life situation, seems to be optimal to achieve an improvement of EC.

5.1. Patients and experimental design

To assess the impact of moderate CR, we recruited 50 obese patients (age 37 ± 11 years, BMI: 37.7 ± 6.1 kg/m^2, 72% women). The study was approved by the institutional Ethics Committee (decision number: 217/11) and all patients submitted their informed consent. The exclusion criteria involved overt diabetes, congestive heart failure, an acute coronary syndrome over the past 6 months, malignant or systemic illness, pregnancy, bariatric surgery, a known eating disorder and a change in body weight greater than 2 kg over the past 3 months. Glucose intolerance and hypertension are very common abnormalities seen in obese patients; therefore we decided to include them in our study. Glucose intolerance was the most common disorder (46%). Therefore, the obese patients were divided into the normoglycemic (N) obese (age 37 ± 12 years, BMI: 36.2 ± 6.1 kg/m^2, 78% women); treated only with a diet (n = 27) and the obese with glucose intolerance (GI) (age 38 ± 10 years, BMI: 38.8 ± 7.6 kg/m^2, 70% women) and treated with a diet and a hypoglycemic drug metformin (n = 23). The results were derived from all 50 obese patients who completed the 8-week mild CR program and as a result of this intervention they reduced their body weight.

The dietary intervention lasted 8 weeks and aimed to produce a 15–30% energy deficit (a reduction by 300–500 kcal/day). The patients' basal metabolic rate (BMR) was calculated according to the Harris-Benedict equation and corrected for physical activity according to WHO criteria [79]. The estimated BMR ranged between 1454 and 2045 kcal/d [79] and all patients displayed low physical activity (physical activity factor: 1.4) [80]. The participants were supervised twice a week by a dietician, who designed individualized dietary plans that supplied energy from similar sources but took into account patients' food preferences. The diet was composed of: 25% fat: saturated 7%; 20–25% protein; 50–55% carbohydrates: complex 45–50%, saccharose <10% (exemplary diet is presented in appendix). To assess only the effect of mild CR, physical activity was not recommended.

5.2. Detected parameters

To minimize diurnal variations, fasting blood samples were always collected between 7.30 and 9.00 am. Samples of serum were aliquoted and stored at −80°C until assayed. Before and after CR we measured the following parameters:

- mediators of ECs function (sICAM-1, sVCAM-1, sE-selectin, TM, vWF, PAI-1, ADMA, NO);
- proliferation, migration and invasion using endothelial cell culture *in vitro* after exposition to medium supplemented with 20% serum taken before and after CR;
- adipokines (leptin, adiponectin, vaspin, rezistin, TNF-α, Il-6);
- angiogenic factors (VEGF, bFGF, Ang-1, IGF-1, Il-8, MMP-2, MMP-9);
- angiostatic factors (Ang-2, endostatin, TSB-1, TIMP-1, INF-γ, IP-10);
- oxidative stress (TAS—total antioxidant status, SOD—superoxide dismutase, catalase, ROS production by ECs *in vitro*);
- fat content;
- homeostatic model of assessment of insulin resistance (HOMA-IR).

5.3. Methods

Using the *in vitro* culture (HUVEC lineEA.hy926), we evaluated endothelial pro-angiogenic processes, such as proliferation, migration and invasion.

http://dx.doi.org/10.5772/intechopen.72624

- Cell proliferation was measured using an MTT assay (methylthiazol tetrazolium assay) [81]. Briefly, monolayers of 2×10^4 ECs were exposed to standard medium (M199, Sigma, USA) supplemented with 20% serum taken before and after CR for 24 h in hypoxic condition (1% O_2). After the exposition, cells were incubated in a medium containing 1.25 mg/ml of the MTT salt (3-[4,5-dimethylthiazol-2-yl]-2,5-diphenyl-tetrazolium bromide) for 4 h at 37°C. The active mitochondrial dehydrogenases metabolized the conversion of MTT salt [82]. The generated formazan product was dissolved with the acidic solution of sodium dodecyl sulfate and N,N-dimethylformamide. Absorbance of the converted dye was recorded at 595 nm with a reference wavelength of 690 nm.
- Migration and invasion were tested using Boyden chamber (Cultrex Kit, USA). Briefly, ECs were grown to 80% confluency in a culture medium. Then the cells were harvested, resuspended in serum-free medium and place in an upper migration chamber (5×10^4 cell/100 μl). To detect cell migration, this chamber was coated only with assay buffer in the contrary to invasion process where this surface was coated with basement membrane extracts. Cells were then stimulated for 24 h in hypoxic condition (1% O_2) with standard medium supplemented with 20% serum taken before and after CR placed in the lower chamber. Migrated cells were detached and treated with calcein AM in the lysis buffer. Fluorescence of cell lysates was measured using 480 and 520 nm wavelengths for excitation and emission, respectively.
- Generation of ROS by endothelial cells treated with standard medium supplemented with 20% serum taken before and after CR for 24 h was assessed by labeling with 2′,7′-dichlorodihydrofluorescein diacetate (H_2DCFDA, Molecular Probes, USA) that is trapped inside the cells and activated by intracellular ROS. Briefly, following the exposure to medium, 2×10^4 cells were loaded with 10 μM H_2DCFDA for 30 min and then treated with the lysis buffer. Fluorescence emitted by cell lysates was measured using wavelengths of 485 and 535 nm for excitation and emission, respectively [83].
- To detect serum factors we used the immunoassays from R&D Systems (USA).
- Nitric oxide and TAS were measured by colorimetric assays from R&D Systems (USA) and Cayman (USA), respectively.
- SOD and catalase were tested using enzymatic tests from Cayman (USA).
- Fat content was estimated by bioelectrical impedance analysis (Tanita/Acern, Japan).
- Homeostasis model assessment (HOMA-IR)—an index of insulin resistance was measure using the following equation: fasting insulinemia (mU/ml) × fasting glycemia mg/dl)/405 [84].

5.4. Statistical analysis

Statistical analysis was performed using GraphPad Prism™ 6.00 (GraphPad Software Inc., San Diego, California). The Wilcoxon test and the Mann-Whitney test were used for comparing paired and unpaired data, respectively. The data were also analyzed with repeated measures analysis of variance using a post hoc test for multiple comparisons. Associations between variables were assessed with the Spearman correlation. The level of significance was set at $p < 0.05$.

5.5. Results

Moderate CR induced a reduction of the anthropometric measurements and angiogenic adipokines in all subjects (leptin, Il-6 and TNF-α) (**Figure 7A** and **B**). The largest decrease was achieved in TNF-α concentration in normoglycemic obese patients (N: −66 ± 5% vs. GI: −38 ± 7%) Similarly, a decrease in fat mass was greater in obese patients with a normal glucose profile (N: −10.4 ± 2.1% vs. GI: −8.7 ± 3.3%). CR also decreased the percentage of patients with life-threatening obesity from 34 to 18%. Actually, more beneficial changes in lipids and carbohydrates parameters were observed in normoglycemic obese subjects (HOMA-IR: N: −27 ± 4% vs. GI: −8 ± 2%; cholesterol: N: −9 ± 5% vs. GI: −1.5 ± 1%; triglycerides: N: −24 ± 9% vs. GI: −7 ± 4%). CR was less effective in the obese with GI, certainly because of a higher percentage of patients with life-threatening obesity (GI: 52% vs. N: 34%). Dietary treatment significantly reduced the pro-angiogenic (VEGF: −11 ± 6%, bFGF: −35 ± 10%, Ang-1: −18 ± 9%) and angiostatic (endostatin: −126 ± 5%, IP-10: −76 ± 14%, IFN-gamma: −74 ± 17%) factors, especially in normoglycemic patients (**Figure 7A** and **B**). In the obese with GI, CR reduced only two angiogenic parameters of 13 analyzed (angiostatin-1: −27 ± 7%, endostatin: −8 ± 2%). This group was also characterized by a higher concentration of VEGF (+105 ± 12%), IFN-gamma (+225 ± 24%), IP-10 (+103 ± 25%) and lower IGF-1 (−49 ± 15%) after the treatment when compared to the normoglycemic obese. It should be emphasized that, at baseline, the GI group was characterized by a higher concentration of VEGF (+93 ± 18%) and lower IP-10 (−45 ± 13%). Additionally, the decrease in pro-angiogenic leptin and bFGF was positively correlated with the reduction of anthropometric measurements (body mass, BMI, WC (waist circumference) and fat mass) after dietary intervention. CR in both tested groups, in a comparable way, reduced pro-inflammatory markers of endothelial activation (sICAM-1 in both groups −5 ± 1.5%; sE-selectin: N: −21 ± 4% vs. GI: −42 ± 10%) and ADMA (N: −35 ± 5% vs. GI: −37 ± 10%), but did not change the production of NO (**Figure 7A** and **B**). The changes in coagulation and fibrinolisis parameters were far less pronounced especially in obese patients with GI. Mild CR was only partially effective in reducing oxidative stress by increasing SOD in obese normoglycemic patients. The culture medium supplemented with serum obtained from obese patients, before and after CR, modified endothelial function essential for angiogenesis. We have documented an increase in endothelial proliferation and a decrease in endothelial migration and invasion after 8 weeks of CR under hypoxic condition. These observations were less pronounced in the obese with GI (**Figure 7A** and **B**).

5.6. Discussion

Eight weeks of moderate CR reduced the anthropometric measurements (BMI, body weight and fat mass), pro-angiogenic and pro-inflammatory adipokines such leptin, Il-6 and TNF-α in all obese patients. Additionally, in both tested groups (i.e. in normoglycemic and in glucose intolerance participants), CR in a comparable way, reduced pro-inflammatory markers of endothelial activation (sICAM-1 and sE-selectin), inhibitor of eNOS—ADMA, but did not change the production of NO. Worth emphasizing is that more beneficial changes were observed in normoglycemic obese. We have observed: (i) the improvement of laboratory tests assessing carbohydrate and lipid profile (especially HOMA), (ii) reduced level of many angiogenic and angiostatic factors and (iii) modification of angiogenic properties of EC. Moderate

http://dx.doi.org/10.5772/intechopen.72624

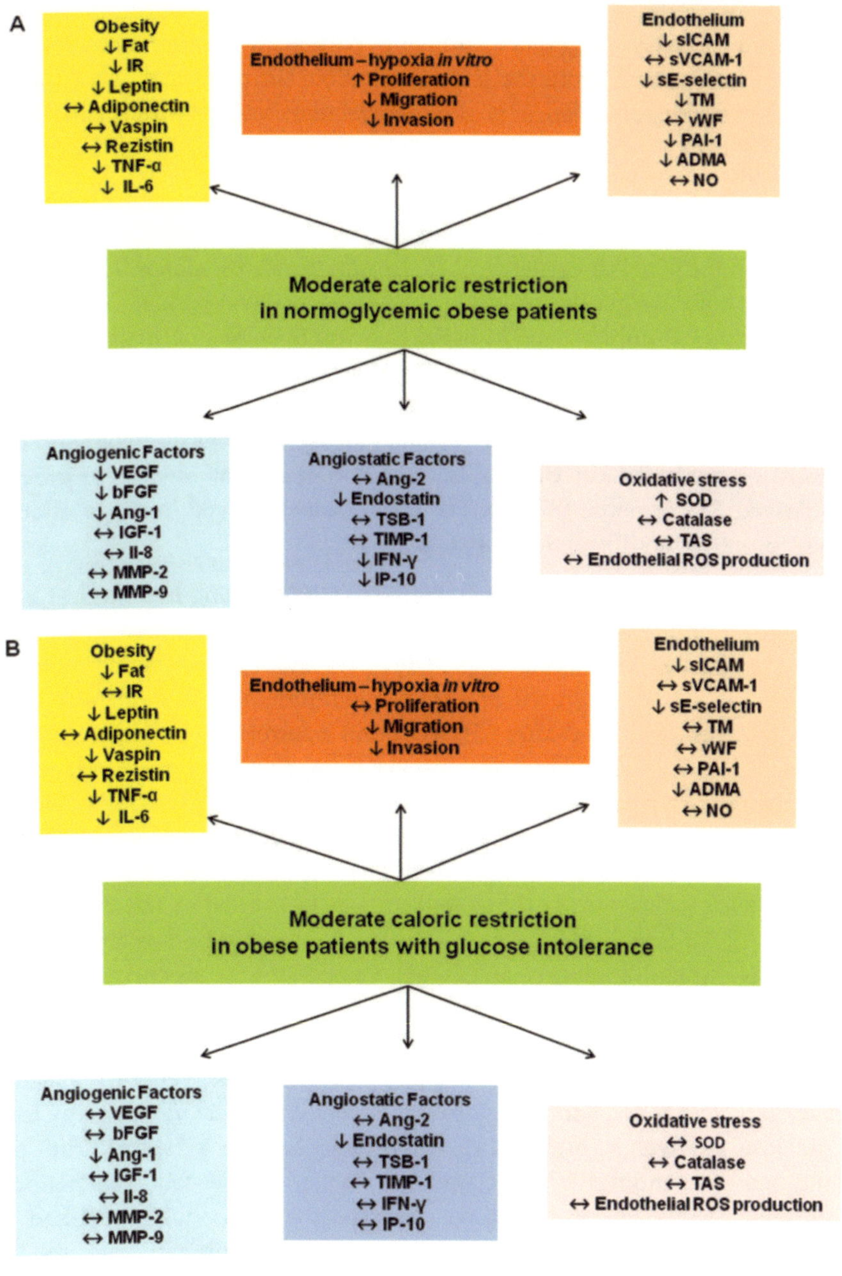

Figure 7. Effect of moderate caloric restriction in (A) obese normoglycemic patients, (B) obese patients with glucose intolerance. *Abbreviations*: IR, insulin resistance; Il-6, interleukin 6; TNF-alpha, tumor necrosis factor-alpha; sICAM-1, soluble form of intercellular cell adhesion molecule-1; sVCAM-1, soluble form of vascular cell adhesion molecule-1; sE-selectin, soluble form of selectin E; TM, thrombomodulin; vWF, von Wilebrand factor; PAI-1, plasminogen activator inhibitor-1; ADMA, asymmetric dimethylarginine; NO, nitric oxide; VEGF, vascular endothelial growth factor; bFGF, basic fibroblast growth factor; Ang-1, angiopoetin 1; IGF-1, insulin-like growth factor 1; Il-8, interleukin 8; MMP, metalloproteinase; Ang-2, angiopoetin 2; TBS-1, thrombospondin-1; TIMP, tissue inhibitor of metalloproteinase; INF-γ, interferon γ; IP-10, interferon-inducible protein; ↔, without changes.

CR has probably not exerted as many beneficial effects in the obese patients with GI because this group was characterized by a greater number of patients with life-threatening obesity. The parameters of oxidative stress were the least susceptible for modification by moderate CR. Additionally, we have documented a positive correlation with the reduction of all tested anthropometric measurements after dietary intervention and a decrease in pro-angiogenic leptin and bFGF.

Weight reduction in obese people is not easy to achieve due to the difficulty in maintaining a dietary regimen and the usual co-existence of IR. Insulin resistance makes it harder for patients to lose unnecessary body weight by hindering glucose utilization by the muscles and liver [85]. There is no doubt that CR improves endothelial function [7–9, 68], particularly the concentration of adhesive molecules, pro-inflammatory cytokines and NO production [7, 8, 66]. It is well documented that changes in NO production by endothelium is triggered by diet are generally related to changes in weight loss [7, 8, 67], plasma glucose concentration [68] and duration of CR [86]. However, a short-term dietary intervention does not always improve vascular endothelial-derived NO response [87, 88]. The parameters involved in coagulation and fibrinolysis are less prone to modification [7, 66, 67].

An important issue is whether even a small degree of CR, resulting in a modest loss of body weight, will improve endothelial function. To investigate this, it is necessary to find a parameter that is sensitive enough to reflect an improvement of endothelial function even with only a slight weight loss. Using ECs cultured *in vitro* in medium supplemented with serum taken from the obese patients before and after CR, we found a correlation between EC proliferation and weight loss after CR. This effect was especially apparent in male subjects [78]. The mechanisms underlying changes in EC angiogenic properties in response to dietary intervention are difficult to define unequivocally. They are probably context-dependent. In addition to the effects exerted by leptin and adiponectin through their similar receptors [59] and the effect of sex hormones [89, 90], changes in EC metabolism may be exerted by the alteration of energy homeostasis [91, 92]. Various metabolic pathways are now recognized as contributing significantly to obesity-associated angiogenesis [93, 94]. Proliferation is an energy-consuming process, it is tempting to hypothesize that the magnitude of serum-induced endothelial growth response reflects a tendency for conserving energy during CR. Interesting observations have recently been published by Reinhardt et al. [91, 92]. They observed that patients with a "thrifty" phenotype (economic and energy saving) could distribute more energy for cell proliferation and lose less weight during CR, while patients with a "spendthrift" phenotype (wasteful and energy spending) would spend less energy for the cell proliferation and lost more weight after CR [91]. Accordingly, we observed that individuals who had lost more weight exhibited a decrease in cell proliferation (for quantitative data see [78]). We documented that a moderate CR in obese subjects changes the endothelial genes expression profile involved in the cell cycle [78]. Similarly, Ellsworth et al. have recently revealed significant changes in peripheral blood gene expression patterns, including those involved in cell cycle in obese patients undergoing intensive long-term lifestyle modifications. Observed changes occurred only in patients who achieved considerable weight loss (>10%) over 1 year, but not in participants with minimal weight loss [65]. As the authors emphasized, the mechanism by which a CR protects the function of capillaries remains unexplained. It certainly improves many of the endothelial functions essential for angiogenesis, such as proliferation, tube formation and prevents against apoptosis and aging [74], Csiszar et al. explained that the reduction of oxidative stress and inflammation would primarily improve EC functions. Dietary intervention drives a change in the concentration of many neuroendocrine factors, which reach the capillary ECs from the bloodstream and initiate a variety of cytoprotective processes [77].

We have measured 13 factors involved in angiogenesis (angiogenic/angiostatic). Reducing AT after the dietary treatment makes it less demanding for the factors necessary for angiogenesis. Dietary restriction led to a decrease in the concentration of three pro-angiogenic factors (VEGF, bFGF and Ang-1) and three angiostatic factors (endostatin, IP-10 and IFN-γ) in normoglycemic obese subjects. In obese patients with GI, CR reduced only 2 parameters involved in the angiogenesis process, out of 13 analyzed (Ang-1, endostatin). Glucose intolerance in obese people adversely affects the angiogenesis process. This has been confirmed by Nathan et al. where the lower adhesion, migration and tubular structure formation in endothelium were observed compared to the normoglycemic control group [95].

One of the most important factors in the angiogenesis process that stimulates migration and EC proliferation is VEGF [29]. Miyazawa-Hoshimoto et al. have demonstrated a positive correlation between serum VEGF levels and anthropometric parameters of obese persons, which indicates that visceral fat is the most important factor that determines the VEGF concentration in obesity. We have also observed that obese patients with high BMI and fat mass (particularly obese with GI) exhibit elevated VEGF level at baseline when compared with normoglycemic obese; nevertheless, CR did not reduce the level of VEGF. Weight reduction might decrease VEGF concentration [96], however, this effect is not always achieved [52, 75, 97]. We have observed a decline in VEGF level only in the normoglycemic obese. Higher VEGF level is characteristic for the obese with GI when compared with the normoglycemic patients [52, 98]. Insulin stimulates VEGF production in vascular ECs [99] and in adipocytes [100] by stimulating the HIF-1α expression [29]. The authors emphasize that insulin is a potent mitogen, and its stimulatory effect on VEGF production and proliferation is already present at physiological concentrations [29, 100]. EC proliferation after CR was higher in the normoglycemic obese and was not observed in patients with GI despite significantly higher insulin and VEGF concentrations. Severe obese patients with glucose intolerance treated with metformin and/or moderate CR not always reduced insulin concentration and HOMA levels [101, 102]. EC proliferation in obese subjects is complex and cannot be explained by the effects of typical angiogenic factors as elevated level of insulin and VEGF [78]. Yamagishi et al. performed an experiment showing that, despite higher VEGF level following insulin stimulation, no increase in VEGF receptor-mediated EC proliferation was observed. They concluded that this effect may hamper the response to pro-angiogenic VEGF in patients with hyperinsulinemia [99]. Recent work by Aplin and Nicosia also confirms the decline in expression of VEGF receptors in the EC under hypoxia [30]. Experiment done by Csiszar et al. using nonhuman primate *Macaca mulatta* after 10 years of CR showed similar observation [74].

bFGF is the subsequent crucial angiogenic factor modified by weight loss [78, 96]. The correlation between bFGF and abdominal obesity is obscure [40, 41], nevertheless we observed a positive correlation between the decrease in bFGF and the reduction in body mass, fat mass,

BMI and waist circumference. bFGF changes endothelial angiogenic properties [38]. The correlation between bFGF and MMPs in an endothelial culture medium suggests that the expression of MMPs is critical for the migration and invasiveness of cells in the formation of new blood vessels [39]. The significant lowering of bFGF in patients treated with a diet alone was probably one of the most important factors that contributed to the decreased migration and invasiveness of EC after the intervention.

Endostatin inhibits the proliferation, migration, adhesion and ability to form the tubes by altering the action of VEGF and bFGF. It blocks multiple signaling pathways (TNF-α, NF-κB, adhesion and clotting) [47]. The elevated endostatin concentrations are characteristic of overweight patients [37]. Eight weeks of moderate CR was enough to decrease endostatin concentration in both obese groups. It is worth to emphasize that endostatin was the only angiostatic parameter modified by CR in obese patients with GI.

Ang-1 and Ang-2 control the maturation and stabilization of blood vessels [42, 48] and by that means regulate AT growth [48]. Dietary restrictions reduce their concentration [75]. Ang-1 was the only angiogenic parameter that was reduced in obese patients with GI. Since Ang-1 stimulates proliferation and migration, its reduced concentration after CR could also be responsible for diminished endothelial angiogenic function observed *in vitro*. Ang-2 is synthesized almost exclusively by ECs cells during vascular remodeling [103]. It destabilizes the vascular wall to facilitate the action of other pro-angiogenic factors [104]. The mechanism of angiopoietins' action is not fully understood. Ang-2 has dual pro- and anti-angiogenic properties. It is believed that Ang-2 acts via a Tie-2 receptor as its antagonist, when Ang-1 is not available or acts independently without a Tie-2 receptor [105]. Higher level of Ang-2 is observed in patients with type 2 diabetes [106] as a hyperglycemia effect [107]. It has been suggested that elevated concentrations of Ang-2 and hyperglycemia may promote abnormal neovascularization and endothelial dysfunction, which in turn leads to diabetic micro- and macroangiopathy [108].

IP-10 is a chemotactic factor for T cells, produced by various cells such as monocytes, ECs, fibroblasts, in response to IFN-γ stimulation [50]. Dalmas et al. show higher blood levels of IP-10 in obese patients, without any differences between diabetic and non-diabetic patients [52]. The group of obese patients with GI was characterized by a lower IP-10 (−45%) at baseline. CR reduced the IP-10 concentration by 76% only in the normoglycemic obese. The 10-year follow-up of patients with type 2 diabetes in the MONICA/KORA clinical trial suggests that the IP-10 protein is one of the risk factors for the clinical development of diabetes [109] and its concentration could be lowered by CR and lifestyle modification [110].

Infiltrating of immune cells in AT is an important factor leading to inflammation and IR [6] Interferon-γ is known to change the macrophage phenotype to more pro-inflammatory (M1) [53]. Patients with GI had a higher IFN-γ concentration after CR. Higher fat content and stronger stimulation by macrophage-derived IFN-γ were the important factors for higher concentrations of pro-inflammatory adipokines after the experiment (higher TNF-α after CR). Obese individuals usually have elevated IFN-γ levels, particularly patients with central obesity [54]. Diet intervention significantly decreased IFN-γ levels in the normoglycemic obese (−74%). Although plasma concentrations of IP-10 and IFN-γ in the obese with GI after CR were significantly higher when compared with the normoglycemic obese, the diet did not change their concentrations. It is well known that hyperglycemia in diabetic patients significantly modifies the immune response, particularly the humoral immunity [12]. Higher levels of IP-10 and IFN-γ seen in the obese with GI, may reflect a different immune response observed in this group.

Metformin is one of the oldest commonly used oral hypoglycemic drugs, which does not affect insulin secretion. It functions omnidirectionally on various cells [85, 111], reducing the risk of CVD by improving blood vessels, vascular endothelium or decreasing inflammatory markers [85]. Animal models and *in vitro* experiments showed the anti-angiogenic effect of metformin and emphasized its beneficial role which goes far beyond lowering the glucose level [112, 113]. Endothelium treated with metformin alters the secretion profile of angiogenic and angiostatic factors [112]. Moreover, metformin protects the myocardium against hypoxia. The cardioprotective effect of metformin is the result of the reduced oxidative stress and bFGF level, which are responsible for hypertrophy and myocardial fibrosis [111]. The ability to reduce bFGF concentration is one of metformin's anti-tumor activities additional to its inhibitory effect on the migration and proliferation of both endothelial and tumor cells [112, 113]. Our obese patients treated with CR and metformin had tendency for higher anthropometric parameters (more patients with life-threatening obesity), additionally more patients had treated hypertension. The angiogenic mediators and endothelial cell function were significantly less modified by moderate CR in compare with nomoglycemic patients treated only with diet.

6. Conclusions

AT remodeling is pathologically accelerated in an obese state due to local hypoxia leading to reduced angiogenesis, severe immune cell infiltration with subsequent pro-inflammatory responses and additional deterioration of EC functions. It is believed that EC dysfunction in obesity can be reduced by CR. Moderate CR reflects a real-life situation and could be optimal to achieve an improvement in EC. Our observations suggest that a moderate CR can improve several parameters of EC function, especially those involved in angiogenesis. It also improves anthropometric and metabolic measurements, but does not significantly strengthen the antioxidant status. The *in vitro* model shows how various circulating factors, induced by CR, affect the endothelial proliferation, migration and invasiveness. This process is a result of a reduction of inflammation and a modification of angiogenic and angiostatic factors. Additionally, in patients with glucose intolerance, it is also caused by potential anti-angiogenic properties of metformin. The obtained results are particularly pronounced in the normoglycemic obese, and to a lesser extent in the obese with GI and IR, who may have an adverse impact on AT remodeling, the cardiovascular system and might have an increased risk of obesity-associated cancer diseases.

Acknowledgements

The author would like to thank the following researchers: Prof. Marian Grzymisławski, Dr Ewelina Swora-Cwynar and Dr Alina Kanikowska from the Department of Internal Medicine, Metabolic Diseases, and Dietetics, Poznań University of Medical Sciences, Poland and Prof. Janusz Witowski, Dr Natasza Czepulis, Dr inż. Joanna Łuczak from the Department of

Pathophysiology, Poznań University of Medical Science, Poland, for their involvement in this medical project. This project was financially supported by Grant NCN-NN404 151340 from the Polish Ministry of Science and Higher Education—National Science Centre Poland.

Conflict of interest

The author do not declare the conflict of interest.

A. Appendix and nomenclature: Exemplary diet

Diet plan

The energy supply was set at 1500 kcal

Meal	Hours	Share of energy supply (%)	Caloric value (kcal)
I breakfast	7:00–8:00	20	300
II breakfast	10:00–11:00	20	300
Lunch	13:00–14:00	10	150
Snack	16:00–17:00	30	450
Dinner	18:30–19:30	20	300

Exemplary menu 1500 kcal—version 1

I breakfast—330 kcal

Italian sandwich "Caprese"

- 1 wholemeal roll (80 g)
- 1 small tomato
- Cottage cheese (50 g)
- Fresh basil
- 2 teaspoons of olive oil (10 g)
- Black pepper

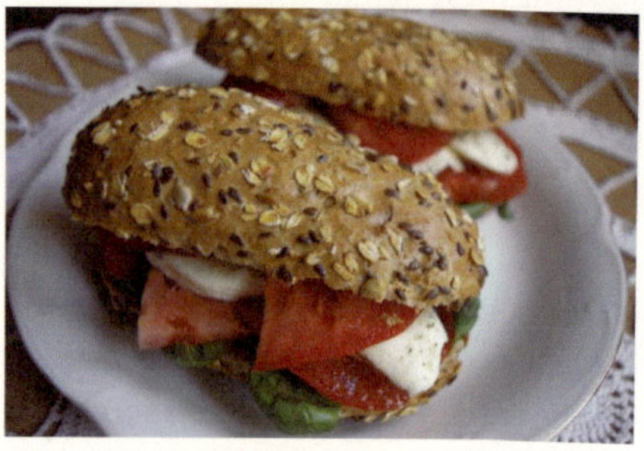

II breakfast—310 kcal

Sandwich with egg and radishes

- 2 slice of wholemeal bread (80 g)
- 1 teaspoon of butter (5 g)
- Lettuce

http://dx.doi.org/10.5772/intechopen.72624

- 1 boiled egg
- A few radishes

Tomato juice—small bottle (300 ml)

Lunch—440 kcal

Italian spaghetti—1 portion

Spaghetti should be boiled *al dente.*

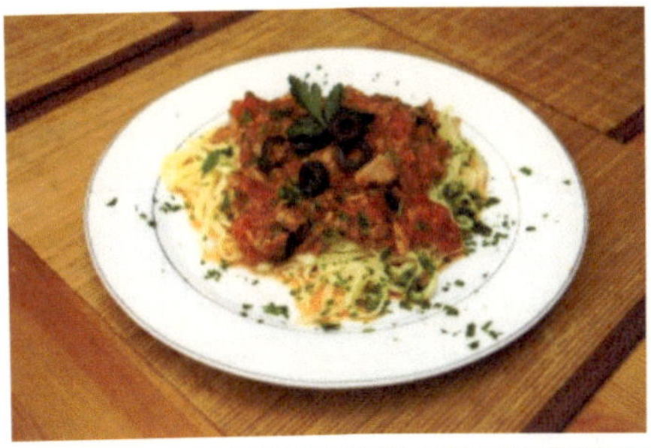

Ingredients for 3 potions:

- 250 g wholemeal pasta
- 1 cane of tomatoes or fresh tomatoes
- 1 chicken breast (200 g)
- 10 capers
- 10 black olives
- 1 small onion
- 2 cloves of garlic
- Olive oil (1 spoon)
- Fresh parsley (2 spoons)
- Pepper, basil

Snack—160 kcal

Natural yogurt—2% fat (180–200 g) with 1 spoon of wheat bran.

Tangerines (2 medium size—150 g)

Dinner—290 kcal

Tuna salad with parsley sauce (1 portion)

1 slice of wholemeal bread (40 g)

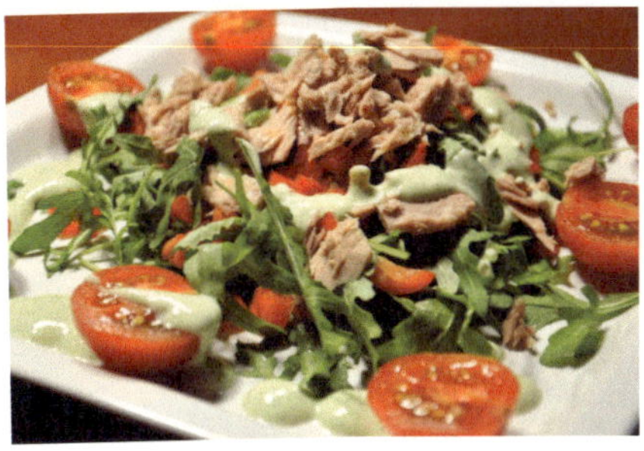

- Rucola salad
- 100 g cocktail tomatoes
- 1/3 red pepper
- Canned tuna in its own sauce (50 g—2 spoons)
- Natural yogurt 2% fat (75 g—3 spoons)

- Sunflower seeds (15 g—3 teaspoons)
- Parsley
- Lemon juice

Exemplary menu 1500 kcal—version 2

I breakfast—330 kcal.

Sandwich with ham and vegetables

- 1 slice of ray bred (40 g)
- Butter (1 teaspoon)
- Lettuce
- 1 slice of chicken ham (20 g)
- Small tomato (100 g)
- 1–2 small cucumbers

Natural yogurt 2% fat (400 g)

II breakfast—280 kcal

Cottage cheese

- Cottage cheese—3% fat (150 g)
- A few radishes (chopped or grated)
- Sunflower seeds (1 spoon)

1 slice of ray bread (40 g)

Lunch—440 kcal.

Asparagus cream soup—1 portion

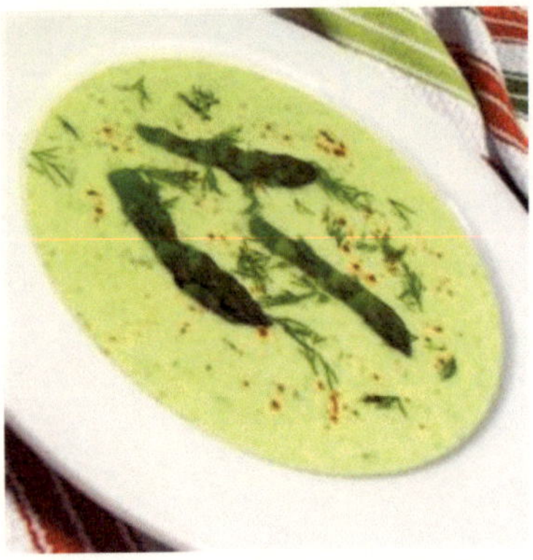

Ingredients for 4 portions

- 1 bunch of green asparagus
- 1 zucchini
- 1 clove of garlic
- 1 onion
- 1 liter of bullion
- Olive oil (2 spoons)
- Pepper
- 1–2 teaspoons of lemon juice
- pine nuts/ almond flakes (4 teaspoons)
- cream cheese or natural yoghurt (4 teaspoons)

http://dx.doi.org/10.5772/intechopen.72624

1 wholemeal roll (80 g) or 2 slices of rye bread with butter (1 teaspoon)

1 orange (350 g) or ½ pomelo

Snack—160 kcal

Oatmeal with dried plums (49 g)

Dinner—290 kcal

Salad with baked pepper and tomatoes

- 1 green or yellow pepper baked in the oven and peeled
- 1 big tomato (200 g)
- 1 spoon of olive oil or sunflower oil
- 1 spoon of chopped lettuce
- 1 spoon of chopped celery leaves
- Pepper

Sandwich with ham

- 1 slice of ray bread (40 g)
- 2 slices of chicken ham (40 g)

Author details

Katarzyna Korybalska

Address all correspondence to: koryb@ump.edu.pl

Pathophysiology Department, Poznań University of Medical Science, Poznań, Poland

References

[1] Kaplan NM. The deadly quartet. Upper-body obesity, glucose intolerance, hypertriglyceridemia, and hypertension. Archives of Internal Medicine. 1989;**149**:1514-1520

[2] Higgins M, Kannel W, Garrison R, Pinsky J, Stokes J III. Hazards of obesity—The Framingham experience. Acta Medica Scandinavica. Supplementum. 1988;**723**:23-36

[3] Rosen ED, Spiegelman BM. What we talk about when we talk about fat. Cell. 2014; **156**:20-44

[4] Avogaro A, De Kreutzenberg SV. Mechanisms of endothelial dysfunction in obesity. Clinica Chimica Acta. 2005;**360**:9-26

[5] Van dV, Pauwels B, Boydens C, Decaluwe K. Adipocytokines in relation to cardiovascular disease. Metabolism. 2013;**62**:1513-1521

[6] Sun K, Kusminski CM, Scherer PE. Adipose tissue remodeling and obesity. The Journal of Clinical Investigation. 2011;**121**:2094-2101

[7] Hamdy O, Ledbury S, Mullooly C, Jarema C, Porter S, Ovalle K, Moussa A, Caselli A, Caballero AE, Economides PA, Veves A, Horton ES. Lifestyle modification improves endothelial function in obese subjects with the insulin resistance syndrome. Diabetes Care. 2003;**26**:2119-2125

[8] Joris PJ, Zeegers MP, Mensink RP. Weight loss improves fasting flow-mediated vasodilation in adults: A meta-analysis of intervention studies. Atherosclerosis. 2014;**239**:21-30

[9] Sciacqua A, Candigliota M, Ceravolo R, Scozzafava A, Sinopoli F, Corsonello A, Sesti G, Perticone F. Weight loss in combination with physical activity improves endothelial dysfunction in human obesity. Diabetes Care. 2003;**26**:1673-1678

[10] Alexopoulos N, Katritsis D, Raggi P. Visceral adipose tissue as a source of inflammation and promoter of atherosclerosis. Atherosclerosis. 2014;**233**:104-112

[11] Kwon H, Pessin JE. Adipokines mediate inflammation and insulin resistance. Frontiers in Endocrinology. 2013;**4**:71

[12] Ouchi N, Parker JL, Lugus JJ, Walsh K. Adipokines in inflammation and metabolic disease. Nature Reviews. Immunology. 2011;**11**:85-97

[13] Kajimura S, Seale P, Spiegelman BM. Transcriptional control of brown fat development. Cell Metabolism. 2010;**11**:257-262

[14] Snijder MB, Dekker JM, Visser M, Yudkin JS, Stehouwer CD, Bouter LM, Heine RJ, Nijpels G, Seidell JC. Larger thigh and hip circumferences are associated with better glucose tolerance: The Hoorn study. Obesity Research. 2003;**11**:104-111

[15] Snijder MB, Visser M, Dekker JM, Seidell JC. Re: "Changes in body weight and body fat distribution as risk factors for clinical diabetes in US men". American Journal of Epidemiology. 2004;**160**:1133-1134

[16] Grauer WO, Moss AA, Cann CE, Goldberg HI. Quantification of body fat distribution in the abdomen using computed tomography. The American Journal of Clinical Nutrition. 1984;**39**:631-637

[17] Krotkiewski M, Bjorntorp P, Sjostrom L, Smith U. Impact of obesity on metabolism in men and women. Importance of regional adipose tissue distribution. The Journal of Clinical Investigation. 1983;**72**:1150-1162

[18] Lumeng CN, Bodzin JL, Saltiel AR. Obesity induces a phenotypic switch in adipose tissue macrophage polarization. The Journal of Clinical Investigation. 2007;**117**:175-184

[19] Apovian CM, Bigornia S, Mott M, Meyers MR, Ulloor J, Gagua M, McDonnell M, Hess D, Joseph L, Gokce N. Adipose macrophage infiltration is associated with insulin resistance

and vascular endothelial dysfunction in obese subjects. Arteriosclerosis, Thrombosis, and Vascular Biology. 2008;**28**:1654-1659

[20] Carmeliet P. Angiogenesis in health and disease. Nature Medicine. 2003;**9**:653-660

[21] van HV, Koolwijk P. Endothelial sprouting and angiogenesis: matrix metalloproteinases in the lead. Cardiovascular Research. 2008;**78**:203-212

[22] Corvera S, Gealekman O. Adipose tissue angiogenesis: Impact on obesity and type-2 diabetes. Biochimica et Biophysica Acta. 2014;**1842**:463-472

[23] Lemoine AY, Ledoux S, Queguiner I, Calderari S, Mechler C, Msika S, Corvol P, Larger E. Link between adipose tissue angiogenesis and fat accumulation in severely obese subjects. The Journal of Clinical Endocrinology and Metabolism. 2012;**97**:E775-E780

[24] Lemoine AY, Ledoux S, Larger E. Adipose tissue angiogenesis in obesity. Thrombosis and Haemostasis. 2013;**110**:661-668

[25] Michiels C, Arnould T, Remacle J. Endothelial cell responses to hypoxia: Initiation of a cascade of cellular interactions. Biochimica et Biophysica Acta. 2000;**1497**:1-10

[26] Trayhurn P. Hypoxia and adipose tissue function and dysfunction in obesity. Physiological Reviews. 2013;**93**:1-21

[27] Lolmede K, Durand de Saint Front V, Galitzky J, Lafontan M, Bouloumie A. Effects of hypoxia on the expression of proangiogenic factors in differentiated 3T3-F442A adipocytes. International Journal of Obesity and Related Metabolic Disorders. 2003;**27**:1187-1195

[28] Ribatti D, Vacca A, Nico B, Presta M, Roncali L. Angiogenesis: Basic and clinical aspects. Italian Journal of Anatomy and Embryology. 2003;**108**:1-24

[29] Forsythe JA, Jiang BH, Iyer NV, Agani F, Leung SW, Koos RD, Semenza GL. Activation of vascular endothelial growth factor gene transcription by hypoxia-inducible factor 1. Molecular and Cellular Biology. 1996;**16**:4604-4613

[30] Aplin AC, Nicosia RF. Hypoxia paradoxically inhibits the angiogenic response of isolated vessel explants while inducing overexpression of vascular endothelial growth factor. Angiogenesis. 2016;**19**:133-146

[31] Matsushita H, Morishita R, Nata T, Aoki M, Nakagami H, Taniyama Y, Yamamoto K, Higaki J, Yasufumi K, Ogihara T. Hypoxia-induced endothelial apoptosis through nuclear factor-kappaB (NF-kappaB)-mediated bcl-2 suppression: In vivo evidence of the importance of NF-kappaB in endothelial cell regulation. Circulation Research. 2000;**86**:974-981

[32] Cines DB, Pollak ES, Buck CA, Loscalzo J, Zimmerman GA, McEver RP, Pober JS, Wick TM, Konkle BA, Schwartz BS, Barnathan ES, McCrae KR, Hug BA, Schmidt AM, Stern DM. Endothelial cells in physiology and in the pathophysiology of vascular disorders. Blood. 1998;**91**:3527-3561

[33] Halberg N, Khan T, Trujillo ME, Wernstedt-Asterholm I, Attie AD, Sherwani S, Wang ZV, Landskroner-Eiger S, Dineen S, Magalang UJ, Brekken RA, Scherer PE. Hypoxia-inducible

factor 1alpha induces fibrosis and insulin resistance in white adipose tissue. Molecular and Cellular Biology. 2009;**29**:4467-4483

[34] Trayhurn P, Wang B, Wood IS. Hypoxia in adipose tissue: A basis for the dysregulation of tissue function in obesity? The British Journal of Nutrition. 2008;**100**:227-235

[35] Rupnick MA, Panigrahy D, Zhang CY, Dallabrida SM, Lowell BB, Langer R, Folkman MJ. Adipose tissue mass can be regulated through the vasculature. Proceedings of the National Academy of Sciences of the United States of America. 2002;**99**:10730-10735

[36] Nishimura S, Manabe I, Nagasaki M, Hosoya Y, Yamashita H, Fujita H, Ohsugi M, Tobe K, Kadowaki T, Nagai R, Sugiura S. Adipogenesis in obesity requires close interplay between differentiating adipocytes, stromal cells, and blood vessels. Diabetes. 2007;**56**: 1517-1526

[37] Silha JV, Krsek M, Sucharda P, Murphy LJ. Angiogenic factors are elevated in overweight and obese individuals. International Journal of Obesity. 2005;**29**:1308-1314

[38] Montesano R, Vassalli JD, Baird A, Guillemin R, Orci L. Basic fibroblast growth factor induces angiogenesis in vitro. Proceedings of the National Academy of Sciences of the United States of America. 1986;**83**:7297-7301

[39] Tsuboi R, Sato Y, Rifkin DB. Correlation of cell migration, cell invasion, receptor number, proteinase production, and basic fibroblast growth factor levels in endothelial cells. The Journal of Cell Biology. 1990;**110**:511-517

[40] Seida A, Wada J, Kunitomi M, Tsuchiyama Y, Miyatake N, Fujii M, Kira S, Takahashi K, Shikata K, Makino H. Serum bFGF levels are reduced in Japanese overweight men and restored by a 6-month exercise education. International Journal of Obesity and Related Metabolic Disorders. 2003;**27**:1325-1331

[41] Zimering MB, Anderson RJ, Luo P, Moritz TE. Plasma basic fibroblast growth factor is correlated with plasminogen activator inhibitor-1 concentration in adults from the Veterans Affairs Diabetes Trial. Metabolism. 2008;**57**:1563-1569

[42] Folkman J. Angiogenesis and angiogenesis inhibition: An overview. EXS. 1997;**79**:1-8

[43] Fontana L, Klein S. Aging, adiposity, and calorie restriction. JAMA. 2007;**297**:986-994

[44] Bagavandoss P, Wilks JW. Specific inhibition of endothelial cell proliferation by thrombospondin. Biochemical and Biophysical Research Communications. 1990;**170**: 867-872

[45] Varma V, Yao-Borengasser A, Bodles AM, Rasouli N, Phanavanh B, Nolen GT, Kern EM, Nagarajan R, Spencer HJ II, Lee MJ, Fried SK, McGehee RE Jr, Peterson CA, Kern PA. Thrombospondin-1 is an adipokine associated with obesity, adipose inflammation, and insulin resistance. Diabetes. 2008;**57**:432-439

[46] Cho HH, YJ KIM, Kim JT, Song JS, Shin KK, Bae YC, Jung JS. The role of chemokines in proangiogenic action induced by human adipose tissue-derived mesenchymal stem cells

in the murine model of hindlimb ischemia. Cellular Physiology and Biochemistry. 2009;**24**:511-518

[47] Rehn M, Veikkola T, Kukk-Valdre E, Nakamura H, Ilmonen M, Lombardo C, Pihlajaniemi T, Alitalo K, Vuori K. Interaction of endostatin with integrins implicated in angiogenesis. Proceedings of the National Academy of Sciences of the United States of America. 2001;**98**:1024-1029

[48] Dallabrida SM, Zurakowski D, Shih SC, Smith LE, Folkman J, Moulton KS, Rupnick MA. Adipose tissue growth and regression are regulated by angiopoietin-1. Biochemical and Biophysical Research Communications. 2003;**311**:563-571

[49] Pasarica M, Sereda OR, Redman LM, Albarado DC, Hymel DT, Roan LE, Rood JC, Burk DH, Smith SR. Reduced adipose tissue oxygenation in human obesity: Evidence for rarefaction, macrophage chemotaxis, and inflammation without an angiogenic response. Diabetes. 2009;**58**:718-725

[50] Dufour JH, Dziejman M, Liu MT, Leung JH, Lane TE, Luster AD. IFN-gamma-inducible protein 10 (IP-10; CXCL10)-deficient mice reveal a role for IP-10 in effector T cell generation and trafficking. Journal of Immunology. 2002;**168**:3195-3204

[51] Sindhu S, Thomas R, Shihab P, Sriraman D, Behbehani K, Ahmad R, Obesity I. A positive modulator of IL-6R and IL-6 expression in the subcutaneous adipose tissue: Significance for metabolic inflammation. PLoS One. 2015;**10**:e0133494

[52] Dalmas E, Rouault C, Abdennour M, Rovere C, Rizkalla S, Bar-Hen A, Nahon JL, Bouillot JL, Guerre-Millo M, Clement K, Poitou C. Variations in circulating inflammatory factors are related to changes in calorie and carbohydrate intakes early in the course of surgery-induced weight reduction. The American Journal of Clinical Nutrition. 2011;**94**:450-458

[53] O'Rourke RW, Metcalf MD, White AE, Madala A, Winters BR, Maizlin II, Jobe BA, Roberts CT Jr, Slifka MK, Marks DL. Depot-specific differences in inflammatory mediators and a role for NK cells and IFN-gamma in inflammation in human adipose tissue. International Journal of Obesity. 2009;**33**:978-990

[54] Schmidt FM, Weschenfelder J, Sander C, Minkwitz J, Thormann J, Chittka T, Mergl R, Kirkby KC, Fasshauer M, Stumvoll M, Holdt LM, Teupser D, Hegerl U, Himmerich H. Inflammatory cytokines in general and central obesity and modulating effects of physical activity. PLoS One. 2015;**10**:e0121971

[55] Sumarac-Dumanovic M, Jeremic D, Pantovic A, Janjetovic K, Stamenkovic-Pejkovic D, Cvijovic G, Stevanovic D, Micic D, Trajkovic V. Therapeutic improvement of glucoregulation in newly diagnosed type 2 diabetes patients is associated with a reduction of IL-17 levels. Immunobiology. 2013;**218**:1113-1118

[56] Bakker W, Eringa EC, Sipkema P, Van HV. Endothelial dysfunction and diabetes: Roles of hyperglycemia, impaired insulin signaling and obesity. Cell and Tissue Research. 2009;**335**:165-189

[57] Hanzu FA, Palomo M, Kalko SG, Parrizas M, Garaulet M, Escolar G, Gomis R, Az-Ricart M. Translational evidence of endothelial damage in obese individuals: Inflammatory and prothrombotic responses. Journal of Thrombosis and Haemostasis. 2011;**9**:1236-1245

[58] Rutkowski JM, Davis KE, Scherer PE. Mechanisms of obesity and related pathologies: The macro- and microcirculation of adipose tissue. The FEBS Journal. 2009;**276**:5738-5746

[59] Adya R, Tan BK, Randeva HS. Differential effects of leptin and adiponectin in endothelial angiogenesis. Journal of Diabetes Research. 2015;**2015**:648239

[60] Mastronardi CA, WH Y, McCann SM. Resting and circadian release of nitric oxide is controlled by leptin in male rats. Proceedings of the National Academy of Sciences of the United States of America. 2002;**99**:5721-5726

[61] Brakenhielm E, Veitonmaki N, Cao R, Kihara S, Matsuzawa Y, Zhivotovsky B, Funahashi T, Cao Y. Adiponectin-induced antiangiogenesis and antitumor activity involve caspase-mediated endothelial cell apoptosis. Proceedings of the National Academy of Sciences of the United States of America. 2004;**101**:2476-2481

[62] Mahadev K, Wu X, Donnelly S, Ouedraogo R, Eckhart AD, Goldstein BJ. Adiponectin inhibits vascular endothelial growth factor-induced migration of human coronary artery endothelial cells. Cardiovascular Research. 2008;**78**:376-384

[63] Hursting SD, Dunlap SM, Ford NA, Hursting MJ, Lashinger LM. Calorie restriction and cancer prevention: A mechanistic perspective. Cancer & Metabolism. 2013;**1**:10

[64] Ungvari Z, Parrado-Fernandez C, Csiszar A. De CR: Mechanisms underlying caloric restriction and lifespan regulation: Implications for vascular aging. Circulation Research. 2008;**102**:519-528

[65] Ellsworth DL, Mamula KA, Blackburn HL, McDyer FA, Jellema GL, Van LR, Costantino NS, Engler RJ, Vernalis MN. Importance of substantial weight loss for altering gene expression during cardiovascular lifestyle modification. Obesity (Silver Spring). 2015;**23**:1312-1319

[66] Egert S, Baxheinrich A, Lee-Barkey YH, Tschoepe D, Wahrburg U, Stratmann B. Effects of an energy-restricted diet rich in plant-derived alpha-linolenic acid on systemic inflammation and endothelial function in overweight-to-obese patients with metabolic syndrome traits. The British Journal of Nutrition. 2014;**112**:1315-1322

[67] Hankey CR, Lean ME, Lowe GD, Rumley A, Woodward M. Effects of moderate weight loss on anginal symptoms and indices of coagulation and fibrinolysis in overweight patients with angina pectoris. European Journal of Clinical Nutrition. 2002;**56**: 1039-1045

[68] Raitakari M, Ilvonen T, Ahotupa M, Lehtimaki T, Harmoinen A, Suominen P, Elo J, Hartiala J, Raitakari OT. Weight reduction with very-low-caloric diet and endothelial function in overweight adults: Role of plasma glucose. Arteriosclerosis, Thrombosis, and Vascular Biology. 2004;**24**:124-128

http://dx.doi.org/10.5772/intechopen.72624

[69] Watroba M, Szukiewicz D. The role of sirtuins in aging and age-related diseases. Advances in Medical Sciences. 2016;**61**:52-62

[70] Wolin KY, Colditz GA. Can weight loss prevent cancer? British Journal of Cancer. 2008;**99**:995-999

[71] Sjostrom L, Gummesson A, Sjostrom CD, Narbro K, Peltonen M, Wedel H, Bengtsson C, Bouchard C, Carlsson B, Dahlgren S, Jacobson P, Karason K, Karlsson J, Larsson B, Lindroos AK, Lonroth H, Naslund I, Olbers T, Stenlof K, Torgerson J, Carlsson LM. Effects of bariatric surgery on cancer incidence in obese patients in Sweden (Swedish Obese Subjects Study): A prospective, controlled intervention trial. The Lancet Oncology. 2009;**10**:653-662

[72] Folkman J, Long DM Jr, FF B. Growth and metastasis of tumor in organ culture. Cancer. 1963;**16**:453-467

[73] Tinahones FJ, Coin-Araguez L, Mayas MD, Garcia-Fuentes E, Hurtado-del-Pozo C, Vendrell J, Cardona F, Calvo RM, Obregon MJ, El Bekay R. Obesity-associated insulin resistance is correlated to adipose tissue vascular endothelial growth factors and metalloproteinase levels. BMC Physiology 2012;**12**:4

[74] Csiszar A, Sosnowska D, Tucsek Z, Gautam T, Toth P, Losonczy G, Colman RJ, Weindruch R, Anderson RM, Sonntag WE, Ungvari Z. Circulating factors induced by caloric restriction in the nonhuman primate *Macaca mulatta* activate angiogenic processes in endothelial cells. The Journals of Gerontology. Series A, Biological Sciences and Medical Sciences. 2013;**68**:235-249

[75] Cullberg KB, Christiansen T, Paulsen SK, Bruun JM, Pedersen SB, Richelsen B. Effect of weight loss and exercise on angiogenic factors in the circulation and in adipose tissue in obese subjects. Obesity (Silver Spring). 2013;**21**:454-460

[76] Higami Y, Barger JL, Page GP, Allison DB, Smith SR, Prolla TA, Weindruch R. Energy restriction lowers the expression of genes linked to inflammation, the cytoskeleton, the extracellular matrix, and angiogenesis in mouse adipose tissue. The Journal of Nutrition. 2006;**136**:343-352

[77] Csiszar A, Labinskyy N, Jimenez R, Pinto JT, Ballabh P, Losonczy G, Pearson KJ, de Cabo R, Ungvari Z. Anti-oxidative and anti-inflammatory vasoprotective effects of caloric restriction in aging: Role of circulating factors and SIRT1. Mechanisms of Ageing and Development. 2009;**130**:518-527

[78] Korybalska K, Swora-Cwynar E, Luczak J, Kanikowska A, Czepulis N, Rutkowski R, Breborowicz A, Grzymislawski M, Witowski J. Association of endothelial proliferation with the magnitude of weight loss during calorie restriction. Angiogenesis. 2016;**19**:407-419

[79] Harris JA, Benedict JA. Biometric studies of basal metabolism in man. Carnegie Institute of Washington DC. 1919

[80] Baecke JA, Burema J, Frijters JE. A short questionnaire for the measurement of habitual physical activity in epidemiological studies. The American Journal of Clinical Nutrition. 1982;**36**:936-942

[81] Mosmann T. Rapid colorimetric assay for cellular growth and survival: Application to proliferation and cytotoxicity assays. Journal of Immunological Methods. 1983;**65**:55-63

[82] Carmichael J, DeGraff WG, Gazdar AF, Minna JD, Mitchell JB. Evaluation of a tetrazolium-based semiautomated colorimetric assay: Assessment of chemosensitivity testing. Cancer Research. 1987;**47**:936-942

[83] Ksiazek K, Piwocka K, Brzezinska A, Sikora E, Zabel M, Breborowicz A, Jorres A, Witowski J. Early loss of proliferative potential of human peritoneal mesothelial cells in culture: The role of p16INK4a-mediated premature senescence. Journal of Applied Physiology (1985). 2006;**100**:988-995

[84] Wallace TM, Levy JC, Matthews DR. Use and abuse of HOMA modeling. Diabetes Care. 2004;**27**:1487-1495

[85] Lau DC, Teoh H. Impact of current and emerging glucose-lowering drugs on body weight in type 2 diabetes. Canadian Journal of Diabetes. 2015;**39**(Suppl 5):S148-S154

[86] Seligman BG, Polanczyk CA, Santos AS, Foppa M, Junges M, Bonzanini L, Nicolaidis G, Camey S, Lopes AL, Sehl P, Duncan BB, Clausell N. Intensive practical lifestyle intervention improves endothelial function in metabolic syndrome independent of weight loss: A randomized controlled trial. Metabolism. 2011;**60**:1736-1740

[87] Brook RD, Bard RL, Glazewski L, Kehrer C, Bodary PF, Eitzman DL, Rajagopalan S. Effect of short-term weight loss on the metabolic syndrome and conduit vascular endothelial function in overweight adults. The American Journal of Cardiology. 2004;**93**:1012-1016

[88] Wycherley TP, Brinkworth GD, Noakes M, Buckley JD, Clifton PM. Effect of caloric restriction with and without exercise training on oxidative stress and endothelial function in obese subjects with type 2 diabetes. Diabetes, Obesity & Metabolism. 2008;**10**: 1062-1073

[89] Cai J, Hong Y, Weng C, Tan C, Imperato-McGinley J, Zhu YS. Androgen stimulates endothelial cell proliferation via an androgen receptor/VEGF/cyclin A-mediated mechanism. American Journal of Physiology. Heart and Circulatory Physiology. 2011;**300**: H1210-H1221

[90] Morales DE, McGowan KA, Grant DS, Maheshwari S, Bhartiya D, Cid MC, Kleinman HK, Schnaper HW. Estrogen promotes angiogenic activity in human umbilical vein endothelial cells in vitro and in a murine model. Circulation. 1995;**91**:755-763

[91] Reinhardt M, Thearle MS, Ibrahim M, Hohenadel MG, Bogardus C, Krakoff J, Votruba SB, Human Thrifty A. Phenotype associated with less weight loss during caloric restriction. Diabetes. 2015;**64**:2859-2867

[92] Whitfield ML, George LK, Grant GD, Perou CM. Common markers of proliferation. Nature Reviews. Cancer. 2006;**6**:99-106

[93] Renehan AG, Zwahlen M, Egger M. Adiposity and cancer risk: New mechanistic insights from epidemiology. Nature Reviews. Cancer. 2015;**15**:484-498

[94] Vandekeere S, Dewerchin M, Carmeliet P. Angiogenesis revisited: An overlooked role of endothelial cell metabolism in vessel sprouting. Microcirculation. 2015;**22**:509-517

[95] Nathan AA, Tej MA, Chitiprolu M, Rangan S, Mohan V, Harish R, Anand SB, Dixit M. Impaired glucose tolerance alters functional ability of peripheral blood-derived mononuclear cells in Asian Indian men. Diabetes & Vascular Disease Research. 2015;**12**:13-22

[96] Miyazawa-Hoshimoto S, Takahashi K, Bujo H, Hashimoto N, Saito Y. Elevated serum vascular endothelial growth factor is associated with visceral fat accumulation in human obese subjects. Diabetologia. 2003;**46**:1483-1488

[97] Ersoy C, Kiyici S, Budak F, Oral B, Guclu M, Duran C, Selimoglu H, Erturk E, Tuncel E, Imamoglu S. The effect of metformin treatment on VEGF and PAI-1 levels in obese type 2 diabetic patients. Diabetes Research and Clinical Practice. 2008;**81**:56-60

[98] Blann AD, Belgore FM, McCollum CN, Silverman S, Lip PL, Lip GY. Vascular endothelial growth factor and its receptor, Flt-1, in the plasma of patients with coronary or peripheral atherosclerosis, or Type II diabetes. Clinical Science (London, England). 2002;**102**:187-194

[99] Yamagishi S, Kawakami T, Fujimori H, Yonekura H, Tanaka N, Yamamoto Y, Urayama H, Watanabe Y, Yamamoto H. Insulin stimulates the growth and tube formation of human microvascular endothelial cells through autocrine vascular endothelial growth factor. Microvascular Research. 1999;**57**:329-339

[100] Mick GJ, Wang X, McCormick K. White adipocyte vascular endothelial growth factor: Regulation by insulin. Endocrinology. 2002;**143**:948-953

[101] Krysiak R, Gdula-Dymek A, Okopien B. Effect of metformin on selected parameters of hemostasis in fenofibrate-treated patients with impaired glucose tolerance. Pharmacological Reports. 2013;**65**:208-213

[102] Razny U, Kiec-Wilk B, Polus A, Goralska J, Malczewska-Malec M, Wnek D, Zdzienicka A, Gruca A, Childs CE, Kapusta M, Slowinska-Solnica K, Calder PC, Mbinska-Kiec A. Effect of caloric restriction with or without n-3 polyunsaturated fatty acids on insulin sensitivity in obese subjects: A randomized placebo controlled trial. BBA Clinical. 2015;**4**:7-13

[103] Maisonpierre PC, Suri C, Jones PF, Bartunkova S, Wiegand SJ, Radziejewski C, Compton D, McClain J, Aldrich TH, Papadopoulos N, Daly TJ, Davis S, Sato TN, Yancopoulos GD. Angiopoietin-2, a natural antagonist for Tie2 that disrupts in vivo angiogenesis. Science. 1997;**277**:55-60

[104] Fiedler U, Reiss Y, Scharpfenecker M, Grunow V, Koidl S, Thurston G, Gale NW, Witzenrath M, Rosseau S, Suttorp N, Sobke A, Herrmann M, Preissner KT, Vajkoczy P, Augustin HG. Angiopoietin-2 sensitizes endothelial cells to TNF-alpha and has a crucial role in the induction of inflammation. Nature Medicine. 2006;**12**:235-239

[105] Felcht M, Luck R, Schering A, Seidel P, Srivastava K, Hu J, Bartol A, Kienast Y, Vettel C, Loos EK, Kutschera S, Bartels S, Appak S, Besemfelder E, Terhardt D, Chavakis E, Wieland T, Klein C, Thomas M, Uemura A, Goerdt S, Augustin HG. Angiopoietin-2 differentially regulates angiogenesis through TIE2 and integrin signaling. The Journal of Clinical Investigation. 2012;**122**:1991-2005

[106] Lim HS, Lip GY, Blann AD. Angiopoietin-1 and angiopoietin-2 in diabetes mellitus: Relationship to VEGF, glycaemic control, endothelial damage/dysfunction and atherosclerosis. Atherosclerosis. 2005;**180**:113-118

[107] Lieb W, Zachariah JP, Xanthakis V, Safa R, Chen MH, Sullivan LM, Larson MG, Smith HM, Yang Q, Mitchell GF, Vita JA, Sawyer DB, Vasan RS. Clinical and genetic correlates of circulating angiopoietin-2 and soluble Tie-2 in the community. Circulation. Cardiovascular Genetics. 2010;**3**:300-306

[108] Rasul S, Reiter MH, Ilhan A, Lampichler K, Wagner L, Kautzky-Willer A. Circulating angiopoietin-2 and soluble Tie-2 in type 2 diabetes mellitus: A cross-sectional study. Cardiovascular Diabetology. 2011;**10**:55

[109] Herder C, Baumert J, Thorand B, Martin S, Lowel H, Kolb H, Koenig W. Chemokines and incident coronary heart disease: Results from the MONICA/KORA Augsburg case-cohort study, 1984-2002. Arteriosclerosis, Thrombosis, and Vascular Biology. 2006;**26**: 2147-2152

[110] Wong E, Freiberg M, Tracy R, Kuller L. Epidemiology of cytokines: The Women On the Move through Activity and Nutrition (WOMAN) Study. American Journal of Epidemiology. 2008;**168**:443-453

[111] Viollet B, Guigas B, Sanz GN, Leclerc J, Foretz M, Andreelli F. Cellular and molecular mechanisms of metformin: An overview. Clinical Science (London, England). 2012;**122**: 253-270

[112] Dallaglio K, Bruno A, Cantelmo AR, Esposito AI, Ruggiero L, Orecchioni S, Calleri A, Bertolini F, Pfeffer U, Noonan DM, Albini A. Paradoxic effects of metformin on endothelial cells and angiogenesis. Carcinogenesis. 2014;**35**:1055-1066

[113] Tan BK, Adya R, Chen J, Farhatullah S, Heutling D, Mitchell D, Lehnert H, Randeva HS. Metformin decreases angiogenesis via NF-kappaB and Erk1/2/Erk5 pathways by increasing the antiangiogenic thrombospondin-1. Cardiovascular Research. 2009;**83**:566-574

Chapter 12

Pulmonary Vascular Endothelial Cells

Joyce N. Gonzales and Alexander D. Verin

Additional information is available at the end of the chapter

http://dx.doi.org/10.5772/intechopen.76995

Abstract

Pulmonary vascular endothelial cells (ECs) line the surface of the lung vasculature and accommodate the various levels of blood flow. Pulmonary endothelium is a critical regulator of vascular homeostasis by inhibiting coagulation of the blood. The ECs bind tissue factor pathway inhibitors (TFPI), modulate hemostasis with opposing effects such as antiplatelet, anticoagulant and fibrinolytic properties. Lung endothelium regulates synthesis and metabolism of vasoactive compounds such as nitric oxide and endothelin-1, both potent regulators of vascular tone. Cytokines, chemokines, interleukins, adhesion molecules, and growth factors can be secreted by pulmonary ECs with positive and adverse effects. Pulmonary endothelium exhibits heterogeneity with diverse expression of molecules and specific differences in signaling induced by various infections such as Gram-positive bacteria. The distinction of macro or microvascular endothelium occurs from the larger vessels to small capillaries in the lung alveoli system. Lectin-binding patterns discriminate between pulmonary artery and pulmonary microvascular capillary endothelium. The lung is one of the body's organs with the highest expression of vascular endothelial growth factor that stimulates small vessel formation of the microvascular endothelium. Acute respiratory distress syndrome and acute chest syndrome in sickle cell disease are two prototypes of devastating diseases caused by pulmonary EC dysfunction.

Keywords: pulmonary endothelial cells, pulmonary microvascular endothelial cells, pulmonary macrovascular endothelial cells, ARDS, Acute Chest Syndrome, Endothelial cell dysfunction

1. Introduction

Endothelial cells (ECs) line the interior surface of blood cells and lymphatic vessels forming an interface between circulating blood or lymph in the lumen and the vessel wall. ECs are a thin layer of squamous cells. The vascular EC line the entire circulatory system from the large vessels to the smallest capillaries, thereby accommodating various levels of blood flow from the turbulent high pressures from large vessels entering and leaving the heart as well as small vessels such as that of the minute capillaries of the lungs, liver, kidneys, and the moderate vessels throughout the body. ECs from different blood vessels and microvascular ECs from different tissues have distinct and characteristic gene expression profiles. Pervasive differences in gene expression patterns distinguish the EC of large vessels from microvascular ECs [1].

2. Pulmonary endothelial cell dysfunction

Vascular endothelium is a critical regulator of vascular homeostasis. All EC inhibit coagulation of the blood. ECs bind tissue factor pathway inhibitors (TFPIs) that prevent the initiation of coagulation by blocking the actions of the factor (f) VIIa tissue factor (TF) complex [2]. Like other ECs, lung ECs modulate hemostasis with sometimes opposing effects such as antiplatelet, anticoagulant, and fibrinolytic properties; yet after injury or activation ECs are capable of exerting procoagulant functions. The balance between endothelial anti and prothrombotic activities determines whether thrombus formation, propagation, or dissolution occurs [3]. An intact endothelium in a healthy vessel inhibits the adhesion of platelets, platelet activation, and aggregation and adhesion of platelets and leucocytes to vessel wall through the release of nitric oxide (NO) [4]. On the other hand, injury or activation of ECs results in a procoagulant phenotype that contributes to localized clot formation.

Activation of the coagulation cascade is one of the early occurring events in lung injury, and it is initiated via the extrinsic pathway [5]. Endothelium activated by inflammation and/or injury releases the procoagulant molecule TF which binds with circulating coagulation fVII to form a TF/fVIIa complex that cleaves fIX and thrombin. (**Figure 1**). Thrombin further activates platelets

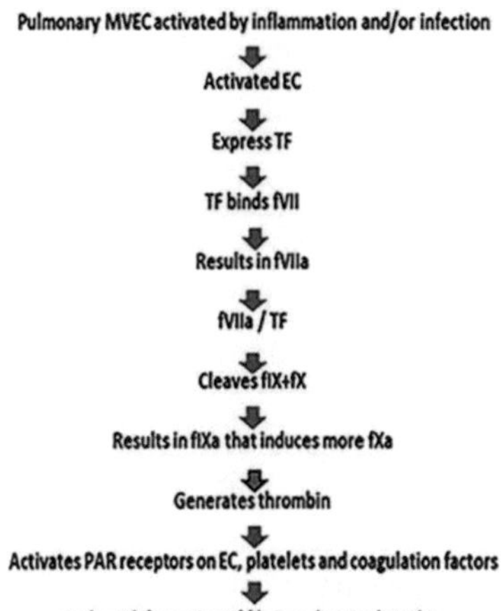
Pulmonary MVEC activated by inflammation and/or infection
Activated EC
Express TF
TF binds fVII
Results in fVIIa
fVIIa / TF
Cleaves fIX+fX
Results in fIXa that induces more fXa
Generates thrombin
Activates PAR receptors on EC, platelets and coagulation factors
Cycle with formation of fibrin and more thrombin

Figure 1. Schematic representation of pulmonary microvascular endothelial cells (MVEC) activated by inflammation and/or injury following release of the pro-coagulant molecule TF which binds with circulating coagulation factor VII (fVII) to form a TF/fVIIa complex that cleaves fIX, and generates thrombin.

and coagulation factors in the intrinsic coagulation pathway generating more thrombin and formation of a fibrin mesh. The adhesion of platelets is facilitated by von Willebrand factor (vWF). vWF is a product of normal EC and is not synthesized after endothelial injury. The clotting pathway is also induced by cytokines such as tumor necrosis factor alpha (TNF-α) or interleukin 1 (IL-1) or bacterial endotoxin such as lipopolysaccharide (LPS) to secrete TF which activates the extrinsic clotting pathway [3]. In a tightly regulated system, the proteases and molecules of the coagulation cascade can be inhibited by circulating protease inhibitors, such as antithrombin, heparin cofactor II, TF pathway inhibitor and C1 inhibitor. These bind with the active sites of proteases, thereby inactivating them. In addition, coagulation factors can be degraded through activation of the protein C and protein S complex, synthesized by ECs as a cofactor that is then catalyzed by the presence of thrombomodulin and endothelial protein C receptor (EPCR). Other pathways of coagulation factor degradation are disintegrin and metalloproteinase with a thrombospondin type 1 motif, member 13 (ADAMTS13). ADAMTS13 cleaves the multimeric strands of vWF, thereby disrupting platelet adhesion. ECs synthesize tissue plasminogen activator (t-PA), promoting fibrinolytic activity to clear fibrin deposits from endothelial surfaces [3, 6]. Thrombin also binds to its protease activated receptor-1 (PAR-1) and induces a signaling cascade resulting in EC junctional gaps that lead to increased endothelial permeability [7].

Lung ECs also regulate the synthesis and metabolism of vasoactive compounds such as nitric oxide (NO) and endothelin-1 (ET-1), potent regulators of pulmonary vascular tone [8]. EC-derived NO, synthesized by the endothelial nitric oxide synthase (eNOS) from the precursor L-arginine, regulates the healthy endothelium. Antithrombotic effects of EC-derived NO are likely related to release of prostaglandin I_2 and inhibition of plasminogen activator inhibitor-1 (PAI-1), a prothrombotic protein [6, 9].

The enzyme eNOS depends on intracellular calcium (Ca^{2+}) level. In response to a rise in EC intracellular Ca^{2+} eNOS catalyzes the production of NO. The Ca^{2+}-dependent eNOS synthesizes small amounts of NO until the Ca^{2+} levels decrease. This Ca^{2+}-dependent eNOS provides the basal release of NO and is sufficient to inhibit the adhesion and activation of platelets providing homeostasis in unstimulated ECs [10].

Cytokines are small soluble proteins that are important in cell signaling and can change the behavior or properties of cells. Cytokines can be secreted by many cells including pulmonary ECs [11]. Cytokines can be grouped into families including the interferons, the chemoattractants (chemokines), the tumor necrosis factors (TNFs), the interleukins (IL-2, IL-3, IL-4 etc.), the epidermal growth factor family (EGF) and transforming growth factors-alpha and beta (TGF-α and β), the growth factors include vascular endothelial growth factor (VEGF and others) that are important in vasculogenesis and angiogenesis. The VEGF family of growth factors restores the oxygen supply to tissues in hypoxic conditions [12].

Pulmonary EC express adhesion molecules and pro and anti-inflammatory cytokines and are intricately involved in inflammatory processes [12, 13]. It was shown that there is a central role via the sphingosine-1-phosphate (S1P) receptor in pulmonary endothelium for regulating an excessive pro-inflammatory cytokine and chemokine production in an influenza virus-induced cytokine storm [14]. A deficiency of alpha 1-antitrypsin (A1AT), a protein that has been shown to trigger an inflammatory response leading to increased circulating concentrations of pro-inflammatory cytokines such as TNF-α from ECs. In A1AT, cytokines activate their receptors and stimulate nuclear factor kappa-light-chain-enhancer of activated B cells (NF-kB) activity and nuclear factor of kappa light polypeptide gene enhancer in B-cells inhibitor (IkBα), a regulatory protein that inhibits NF-kB degradation. The translocation of NF-kB increases the transcription of inflammatory genes, including an increased secretion of TNF-α from ECs [15]. The role of pulmonary EC cytokines has also been shown in the pathology of lung fibrosis where numerous cytokines have been implicated in pathogenesis including TGF-β, TNF-α, ET-1 and IL-1 and IL-8 [16].

ECs participate in the control of the adhesion and migration of inflammatory cells and the exchange of fluid from the vasculature into damaged tissue. Resting ECs do not interact with leukocytes; however, they store proteins such as P-selectin and chemokines in specialized secretory vesicles called Weibel-Palade bodies (WPBs) in microvascular ECs for interaction with leukocytes when needed [17]. ICAM-1 and E-selectin mediate the firm adhesion to ECs and are an obligatory step in neutrophil migration as neutrophils initially adhere to ECs, then migrate through the EC barrier [18]. Resting ECs also suppress the transcription of other adhesion molecules such as E-selectin, vascular cell-adhesion molecule 1 (VCAM) and intercellular adhesion molecule 1 (ICAM-1) [2]. Upon EC activation, the resulting inflammation is characterized by tissue infiltration of neutrophils, followed by macrophages [19, 20].

EC activation can be induced by endotoxin, cytokines and chemokines, and viruses and bacterial pathogens, all of which can activate NF-kB resulting in modulation of EC synthesis of pro-inflammatory cytokines and chemokines. When stimulated, the endothelium displays increased adhesiveness for monocytes, lymphocytes, and granulocytes mediated by endothelial leukocyte adhesion molecules such as ICAM-1, VCAM-1 and E-selectin. The secretion of inflammatory cytokines and of leukocyte specific chemo attractants such al IL-8 and MCP-1 also contributes to leukocyte recruitment during inflammatory responses [21]. In general, human endothelium can express a broad spectrum of pro-and anti-inflammatory cytokines, including IL-1, IL-5, IL-6 and IL-8, MCP-1 (monocyte chemotactic protein-1), CSFs (colony-stimulating factors), GM-CSF (granulocyte/macrophage CSF), G-CSF (granulocyte CSF), M-CSF (macrophage CSF), PDGF, and VEGF [12].

2.1. Pulmonary endothelial cell heterogeneity

ECs from various organs have distinctive vascular responses to chemokines, cytokines, and adhesions molecules and exhibit unique functional properties [22, 23]. Phenotypic heterogeneity among ECs may account for important organ-specific behaviors [24]. The unique features of pulmonary ECs allow them to function at multiple basic levels such as function as a dynamic barrier critical for lung gas exchange and the regulation of fluid and solute passage between the blood and interstitial compartments in the lung [25].

Pulmonary endothelium exhibits a high expression of adhesion molecules which contribute to the margination of the large intravascular pool of leucocytes in the lung [26]. Adhesion molecules are expressed by activated ECs in a sequential manner. Cytokines activate E-selectin promoter, which induces E-selectin and a prolonged contact among leukocytes, causing them to roll along the endothelium [27]. Other selectins such as platelet endothelial cell adhesion molecule (PECAM, CD31), ICAM-1, and the inducible VCAM-1 are all essential to the subsequent firm attachment of leukocytes to and migration through the endothelium. Many studies of lung EC expression of molecules, including adhesion molecules, were initially accomplished on human pulmonary artery EC (HPAEC) or even human umbilical vein EC (HUVEC) due to the availability of these cells for culture. However, more recently there is a recognition that there are differences between the expression of pulmonary macrovascular and microvascular EC. For example, the study of adhesion molecules of macrovascular large vessel cells cannot be extrapolated to microvascular capillary cells. In vitro study of HPAEC is not comparable to study of the pulmonary microvasculature in vivo or in vitro [27].

Gram-positive bacterial pathogens cause lung inflammation and alterations in lung ECs. In macrovascular ECs, pharmacological inhibition of Rho kinase with the Rho kinase (ROCK) inhibitor Y27632 significantly suppressed p38 mitogen-activated protein kinase (MAPK) cascade activation, while inhibition of p38 MAPK with specific inhibitor p38α and β, SB203580 had no effect on Rho activation [28]. In contrast, inhibition of p38 MAPK in microvascular ECs suppressed lipoteichoic acid and peptidoglycan (LTA/PepG), found on the cell wall of Gram-positive bacteria induced activation of Rho, while Rho inhibitor suppressed activation of p38 MAPK [28]. These results demonstrate cell type-specific differences in signaling induced by *Staphylococcus aureus* derived pathogens in pulmonary endothelium. Thus, although Gram-positive bacterial compounds caused barrier dysfunction in both ECs types, it was induced by different patterns of crosstalk between Rho, p38 MAPK, and NFκB signaling [28].

The distinction of macro or microvascular endothelium is between those from the larger vessels to the small capillaries that feed the entire alveolar system in the lung [29]. Lectin-binding pattern discriminates between PAEC and Pulmonary microvascular EC (MVEC), and lectin protein agglutinins isolated from plant or animal sources are often used for distinguishing between cell phenotypes [23, 30]. It was identified that *Helix pomatia* (an agglutinin from the *Helix pomatia* snail) (HPA) and *Griffonia* lectins (a lectin from Bandeiraea simplicifolia (BS I), these lectins are isolated from a variety of natural sources including plants, mollusks, fish eggs) differentially bind to macro and microvascular EC. HPA preferentially binds macrovascular endothelium whereas BS I preferentially binds to microvascular endothelium (**Figure 2**) [31]. In cell culture experiments investigating diseases such as acute respiratory distress syndrome (ARDS), pulmonary edema, or acute chest syndrome in sickle cell disease (SCD), the distinction of macro versus microvascular cells could be important.

Majority of studies in the lung have been performed on macrovascular ECs from the HPAEC, bovine PAEC or human umbilical AEC. HPAEC are used to study various diseases of the lung involved in endothelial dysfunction such as hypoxia, inflammation, and environmental stresses. It was shown in one study in macrovascular HPAEC that thrombin induces protein kinase C (PKC)-dependent ezrin, moesin, radixin (ERM) phosphorylation on critical threonine residues ERM and translocation of phosphorylated ERM to the EC periphery and that the ERM proteins play differential roles in thrombin-induced modulation of EC permeability [32]. The results in this study are important to the knowledge of the EC barrier in the lung diseases; however, the critical EC in ARDS, pulmonary edema, and ACS are the pulmonary microvascular endothelial cells (PMVEC), and it is unclear if the results would be similar as our understanding of the molecular regulation of PMVEC permeability is incomplete [33].

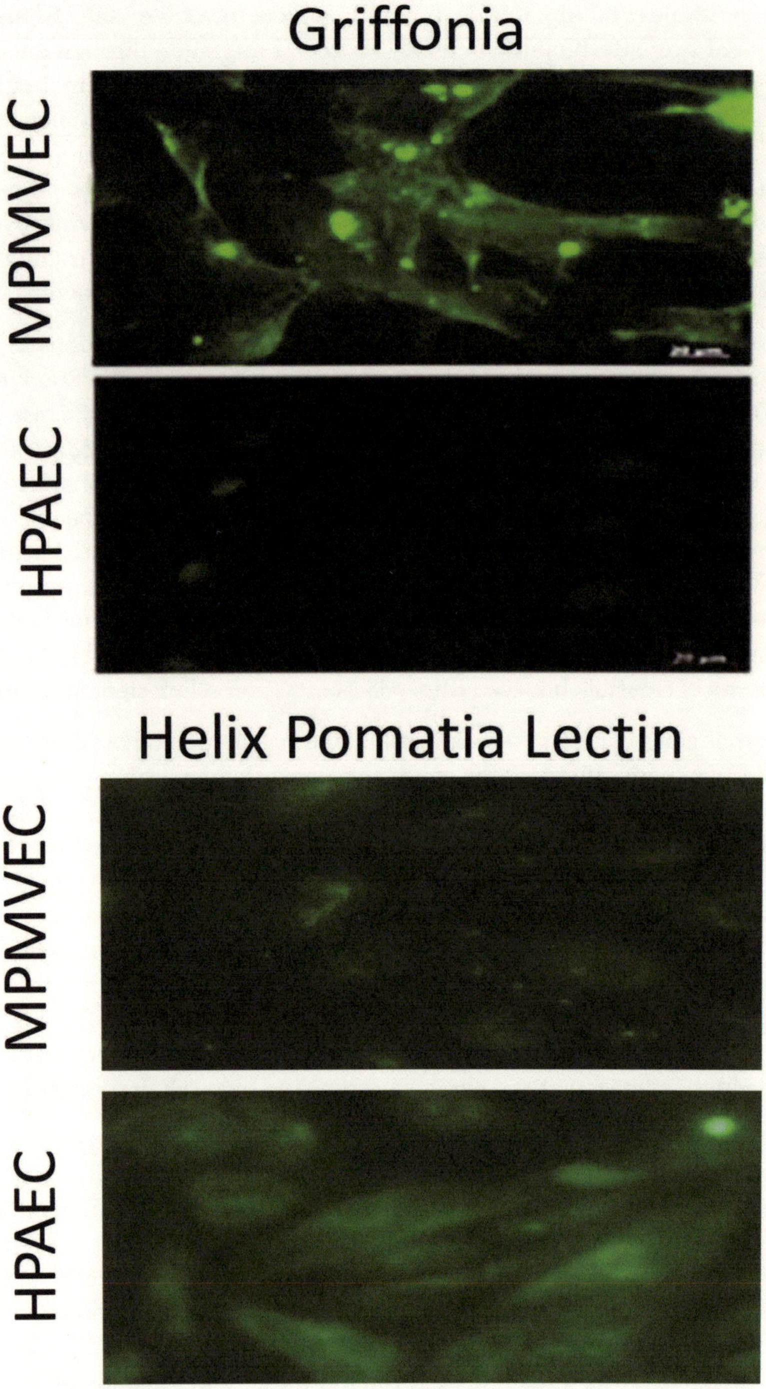

Figure 2. Lectin immunocytochemistry is used to identify pulmonary microvascular cells (top, Griffonia) compared to pulmonary macrovascular cells bottom, (*Helix pomatia* Lectin). ECs were cultured at 37°C in complete endothelial growth basal medium-2 until confluent. Endothelial cells were isolated from murine lungs or human pulmonary artery EC were used and stained with either *Top-Griffonia* to identify microvascular EC and compared to HPAEC or *Bottom-Helix pomatia* stain to identify human pulmonary macrovascular EC.

http://dx.doi.org/10.5772/intechopen.76995

In another in vitro study comparing MVEC and PAECs, metabolic requirements for growth were studied in rat pulmonary cells. It was found that PMVEC populations had a higher metabolic function and grow faster than PAEC. PMVEC consumed threefold more glucose in cell culture over comparable time frame than PAECs. PMVECs but not PAECs generated a lactic acidosis, higher ATP concentrations, and lower oxygen consumption than PAECs [34]. The hydraulic conductance of rat PMVEC and PAEC were compared to study lung EC permeability, such as may occur in pulmonary edema to hydraulic stress. The results of these studies indicated dramatic differences in the baseline hydraulic responses to hydrostatic pressure between the two phenotypes with PAEC values averaged 22 times higher than PMVEC in new monolayers. It was speculated that the dramatic differences in PMVEC and RPAEC may be due to different embryologic origins, being derived respectively by vasculogenesis and angiogenesis [35]. The same group investigated the role of cytosolic calcium (Ca2+) in rat PMVECs and PAECs; they found that Thapsigargin (a non-competitive inhibitor of the sarco/endoplasmic reticulum Ca^{2+} ATPase) produced higher Ca2+ levels in PAECs than in PMVECs and increased permeability in PAEC but not in PMVEC monolayers. The significance is that whereas increased Ca2+ promotes permeability in PAECs it is not sufficient in PMVECs which show an apparent uncoupling of Ca2+ signaling pathways or dominant Ca2+ – independent mechanisms for controlling cellular gap formation and permeability [25].

Macrovascular ECs more abundantly express eNOS and generate more NO than do microvascular ECs [23, 30]. NOS and inducible NOS (iNOS) production in rat pulmonary macrovascular EC was shown to be greater than rat pulmonary microvascular ECs when cell cultures were stimulated with various combinations of TNF-α, interferon gamma (IFN-), and LPS, suggesting that differences between ECs populations may be substantial [24].

HPAEC are also useful to investigate the effects of various compounds and drugs. Other EC types such as human umbilical artery (HUVEC) or bovine pulmonary artery cells (BPAECs) have also been used previously due to their dependable, more robust nature and commercial availability.

2.2. Pulmonary microvascular endothelial cells

Pulmonary microvascular ECs (MVECs) are an active and dynamic layer of cells in the most delicate portion of the lung at the alveolar level (**Figure 3**) where they function to exert both specific and general endothelial function. In the microvascular circulation, the arteries are less than 70 μm in diameter, are nonmuscular arterioles, and extend into the alveolar capillaries. The walls of capillaries are composed of a single layer of MVECs. The general function of lung EC include regulation of systemic blood flow, tissue perfusion thorough changes in vessel diameter and vascular tone, performed in conjunction with underlying smooth muscle cells and pericytes [6] (**Figure 4**). The pulmonary microcirculation is less permeable to protein and water flux as compared to large pulmonary vessels [26]. Experiments have shown that the MVECs form a tighter barrier compared to the macrovascular barrier while showing less permeability to sucrose and albumin compared to macrovascular EC [36]. Lung injury or inflammation are associated with activation of mediators or secretion of cytokines that induce a prolonged increase in paracellular permeability and vessel wall leakiness. Endothelial barrier properties are known to be strictly dependent on the integrity of endothelial adherens and tight junctions [37]. The

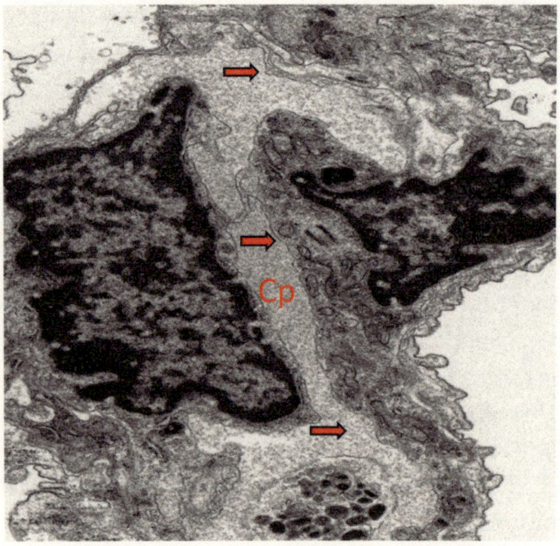

Figure 3. Transmission electron micrograph of a mouse alveolar capillary (Cp) with microvascular endothelial (EC) lining (arrows). Source is mouse alveoli from authors (JG) collection of images processed in the vascular biology laboratory, Augusta University health, electron microscope Core Laboratory (Libby Perry and Brendan Marshall PhD).

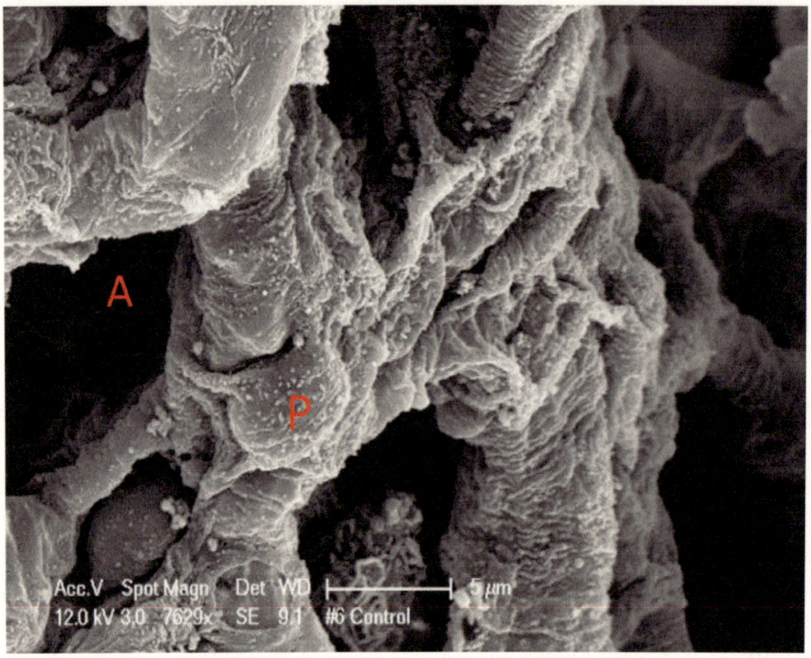

Figure 4. Scanning micrograph of mouse alveoli (a) and vessel with pericyte (P) surrounding the alveolar lining. Source is mouse alveoli from authors (JG) collection of images processed in the vascular biology laboratory, Augusta University health, electron microscope Core Laboratory (Libby Perry and Brendan Marshall PhD).

inter-endothelial junctions consist of adherens, tight and gap junctional complexes, and promote adhesion of opposing cells in the monolayer of microvascular ECs [38]. Microvascular EC gene clusters include genes related to lipid transport and metabolism [3].

The lung is one of the body's organs with the highest expression of VEGF [39]. VEGF stimulates small vessel formation of MVEC and is an essential component of the angiogenic process and MVECs survival. VEGF signaling orchestrates capillary development along the basement membrane of airway epithelium [23]. Excessive VEGF expression has a broad impact on ECs including vascular permeability increase [39]. VEGF can be induced by hypoxia-inducible factor (HIF) in cells under hypoxic conditions. Gene studies evaluating VEGF have shown a higher level of expression of actin binding proteins—Lin11, Isl-1 and Mec-3 (LIM) proteins 1, actinin-associated LIM protein, Arginase (Arg) binding protein 2, Slingshot, vav3, myosin IB, myosin 5C, myosin7A, and myosin light chain kinase in the microvascular ECs [3, 40]. These are proteins that play important roles in basic biological processes including cytoskeleton organization. This increase in cytoskeletal protein expression may be related to the ability of MVECs to undergo extensive cytoskeletal remodeling and migration during angiogenesis [3]. VEGF increases permeability by at least two different pathways: one, involving proto-oncogene (Raf-1), mitogen-activated protein kinase/ERK kinase (MEK), and extracellular signal-regulated kinases 1,2 (ERK); and the other involving endothelial nitric oxide synthase (eNOS). Protein kinase C (PKC) is a mediator of VEGF-induced ERK-1/2 phosphorylation and hyperpermeability which increases permeability via increased NO production [33]. Endothelin-1 (ET-1) is known to play a pathogenic role in pulmonary arterial hypertension (PAH). VEGF may have beneficial effects by decreasing ET-1 production in HLMVEC thereby modulating endothelin production in PAH [41].

Microvascular ECs are known to produce macrophage inflammatory protein-1beta (MIP-1β) and MIP-2 (the mouse equivalent to human interleukin-8) in the lung which act as major chemotactic factors responsible for the recruitment of neutrophils into the alveolar spaces during inflammation or infection [22, 41].

2.3. Pulmonary endothelial cells in ARDS and pneumonia

ARDS is a severe lung inflammatory disorder with a declining but still unacceptably high.

Mortality (25–46%) [42, 43]. The healthy alveolar-capillary barrier is formed by the microvascular endothelium, the alveolar epithelium, and the basement membrane. The homogeneous pulmonary microvasculature layer of ECs lining the pulmonary circulation forms a tight barrier [44]. The EC barrier dysfunction that occurs in acute lung injury is tightly linked to agonist-induced cytoskeletal remodeling resulting in the disruption of cell–cell contacts, paracellular gap formation, and EC barrier compromise [45, 46]. Tight junctions are formed by the fusion of the outer layers of the plasma membranes and are comprised of occludins, claudins, and junctional adhesion molecules that in turn bind to other protein partners in the actin cytoskeleton [8, 36]. Integrity of adherens junctions (AJs) is critical in regulating paracellular permeability and disruption of VE-cadherin homophilic adhesions leads to excessive accumulation of fluid in the interstitial space and is associated with inflammation, atherogenesis, and acute lung injury [38]. AJs are composed of VE-cadherin and its cytoplasmic binding partners: α-, β- γ-, p120 catenins, which link AJs to the actin cytoskeleton. The assembly of the VE-cadherin-catenin complex is regulated by phosphorylation, and their dissociation leads to cytoskeletal changes and loss of cohesive structure required for an intact EC barrier [36]. Therefore, the complex network of cytoskeletons is critical in the EC barrier regulation.

On the cellular level, in ARDS, there is increased pulmonary capillary EC permeability and fluid leakage into the pulmonary parenchyma that is followed by neutrophils, cytokines, and an acute inflammatory response [47]. Adhesion molecule upregulation on the vascular endothelium of the lung results from the systemic inflammatory cascade that occurs in EC activation. In fact, the expression of molecules that mediate adhesion and signaling of leukocytes is nearly synonymous with endothelial activation [48]. When ECs are activated by toxins such as LPS, other bacterial toxins, viral infections, thrombin or hypoxia, the ECs release cytokines such as TNF-α, IL-1ß or IL-8, and a shift toward a pro-inflammatory phenotype occurs [36]. There is a consecutive expression of adhesion molecules, including PECAM (CD-31), ICAM–1, VCAM, and E selectin, that plays a central role in the leukocyte endothelial adhesion. These adhesion molecules are responsible for recruiting and directing leukocytes to the sites of inflammation.

Muller et al. analyzed the autopsy lung specimen ECs for PECAM (CD-31), ICAM–1 in patients with Gram-negative sepsis-induced ARDS and found these adhesion molecules strongly expressed compared to normal lung autopsy specimen [49]. Another study demonstrated that blockade of the VCAM-1 receptor on the pulmonary vascular endothelium diminishes lung injury in established pancreatitis-induced ARDS [50]. In our own unpublished data, mice with lung injury induced by LPS and Gram-positive toxin, pneumolysin, an attenuation of ICAM-1 by a low-anticoagulant heparin, has been shown to attenuate neutrophils and acute lung injury (data not published). Neutrophil recruitment into the lung is the hallmark of acute lung injury (ALI) [51]. Neutrophils enter the interstitial spaces by rolling on the endothelium, and this is mediated by the selectins. The neutrophils adhere to the endothelium and affect the endothelial cytoskeleton inducing remodeling of the tight junctions and further facilitating the transmigration of neutrophils [51].

Once activated, ECs display recruited neutrophils in ARDS; there is considerable evidence that pro-and anti-inflammatory cytokines and chemokines play a major role in the pathogenesis of acute lung injury from sepsis and pneumonia [51]. There is a complex network of inflammatory cytokines and chemokines that play a major role in mediating, amplifying, and perpetuating the lung injury process. The pro-inflammatory cytokines IL–1 beta and TNF-α have been located in bronchoalveolar lavage fluid (BALF) from ARDS patients [52]. In influenza, early induction of the cytokines IFN-α, TNF-α, IL-1α, and IL-6 and the chemokines CCL2, CCL3, CXCL2 (IL-8), and CXCL10 are associated with clinical symptoms and morbidity in humans [14, 53, 54]. Simultaneous production of anti-inflammatory cytokines can counteract pro-inflammatory cytokine effects and modify the intensity of the inflammatory process in ARDS [52].

There is a search for biomarkers in ARDS to assess the activation and dysfunction of ECs. One marker may be endothelial progenitor cells (EPCs) as a marker of EC dysfunction and damage. It has been reported that there is an association between the EPC count and survival in ARDS [55]. The cells are present at very low levels in normal patients, but the number of EPCs increased significantly in conditions associated with vascular damage such as ARDS. In the study of Moussa et al. [56], EPC counts were increased in patients with moderate and severe ARDS compared with non-ARDS patients [56]. Higher EPC counts were also found in non-survivors of ARDS in this same study [56]. Other promising biomarkers are angiopoietin–2

http://dx.doi.org/10.5772/intechopen.76995

(Ang-2), an endothelial growth factor. Ang-2, a mediator of pulmonary vascular permeability, binds to the tyrosine kinase receptor and plays a key role in endothelial junctional integrity [57]. Ang–2 levels have been shown to be higher in ARDS patients than in patients with hydrostatic pulmonary edema [58]. Increased levels have also been linked with the severity and mortality of ARDS [58]. Stimulation of PMVEC with IL–8 leads to cytoskeletal reorganization and cell retraction which in turn leads to gap formation between cells and IL-8 levels that are higher in non-survivors of ARDS [59]. Studies for biomarkers are ongoing with the potential that the EC biomarkers will aid in the diagnosis of acute lung injury.

2.4. Endothelial cells in acute chest syndrome in sickle cell disease

Sickle cell disease (SCD) is an inherited red blood cell disorder that affects millions of people throughout the world and in most common among those whose ancestors came from sub-Saharan Africa, Spanish-speaking regions in the Western hemisphere, Saudi Arabia, India, and Mediterranean countries [60]. SCD is caused by a mutant β-globin gene that substitutes valine for glutamic acid at position 6 in the β-globin chain of hemoglobin A. The resultant hemoglobin is called hemoglobin S and is characterized by red blood cells (RBCs) that are crescent or sickle shaped rather than the normal rounded disc shape [61]. One of the most common forms of acute pulmonary disease associated with morbidity and mortality in SCD is acute chest syndrome (ACS). Hypoxia induces abnormal hemoglobin S polymerization and RBC sickling, and the abnormal cells are rigid and unable to pass through narrow capillaries leading to vessel occlusion and ischemia [62]. ACS is the most common form of acute pulmonary disease associated with SCD. ACS is diagnosed by a new infiltrate on chest x-ray that is consistent with alveolar consolidation triggered by infection, fat embolization, or pulmonary sequestration of sickled erythrocytes [61, 62]. The patient experiences chest pain, fever, tachypnea, wheezing, or cough. Under hypoxic and infectious conditions, cell–cell junctions can be destabilized causing the passage of systemic inflammatory mediators into the lungs, producing pulmonary edema; in this sense, ACS is similar to ARDS [61, 62]. Other pathologies include alterations in activated EC metabolic functions that may contribute to the vaso-occlusive events in ACS [63]. The balance between vasoconstriction and vasodilation in ACS may be altered. The ET-1 gene is upregulated in the lung and is released by activated lung ECs in response to hypoxia and reduced NO bioavailability [64, 65]. In a transgenic mouse model consistent with chronic organ lesions, tissue lesions, and acute vaso-occlusive events analogous to human SCD, SAD mice [S(β6val) Antilles (β23lle) D-Punjab(β121Gln)] [66], it was found that ET-1 is produced at a higher level in the pulmonary MVEC of SAD mice than wild type (WT) mice. Further, in the SAD mice, bosentan, an ET receptor antagonist, was shown to prevent death of SAD mice exposed to a severe hypoxic challenge [64].

Painful vaso-occlusive crisis (VOC), one of the major and specific manifestations of SCD, is the most debilitating manifestation of SCD [67]. In VOC, the circulation of blood vessels is obstructed by sickled red blood cells causing ischemic injury and severe pain. Sickling and/or hypoxia associated with VOC in SCD may shift the balance of endothelial vasodilator and vasoconstrictor response in favor of vasoconstriction [68]. The study of Hammerman et al. [63] measured NO products from cultured pulmonary ECs exposed to red blood cells and/or plasma from SCD patients during VOC [63]. Exposure to the plasma from SCD patients during VOC increased total NO production by both macro and microvascular lung ECs [63]. However, these increases were not accompanied by changes in eNOS or iNOS expression. Based on their findings, the authors suggested that altered NO production might contribute to the pathogenesis of ACS [63].

The vascular inflammation and increased thrombotic activity known to occur in patients with ACS in SCD may be associated with platelet activation of ECs through CD40, a platelet associated pro-inflammatory molecule that promotes ECs activation and is known to be elevated in the circulation of SCD patients [69]. Cluster of differentiation (CD)40, a protein found on antigen-presenting cells and its ligand (L), a protein receptor, are members of the TNF superfamily of molecules. The binding of CD40 to the endothelial cell induces a variety of downstream effects and initiates a variety of immune and inflammatory responses including the production of reactive oxygen species (ROS), chemokines, and cytokines and the expression of adhesion molecules such as E-selectin, ICAM-1 and VCAM-1. The inflammatory response then fosters recruitment of leukocytes around the EC [69]. Furthermore, the ROS generated by CD40L antagonizes NO synthesis and additionally promotes EC dysfunction [69]. A cohort of SCD patients was evaluated for the association of CD40L and inflammation with SCD clinical complications including ACS [69]. It was found that plasma CD40L was associated with ACS and that SCD patients with a lifetime history of ACS presented with significantly higher plasma CD40L than in SCD patients that had never experienced an episode of ACS [70]. Thrombospondin (TSP-1), also a platelet derived protein that activates ECs was found in the same study to correlate with increased ACS ECs activation of cytokines and chemokines [70].

One of the factors that have been identified in ACS is increased adherence between sickled red blood cells (RBC) and ECs [71]. Some investigators interpret abnormal endothelial adhesion as evidence of a pro-inflammatory state [72]. The pro-inflammatory state in SCD is associated with endothelial damage, increased production of ROS, hemolysis, and increased production of pro-inflammatory cytokines [73]. Transgenic SCD mice have been used to study the inflammatory responses that occur in SCD in many organs including the lung. The transgenic mice models have an active inflammatory response similar to human SCD patients [74]. Adhesion molecules VCAM, ICAM and PECAM have been shown to be upregulated in LPS-treated normal and transgenic-treated lungs [74]. IL-6 and NF-kB expressions were also increased in the lungs of transgenic SCD mice suggesting a vigorous inflammatory response with activated macro and microvascular ECs in the lungs [74]. LPS challenge is associated with increased mortality and increased levels of serum and BALF cytokines TNF-α, IL-1β and VCAM-1 in sickle mice compared with control subjects [72].

The role of the lung ECs and their interactions with sickle RBCs depend on multiple factors including the presence of inflammatory cells, cytokines, reactive oxygen species, hypoxic stress and infection that augment sickle cells' and white blood cells' (WBC) adherence to the endothelium. ACS is associated with infections, pneumonia, and fever, and in this setting, there is activation of pro-inflammatory factors such as cytokines that further activate the ECs and promote changes in vascular tone and permeability, anticoagulant-procoagulant balance, and leukocyte trafficking in the lungs of the SCD patient [74].

http://dx.doi.org/10.5772/intechopen.76995

3. Conclusion

Endothelial cells are an active component of the lung and line the large and small vessels of the lung. They all engage in forming a barrier separation but also are an active constituent in the healthy and diseased lungs. The pulmonary ECs manifest disruption and breakdown under abnormal conditions such as hypoxia and infection and pathologic conditions such as infection, ARDS, and ACS. The ongoing research in pulmonary ECs has highlighted the significance of pulmonary microvascular and macrovascular EC in health and disease with continuing focus toward improving morbidity and mortality of disease involving the pulmonary microvasculature.

Acknowledgements

The authors work is generously supported by the Hemoglobinopathy Translational Research Core (HTRC) support (JG) and Dr. Madaio, and the Augusta University Health Medical Center, Department of Medicine (JG), NIH grant HL101902 (ADV). We also thank Dr. Anita Kovacs-Kasa for her work in pulmonary microvascular cell immunocytochemistry figure and the Augusta University Health Vascular Biology Center Electron Microscope Imaging Center, Dr. Brendan Marshall and Libby Perry.

Conflict of interest

We declare no author has any disclosure or conflict of interest for any product or result in this manuscript.

Research support

This work was supported by the generous support of Dr. Madaio, and the Augusta University Health Department of Medicine (JG), NIH grant HL101902 (ADV).

Author details

Joyce N. Gonzales[1,2]* and Alexander D. Verin[1,2]

*Address all correspondence to: jgonzales@augusta.edu

1 Vascular Biology Center, Augusta University Health, Augusta, GA, USA

2 Division of Pulmonary and Critical Care Medicine, Department of Internal Medicine, Georgia Regents University, Augusta, GA, USA

References

[1] Cho JT, Guay-Woodford LM. Heterozygous mutations of the gene for Kir 1.1 (ROMK) in antenatal Bartter syndrome presenting with transient hyperkalemia, evolving to a benign course. Journal of Korean Medical Science. 2003;**18**(1):65-68

[2] Pober JS, Sessa WC. Evolving functions of endothelial cells in inflammation. Nature Reviews. Immunology. 2007;**7**(10):803-815

[3] Simionescu N, Simionescu M, editors. Endothelial Cell Dysfunctions. New York: Plenum Press; 1992. p. 565

[4] Bauer V, Sotníková R. Nitric oxide--the endothelium-derived relaxing factor and its role in endothelial functions. General Physiology and Biophysics. 2010;**29**(4):319-340

[5] Chambers RC. Procoagulant signalling mechanisms in lung inflammation and fibrosis: Novel opportunities for pharmacological intervention? British Journal of Pharmacology. 2008;**153**(Suppl 1):S367-S378

[6] Yau JW, Teoh H, Verma S. Endothelial cell control of thrombosis. BMC Cardiovascular Disorders. 2015;**15**(1):1-11. Available from: http://bmccardiovascdisord.biomedcentral.com/articles/10.1186/s12872-015-0124-z

[7] Singh I, Knezevic N, Ahmmed GU, Kini V, Malik AB, Mehta D. Galphaq-TRPC6-mediated Ca2+ entry induces RhoA activation and resultant endothelial cell shape change in response to thrombin. The Journal of Biological Chemistry. 2007;**282**(11):7833-7843

[8] Millar FR, Summers C, Griffiths MJ, Toshner MR, Proudfoot AG. The pulmonary endothelium in acute respiratory distress syndrome: Insights and therapeutic opportunities. Thorax. 2016;**71**(5):462-473

[9] Landmesser U, Hornig B, Drexler H. Endothelial function: A critical determinant in atherosclerosis? Circulation. 2004;**109**(21 Suppl 1):II27-II33

[10] Loscalzo J, Freedman J, Inbal A, Keaney JF, Michelson AD, Vita JA. Nitric oxide insufficiency and arterial thrombosis. Transactions of the American Clinical and Climatological Association. 2000;**111**:158-163

[11] Toews GB. Cytokines and the lung. The European Respiratory Journal. 2001;**18**(1):3-17

[12] Kofler S, Nickel T, Weis M. Role of cytokines in cardiovascular diseases: A focus on endothelial responses to inflammation. Clinical Science (London, England : 1979). 2005; **108**(3):205-213

[13] Krishnaswamy G, Kelley J, Yerra L, Smith JK, Chi DS. Human endothelium as a source of multifunctional cytokines: Molecular regulation and possible role in human disease. Journal of Interferon & Cytokine Research. 1999;**19**(2):91-104

[14] Teijaro JR, Walsh KB, Cahalan S, Fremgen DM, Roberts E, Scott F, et al. Endothelial cells are central orchestrators of cytokine amplification during influenza virus infection. Cell. 2011;**146**(6):980-991

[15] Lockett AD, Kimani S, Ddungu G, Wrenger S, Tuder RM, Janciauskiene SM, et al. α_1-antitrypsin modulates lung endothelial cell inflammatory responses to TNF-α. American Journal of Respiratory Cell and Molecular Biology. 2013;**49**(1):143-150

[16] Coker RK, Laurent GJ. Pulmonary fibrosis: Cytokines in the balance. The European Respiratory Journal. 1998;**11**(6):1218-1221

[17] Metcalf DJ, Nightingale TD, Zenner HL, Lui-Roberts WW, Cutler DF. Formation and function of Weibel-Palade bodies. Journal of Cell Science. 2008;**121**(Pt 1):19-27

[18] Liu G, Place AT, Chen Z, Brovkovych VM, Vogel SM, Muller WA, et al. ICAM-1-activated Src and eNOS signaling increase endothelial cell surface PECAM-1 adhesivity and neutrophil transmigration. Blood. 2012;**120**(9):1942-1952

[19] Kadl A, Leitinger N. The role of endothelial cells in the resolution of acute inflammation. Antioxidants & Redox Signaling. 2005;**7**(11-12):1744-1754

[20] Rao RM, Yang L, Garcia-Cardena G, Luscinskas FW. Endothelial-dependent mechanisms of leukocyte recruitment to the vascular wall. Circulation Research. 2007;**101**(3, 3): 234-247

[21] De Caterina R, Libby P, Peng HB, Thannickal VJ, Rajavashisth TB, Gimbrone MA, et al. Nitric oxide decreases cytokine-induced endothelial activation. Nitric oxide selectively reduces endothelial expression of adhesion molecules and proinflammatory cytokines. The Journal of Clinical Investigation. 1995;**96**(1):60-68

[22] Lim Y-C, Garcia-Cardena G, Allport JR, Zervoglos M, Connolly AJ, Gimbrone MA, et al. Heterogeneity of endothelial cells from different organ sites in T-cell subset recruitment. The American Journal of Pathology. 2003;**162**(5):1591-1601

[23] King J, Hamil T, Creighton J, Wu S, Bhat P, McDonald F, et al. Structural and functional characteristics of lung macro- and microvascular endothelial cell phenotypes. Microvascular Research. 2004;**67**(2):139-151

[24] Geiger M, Stone A, Mason SN, Oldham KT, Guice KS. Differential nitric oxide production by microvascular and macrovascular endothelial cells. The American Journal of Physiology. 1997;**273**(1 Pt 1):L275-L281

[25] Kelly JJ, Moore TM, Babal P, Diwan AH, Stevens T, Thompson WJ. Pulmonary microvascular and macrovascular endothelial cells: Differential regulation of Ca2+ and permeability. The American Journal of Physiology. 1998;**274**(5 Pt 1):L810-L819

[26] Pries AR, Kuebler WM. Normal endothelium. Handbook of Experimental Pharmacology. 2006;(176 Pt 1):1-40

[27] Müller AM, Hermanns MI, Cronen C, Kirkpatrick CJ. Comparative study of adhesion molecule expression in cultured human macro- and microvascular endothelial cells. Experimental and Molecular Pathology. 2002;**73**(3):171-180

[28] Wu T, Xing J, Birukova AA. Cell-type-specific crosstalk between p38 MAPK and rho signaling in lung micro- and macrovascular barrier dysfunction induced by Staphylococcus

aureus-derived pathogens. Translational Research, The Journal of Laboratory and Clinical Medicine. 2013;**162**(1):45-55

[29] Lang I, Pabst MA, Hiden U, Blaschitz A, Dohr G, Hahn T, et al. Heterogeneity of microvascular endothelial cells isolated from human term placenta and macrovascular umbilical vein endothelial cells. European Journal of Cell Biology. 2003;**82**(4):163-173

[30] Comhair SAA, Xu W, Mavrakis L, Aldred MA, Asosingh K, Erzurum SC. Human primary lung endothelial cells in culture. American Journal of Respiratory Cell and Molecular Biology. 2012;**46**(6):723-730

[31] Kovas-Kasa M, Verin G. Method for the culture of mouse pulmonary microvascular endothelial cells. Scientific Pages of Pulmonology. 2017;**1**(1):7-18

[32] Adyshev DM, Dudek SM, Moldobaeva N, Kim K, Ma S-F, Kasa A, et al. Ezrin/radixin/moesin proteins differentially regulate endothelial hyperpermeability after thrombin. American Journal of Physiology. Lung Cellular and Molecular Physiology. 2013; **305**(3):L240-L255

[33] Catravas JD, Snead C, Dimitropoulou C, Chang ASY, Lucas R, Verin AD, et al. Harvesting, identification and barrier function of human lung microvascular endothelial cells. Vascular Pharmacology. 2010;**52**(5-6):175-181

[34] Parra-Bonilla G, Alvarez DF, Al-Mehdi A-B, Alexeyev M, Stevens T. Critical role for lactate dehydrogenase a in aerobic glycolysis that sustains pulmonary microvascular endothelial cell proliferation. American Journal of Physiology. Lung Cellular and Molecular Physiology. 2010;**299**(4):L513-L522

[35] Parker JC, Stevens T, Randall J, Weber DS, King JA. Hydraulic conductance of pulmonary microvascular and macrovascular endothelial cell monolayers. American Journal of Physiology. Lung Cellular and Molecular Physiology. 2006;**291**(1):L30-L37

[36] Kása A, Csortos C, Verin AD. Cytoskeletal mechanisms regulating vascular endothelial barrier function in response to acute lung injury. Tissue Barriers. 2015;**3**(1-2):e974448e

[37] Bazzoni G, Dejana E. Endothelial cell-to-cell junctions: Molecular organization and role in vascular homeostasis. Physiological Reviews. 2004;**84**(3):869-901

[38] Komarova Y, Malik AB. Regulation of endothelial permeability via paracellular and transcellular transport pathways. Annual Review of Physiology. 2010;**72**:463-493

[39] Voelkel NF, Vandivier RW, Tuder RM. Vascular endothelial growth factor in the lung. American Journal of Physiology. Lung Cellular and Molecular Physiology. 2006;**290**(2):L209-L221

[40] Bach I. The LIM domain: Regulation by association. Mechanisms of Development. 2000; **91**(1-2):5-17

[41] Star GP, Giovinazzo M, Lamoureux E, Langleben D. Effects of vascular endothelial growth factor on endothelin-1 production by human lung microvascular endothelial cells in vitro. Life Sciences. 2014;**118**(2):191-194

[42] Bellani G, Laffey JG, Pham T, Fan E, Brochard L, Esteban A, et al. Epidemiology, patterns of care, and mortality for patients with acute respiratory distress syndrome in intensive care units in 50 countries. Journal of the American Medical Association. 2016; **315**(8):788-800

[43] Wang CY, Calfee CS, Paul DW, Janz DR, May AK, Zhuo H, et al. One-year mortality and predictors of death among hospital survivors of acute respiratory distress syndrome. Intensive Care Medicine. 2014;**40**(3):388-396

[44] Burns A. Unique structural features that influence neutrophil emigration into the lung. Physiological Reviews. 2003;**83**:309-336

[45] Bogatcheva NV, Verin AD. The role of cytoskeleton in the regulation of vascular endothelial barrier function. Microvascular Research. 2008;**76**(3):202-207

[46] Dudek SM, Garcia JG. Cytoskeletal regulation of pulmonary vascular permeability. Journal of Applied Physiology (Bethesda, Md. : 1985). 2001;**91**(4):1487-1500

[47] Gonzales JN, Lucas R, Verin AD. The acute respiratory distress syndrome: Mechanisms and perspective therapeutic approaches. Austin Journal of Vascular Medicine. 2015;**4**:2(1)

[48] Zimmerman GA, Albertine KH, Carveth HJ, Gill EA, Grissom CK, Hoidal JR, et al. Endothelial activation in ARDS. Chest. 1999;**116**(1 Suppl):18S-24S

[49] Müller AM, Cronen C, Müller K-M, Kirkpatrick CJ. Heterogeneous expression of cell adhesion molecules by endothelial cells in ARDS: Cell adhesion molecules in ARDS. The Journal of Pathology. 2002;**198**(2):270-275

[50] Callicutt CS, Sabek O, Fukatsu K, Lundberg AH, Gaber L, Wilcox H, et al. Diminished lung injury with vascular adhesion molecule-1 blockade in choline-deficient ethionine diet-induced pancreatitis. Surgery. 2003;**133**(2):186-196

[51] Grommes J. Contribution of neutrophils to acute lung injury. Molmed. 2011;**17**(3-4):293-307

[52] Goodman RB, Pugin J, Lee JS, Matthay MA. Cytokine-mediated inflammation in acute lung injury. Cytokine & Growth Factor Reviews. 2003;**14**(6):523-535

[53] Hayden FG, Fritz R, Lobo MC, Alvord W, Strober W, Straus SE. Local and systemic cytokine responses during experimental human influenza a virus infection. Relation to symptom formation and host defense. The Journal of Clinical Investigation. 1998; **101**(3):643-649

[54] Kaiser L, Fritz RS, Straus SE, Gubareva L, Hayden FG. Symptom pathogenesis during acute influenza: Interleukin-6 and other cytokine responses. Journal of Medical Virology. 2001;**64**(3):262-268

[55] Cribbs SK, Martin GS. Stem cells in sepsis and acute lung injury. The American Journal of the Medical Sciences. 2011;**341**(4):325-332

[56] Moussa MD, Santonocito C, Fagnoul D, Donadello K, Pradier O, Gaussem P, et al. Evaluation of endothelial damage in sepsis-related ARDS using circulating endothelial cells. Intensive Care Medicine. 2015;**41**(2):231-238

[57] Agrawal A, Matthay MA, Kangelaris KN, Stein J, Chu JC, Imp BM, et al. Plasma angiopoietin-2 predicts the onset of acute lung injury in critically ill patients. American Journal of Respiratory and Critical Care Medicine. 2013;**187**(7):736-742

[58] Bhandari V, Choo-Wing R, Lee CG, Zhu Z, Nedrelow JH, Chupp GL, et al. Hyperoxia causes angiopoietin 2-mediated acute lung injury and necrotic cell death. Nature Medicine. 2006;**12**(11):1286-1293

[59] Schraufstatter IU, Chung J, Burger M. IL-8 activates endothelial cell CXCR1 and CXCR2 through rho and Rac signaling pathways. American Journal of Physiology. Lung Cellular and Molecular Physiology. 2001;**280**(6):L1094-L1103

[60] Centers for Disease Control and Prevention. Sickle Cell Disease, SCD Homepage. Report No.: www.cdc.gov/ncbddd/sicklecell/data.html

[61] Gladwin MT, Vichinsky E. Pulmonary complications of sickle cell disease. The New England Journal of Medicine. 2008;**359**(21):2254-2265

[62] Umapathy NS, Gonzales J, Makala LH, Xu H, Biddinger P, Pace BS. Impaired pulmonary endothelial barrier function in sickle cell mice. Haematologica. 2017;**102**(1):e26-e29

[63] Hammerman SI, Klings ES, Hendra KP, Upchurch GR, Rishikof DC, Loscalzo J, et al. Endothelial cell nitric oxide production in acute chest syndrome. The American Journal of Physiology. 1999;**277**(4 Pt 2):H1579-H1592

[64] Sabaa N, de Franceschi L, Bonnin P, Castier Y, Malpeli G, Debbabi H, et al. Endothelin receptor antagonism prevents hypoxia-induced mortality and morbidity in a mouse model of sickle-cell disease. The Journal of Clinical Investigation. 2008;**118**(5):1924-1933

[65] Koehl B, Nivoit P, El Nemer W, Lenoir O, Hermand P, Pereira C, et al. The endothelin B receptor plays a crucial role in the adhesion of neutrophils to the endothelium in sickle cell disease. Haematologica. 2017;**102**(7):1161-1172

[66] Trudel M, De Paepe ME, Chrétien N, Saadane N, Jacmain J, Sorette M, et al. Sickle cell disease of transgenic SAD mice. Blood. 1994;**84**(9):3189-3197

[67] Ender KL, Krajewski JA, Babineau J, Tresgallo M, Schechter W, Saroyan JM, et al. Use of a clinical pathway to improve the acute management of vaso-occlusive crisis pain in pediatric sickle cell disease. Pediatric Blood & Cancer. 2014;**61**(4):693-696

[68] Ergul S, Brunson CY, Hutchinson J, Tawfik A, Kutlar A, Webb RC, et al. Vasoactive factors in sickle cell disease: In vitro evidence for endothelin-1-mediated vasoconstriction. American Journal of Hematology. 2004;**76**(3):245-251

[69] Szmitko PE, Wang C-H, Weisel RD, de Almeida JR, Anderson TJ, Verma S. New markers of inflammation and endothelial cell activation: Part I. Circulation. 2003;**108**(16):1917-1923

[70] Garrido VT, Sonzogni L, Mtatiro SN, Costa FF, Conran N, Thein SL. Association of plasma CD40L with acute chest syndrome in sickle cell anemia. Cytokine. 2017;**97**:104-107

[71] Hebbel RP, Yamada O, Moldow CF, Jacob HS, White JG, Eaton JW. Abnormal adherence of sickle erythrocytes to cultured vascular endothelium: Possible mechanism for microvascular occlusion in sickle cell disease. The Journal of Clinical Investigation. 1980;**65**(1):154-160

[72] Holtzclaw JD, Jack D, Aguayo SM, Eckman JR, Roman J, Hsu LL. Enhanced pulmonary and systemic response to endotoxin in transgenic sickle mice. American Journal of Respiratory and Critical Care Medicine. 2004;**169**(6):687-695

[73] Bandeira ICJ, Rocha LBS, Barbosa MC, Elias DBD, Querioz JAN, Freitas MVC, et al. Chronic inflammatory state in sickle cell anemia patients is associated with HBB(*)S haplotype. Cytokine. 2014;**65**(2):217-221

[74] Belcher JD, Bryant CJ, Nguyen J, Bowlin PR, Kielbik MC, Bischof JC, et al. Transgenic sickle mice have vascular inflammation. Blood. 2003;**101**(10):3953-3959

Chapter 13

Smoking, Respiratory Diseases and Endothelial Dysfunction

Vera Nevzorova, Tatiana Brodskaya and
Natalia Zakharchuk

Additional information is available at the end of the chapter

http://dx.doi.org/10.5772/intechopen.73555

Abstract

Vascular endothelium actively participates in inflammatory reactions in the majority of chronic respiratory diseases. Smoking is a major risk factor for bronchopulmonary diseases, and it plays an important role in endothelial dysfunction development. Some experiments prove that aggressive pollutants of tobacco smoke (benzopyrene, peroxynitrite, acrolein, cyanides, peroxides, etc.) can cause direct damage to endothelial cells due to expression of adhesion molecules on their surface and intensification of lipid peroxidation. In turn, oxidized lipoproteins in the tunica intima of the vessel work as attractants for chemotaxis of leukocytes and monocytes that start to produce pro-inflammatory cytokines in big amounts. These processes trigger systemic inflammatory response that leads to irreversible thickening of the vessel walls and deterioration of their mechanical properties. Chronic exposure to tobacco smoke and the products of combustion of tobacco leads to chronic system inflammatory reaction, oxidative stress, endothelial dysfunction and morpho-functional damage of target organs. Nowadays, the connection between chronic obstructive pulmonary disease (COPD) and some cardiovascular and cerebrovascular diseases has been well established. Studying the mechanisms of endothelial dysfunction in brain blood vessels of patients with smoking habits and COPD can be very important for preventing acute vascular events.

Keywords: endothelium, endothelial dysfunction, cardiovascular system, cerebral vessels, smoking, respiratory diseases, COPD

1. Introduction

Vascular endothelium initiates and actively participates in inflammatory reactions in the majority of chronic respiratory diseases. Endothelial dysfunction (ED) that develops as clinically manifested disruptions of endothelium-dependent vasomotor reactions on local and systemic levels related with inflammation of different genesis should be regarded as a major segment of the cardiorespiratory continuum. Endothelium can autonomously produce at least 20 biologically active substances that are synthesized and released depending on current functional requirements. Endothelium functions create a balance of regulatory substances that determine the whole operation of interaction and control system (**Figure 1**). They include factors that are responsible for contraction and relaxation of smooth muscles in vessel walls, coagulation and fibrinolysis, control of cell proliferation and apoptosis, regulating the reaction to foreign substances and facilitating interaction with lymph vessels and drainage.

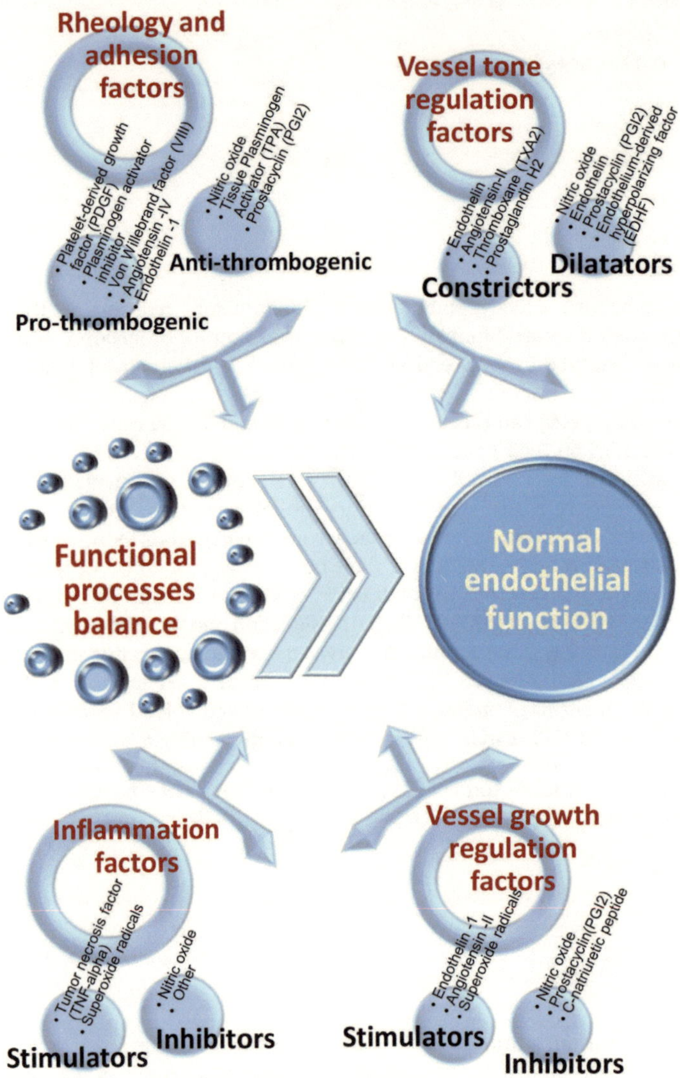

Figure 1. Functional processes balance in normal endothelial function.

http://dx.doi.org/10.5772/intechopen.73555

Today there is a substantial amount of evidence proving the endothelium involvement in development of local and systemic damage from tobacco smoke that is an indisputable cause of chronic respiratory diseases, such as chronic obstructive pulmonary disease (COPD), some phenotypes of asthma, idiopathic pulmonary fibrosis and so on [2, 7, 8, 20]. The correlation between the intensity of tobacco smoking and rapid decline in lung function is a proven fact. According to WHO, tobacco smokers experience sudden death five times more frequently than non-smokers [1]. The mechanisms of damage done to the blood vessels induced by tobacco combustion products have not been studied extensively at the moment, even though it is accepted that tobacco does not have any exclusive ways of producing vascular damage. Nicotine being the main component of tobacco smoke stimulates catecholamine release leading to stimulation of β1 and β2 adrenoreceptors. Nicotine induces a degradation of nitric oxide (NO) [2]. NO induces vasodilation by stimulating soluble guanylate cyclase (GC) to produce cyclic guanosine monophosphate (cGMP) [3]. Thus, nicotine causes change of reactions during vasodilatation. Apart from nicotine, tobacco smoke includes 4000 chemical substances, 100 of them having various toxic effects along with antigenic, cytotoxic, mutagenic and carcinogenic properties [4, 5]. They are able to interfere with cellular structure and processes of intercellular signaling by stimulating apoptosis, lipid peroxidation in cellular membrane, DNA and RNA strings' rupture and mitochondrial respiratory chain disruption. Tobacco smoke components are not the only factors directly responsible for stimulating and damaging endothelium in case of respiratory diseases; there are also endogenous factors, such as cellular and non-cellular inflammation mediators, bacterial toxins, immune complexes, hypoxemia, free radicals and shear stress alteration in endothelium [6–12].

In general, the sequence of events altering functional properties of endothelium can be described as follows. Damaging factors (different in nature, intensity and length) activate and/or damage endothelium gradually exhausting its compensation abilities and leading to abnormal (altered) response to the same damaging factors and even to regular stimuli. It results in prolonged vasoconstriction, higher adhesion and clotting level, weakened barrier function, intensification of cellular proliferation and some other consequences with certain clinical symptoms: vascular hypertension, swelling, vascular remodeling and so on. In addition, some effects, including those related to renin-angiotensin system and endothelial involvement in inflammation process, are both local and systemic nature.

2. Respiratory diseases and cerebral vascular endothelial dysfunction

According to modern conceptions, the central nervous system is an important participant in the pathogenesis of a number of chronic respiratory diseases, including those having a nicotine-associated nature. An important regulator of hemoperfusion of the brain is the vascular endothelium [8]. There are specific endothelium-dependent reactions in the arteries of the brain [9, 15]. Cerebral autoregulation maintains constant blood flow (CBF) through the brain in spite of changing mean arterial pressure. Autoregulation of cerebral blood flow consists of mechano- and chemoregulation. Chemoregulation is in direct correlation to the serum level of carbon dioxide and is, contrary to mechanoregulation, independent of changes in mean arterial pressure.

Mechanoregulation depends on transmural pressure gradient and endothelial vasodilatation. Mechanoregulation has been shown to be the main supervisory mechanism of CBF. However, it is well established that endothelial vasodilatation of greater arteries is much more pronounced in cerebral vasculature than elsewhere. Proper endothelial function is of crucial importance in regulation in many vascular beds. Dysfunctional cerebral endothelium releases less endothelial NO. As a consequence, relaxation of smooth muscle cells of small arteries is disturbed. Studies in animals and humans have revealed that mechanoregulation is not compromised even in older age and pathological conditions harming endothelium. On the contrary, outcomes of many studies and clinical reports confirm the dependency of chemoregulation of CBF on vascular endothelial integrity. Reduced chemoregulation was found in patients with dysfunctional cerebral endothelium [9]. The development of cognitive disorders recognized by experts as a typical systemic manifestation of the disease remains insufficiently investigated so far in the pathogenesis of nicotine-associated respiratory diseases and in particular COPD [10, 11, 16, 17]. It has been proven that one of the manifestations of vascular dysfunction can be a violation of the regional correspondence of the blood flow, which has a significant effect on the further course of the disease [12, 13, 18, 19]. According to research, a complex cascade of teratogenesis in respiratory diseases initiates acute and chronic hypoxemia and, in severe cases, hypercapnia. In turn, cerebral dysfunction in COPD can be a factor in the violation of respiratory and vasomotor reactivity in response to hypercapnia due to a decrease in the sensitivity of central chemoreceptors to it. It is known that central chemoreceptors represent up to 80% of the total chemo-sensitivity of the organism to carbon dioxide [4, 5]. The consequence of the violation of central vasomotor control is inadequate blood supply to various areas, including the brain itself [4, 5, 15]. Not being invalidating, violations of the central nervous system significantly affect the ability to work and social activity of patients. The main consequence of the violation of brain perfusion in these patients is the violation of the integral function of the central nervous system, which results in inadequate blood supply to various areas, including the brain [5, 7, 9]. This becomes the closing link of a peculiar "vicious circle" of regional vascular dysfunctions. **Figure 2** shows the place and role of functional imbalance of endothelium-dependent mechanisms in the pathogenesis of respiratory diseases.

2.1. Effect of tobacco smoke components on vascular function

Consequences and mechanisms of tobacco combustion products damaging vascular bed still require more research. Tobacco smoking is known to cause ED [19, 21] that has its peculiarities depending on the intensity and time of exposure as well as characteristics of the arteries. For instance, one of the crucial characteristics of cerebral blood circulation is a high level of autonomous self-regulation providing relative independence of cerebral hemodynamics from shifts in systemic circulation. Short-term exposure to tobacco smoke results in damage from its toxins on vascular endothelium and activation of sympathoadrenal system. [22]. Chronic exposure to tobacco smoke leads to a lower level of endothelial NO synthase (eNOS) activity and NO synthesis, adhesion molecules expression on the surface of endothelial cells, protein kinase C (PKC) activation and intensification of lipid peroxidation followed by persistent remodeling of the vascular wall [23, 24]. Some experiments describe development of endothelial dysfunction of cerebral and conductance arteries in mice exposed to tobacco smoke that was characterized by significant intensification and predominance of constricting activity of

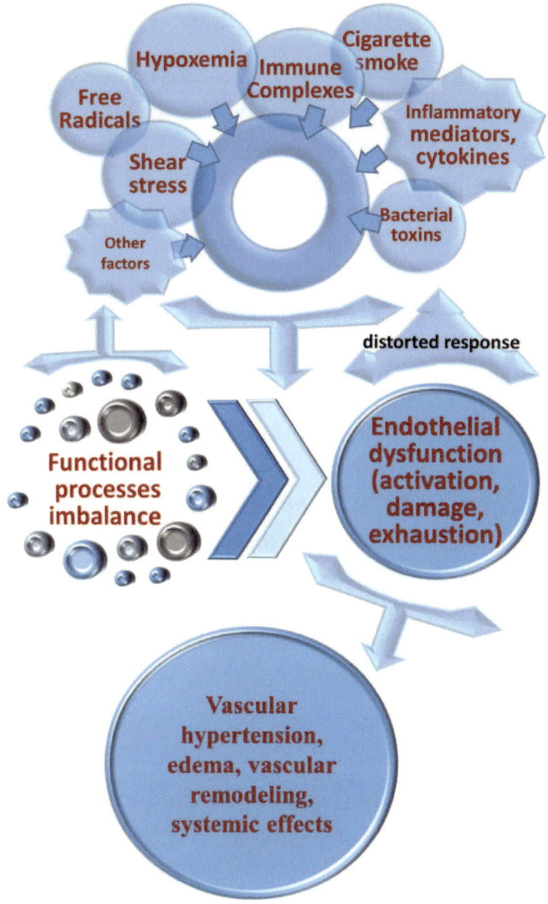

Figure 2. Functional processes imbalance due to endothelial dysfunction in respiratory diseases.

arteries, as well as abnormal reduction of cerebral arterial vasodilatory reserve along with asymmetric increase of carotid artery constriction [11, 14]. Apart from endothelial dysfunction and alterations of vasomotor reactions in response to tobacco smoking, some experiments revealed a connection between long-term exposure to tobacco smoke and irreversible changes in large arteries, such as wall thickening and deterioration of their mechanical properties [24, 25]. At the same time, smoke-exposed rats showed elevated levels of elastase and progressing degenerative changes of thoracic and abdominal aorta accompanied by a lower quality of their elastic and mechanical properties [26]. Some researches show that smoking increases risk of development of abdominal aortic aneurysm (AAA). For example, AAA growth rate was lower in those with low ankle/brachial pressure index and diabetes but higher for current smokers. No other factor (including lipids and blood pressure) was associated with AAA growth. [27]. Current smokers were 7.6 times more likely to have an AAA than non-smokers. Ex-smokers were 3.0 times more likely to have an AAA than non-smokers. Duration of smoking was significantly associated with an increased risk of AAA, and there was a clear linear dose response relationship with the duration of smoking; each year of smoking increased the relative risk of AAA by 4% [28].

2.2. Carotid arteries condition in COPD depending on the smoking status

COPD is considered to be systemic pathology with multiple extrapulmonary effects that define patients' prognosis and quality of life. Smoking plays a significant part in COPD pathogenesis. Chronic exposure to tobacco smoke works as an integral agent between topical changes of bronchopulmonary system and systemic pro-inflammatory activation with development of oxidative stress, endothelial dysfunction and progressing morphofunctional damage of target organs. Today, the connection of COPD and some cardiovascular and cerebrovascular diseases with atherosclerotic vascular damage has been proven [29, 30]. Atherosclerosis of conductance cerebral arteries also might be both the reason for chronic brain ischemia and a sign of severe alterations in brain blood circulation.

An important indicator of atherosclerosis is thickening of intima-media complex of carotid arteries and development of atherosclerotic plaques that serve as markers for high risk of developing ischemic heart disease and stroke, as shown by the data from the Cardiovascular Health Study and Rotterdam Study [31]. Implementation of different imaging methods has significantly broadened the horizons of atherosclerosis diagnostics. One of the methods is ultrasound scanning of brain vessels that has some advantages, like providing extensive information, non-invasiveness of the procedure, accessibility and relatively low cost. Also, this method allows to get information about structural characteristics of atherosclerotic plaques, velocity and spectral parameters of the blood flow [32]. Nowadays there is an ongoing search for general risk factors and development mechanisms of cardiovascular and cerebrovascular pathology in COPD.

Using transcranial Doppler ultrasound (Nicolet Companion Biomedikal, the USA), we evaluated some parameters of cerebral hemodynamics. The research included 75 COPD patients (aged 54.81 ± 8.36 years) who smoke. The control group consisted of 20 healthy volunteers of comparable gender and age. Using carotid duplex ultrasound (MyLab 50 Esaote, Italy), we measured intima-media thickness (IMT) of the common carotid arteries (CCA) and middle cerebral arteries (MCA). We found thickening of the intima-media complex in the majority of COPD patients who smoke (**Figure 3**). Apart from that, one-third of the examined patients had atherosclerotic plaques in the CCA bifurcation area and internal carotid artery mouth that led to artery stenosis in up to 22.5 ± 4.2% of cases. Parameters of velocity are presented in **Tables 1** and **2**.

Some papers present convincing data on direct connection between COPD patients with carotid atherosclerosis and air flow velocity shown by spirometry [34–36]. COPD patients are more likely to have unstable atherosclerotic plaques with big lipid nuclei. These changes are visible even in patients with a mild case of COPD. Lahousse et al. have discovered that atherosclerotic plaques are very common for COPD patients in 60% of non-smoking patients and 80% of smokers [36]. Atherosclerotic plaques in case of COPD have a high risk of rupture even for patients with a very mild case of airway obstruction, while smoking only increases that risk [37]. Unstable atherosclerotic plaques with big lipid nuclei appear early in COPD and explain the doubling of mortality rates from cardiovascular diseases in this group of patients [38]. Animal tests show that systemic inflammation in COPD releases pro-inflammatory

http://dx.doi.org/10.5772/intechopen.73555

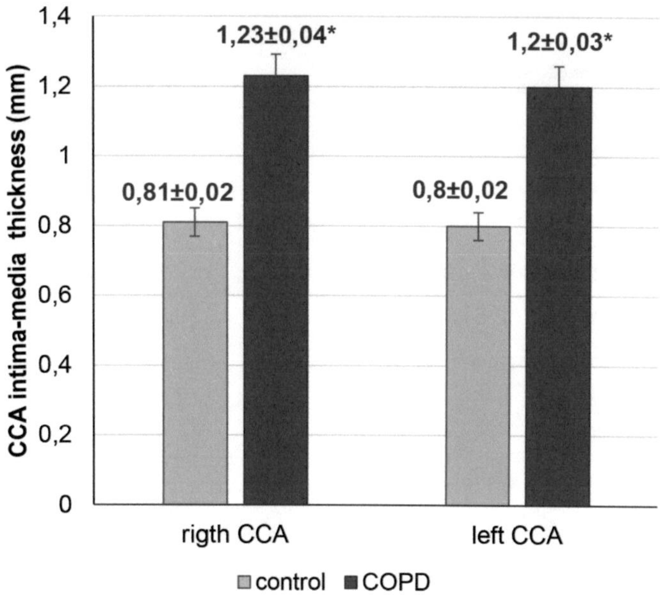

Figure 3. The thickness of the intima-media complex in the common carotid arteries in COPD patients and healthy people according to the data of ultrasound duplex scanning (mean ± SD, *p < 0.05 in comparison with the control group; t-test analysis was used to assess the differences in the values). CCA: common carotid artery. Explanations are in the text.

mediators that facilitate inflammatory cells migration into atherosclerotic plaques, increasing the level of lipids there and thus creating unstable plaques [39].

Exposure to smoke induces a significant thickening of intima-media complex in conductance arteries, atherosclerotic plaques in the CCA bifurcation area and internal carotid artery mouth

Parameter	Control (healthy people, N = 20)	COPD and smoking (patients, N = 75)
Peak systolic velocity in the right CCA, cm/s	71.5 ± 7.3	53.1 ± 5.5*
Mean velocity in the right CCA, cm/s	38.2 ± 4.0	27.4 ± 3.1*
End diastolic velocity in the right CCA, cm/s	18.4 ± 1.6	14.9 ± 1.5*
Peak systolic velocity in the left CCA, cm/s	72.9 ± 8.1	53.9 ± 5.2*
Mean velocity in the left CCA, cm/s	37.9 ± 3.9	27.3 ± 3.1*
End diastolic velocity in the left CCA, cm/s	18.8 ± 1.7	15.1 ± 1.4*
Pulsatility index in the right CCA	2.02 ± 0.24	1.39 ± 0.13*
Pulsatility index in the left CCA	2.04 ± 0.25	1.50 ± 0.16*
Resistance index in the right CCA	0.75 ± 0.04	0.71 ± 0.06
Resistance index in the left CCA	0.74 ± 0.05	0.70 ± 0.06

Data are presented as mean ± SD. *p < 0.05 (t-test analysis was used to assess the differences in the values) in comparison with the control group. COPD is chronic obstructive pulmonary disease and CCA is common carotid artery.

Table 1. Blood flow parameters from transcranial dopplerography in the common carotid artery.

Parameter	Control (healthy people, N = 20)	COPD and smoking (patients, N = 75)
Peak systolic velocity in the right MCA, cm/s	95.8 ± 11.1	91.2 ± 10.6
Mean velocity in the right MCA, cm/s	56.1 ± 4.1	48.2 ± 3.2*
End diastolic velocity in the right MCA, cm/s	49.8 ± 3.9	46.7 ± 3.0
Peak systolic velocity in the left MCA, cm/s	93.8 ± 9.8	85.2 ± 8.8
Mean velocity in the left MCA, cm/s	56.0 ± 4.6	44.8 ± 3.3*
End diastolic velocity in the left MCA, cm/s	49.2 ± 4.0	44.4 ± 3.7
Pulsatility index in the right MCA	0.82 ± 0.04	0.93 ± 0.05*
Pulsatility index in the left MCA	0.81 ± 0.04	0.93 ± 0.04*
Resistance index in the right MCA	0.47 ± 0.03	0.50 ± 0.03
Resistance index in the left MCA	0.46 ± 0.03	0.49 ± 0.04

Data are presented as mean ± SD. *$p < 0.05$ (t-test analysis was used to assess the differences in the values) in comparison with the control group. COPB is chronic obstructive pulmonary disease and MCA is middle carotid artery.

Table 2. Blood flow parameters from transcranial dopplerography in the middle cerebral artery.

that leads to partial artery stenosis [33]. Long-term exposure to toxic products of tobacco combustion causes hypertrophy of smooth muscle cells, disorganization of arterial myoelastic tissue, faster lipid peroxydation leading to thickening of vessel walls, deterioration of their mechanic properties and atherogenesis [23, 40]. It results in the lower level of arterial elasticity, excessive rigidity of vessel walls with loss of their damping properties in response to fluctuations of systemic arterial pressure and other effects of situational hemodynamic stresses, thus, increasing the risk of arterial hypertension and worsening the prognosis for the course of the disease [41].

Structural deterioration of conductance arteries causes alterations in blood flow velocity. At the same time, the resistance of peripheral vessels and elastic properties of vessel wall decrease which is indicated by lower pulsation index and, to a lesser extent, resistance index [33].

Our studies of blood flow in conductance and extracerebral arteries using transcranial dopplerography showed reduced velocity of blood flow in common carotid arteries and medial cerebral arteries (**Tables 1** and **2**). More significant changes of cerebral hemodynamics were found in the medium velocity of blood flow. There was also a significant drop in pulsation index and slight reduction of resistance index (**Tables 1** and **2**), as it has been shown earlier [33].

Unlike CCAs, MCAs in patients with COPD demonstrate increased peripheral resistance indexes (**Table 2**).

Brain arteries are frequently considered to be a system comprising interrelated but independent segmental effectors [42, 43]. According to the conducted research, MCAs mostly have vasospastic reactions that are reflected in the increase of both indexes characterizing peripheral resistance level, that is, pulsatility index and resistance index. Also, MCAs in the COPD group show lower velocity of blood flow, but they are 2–3 times less pronounced than in CCAs and have significant differences only in the medium velocity parameter. Since the ultimate goal of myogenic response of conductance arteries is to maintain stable blood flow along the whole regional vascular network [44], the discovered reduction in deviations of blood flow velocity in MCAs from the control values is quite logical, unlike in case of the CCA results.

It is important to note that slower blood flow velocity and higher peripheral resistance indexes in the MCAs mostly indicate not the transformation of elastic properties of the vessel but a shift from a dilatatory function of the endothelium to a constricting one which is common for distributional sector of blood circulation in pia matter [13, 42]. Such significant change in pial arteries reaction can be an indicator of endothelial dysfunction resulting from a sequence of biochemical processes triggered by toxic influence of tobacco smoke components and being a product of systemic inflammatory response that suppresses endothelial production of vasodilators, including NO [24].

An important indicator of cerebrovascular hemodynamics is the reaction of small pial and precortical arteries that are extremely sensitive to brain blood flow alterations [42]. Breath-holding test (hypercapnic test) and hyperventilation test (hyperoxia test) allow to calculate the indexes of endothelium-dependent reaction of those vessels in terms of their dilatatory and constricting functions, respectively [45, 46]. The obtained results show an existing imbalance of endothelial vasomotor activity in small pial and cerebral vessels where vasospastic reactions are intensified with unchanged or slightly reduced endothelial dilatation ability of these vessels in patients with smoking-induced COPD (**Figure 4**) [33]. The value of vascular responsiveness index (VRI) was calculated as: VRI = $(Vps_2 - Vps_1)/Vps_1 \times 100\%$, Vps_1 is peak systolic velocity in the MCA under investigation and Vps_2 is peak systolic velocity in the MCA after

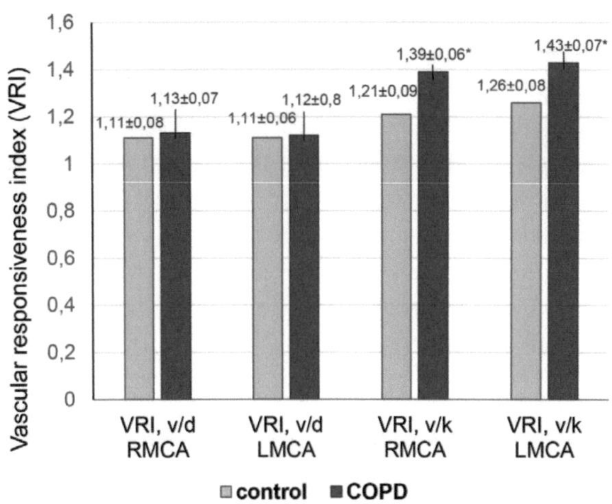

Figure 4. Vascular responsiveness index (VRI) in COPD patients and healthy patients assessed by ultrasound duplex scanning (mean ± SD, *$p < 0.05$ in comparison with the control group; t-test analysis was used to assess the differences in the values). VRI v/d is cerebral reactivity index to vasodilation, VRI v/c is cerebral reactivity index to vasoconstriction, RMCA is right middle cerebral artery and LMCA is left middle cerebral artery. Explanations are in the text.

the appropriate tests. One of the hyperoxic vasoconstriction mechanisms can be NO inactivation by superoxide anions resulting from superoxygenation [24, 47]. As a result of those processes, vasorelaxant effect of NO weakens; perfusion reserve and self-regulation potential of resistance vessels are reduced while the risks of cerebrovascular pathology become higher [48].

At the same time, in the precortical arterioles, the production of vasodilator increases as an adaptive physiological process. It leads to a vasodilatation, increase in diameter of vessels that promotes improvement of brain perfusion as an adaptive mechanism [42]. If this does not happen, the conditions for acute and chronic hemodynamic disorders start to develop. At the moment, enough data have been collected to prove the close connection between one's smoking history and frequency of cerebrovascular events, lacunar strokes, vascular dementia and cognitive deficiency [49–51].

2.3. Vasomotor function of cerebral vessels in tobacco smoking

An important feature of cerebral blood circulation is a high level of autonomous self-regulation that provides relative independence and protection for cerebral hemodynamics from shifts in systemic blood circulation. Observation has shown that smoking is an independent risk factor of ischemic stroke for both men and women [50]. We may assume that there is an integrating development mechanism of systemic vascular dysfunction in chronic tobacco smoking that is also responsible for damaging brain vessels. Cerebral blood flow disruption is known to be initiated by the failing self-regulation mechanism, and its vulnerability grows if functional and morphological integrity of endothelium is damaged. Meta-analysis of 22 researches showed that chronic tobacco smoking can double the relative risk of ischemic stroke [50]. Endothelial dysfunction is suggested to be a part of pathological cascade of vascular remodeling influenced by tobacco smoking [52].

In order to study vasomotor activity of endothelium in arteries exposed to chronic tobacco smoke in vivo, many experiments have been designed in rats [53–55]. Considering the similarities between rats and humans in terms of Willis' circle structure and its topography as well as anatomical likeness, the use of these animals is objectively relevant for modeling different pathologies in brain vessels with subsequent extrapolation of the result to humans. Since it is impossible to use non-invasive dopplerography in rats, invasive method had to be used when the rats were injected with vasodilators and vasoconstrictors. Afterwards, the diameter changes in cerebral arteries affected by pharmacological stimuli were studied with magnetic resonance imaging (MRI) brain scanning (**Figure 5**).

To assess endothelial function of cerebral arteries we used pharmacological tests that proved to be a highly efficient and specific means for studying endothelium-dependent and endothelium-independent mechanisms of the vasomotor activity regulation. The selected pharmacological agents have well-known action modes and certain points of application allowing to assess the mechanisms of vasomotor reaction development.

The study was conducted on the middle cerebral artery of mature male Wistar rats weighing 180–200 g that were divided into a control group (n = 10) and experimental group (n = 10), respectively. The animals from the control group were breathing regular atmospheric air, while

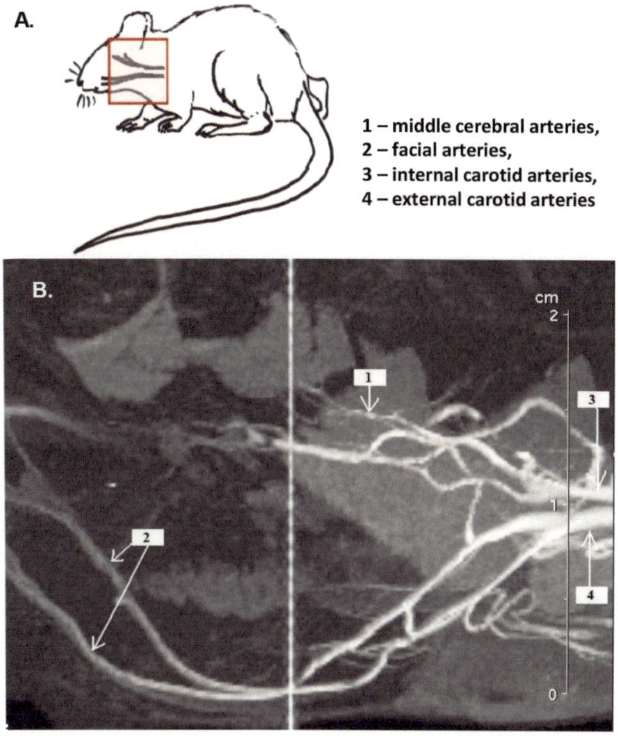

Figure 5. The chart (A) and a MRI tomographic image (B) of the cerebral arteries in the sagittal plane in rats (chronic tobacco smoke model, experimental group). Chart A shows a contour of the tomographic scan area. Arrows in tomographic image point to approximate locations of the measurements of the arteries indicated by numbers: 1: Middle cerebral arteries, 2: Facial arteries, 3: Internal carotid arteries, 4: External carotid arteries. Explanations are in the text.

experimental group was exposed to inhaling tobacco smoke for 6 months to create chronic tobacco smoke model (method by Zheng et al.) [56]. Rats of experimental group were placed in a special chamber for inhalation, where they were exposed to tobacco smoke for 1 h in the morning and 1 h in the daytime, 7 days in a week, for 36 weeks. Then, using MRI of the brain, the level of change in the cerebral arteries diameter after pharmacological stimuli was assessed. This method was used for investigating endothelium-dependent vasodilatation (EDVD) after the acetylcholine (ACh) injection, endothelium-independent vasodilatation (EIVD) after the nitroglycerin injection, endothelium-dependent vasoconstriction (EDVC) after the N-monomethyl-L-arginine (L-NMLA) injection and endothelium-independent vasoconstriction (EIVC) after the norepinephrine injection. Cerebral vascular reactivity index (CVRI) was used to describe vasomotor function of the endothelium. CVRI was calculated using the formula: CVRI = (d2-d1):(d3-d1), where d1 is the the initial diameter of the artery, d2 is diameter of the artery EDVD and d3 is the diameter of the artery EDVC. Brain MRI was performed on the scanner for experimental studies "PharmaScan US 70/16" (Bruker, Germany).

The study showed vascular dysfunction in cerebral blood circulation of animals chronically exposed to tobacco smoke [57]. Data indicating vasomotor function of brain arteries in rat smokers are presented in **Table 3**.

Descriptor	Control (rats, N = 10)	Tobacco smoking (rats, N = 12)
EDVD, %	+11.89 ± 0.98	−0.64 ± 0.02*
EIDVD, %	+17.84 ± 1.25	+ 8.64 ± 0.76*
EDVC, %	−6.31 ± 0.14	+5.95 ± 0.34*
EIDVC, %	−4.83 ± 0.12	−11.2 ± 1.01*

Data are presented as mean ± SD. *$p < 0.05$ (t-test analysis was used to assess the differences in the values) in comparison with the control group. EDVD, endothelium-dependent vasodilation; EIDVD, endothelium-independent vasodilation; EDVC, endothelium-dependent vasoconstriction; EIDVC, endothelium endothelium-independent vasoconstriction; %, percent change after the appropriate tests.

Table 3. Vasomotor function of cerebral arteries in smoking.

Pharmacological tests caused expected endothelium-dependent and endothelium-independent vasodilation in healthy rats proving that NO synthase and GC mechanisms of vascular endothelium dilation remained intact [57].

At the same time, our results showed significant differences in vasomotor reactions of rats exposed to tobacco smoking. ACh stimulates eNOS causing NO secretion that results in pronounced EDVD [58]. Our results showed that the control group of rats exhibited an expected, sufficient level of EDVD in their brain vessels. Furthermore, arterial diameter increased by more than 10% of the original level in healthy rats indicating that the Enos-mediated mechanism of vasodilation remained intact (**Table 3**).

Alternatively, the group of smokers had pathological vasospastic reactions after ACh administration (**Table 3**). The reason might be related to functional damage of vascular endothelium. Some experiments showed that chronic exposure to tobacco smoke causes NO deficiency and weaker activity of eNOS [59, 60]. Based on previous mechanistic reports [53–55], we can assume that there is an NO deficiency and lower level of endothelial eNOS activity in our model of tobacco smoking that indicates substantial damage of eNOS mechanism and thus impaired vasodilation.

Apart from the eNOS mechanism of vasodilation, there is also another one involving GC. NO molecule is a highly active radical due to its unpaired electron. Its chemical properties allow it to access vascular myocytes and activate intracellular GC without any receptors. As a result, the cell concentration of cGMP becomes higher, and smooth muscle cells relax [61, 62]. GC mechanism of vasodilation was studied by injecting rats with nitroglycerin as the NO donor. The control group of rats had an expected level of EIDVD induced by nitroglycerin. In addition, arterial diameter increases by more than 15% of the original level indicates that GC endothelium-independent mechanism of vasodilation in healthy rats remained intact [63]. Chronic smokers' group had insufficient vasodilation after the same stimulation that indicates damages in both eNOS and GC mechanisms of vasodilation in animal smokers. Some authors believe that weaker response of vascular smooth muscle cells to nitrovasodilators might be initiated by hypoxia that exists in long-term smoking [52, 64–66].

Analysis of the constricting section in the smokers' group shows pathological vasodilation in response to L-NMMA constrictor administration and pronounced constriction after norepinephrine injection [57]. L-NMMA test allows us to evaluate consistency of adrenergic mechanisms of vascular tone regulation and endothelium-dependent vasoconstriction [57]. L-NMMA directly inhibits eNOS and indirectly inhibits inducible NOS (iNOS). Its injection helps to reduce NO production in endothelial cells and abolishes the NO-dependent dilation of vessels [67, 68].

At any specific time, vascular tone is defined by the balance of constricting and dilating influence on vascular smooth muscle cells. VRI of vasodilation in the smokers' group was 15 times lower than required (VRI for the control group is 1.88 ± 0.11; VRI for the smokers' group is 0.12 ± 0.08; $p < 0.001$) that indicates a significant damage of endothelial vasomotor function due to predominant pathological constricting reactions (**Figure 6**).

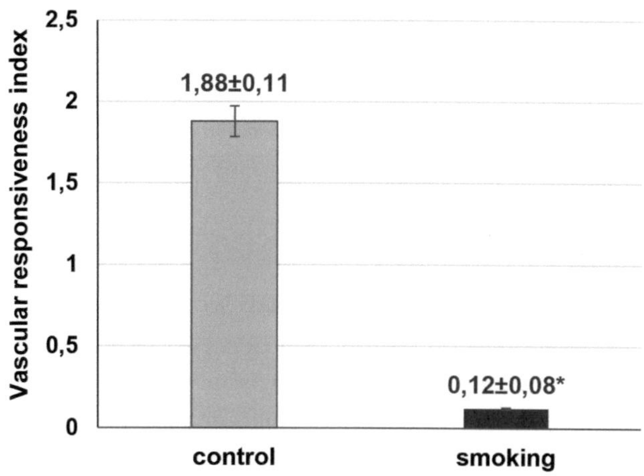

Figure 6. Vascular responsiveness index (VRI) of cerebral arteries in rats obtained by MRI scanning (chronic tobacco smoke model, experimental group, results are presented as mean ± SD, *$p < 0.05$ in comparison with the control group; t-test analysis was used to assess the differences in the values).

3. Conclusion

Endothelium initiates and modulates the main pathomorphological processes of chronic respiratory diseases. In particular, endothelium activation is an important factor of initiation, development and persistence of inflammation and vessels and tissue remodeling; it contributes to lymph circulation dysfunction and development of systemic effects. Endothelial cells of different vessels are morphologically and functionally oriented toward optimal regulation of organs' blood supply by synthesizing and releasing locally acting mediators. Pathology of endothelial cells can develop selectively: the cells are sensitive to hypoxia, tobacco smoke influence, products of inflammatory response, peroxidation, ischemic disorders, swelling and so on. Vessel remodeling usually starts as adaptation to hemodynamic changes or activity of tissue and circulating humoral factors. Long-term adaptation is replaced by vessel structure deterioration as a response to damaging factors, including toxic components of tobacco smoke and metabolites and atherogenic factors or changes of hemodynamic load. Cognitive dysfunction in cases of chronic nicotine-associated diseases is recognized by the majority of medical experts as one of the systemic symptoms of such diseases and a big medical and socioeconomic challenge. Studying the peculiarities of endothelium dysfunction caused by chronic exposure to tobacco smoke is relevant for finding a way of treating progressing cognitive deficiency and developing personalized methods of preventing acute vascular events.

Author details

Vera Nevzorova, Tatiana Brodskaya* and Natalia Zakharchuk

*Address all correspondence to: brodskaya@mail.ru

Pacific State Medical University, Vladivostok, Russia

References

[1] http://www.who.int/mediacentre/factsheets/fs339/en/

[2] How Tobacco Smoke Causes Disease: The Biology and Behavioral Basis for Smoking-Attributable Disease: A Report of the Surgeon General. Atlanta (GA): Centers for Disease Control and Prevention (US); 2010. 6, Cardiovascular Diseases. PMID: 21452462. Available from: https://www.ncbi.nlm.nih.gov/books/NBK53012/

[3] Kukovetz WR, Holzmann S, Romanin C. Mechanism of vasodilation by nitrates: Role of cyclic GMP. Cardiology 1987;**74**(Suppl 1):12-19. PMID: 2886220

[4] Benowitz NL. Pharmacology of nicotine: Addiction, smoking-induced disease, and therapeutics. Annual Review of Pharmacology and Toxicology. 2009;**49**:57-71. DOI: 10.1146/annurev.pharmtox.48.113006.094742

[5] Rabinoff M, Caskey N, Rissling A, Park C. Pharmacological and chemical effects of cigarette additives. American Journal of Public Health. 2007;**97**(11):1981-1991. DOI: 10.2105/AJPH.2005.078014

[6] Baluk P, Tammela T, Ator E, Lyubynska N, Achen MG, Hicklin DJ, Jeltsch M, Petrova TV, Pytowski B, Stacker SA, Ylä-Herttuala S, Jackson DG, Alitalo K, McDonald DM. Pathogenesis of persistent lymphatic vessel hyperplasia in chronic airway inflammation. Journal of Clinical Investigation. 2005;**115**:247-257. DOI: 10.1172/JCI22037

[7] Brodskaya TA, Nevzorova VA, Geltser BI, Motkina EV. Endothelial dysfunction and respiratory disease. Terapevticheskij arkhiv. 2007;**3**:76-84. PMID: 17526203

[8] Harkness LM, Ashton AW, Burgess JK. Asthma is not only an airway disease, but also a vascular disease. Pharmacology and Therapeutics. 2015;**148**:17-33. DOI: 10.1016/j.pharmthera.2014.11.010

[9] Pretnar-Oblak J. Cerebral endothelial function determined by cerebrovascular reactivity to L-arginine. BioMed Research International. 2014;**2014**:8. DOI: 10.1155/2014/601515

[10] Goldenberg NM, Kuebler WM. Endothelial cell regulation of pulmonary vascular tone, inflammation, and coagulation. Comprehensive Physiology. 2015;**5**(2):531-559. DOI: 10.1002/cphy.c140024

[11] Brodskaya TA, Geltser BI, Nevzorova VA. Arterial Stiffness and Respiratory Diseases (Pathophysiological Mechanisms and Clinical Significance). Vladivostok: Dalnauka; 2008. 248 p. ISBN 978-5-8044-0928-0

[12] Vukic Dugac A, Ruzic A, Samarzija M, Badovinac S, Kehler T, Jakopovic M. Persistent endothelial dysfunction turns the frequent exacerbator COPD from respiratory disorder into a progressive pulmonary and systemic vascular disease. Medical Hypotheses. 2015;**84**(2):155-158. DOI: 10.1016/j.mehy.2014.11.017

[13] Chertok VM, Kotsyuba AE. Endothelial (intimal) mechanism of cerebral hemodynamics regulation: Changing views. Pacific Medical Journal. 2012;**2**:17-26

[14] Geltser BI, Brodskaya TA, Kotelnikov VN, Agafonova IG, Lukyanov PA. Endothelial dysfunction of cerebral and major arteries during chronic obstructive disease. Experimental Biology and Medicine. 2007;**144**(6):768-771. DOI: 10.1007/s10517-007-0427-x

[15] Paulson OB, Strandgaard S, Edvinsson L. Cerebral autoregulation. Cerebrovascular and Brain Metabolism Reviews. 1990;**2**:161-192. PMID: 2201348

[16] Dodd J, Getov S, Jones P. Cognitive function in COPD. The European Respiratory Journal. 2010;**35**(4):913-922. DOI: 10.1183/09031936.00125109

[17] Singh B, Mielke M, Parsaik A, Cha R, Roberts R, Scanlon P, Geda Y, Christianson T, Pankratz S, Petersen R. A prospective study of chronic obstructive pulmonary disease and the risk for mild cognitive impairment. JAMA Neurology. 2014 May;**71**(5):581-588. DOI: 10.1001/jamaneurol.2014.94

[18] Krebs R, Tikkanen JM, Nykänen AI, Wood J, Jeltsch M, Ylä-Herttuala S, Koskinen PK, Lemström KB. Dual role of vascular endothelial growth factor in experimental obliterativ bronchiolitis. American Journal of Respiratory and Critical Care Medicine. 2005;**171**:1421-1429. DOI: 10.1164/rccm.200408-1001OC

[19] Nevzorova VA, Brodskaya TA, Golotina OV, Shekunova OI. Cardiovascular Dysfunction in Chronic Obstructive Pulmonary Disease and Ischemic Heart Disease (Functional Metabolic Parallels). Vladivostok: Dalnauka; 2015. 160 p. ISBN 978-5-8044-1548-9

[20] Van Lieshout RJ, Macqueen G. Psychological factors in asthma. Allergy, Asthma and Clinical Immunology. 2008;**4**(1):12-28. DOI: 10.1186/1710-1492-4-1-12

[21] Puranik R, Celermajer DS. Smoking and endothelial function. Progress in Cardiovascular Diseases. 2003;**45**:443-458. DOI: 10.1053/pcad.2003.YPCAD13

[22] Mahmud A, Feely J. Effect of smoking on arterial stiffness and pulse pressure. Hypertension. 2003;**41**(1):183-187. PMID: 12511550

[23] Barnoya J, Glantz SA. Cardiovascular effects of secondhand smoke: Nearly as large as smoking. Circulation. 2005;**111**(20):2684-2698. DOI: 10.1161/CIRCULATIONAHA.104.492215

[24] Guo X, Oldham MJ, Kleinman MT, Phalen RF, Kassab GS. Effect of cigarette smoking on nitric oxide, structural, and mechanical properties of mouse arteries. American Journal of Physiology. Heart and Circulatory Physiology. 2006;**291**(5):2354-2361. DOI: 10.1152/ajpheart.00376.2006

[25] Nevzorova V, Vakhrusheva S, Tilik T, Surovenko T, Brodskaya T, Isaeva M. Polymorphism of GSTP1 and EPHX1 genes in smokers and patients with I and II stages of chronic obstructive pulmonary disease. European Respiratory Journal. 2012;**40**(S56):776. DOI: 10.1183/13993003.2012.PA776

[26] Jaldin RG, Castardelli É, Perobelli JE, Yoshida WB, de Castro Rodrigues A, Sequeira JL, Paiva SA. Morphologic and biomechanical changes of thoracic and abdominal aorta in a rat model of cigarette smoke exposure. Annals of Vascular Surgery. 2013;**27**(6):791-800. DOI: 10.1016/j.avsg.2013.03.002

[27] Brady AR, Thompson SG, Fowkes FGR, Greenhalgh RM, Powell JT, UK Small Aneurysm Trial Participants. Abdominal aortic aneurysm expansion: Risk factors and time intervals for surveillance. Circulation. 2004;**110**(1):16-21. DOI: 10.1161/01.CIR.0000133279.07468.9F

[28] Wilmink TBM, Quick CRG, Day NE. The association between cigarette smoking and abdominal aortic aneurysms. Journal of Vascular Surgery. 1999;**30**(6):1099-1105

[29] Hunninghake DB. Cardiovascular disease in chronic obstructive pulmonary disease. Proceedings of the American Thoracic Society. 2005;**2**(1):44-49. DOI: 10.1513/pats.200410-050SF

[30] Sin DD, Man SFP. Chronic obstructive pulmonary disease as a risk factor for cardiovascular morbidity and mortality. The Proceedings of the American Thoracic Society. 2005;**2**: 8-11. DOI: 10.1513/pats.200404-032MS

[31] Michiel JB, Peter JK, Albert H, Jacqueline W, Monique B. Transcranial doppler hemodynamic parameters and risk of stroke: The Rotterdam study. Stroke. 2007;**38**:2453-2458. DOI: 10.1161/STROKEAHA.107.483073

[32] Grant EG, Benson CB, Moneta GL, Alexandrov AV, Baker JD, Bluth EI, Carroll BA, Eliasziw M, Gocke J, Hertzberg BS, Katanick S, Needleman L, Pellerito J, Polak JF, Rholl KS, Wooster DL, Zierler RE. Carotid artery stenosis: Gray-scale and Doppler US diagnosis —Society of Radiologists in ultrasound consensus conference. Radiology. 2003;**229**:340-346. DOI: 10.1148/radiol.2292030516

[33] Zakharchuk NV, Nevzorova VA, Chertok VM, Sarafanova NS. Effects of chronic tabacco smoking on the cerebral blood flow. Zhurnal Nevrologii i Psikhiatrii Imeni S.S. Korsakova. 2017;**117**(2):124-129. DOI: 10.17116/jnevro201711721124-129

[34] Barr RG, Ahmed FS, Carr JJ, Hoffman EA, Jiang R, Kawut SM, Watson K. Subclinical atherosclerosis, airflow obstruction and emphysema: The MESA lung study. The European Respiratory Journal. 2012;**39**:846-854. DOI: 10.1183/09031936.00165410

[35] Iwamoto H, Yokoyama A, Kitahara Y, Ishikawa N, Haruta Y, Yamane K, Hattori N, Hara H, Kohno N. Airflow limitation in smokers is associated with subclinical atherosclerosis. American Journal of Respiratory and Critical Care Medicine. 2009;**179**:35-40. DOI: 10.1164/rccm.200804-560OC

[36] Lahousse L, Bouwhuijsen Q, Loth D, Joos G, Hofman A, Witteman J, Lugt A, Brusselle G, Stricker B. Chronic obstructive pulmonary disease and lipid core carotid artery plaques in the elderly. The Rotterdam study. American Journal of Respiratory and Critical Care Medicine. 2013;**187**(1):58-64. DOI: 10.1164/rccm.201206-1046OC

[37] Chindhi S, Thakur S, Sarkar M, Negi PC. Subclinical atherosclerotic vascular disease in chronic obstructive pulmonary disease: Prospective hospital-based case control study. Lung India. 2015;**32**(2):137-141. DOI: 10.4103/0970-2113.152624

[38] Ambrosino P, Lupoli R, Cafaro G, Iervolino S, Carone M, Pappone N, Di Minno MND. Subclinical carotid atherosclerosis in patients with chronic obstructive pulmonary disease: A meta-analysis of literature studies. Annals of Medicine. 2017;**49**(6):513-524. DOI: 10.1080/07853890.2017.1311022

[39] Suwa T, Hogg JC, Quinlan KB, Ohgami A, Vincent R, van Eeden SF. Particulate air pollution induces progression of atherosclerosis. Journal of the American College of Cardiology. 2002;**39**:935-942. PMID: 11897432

[40] Kool M, Hoeks A, Struijker Boudier H, Reneman R, Van Bortel L. Short- and long-term effects of smoking on arterial wall properties in habitual smokers. Journal of the American College of Cardiology. 1993;**22**:1881-1886. DOI: 10.1016/0735-1097(93)90773-T

[41] Macnee W, Maclay J, McAllister D. Cardiovascular injury and repair in chronic obstructive pulmonary disease. Proceedings of the American Thoracic Society. 2008;**5**(8):824-833. DOI: 10.1513/pats.200807-071TH

[42] Chertok VM, Kotsyuba AE. Age-associated characteristics of vasomotor regulation of the pia mater arteries in rats. Bulletin of Experimental Biology and Medicine. 2010;**149**(3):364-368. DOI: 10.1007/s10517-010-0947-7

[43] Zakharchuk NV, Chertok VM, Nevzorova VA, Gonchar EY. Effect of chronic tobacco smoking on the tachykinin receptors distribution in the rats pial arteries. Bulletin of Experimental Biology and Medicine. 2017;**3**:290-293

[44] Alexandrin V, Alexandroff P. The model of a myogenic response of pial arterioles. Regional Haemodynamics and Microcirculation. 2003;**1**(5):73-76

[45] Moreton FC, Dani KA, Goutcher C, O'Hare K, Muir KW. Respiratory challenge MRI: Practical aspects. NeuroImage: Clinical. 2016;**11**:667-677. DOI: 10.1016/j.nicl.2016.05.003

[46] Thomas BP, Liu P, Aslan S, King KS, van Osch MJ, Lu H. Physiologic underpinnings of negative BOLD cerebrovascular reactivity in brain ventricles. NeuroImage. 2013;**83**:505-512. DOI: 10.1016/j.neuroimage.2013.07.005

[47] Demchenko I, Moskvin A, Zhiliaev S, Alekseeva O, Postnikova T, Krivchenko A. Effect of nitric oxide/endothelin interaction on hyperoxic vasoconstriction. Russian Journal of Physiology. 2011;**97**(6):609-618. PMID: 21874873

[48] Gorshkova O, Lensman M, Artem'eva A, Dvoretsky D. Dynamics of pial vessels reactivity after brief cerebral ischemia. Journal of Regional Haemodynamics and Microcirculation. 2015;**14**(1):74-78

[49] Kurth T, Kase C, Berger K, Schaeffner E, Buring J, Gaziano J. Smoking and the risk of hemorrhagic stroke in men. Stroke. 2003;**34**:1151-1155. DOI: 10.1161/01.STR.0000065200.93070.32

[50] Shinton R, Beevers G. Meta-analysis of relation between cigarette smoking and stroke. BMJ. 1989;**298**:789-794. DOI: 10.1136/bmj.298.6676.789

[51] Mazzone P, Tierney W, Hossain M, Puvenna V, Janigro D, Cucullo L. Pathophysiological impact of cigarette smoke exposure on the cerebrovascular system with a focus on the blood-brain barrier: Expanding the awareness of smoking toxicity in an underappreciated area. International Journal of Environmental Research and Public Health. 2010;**7**:4111-4126. DOI: 10.3390/ijerph7124111

[52] Papamichael CM, Aznaouridis KA, Stamatelopoulos KS, Karatzis EN, Protogerou AD, Papaioannou TG, Lekakis JP, Mavrikakis ME. Endothelial dysfunction and type of cigarette smoked: The impact of 'light' versus regular cigarette smoking. Vascular Medicine. 2004;**9**:103-105. DOI: 10.1191/1358863x04vm529oa

[53] Cao L, Zhang Y, Cao YX, Edvinsson L, Xu CB. Cigarette smoke upregulates rat coronary artery endothelin receptors in vivo. PLoS One. 2012;**7**(3):e33008. DOI: 10.1371/journal.pone.0033008

[54] Xu CB, Lei Y, Chen Q, Pehrson C, Larsson L, Edvinsson L. Cigarette smoke extracts promote vascular smooth muscle cell proliferation and enhances contractile responses in the vasculature and airway. Basic & Clinical Pharmacology & Toxicology. 2010;**107**(6):940-948. DOI: 10.1111/j.1742-7843.2010.00610.x

[55] Rahman MM, Elmi S, Chang TK, Bai N, Sallam NA, Lemos VS, Moien-Afshari F, Laher I. Increased vascular contractility in isolated vessels from cigarette smoking rats is mediated by basal endothelin release. Vascular Pharmacology. 2007;**46**:35-42. DOI: 10.1016/j.vph.2006.06.006

[56] Zheng H, Liu Y, Huang T, Fang Z, Li G, He S. Development and characterization of a rat model of chronic obstructive pulmonary disease (COPD) induced by sidestream cigarette smoke. Toxicology Letters. 2009;**189**(3):225-234. DOI: 10.1016/j.toxlet.2009.06.850

[57] Nevzorova VA, Zakharchuk NV, Agafonova IG, Belushkina TR, Gilifanov EA. Endothelium-dependent and endothelium-independent cerebral vessels reactions in a chronic smoking model. International Journal of Biomedicine. 2011;**2**:103-107

[58] Furchgott RF, Zawadzki JV. The obligatory role of endothelial cells in the relaxation of arterial smooth muscle by acetylcholine. Nature. 1980;**288**:373-376. DOI: 10.1038/288373a0

[59] Zeiher AM, Schachinger V, Minnes J. Long-term cigarette smoking impairs endothelium independent coronary arterial vasodilator function. Circulation. 1995;**92**:1094-1100. PMID: 7648652

[60] Celermajer DS, Adams MR, Clarkson P, Robinson J, McCredie R, Donald A, Deanfield JE. Passive smoking and impared endothelium-dependent arterial dilatation in healthy young adults. The New England Journal of Medicine. 1996;**334**(3):150-154. DOI: 10.1056/NEJM199601183340303

[61] Vane JR, Anggård EE, Botting RM. Regulatory functions of the vascular endothelium. New England Journal of Medicine. 1990;**323**(1):27-36. DOI: 10.1056/NEJM199007053230106

[62] Busse R, Mulsch A, Fleming I, Hecker M. Mechanisms of nitric oxide release from the vascular endothelium. Circulation. 1993;**87**(Suppl.V):18-26

[63] Marin J, Rodriges-Martinex MA. Role of vascular nitric oxide in physiological and pathological conditions. Pharmacology & Therapeutics. 1997;**75**(2):111-134. PMID: 9428001

[64] Celermajer DS, Sorensen KE, Georgakopoulos D, Bull C, Thomas O, Robinson J, Deanfield JE. Cigarette smoking is associated with dose-related and potentially reversible impairment of endothelium-dependent dilation in healthy young adults. Circulation. 1993;**88**(5 Pt 1):2149-2155. PMID: 8222109

[65] Dupuy PM, Lançon JP, Françoise M, Frostell CG. Inhaled cigarette smoke selectively reverses human hypoxic vasoconstriction. Intensive Care Medicine. 1995;**21**(11):941-944. PMID: 8636528

[66] Ferrer E, Peinado VI, Castañeda J, Prieto-Lloret J, Olea E, González-Martín MC, Vega-Agapito MV, Díez M, Domínguez-Fandos D, Obeso A, González C, Barberà JA. Effects of cigarette smoke and hypoxia on pulmonary circulation in the guinea pig. The European Respiratory Journal. 2011 Sep;**38**(3):617-627. DOI: 10.1183/09031936.00105110

[67] Repina N, Brodskaya T, Nevzorova V. Aortic stiffness in European ethnicity persons with arterial hypertension related to smoking. Journal of Hypertension. 2016;**34**(S1):e147. DOI: 10.1097/01.hjh.0000500283.43262.ea

[68] Miyazaki H, Matsuoka H, Cooke JP, Usui M, Ueda S, Okuda S, Imaizumi T. Endogenous nitric oxide synthase inhibitor: A novel marker of atherosclerosis. Circulation. 1999;**99**(9):1141-1146. PMID: 10069780

Chapter 14

Vascular Sympathetic Neurotransmission and Endothelial Dysfunction

Joana Sousa and Carmen Diniz

Additional information is available at the end of the chapter

http://dx.doi.org/10.5772/intechopen.72442

Abstract

Endothelium is an important regulator of vascular tone via release of various endothelium-derived substances. Several studies have reported that endothelium may decrease the release of noradrenaline from vascular postganglionic sympathetic nerves and thus neurogenic vasoconstriction. Endothelium derived-mediators (adenosine and NO) can modify vascular sympathetic neurotransmission and are relevant for vascular homeostasis. This is a relevant issue in terms of vascular homeostasis and, any modification, may lead to a deregulation process and to pathologies. Focus on NO-mediated effects on vascular sympathetic transmission will be done, discriminating the effects ascribed to NO generated by NO synthases located in the different vascular layers. A comparison between mesenteric/tail arteries will also be explored, particularly the relevance of the transsynaptic modulation on noradrenaline release mediated by endothelial NO and adenosine in normotensive/hypertensive vascular tissues. Adenosinergic system, namely adenosine, nucleoside transporters and adenosine receptors, can be influenced by endothelium mediators, namely by NO, causing alterations on the way these players interact with each other. In conditions where endothelium is compromised, a deregulation occurs with an increase in vascular sympathetic neurotransmission (as a consequence of adenosinergic system dynamic alteration). In summary, the impact of endothelial dysfunction on vascular neurotransmission is debated with particular focus on adenosinergic and nitroxidergic system dynamics.

Keywords: endothelium, nitric oxide, adenosine, mesenteric artery, tail artery, sympathetic neurotransmission

1. Introduction

Endothelium has been described to present key roles in the vascular physiology: various endothelium-derived endogenous substances [1], namely contracting (endothelin, prostaglandin

F2a and thromboxane A2) and/or relaxing (prostaglandin I2 and nitric oxide, NO) factors [2, 3] can modulate blood vessel tone. These substances, known as endothelium-derived contracting factors (EDCF) or endothelium-derived relaxing factor (EDRF), can modify the vascular smooth muscle tone directly, acting on smooth muscle cells, or indirectly, by altering sympathetic transmission [4]. Nevertheless, when endothelium integrity and/or function is compromised, such regulation can be impaired. Indeed, evidence suggests that endothelial dysfunction (present an altered NO production and oxidative stress) may contribute to the pathogenesis of hypertension. As a consequence, an increase in peripheral vascular resistance occurs in conditions where endothelium is somehow injured. For example, endothelium dysfunction leads to the enhancement of contractile responses to vasoconstrictor agents [2, 5–8]. Nevertheless, in the literature, there are also innumerous other factors that can also influence endothelium function and, therefore, vascular responsiveness, such as tetrahydrobiopterin (BH4), sex hormones and gender, angiotensin, insulin, vascular endothelial growth factor, vitamin D, adiponectin, uric acid, lipids, oxygen-derived free radicals, aldosterone and epithelial sodium channels.

In this chapter, the impact of endothelial dysfunction on vascular neurotransmission is debated with particular focus on adenosinergic and nitroxidergic system dynamics.

2. Endothelium and vasodilation

The vascular wall is composed of layers that can be identified by their respective morphology and by the different functions exhibited by respective cells which, ultimately, are responsible for the vascular tone, influencing blood pressure. Arteries and veins have a similar structure presenting three layers: intima or endothelium, media or smooth muscle and adventitia.

The tunica intima is the inner and thinnest layer and surrounds the lumen. It is made up of endothelial cells lining the entire vasculature and includes circular elastic bands, the internal elastic lamina. The tunica media, also called muscle layer, is composed of vascular smooth muscle, which helps regulate the size of the lumen and externally present circular elastic bands, the external elastic lamina. This tunica differs between arteries and veins: arteries contain more smooth muscle than the tunica media of their counterpart, the veins, and this allows arteries to constrict and dilate to adjust the volume of blood needed by the tissues that they support. Additionally, the structure of arteries differs between large arteries and resistant arteries: in the first type, arteries present a media with large amount of elastic fibers disposed between smooth muscle cells and the thickness of the vascular wall is thinner than that exhibited by resistant arteries that often have multiple strands of smooth muscle layers. The external layer, adventitia layer is composed of connective tissue allowing the blood vessel to withstand forces acting on the vessel wall and of collagen fibers that anchor the vessel to surrounding tissues.

The endothelium can evoke effects, dilation or contraction of the underlying vascular smooth muscle, by releasing endothelium-derived relaxing factors (EDRF) such as NO or endothelium-derived contracting factors (EDCF) such as endothelin or prostanoids.

2.1. NO effects on vasodilation and endothelial dysfunction

NO is a well-known EDRF that induces vasodilation through the activation of soluble guanylyl cyclase in the vascular smooth muscle cells producing cyclic guanosine monophosphate (therefore, through the signaling pathway that can be represented as NO-cGMP/cGMP-dependent kinases).

It is well accepted that the benefits of NO released from endothelium are compromised in vascular diseases and aging since there is a reduced amount of NO. However, evidence also show that the production of NO can be upregulated, for example, by estrogens, exercise and dietary factors and downregulated by oxidative stress, smoking, pollution and oxidized low-density lipoproteins.

Moreover, when endothelium is dysfunctional, the vasodilation induced by endothelial mediators is impaired and it can even lead to vascular smooth muscle cells contraction. For instance, in aged subjects and in vascular diseases (essential hypertension and diabetes) when the production of NO is compromised, endothelium-dependent contractions are intensified.

NO is produced by three isoforms of NO synthase, presenting a more general distribution in the human body than that initially predicted: neuronal NOS (nNOS), inducible NOS (iNOS) and endothelial NOS (eNOS). nNOS is constitutively expressed in central and peripheral nervous system contributing to regulation of blood pressure, smooth muscle dilation and vasodilation via peripheral nitrergic nerves. iNOS is expressed in several cell types and generates large amounts of NO, which is involved in the pathophysiology of inflammatory diseases, as regulatory effector molecule of the innate immune response and septic shock. eNOS is expressed mainly in endothelial cells and has several vasoprotective and anti-atherosclerotic effects as well as an important role in vascular tone and thus blood pressure regulation.

Many cardiovascular risk factors lead to oxidative stress, eNOS uncoupling and endothelial dysfunction in the vasculature. eNOS generates NO which results from the activity of two domains, the oxygenase domain that convert L-arginine to L-citrulline plus NO and the reductase domain that convert nitrites to NO [9].

As mentioned above, NO production from endothelium can be upregulated or downregulated by a number of factors of which vascular endothelial growth factor (VEGF) can upregulate eNOS. Interestingly, a chronic side effect of VEGF inhibitors is the occurrence of hypertension, suggesting a physiological role for VEGF in maintaining endothelial control of vasomotor tone [10–12]. In humans, in hypertension, VEGF inhibitors may cause increased production of endothelin-1 [13, 14] and reduced vascular response to acetylcholine [15, 16].

Acute and chronic increases in flow as well as the resulting augmentation in shear stress of the blood on the endothelial cells can be altered through Ca^{2+}-dependent and Ca^{2+}-independent pathways. It has been described that Ca^{2+}-independent pathway can increase both the expression and activity of eNOS and thus the release of NO [17]. The role played by the endothelial cells to protect against thrombin and other platelet products by increasing the activity of eNOS has been demonstrated both *in vitro* [18–26] and *in vivo* [27]. Serotonin and adenosine diphosphate are mediators released by aggregating platelets, which may activate eNOS and increase NO production. When endothelium is absent/dysfunctional, vasodilation is no longer observed, and aggregating platelets induce contractions, because they release vasoconstrictors (thromboxane A2 and serotonin). When platelet aggregation occurs in a healthy artery (i.e, with an intact and physiologically active endothelium), serotonin (and ADP) release by the platelets as well as production of thrombin will increase NO release from endothelial cells. Thus, NO will be increased in the vicinity of smooth muscle cells inducing dilation, and consequently, increasing blood flow.

Another important factor influencing NO production relies on the presence of reactive oxygen/nitrogen species (ROS/RNS). Indeed, several enzymes from endothelium can produce superoxide anions such as nicotinamide adenine dinucleotide phosphate oxidase (NOX), xanthine oxidase (XO), cyclooxygenases (COX) and also eNOS but only when there is a deficient supply of substrate or of the cofactor BH4. Under pathophysiological conditions, superoxide anions scavenge NO resulting in the formation of peroxynitrite, reducing considerably the bioavailability of NO. Moreover, ROS can inactivate eNOS through S-glutathionylation. Taken together, these may explain why oxidative stress is often associated with endothelial dysfunction.

Moreover, intake of a number of natural products, such as flavonoids and other polyphenols, favors endothelium-dependent dilations and protects endothelium from dysfunction through increased production of NO. The protective effects of polyphenols against endothelial dysfunction involve increased production of NO in response to endothelium-derived vasodilators resulting from: facilitation of the effects of NO on the vascular smooth muscle cells, increased levels of BH4, calcium-independent phosphorylation of eNOS, antioxidant properties preventing the uncoupling of eNOS, activation of estrogen receptors and upregulation of AMP-activated protein kinase (AMPK) and of NAD(+)-dependent deacetylase (SIRT1) [28–31].

2.2. Influence of NO on another EDRF

Besides its direct role as a vasodilator, NO also modulates the release of other endothelium-derived mediators. Thus, in a number of larger arteries, endothelium-derived hyperpolarization (EDH)-mediated dilations become prominent only when the synthesis of NO is inhibited [32, 33]. Hence, EDH is able to take over, at least temporarily, in the case of 'classical' endothelial dysfunction associated with a loss of NO synthesis, demonstrating strong compensatory efficiency of EDH-mediated responses. Intriguingly, exogenous NO attenuates EDH-mediated responses in coronary arteries *in vitro* [34] and in coronary circulation *in vivo* [35, 36]. Moreover, NO has been shown to exert a negative feedback effect on endothelium-dependent dilation through cGMP-mediated desensitization in isolated coronary arteries [32]. Indeed, clinical studies show that chronic therapy with nitrate, used as a NO donor, in patients with ischemic heart disease does not yield a benefit on mortality [37, 38], confirming the importance of the physiological balance between NO and EDH. Moreover, the amount of NO formed in the endothelial cells controls the release of vasoconstrictor prostanoids [39, 40].

3. Endothelium and sympathetic neurotransmission

The sympathetic nervous system (SNS) is known to play a fundamental role in the short- and long-term regulation of different vascular functions. Vessels contain sympathetic nerves distributed between smooth muscle and adventitia layers [41]. Sympathetic nerve fibers are enveloped in Schwann cells: most nerve fibers travel through individual channels in the Schwann cell, but small fibers are sometimes bundled together within a single channel [42]. The SNS signals to dilate or constrict the vessel, changing the lumen size, i.e., regulating vascular tone and, therefore, affecting blood pressure.

Nowadays, it is well established that SNS contributes to the modulation of vascular function and that this relationship is a key factor in the development of cardiovascular diseases. Several factors, such as the renin-angiotensin system, NO, ROS and endothelin, influence this modulation at central and peripheral level [43–45]. Moreover, endothelial function also seems to be regulated by SNS, mainly in the control of vascular tone. Additionally, endothelial dysfunction as well as increase in sympathetic activity has been associated to cardiovascular risk factors and disease. For example, in studies carried out in healthy subjects, an increase in sympathetic activity was associated with a decrease in endothelial function [46] Moreover, in humans, stiffness of large artery was also associated with an increased activity of SNS [47]. On the other hand, large artery stiffness can interfere with autonomic regulation by impairing carotid baroreflex sensitivity [48].

The influence of endothelium in noradrenaline release has also been previously demonstrated [49, 50]. This conclusion was obtained not only in arteries without endothelium but also in a model of endothelial dysfunction (i.e, essential hypertensive arteries), which is shown in **Table 1**. This type of information can be obtained from experiments where synapse events are mimicked allowing the evaluation of putative players able to alter neurotransmitter release from the nerves. Indeed, in such experiments, the use of selective pharmacological tools, such as agonists/antagonists of receptors or of activators/inhibitors of proteins or enzymes, can reveal their respective role in the neurotransmission dynamic. For instance, in experiments where rat vascular tissues, preincubated with [^{3}H]-noradrenaline, are electrically stimulated (5 Hz, 100 pulses, 1 ms, 50 mA), the release of ^{3}H is induced (which mimics a physiological depolarization) and can be measured by liquid scintillation spectrometry. In addition, by altering the receptors or proteins activated (with pharmacological tools), it is possible to evaluate the activity/role of a specific player in neurotransmitter release (please see previous articles from our group where the methodology is described in detail [49, 51, 52]). For example, in **Table 1**, data refer to tissues that were stimulated twice at 30-min interval: outflow (b_n) refers to the 5-min period immediately before each stimulation period. The electrically evoked tritium overflow (S_n) was calculated by subtracting the estimated basal outflow from total outflow observed during and in the 25-min period subsequent to S_1 and expressed as a percentage of the tissue ^{3}H content at the onset of stimulation. Two animal models have been used: spontaneously hypertensive rats (SHR), a well-established model of essential hypertension [53, 54], and the respective controls, the Wistar Kyoto (WKY) rats. Moreover, in WKY animals, some arteries were endothelium denuded. The influence of these conditions on the release of S_1 was evaluated, and the results are presented in **Table 1**.

The results in this table show that the outflow observed in the endothelium-denuded vascular tissue is lower than that obtained in intact tissue. Also, the S_2 values obtained in the endothelium-denuded arteries are altered, with values higher than those observed in intact tissues. These data reveal the importance of a healthy endothelium to the sympathetic neurotransmission homeostasis, once it seems to present a transsynaptic influence mediated by endothelium. In pathological conditions, this influence can be impaired augmenting the amount of noradrenaline release and causing vasoconstriction.

	Basal outflow (b_1) (fractional rate of outflow; min^{-1})	Evoked Overflow (S_1) (% of tissue tritium content)	S_2/S_1	n
Mesenteric artery				
WKY				
Endothelium intact	0.065 ± 0.004	0.202 ± 0.016	1.054 ± 0.038	12
Endothelium denuded	0.081 ± 0.002*	0.329 ± 0.036*	1.002 ± 0.026	12
SHR				
Endothelium intact	0.073 ± 0.003*	0.310 ± 0.041*	1.013 ± 0.031	10
Tail artery				
WKY				
Endothelium intact	0.084 ± 0.004	0.217 ± 0.012	0.932 ± 0.037	18
Endothelium denuded	0.069 ± 0.002*	0.317 ± 0.049*	0.929 ± 0.039	14
SHR				
Endothelium intact	0.063 ± 0.002*	0.259 ± 0.016*	1.034 ± 0.096	14

Tissue preparations of mesenteric and tail arteries from WKY and SHR animals were pre-incubated with [^{3}H]-noradrenaline for 40 min. After pre-incubation with [^{3}H]-noradrenaline, tissues were superfused with [^{3}H]-noradrenaline free medium containing desipramine (400 nM). Values presented are means ± SEM, and n denotes the number of tissue preparations. Significant differences from WKY intact arteries: $^*P < 0.05$.

Table 1. Basal tritium outflow (b_1), electrically evoked tritium overflow (S_1) and S_2/S_1 ratios from normotensive (WKY) and hypertensive (SHR) vessels of the rat.

Several substances produced in endothelial cells, such as NO, adenosine, ROS and/or RNS (e.g. peroxides, superoxide, hydroxyl radical, and singlet oxygen) and prostaglandins can influence sympathetic transmission [55, 56]. Also, the activity of some enzymes, such as adenosine kinase, adenosine deaminase, NOX, XO and COX, can be altered leading to changes in the bioavailability of their respective products, influencing, indirectly, sympathetic neurotransmission.

3.1. NO and vascular neurotransmission

There is evidence demonstrating that NO can modulate sympathetic neurotransmission modifying vascular smooth muscle tone, in various vascular beds, such as in coronary [57, 58], mesenteric [50, 59, 60] and pulmonary arteries [61–63]. Indeed, and as illustrated in **Figure 1**, a NO donor, DEA-NONOATE (10 μM) altered noradrenaline release (measured as explained above, i.e., by determining the amount of ^{3}H overflow using liquid scintillation spectrometry) in differential mode depending on the vascular territory: an increase of noradrenaline release occurs in tail artery contrasting to mesenteric territory where noradrenaline release is reduced.

Another relevant data are related with NO source, i.e., the type of NOS that generates NO (**Figure 1**): in tail arteries, NO production is ascribed mainly to eNOS isoform, particularly to

http://dx.doi.org/10.5772/intechopen.72442

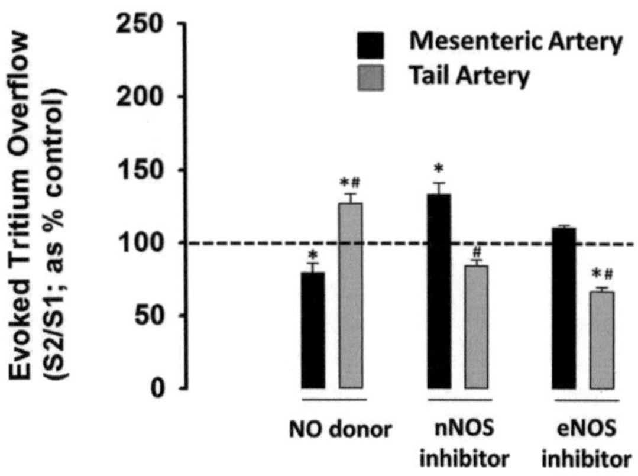

Figure 1. Influence of NOS inhibitors on vascular sympathetic transmission in mesenteric and tail rat arteries. Effect elicited by the NO donor, DEA-NONOate (10 μM), and the interaction exerted by the Nω-propyl-L-arginine hydrochloride, a specific neuronal NOS (nNOS) inhibitor (100 nM), and L-NIO dihydrochloride, a specific endothelial NOS (eNOS) inhibitor (500 nM), on the electrically evoked tritium overflow. Values are mean ± SEM from 5 to 12 artery segments. Significant differences from the appropriate control: $^{*}P < 0.05$ and from mesenteric artery: $^{\#}P < 0.05$ (ANOVA followed by post-hoc Holm-Sidak's multicomparisons t-test).

eNOS oxygenase domain with residual activity of the eNOS reductase domain [50], while in mesenteric arteries, nNOS, with both reductase and oxygenase domains being equally active, seems to be the most relevant isoform producing NO.

These differences in vascular neurotransmission elicited by NO can be explained by the activation of different pathways, leading to opposite outcomes. In resistant arteries, such as tail artery, the well-established NO-cGMP/cGMP-dependent kinases activating voltage-dependent-Ca^{2+} seem to be the predominant pathway [64], leading to vasoconstriction. However, in other vascular territories, such as the mesenteric artery, NO actions, in addition to the classically accepted activation of intracellular cGMP-dependent pathway [65], can also activate cGMP-independent pathways, namely by eliciting an energy decrease in mitochondria (i.e., ATP), particularly with an increase in ATP catabolism, with subsequent adenosine accumulation. Adenosine will then act on presynaptic A_1 receptors causing a reduction in cAMP formation and, consequently, of PKA. Therefore, a reduction of Ca^{2+} channels phosphorylation (by PKA) will occur reducing the intracellular amount of Ca^{2+}. Presynaptically, the amount of intracellular Ca^{2+} is critical for neurotransmission; therefore, lower amounts of calcium will cause a reduction of noradrenaline release and of the postsynaptic signal events triggered by noradrenaline, leading to vasodilation [66].

The location of enzyme isoforms is also relevant: nNOS in mesenteric arteries are located mostly in Schwann cells contrasting to tail arteries where their presence is very scarce (**Figure 2**).

3.2. Adenosine, endothelium and vascular neurotransmission

It is well established that adenosine can act as a physiological neuromodulator through activation of four types of adenosine receptors, A_1, A_{2A}, A_{2B} and A_3 in the vasculature [67]. These receptors present differential affinities for adenosine, with adenosine A_1 receptor requiring lower concentrations to get activated (KdA_1, 0.3–3 nM), followed by A_{2A} receptors with a Kd

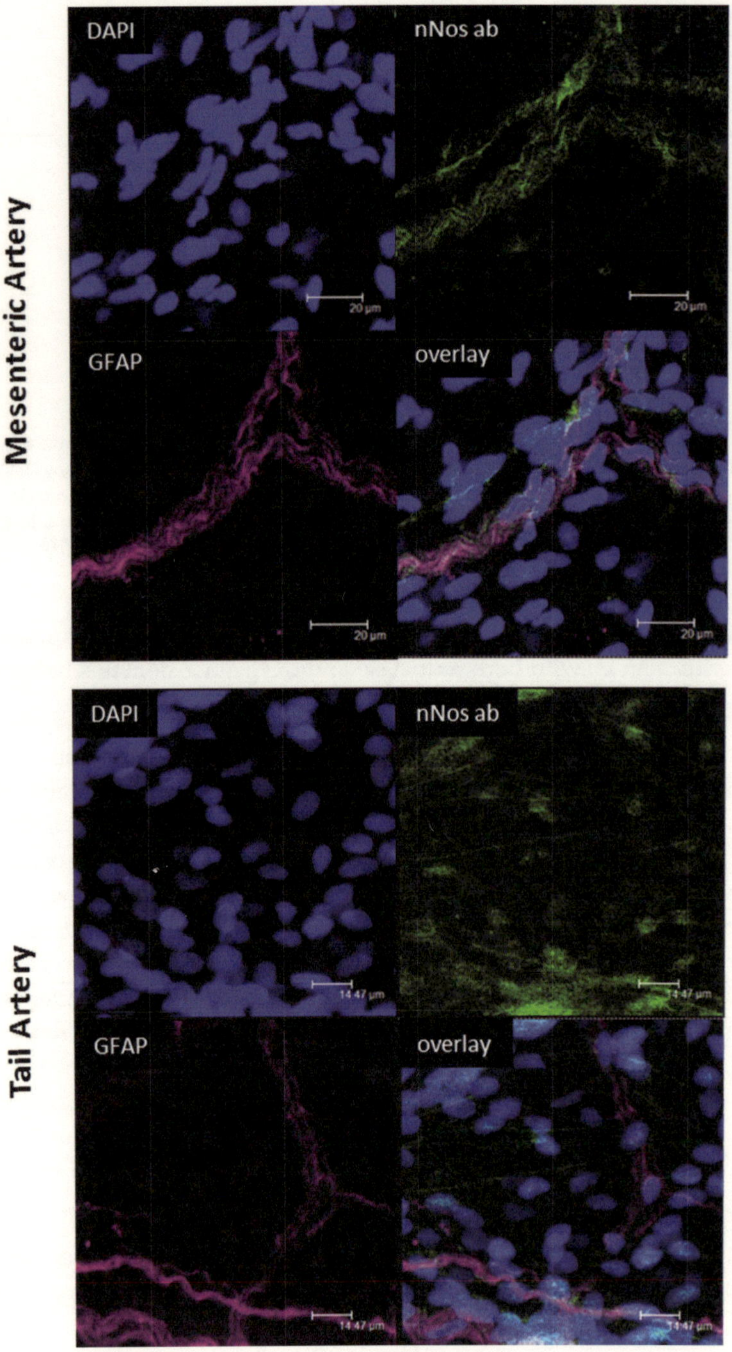

Figure 2. Adventitia mesenteric and tail rat arteries images. Images are representative reconstructions captured with a confocal microscope (Leica SP5 LSCM system fitted with an inverted microscope (x63 oil immersion lens). Stacks of 1-µm-thick serial optical images. Arteries were stained for nNOS (a primary mouse monoclonal anti-NOS1 and a species-specific secondary Alexa 488 antibody), GFAP (a primary rabbit anti-GFAP polyclonal antibody and a species-specific secondary Alexa 647 antibody) and DAPI (nuclear stain).

1–20 nM. Pharmacological studies have also revealed that A_{2B} and A_3 receptors are low affinity receptors for adenosine requiring concentrations higher than 1 μM, although these adenosine receptor subtypes present different Kd (A_3 subtype requires higher concentrations than A_{2B} receptors) [68].

Adenosine, a well-known nucleoside, results from the sequential catabolism of ATP, forming ADP, AMP and adenosine with this later step being mediated by 5′-nucleotidase. Adenosine can then be further converted in inosine by adenosine deaminase or, instead, can be reconverted to AMP by adenosine kinase. In addition to adenosine receptors and adenosine, adenosinergic system is also composed by nucleoside transporters (NTs), which are responsible for nucleoside transport into the cells and vice versa. Some of the NTs in particular some equilibrative nucleoside transporters (ENT)s have already been identified as capable of promoting adenosine transport in vasculature, namely the subtype ENT1 and ENT 4 [69, 70].

In vascular tissues as well as in some diseased states, such as hypertension, the bioavailability of adenosine varies [71], as presented in **Table 2**.

The amount of adenosine present in the vicinity of adenosine receptors depends on the adenosinergic system dynamics which, in turn, can be influenced by innumerous factors, such as NO, ROS, lipid peroxidation, endothelium dysfunction, etc., that can be altered in several pathological conditions, namely in hypertension, diabetes, aging and inflammation.

Another factor related with the relevance of vascular adenosine-mediated effects relies on adenosine receptor subtype distribution in the vasculature. All adenosine receptor subtypes have been identified not only in arteries, such as pulmonary [72], mesenteric [73–77], ear [73], aorta [78] and tail [51, 52, 79–81], but also in veins [75, 82]. In renal vessels, a role of adenosine receptors in sympathetic regulation was also demonstrated [83], conditioning the blood efflux

	Basal outflow (b_1) (pmol/mg of tissue)	Evoked overflow (S_1) (pmol/mg of tissue)	n
Mesenteric artery			
WKY	25.74 ± 2.57	26.47 ± 2.76	5
SHR	75.44 ± 4.22*	77.31 ± 5.47*	5
Tail artery			
WKY	45.64 ± 3.81	49.78 ± 5.29	5
SHR	64.81 ± 5.01*	67.82 ± 4.03*	5

Tissue preparations of mesenteric and tail arteries from WKY and SHR animals were superfused with Krebs-Henseleit. Tissues were stimulated twice at 30-min interval (S_1–S_2; 100 pulses, 5 Hz, 1 ms, 50 mA): b_1 refers to the 5-min period immediately before S_1. The superfusate was collected in 5-min period before and after stimulation, and each sample was heated at 80°C and derivatized using chloroacetaldehyde for 50 min at 70°C in a dry bath incubator. Identification of the ε-adenosine formed in this collected samples was confirmed by a gradient HPLC using a fluorescent detector at 230 nm excitation and 420 nm emission wavelengths. Values presented are means ± SEM of adenosine per mg of tissue, and n denotes the number of tissue preparations. Significant differences from WKY vessels: $^*P < 0.05$.

Table 2. Basal (b_1) and electrically evoked (S_1) adenosine release from sympathetic nerve terminals from normotensive (WKY) and hypertensive (SHR) vessels of the rat.

in the afferent arteriole and, consequently, of renal filtration. In hypertensive arteries and veins, an impairment of the neuromodulation exerted by adenosine A_1 receptors [75–77, 82] was described, contrasting with a preserved adenosine A_{2A} receptor-mediated facilitation of noradrenaline release [75–77]. Note that a redistribution of adenosine A_1 receptors from sympathetic nerves to Schwann cells was reported in hypertensive state while adenosine A_{2A} receptors, in sympathetic nerves, were preserved [77]. Particular relevant information relies on the location of adenosine receptors on the vascular wall layers contributing to the understanding of the functional role ascribed to adenosine receptors.

In endothelium, the four adenosine receptor subtypes have been identified by functional and immunohistochemical assays, for instance in tail artery [80, 84] and aorta [84, 85]. The influence of endothelium in adenosine-mediated responses has been demonstrated, with endogenous adenosine inducing an inhibition on noradrenaline release, through activation of adenosine A_1 receptors, (**Figure 3**, effect of DPCPX, a selective A_1 receptor antagonist). Adenosine availability is a crucial factor (effect demonstrated by pentostatin and α,β-methylene ADP, which inhibit adenosine deaminase and ecto-5′nucleotidase, respectively), conditioning the type of adenosine receptor that is activated. In resistant arteries, this effect is impaired when endothelium is compromised (arteries denuded of endothelium or in essential hypertensive arteries) and, instead, a facilitatory effect mediated by adenosine A_{2A} receptors, revealed by a selective A_{2A} receptor antagonist, the SCH 58261, and by inhibition of adenosine kinase, revealed by an adenosine kinase inhibitor, 5′-iodotubercidin (ITU), and by ecto-5′nucleotidase inhibitor, α,β-methylene ADP, demonstrating the relevance of adenosinergic dynamics both in physiological and pathophysiological contexts, such as in hypertension [49]. The adenosinergic system dynamic is adjusted to the unfavorable conditions created by endothelium injury, with enzymes involved in adenosine formation, such as adenosine deaminase and 5′-nucleotidase operating to promote an increase in the adenosine amount available and favoring the activation of A_{2A} receptors. This occurs despite the efforts of nucleoside transporters to equilibrate the concentration of adenosine between the inner and outer space of cells. In mesenteric arteries, A_{2A} receptor effect is enough to counteract the existing inhibitory tonus mediated by adenosine A_1, but in resistant arteries, the facilitatory effect mediated by A_{2A} receptors (upon noradrenaline release) predominates.

3.3. Interplay between nitroxidergic and other pathways in neurotransmission

NO signaling events, in mesenteric arteries, cause an accumulation of adenosine (as previously described in Section 3.1). This condition may favor adenosine neuromodulation, namely by activation of adenosine A_1 receptors (which is revealed when blockade of A_1 receptors occurs in the presence of the NO donor, DEA-NONOATE; **Figure 4**) in the mesenteric artery. Activation of A_1 receptors leads to a reduction of noradrenaline release, and subsequently, the activation of α_1-adrenoceptors in vascular smooth muscle cells is reduced, leading to vasodilation. In the tail artery, such interplay does not occur, at least in the experimental conditions tested.

The interplay between nitroxidergic and adenosinergic pathways can occur in neurotransmission, with NO promoting the formation of enough amounts of adenosine capable of activating inhibitory A_1 receptors. However, this type of interplay is dependent on the type of vascular bed.

http://dx.doi.org/10.5772/intechopen.72442

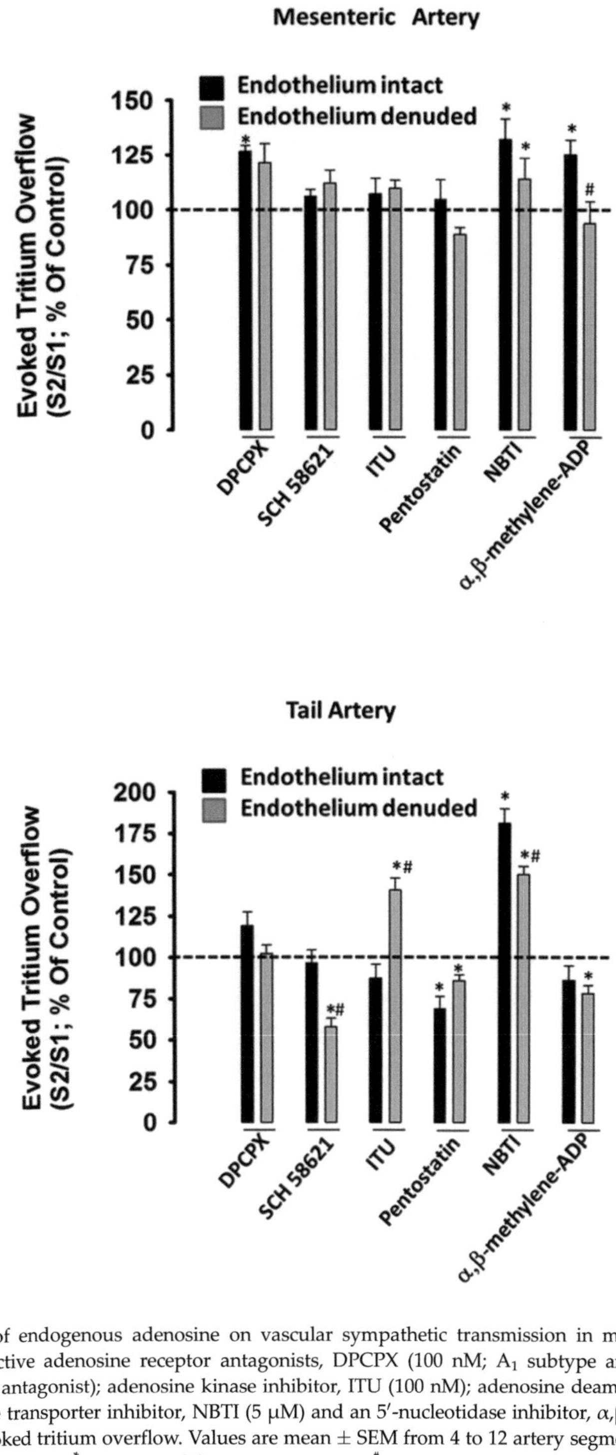

Figure 3. Influence of endogenous adenosine on vascular sympathetic transmission in mesenteric and tail arteries. Interaction with selective adenosine receptor antagonists, DPCPX (100 nM; A_1 subtype antagonist) and SCH 58261 (20 nM; A_{2A} subtype antagonist); adenosine kinase inhibitor, ITU (100 nM); adenosine deaminase inhibitor, Pentostatin (10 μM); a nucleoside transporter inhibitor, NBTI (5 μM) and an 5′-nucleotidase inhibitor, α,β-methylene-ADP (10 μM), on the electrically evoked tritium overflow. Values are mean ± SEM from 4 to 12 artery segments. Significant differences from the appropriate control: $^{*}P < 0.05$ and from intact arteries: $^{\#}P < 0.05$ (ANOVA followed by post-hoc Holm-Sidak's multicomparisons t-test).

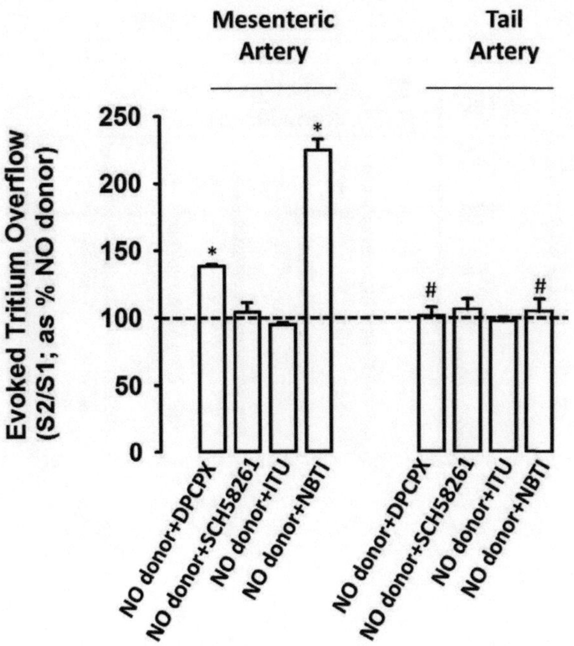

Figure 4. Influence of adenosine A_1 receptor antagonist (DPCPX, 100 nM) and adenosine A_{2A} receptor antagonist (SCH 58261, 20 nM), adenosine kinase inhibitor (ITU, 100 nM) and nucleoside transporter inhibitor (NBTI, 5 μM) in the effect elicited by a nitric oxide donor, DEA-NONOate (10 μM) on the electrically evoked tritium overflow, in mesenteric and tail arteries. Values are mean ± SEM from 4 to 12 artery segments. Significant differences from DEA-NONOate effect alone: $^*P < 0.05$ and from mesenteric artery: $^\#P < 0.05$ (ANOVA followed by post-hoc Holm-Sidak's multicomparisons t-test).

Furthermore, in the cardiovascular system, NO can also interplay with the adrenergic pathway. NO source is, most probably, endothelial since noradrenaline release in the presence of a β-adrenoceptor agonist, isoprenaline (300 nM), caused an increase of noradrenaline release (175.10 ± 13.8%, n = 11), but the increase observed was lower in endothelium-denuded arteries (129.92 ± 13.1%, n = 7). Therefore, these data support the possibility, previously raised by Balligand et al. [86] and by Conti et al. [87], that NO production can lead to an increase in noradrenaline release, as a consequence of adrenergic receptors activation, namely of facilitatory β-adrenoceptors.

4. Current and future developments

In addition to the direct effects exerted by several substances on smooth muscle cells, which can cause vasodilation or vasoconstriction, the evidence that endothelium-derived factors can also influence sympathetic neurotransmission that reinforces the importance of endothelium and of its putative role in pathologies. Indeed, vascular sympathetic neurotransmission and the interplay exerted by endothelium-derived substances are, therefore, relevant in the homeostasis of vascular tone. In pathophysiological conditions, especially when endothelium is injured, their impact on neurotransmission account, at least in part, for the occurring vasoconstriction.

http://dx.doi.org/10.5772/intechopen.72442

NO has been viewed as a vasodilator substance since its direct effect on vascular smooth muscle cells causes dilation. However, NO can influence neurotransmission, and the interplay with adenosinergic and adrenergic pathways altering neurotransmission can, in some cases, cause an increase in noradrenaline release, which consequently will promote vasoconstriction. Therefore, the importance of NO is renewed as well as its ability to interplay with other signaling pathways involving sympathetic regulation such as the adrenergic and adenosinergic ones. Additional information and research on this field are, therefore, required to extend the knowledge on the insights of transsynaptic modulation of vascular neurotransmission. This is particularly important and can be useful to develop new therapeutic strategies, particularly in pathologies or clinical conditions, where the sympathetic system is hyperactivated.

Acknowledgements

This work received financial support from FCT, Fundação para a Ciência e Tecnologia) through project UID/QUI/50006/2013–POCI/01/0145/FEDER/007265 with financial support from FCT/MEC through national funds and co-financed by FEDER, under the Partnership Agreement PT2020. PhD grant [SFRH/BD//2009] supported by FCT. Authors would like to thank Professors Silvia M. Arribas and Maria Carmen González from Department of Physiology, School of Medicine, University Autónoma de Madrid, Spain, for their assistance in the use of the Confocal Microscopy.

Author details

Joana Sousa[1,2] and Carmen Diniz[1,2]*

*Address all correspondence to: cdiniz@ff.up.pt

1 LAQV/REQUIMTE, Faculty of Pharmacy, University of Porto, Portugal

2 Laboratory of Pharmacology, Department of Drug Science, Faculty of Pharmacy, University of Porto, Portugal

References

[1] Furchgott RF, Zawadzki JV. The obligatory role of endothelial cells in the relaxation of arterial smooth muscle by acetylcholine. Nature. 1980;**288**:373-376

[2] Moncada S, Palmer RM, Higgs EA. Nitric oxide: Physiology, pathophysiology, and pharmacology. Pharmacological Reviews. 1991;**43**:109-142

[3] Vanhoutte PM, Mombouli JV. Vascular endothelium: Vasoactive mediators. Progress in Cardiovascular Diseases. 1996;**39**:229-238

[4] Westcott EB, Segal SS. Perivascular innervation: A multiplicity of roles in vasomotor control and myoendothelial signaling. Microcirculation. 2013;**20**:217-238

[5] Stankevicius E, Kevelaitis E, Vainorius E, Simonsen U. Role of nitric oxide and other endothelium-derived factors. Medicina (Kaunas, Lithuania). 2003;**39**:333-341

[6] Torok J. Participation of nitric oxide in different models of experimental hypertension. Physiological Research. 2008;**57**:813-825

[7] Vanhoutte PM. Endothelial dysfunction: The first step toward coronary arteriosclerosis. Circulation Journal. 2009;**73**:595-601

[8] Vanhoutte PM, Shimokawa H, Tang EH, Feletou M. Endothelial dysfunction and vascular disease. Acta Physiologica (Oxford, England). 2009;**196**:193-222

[9] Gautier C, van Faassen E, Mikula I, Martasek P, Slama-Schwok A. Endothelial nitric oxide synthase reduces nitrite anions to NO under anoxia. Biochemical and Biophysical Research Communications. 2006;**341**:816-821

[10] Facemire CS, Nixon AB, Griffiths R, Hurwitz H, Coffman TM. Vascular endothelial growth factor receptor 2 controls blood pressure by regulating nitric oxide synthase expression. Hypertension. 2009;**54**:652-658

[11] Hou HH, Hammock BD, Su KH, Morisseau C, Kou YR, Imaoka S, Oguro A, Shyue SK, Zhao JF, Lee TS. N-terminal domain of soluble epoxide hydrolase negatively regulates the VEGF-mediated activation of endothelial nitric oxide synthase. Cardiovascular Research. 2012;**93**:120-129

[12] Skinner M, Philp K, Lengel D, Coverley L, Lamm Bergstrom E, Glaves P, Musgrove H, Prior H, Braddock M, Huby R, Curwen JO, Duffy P, Harmer AR. The contribution of VEGF signalling to fostamatinib-induced blood pressure elevation. British Journal of Pharmacology. 2014;**171**:2308-2320

[13] Kappers MH, de Beer VJ, Zhou Z, Danser AH, Sleijfer S, Duncker DJ, van den Meiracker AH, Merkus D. Sunitinib-induced systemic vasoconstriction in swine is endothelin mediated and does not involve nitric oxide or oxidative stress. Hypertension. 2012;**59**:151-157

[14] Lankhorst S, Kappers MH, van Esch JH, Danser AH, van den Meiracker AH. Hypertension during vascular endothelial growth factor inhibition: Focus on nitric oxide, endothelin-1, and oxidative stress. Antioxidants & Redox Signaling. 2014;**20**:135-145

[15] Thijs AM, van Herpen CM, Sweep FC, Geurts-Moespot A, Smits P, van der Graaf WT, Rongen GA. Role of endogenous vascular endothelial growth factor in endothelium-dependent vasodilation in humans. Hypertension. 2013;**61**:1060-1065

[16] Mayer EL, Dallabrida SM, Rupnick MA, Redline WM, Hannagan K, Ismail NS, Burstein HJ, Beckman JA. Contrary effects of the receptor tyrosine kinase inhibitor vandetanib on constitutive and flow-stimulated nitric oxide elaboration in humans. Hypertension. 2011;**58**:85-92

[17] Vanhoutte PM, Shimokawa H, Feletou M, Tang EH. Endothelial dysfunction and vascular disease - A 30th anniversary update. Acta Physiologica (Oxford, England). 2017;**219**:22-96

[18] De Mey JG, Claeys M, Vanhoutte PM. Endothelium-dependent inhibitory effects of acetylcholine, adenosine triphosphate, thrombin and arachidonic acid in the canine femoral artery. The Journal of Pharmacology and Experimental Therapeutics. 1982;**222**:166-173

[19] Cohen RA, Shepherd JT, Vanhoutte PM. Inhibitory role of the endothelium in the response of isolated coronary arteries to platelets. Science. 1983;**221**:273-274

[20] Cohen RA, Shepherd JT, Vanhoutte PM. Vasodilatation mediated by the coronary endothelium in response to aggregating platelets. Bibliotheca Cardiologica. 1984;**38**:35-42

[21] Houston DS, Shepherd JT, Vanhoutte PM. Adenine nucleotides, serotonin, and endothelium-dependent relaxations to platelets. The American Journal of Physiology. 1985;**248**:H389-H395

[22] Houston DS, Shepherd JT, Vanhoutte PM. Aggregating human platelets cause direct contraction and endothelium-dependent relaxation of isolated canine coronary arteries. Role of serotonin, thromboxane A2, and adenine nucleotides. The Journal of Clinical Investigation. 1986;**78**:539-544

[23] Shimokawa H, Kim P, Vanhoutte PM. Endothelium-dependent relaxation to aggregating platelets in isolated basilar arteries of control and hypercholesterolemic pigs. Circulation Research. 1988;**63**:604-612

[24] Derkach DN, Ihara E, Hirano K, Nishimura J, Takahashi S, Kanaide H. Thrombin causes endothelium-dependent biphasic regulation of vascular tone in the porcine renal interlobar artery. British Journal of Pharmacology. 2000;**131**:1635-1642

[25] Motley ED, Eguchi K, Patterson MM, Palmer PD, Suzuki H, Eguchi S. Mechanism of endothelial nitric oxide synthase phosphorylation and activation by thrombin. Hypertension. 2007;**49**:577-583

[26] Touyz RM. Regulation of endothelial nitric oxide synthase by thrombin. Hypertension. 2007;**49**:429-431

[27] Shimokawa H, Vanhoutte PM. Angiographic demonstration of hyperconstriction induced by serotonin and aggregating platelets in porcine coronary arteries with regenerated endothelium. Journal of the American College of Cardiology. 1991;**17**:1197-1202

[28] Bieganska-Hensoldt S, Rosolowska-Huszcz D. Polyphenols in preventing endothelial dysfunction. Post®py Higieny i Medycyny Doświadczalnej (Online). 2017;**71**:227-235

[29] Perez-Vizcaino F, Duarte J, Andriantsitohaina R. Endothelial function and cardiovascular disease: Effects of quercetin and wine polyphenols. Free Radical Research. 2006;**40**:1054-1065

[30] Perez-Vizcaino F, Duarte J. Flavonols and cardiovascular disease. Molecular Aspects of Medicine. 2010;**31**:478-494

[31] Yamagata K, Tagami M, Yamori Y. Dietary polyphenols regulate endothelial function and prevent cardiovascular disease. Nutrition. 2015;**31**:28-37

[32] Olmos L, Mombouli JV, Illiano S, Vanhoutte PM. cGMP mediates the desensitization to bradykinin in isolated canine coronary arteries. The American Journal of Physiology. 1995;**268**:H865-H870

[33] Ozkor MA, Quyyumi AA. Endothelium-derived hyperpolarizing factor and vascular function. Cardiology Research and Practice. 2011;**2011**:156146

[34] Bauersachs J, Popp R, Hecker M, Sauer E, Fleming I, Busse R. Nitric oxide attenuates the release of endothelium-derived hyperpolarizing factor. Circulation. 1996;**94**:3341-3347

[35] Nishikawa Y, Stepp DW, Chilian WM. Nitric oxide exerts feedback inhibition on EDHF-induced coronary arteriolar dilation in vivo. American Journal of Physiology. Heart and Circulatory Physiology. 2000;**279**:H459-H465

[36] Shimokawa H, Godo S. Diverse functions of endothelial NO synthases system: NO and EDH. Journal of Cardiovascular Pharmacology. 2016;**67**:361-366

[37] Kojima S, Matsui K, Sakamoto T, Ishihara M, Kimura K, Miyazaki S, Yamagishi M, Tei C, Hiraoka H, Sonoda M, Tsuchihashi K, Shimoyama N, Honda T, Ogata Y, Ogawa H, Japanese Acute I. Coronary syndrome study, long-term nitrate therapy after acute myocardial infarction does not improve or aggravate prognosis. Circulation Journal. 2007;**71**:301-307

[38] Ambrosio G, Del Pinto M, Tritto I, Agnelli G, Bentivoglio M, Zuchi C, Anderson FA, Gore JM, Lopez-Sendon J, Wyman A, Kennelly BM, Fox KA, Investigators G. Chronic nitrate therapy is associated with different presentation and evolution of acute coronary syndromes: Insights from 52,693 patients in the global registry of acute coronary events. European Heart Journal. 2010;**31**:430-438

[39] Banerjee D, Mazumder S, Sinha AK. The role of inhibition of nitric oxide synthesis in the aggregation of platelets due to the stimulated production of thromboxane A2. Blood Coagulation & Fibrinolysis. 2014;**25**:585-591

[40] Sandoo A, van Zanten JJ, Metsios GS, Carroll D, Kitas GD. The endothelium and its role in regulating vascular tone. Open Cardiovascular Medicine Journal. 2010;**4**:302-312

[41] Birch DJ, Turmaine M, Boulos PB, Burnstock G. Sympathetic innervation of human mesenteric artery and vein. Journal of Vascular Research. 2008;**45**:323-332

[42] Saladin KS. Anatomy and Physiology. 6th ed. New YorK: McGraw-Hill; 2011

[43] Zucker IH, Liu JL. Angiotensin II–nitric oxide interactions in the control of sympathetic outflow in heart failure. Heart Failure Reviews. 2000;**5**:27-43

[44] Bruno RM, Ghiadoni L, Seravalle G, Dell'oro R, Taddei S, Grassi G. Sympathetic regulation of vascular function in health and disease. Frontiers in Physiology. 2012;**3**:284

[45] Forstermann U, Sessa WC. Nitric oxide synthases: regulation and function. Eur Heart J. 2012;**33**:829-837 837a-837d

[46] Amiya E, Watanabe M, Komuro I. The relationship between vascular function and the autonomic nervous system. Annals of Vascular Diseases. 2014;**7**:109-119

[47] Parati G, Salvi P. Arterial stiffness and the sympathetic nervous system, in: ME Safar, MF O'Rourke, ED Frohlich (Ed.) Blood Pressure and Arterial Wall Mechanics in Cardiovascular Diseases, Springer, London; 2014

[48] Cao Q, Zhang J, Xu G. Hemodynamic changes and baroreflex sensitivity associated with carotid endarterectomy and carotid artery stenting. Interventional Neurology. 2015;**3**:13-21

[49] Sousa JB, Fresco P, Diniz C. Endothelial dysfunction impairs vascular neurotransmission in tail arteries. Neurochemistry International. 2015;**80**:7-13

[50] Sousa JB, Vieira-Rocha MS, Arribas SM, Gonzalez MC, Fresco P, Diniz C. Endothelial and neuronal nitric oxide activate distinct pathways on sympathetic neurotransmission in rat tail and mesenteric arteries. PLoS One. 2015;**10**:e0129224

[51] Fresco P, Diniz C, Goncalves J. Facilitation of noradrenaline release by activation of adenosine a(2A) receptors triggers both phospholipase C and adenylate cyclase pathways in rat tail artery. Cardiovascular Research. 2004;**63**:739-746

[52] Fresco P, Oliveira JM, Kunc F, Soares AS, Rocha-Pereira C, Goncalves J, Diniz C. A2A adenosine-receptor-mediated facilitation of noradrenaline release in rat tail artery involves protein kinase C activation and betagamma subunits formed after alpha2-adrenoceptor activation. Neurochemistry International. 2007;**51**:47-56

[53] Okamoto K, Aoki K. Development of a strain of spontaneously hypertensive rats. Japanese Circulation Journal. 1963;**27**:282-293

[54] Trippodo NC, Frohlich ED. Similarities of genetic (spontaneous) hypertension. Man and rat. Circulation Research. 1981;**48**:309-319

[55] Reid JJ, Lieu AT, Rand MJ. Interactions between endothelin-1 and other chronotropic agents in rat isolated atria. European Journal of Pharmacology. 1991;**194**:173-181

[56] Wiklund NP, Wiklund CU, Cederqvist B, Ohlen A, Hedqvist P, Gustafsson LE. Endothelin modulation of neuroeffector transmission in smooth muscle. Journal of Cardiovascular Pharmacology. 1991;**17**(Suppl 7):S335-S339

[57] Addicks K, Bloch W, Feelisch M. Nitric oxide modulates sympathetic neurotransmission at the prejunctional level. Microscopy Research and Technique. 1994;**29**:161-168

[58] Schwarz P, Diem R, Dun NJ, Forstermann U. Endogenous and exogenous nitric oxide inhibits norepinephrine release from rat heart sympathetic nerves. Circulation Research. 1995;**77**:841-848

[59] Boerman EM, Segal SS. Depressed perivascular sensory innervation of mouse mesenteric arteries with advanced age. The Journal of Physiology. 2016;**594**:2323-2338

[60] Koyama T, Hatanaka Y, Jin X, Yokomizo A, Fujiwara H, Goda M, Hobara N, Zamami Y, Kitamura Y, Kawasaki H. Altered function of nitrergic nerves inhibiting sympathetic neurotransmission in mesenteric vascular beds of renovascular hypertensive rats. Hypertension Research. 2010;**33**:485-491

[61] Yu M, McAndrew RP, Al-Saghir R, Maier KG, Medhora M, Roman RJ, Jacobs ER. Nitric oxide contributes to 20-HETE-induced relaxation of pulmonary arteries. J Appl Physiol (1985). 2002;**93**:1391-1399

[62] Brassai A, Mako K, Domjanschitz L, Sperlagh B. Lack of prejunctional modulation of noradrenaline release by endogenous nitric oxide in guinea pig pulmonary artery. Neurochemistry International. 2002;**41**:279-283

[63] Vaz-da-Silva MJ, Guimaraes S, Moura D. Adenosine and the endothelium-dependent modulation of 3H-noradrenaline release in the canine pulmonary artery. Naunyn-Schmiedeberg's Archives of Pharmacology. 1995;**352**:640-645

[64] Chen C, Schofield GG. Nitric oxide donors enhanced Ca2+ currents and blocked noradrenaline-induced Ca2+ current inhibition in rat sympathetic neurons. The Journal of Physiology. 1995;**482**(Pt 3):521-531

[65] Martire M, Altobelli D, Cannizzaro C, Preziosi P. Effects of nitric oxide donors on basal and K+−evoked release of [3H]noradrenaline from rat cerebral cortex synaptosomes. European Journal of Pharmacology. 1998;**350**:345-351

[66] Lu Y, Chung HJ, Li Y, Rosenberg PA. NMDA receptor-mediated extracellular adenosine accumulation in rat forebrain neurons in culture is associated with inhibition of adenosine kinase. The European Journal of Neuroscience. 2003;**17**:1213-1222

[67] Ralevic V, Dunn WR. Purinergic transmission in blood vessels. Autonomic Neuroscience. 2015;**191**:48-66

[68] Dunwiddie TV, Masino SA. The role and regulation of adenosine in the central nervous system. Annual Review of Neuroscience. 2001;**24**:31-55

[69] Baldwin SA, Beal PR, Yao SY, King AE, Cass CE, Young JD. The equilibrative nucleoside transporter family, SLC29. Pflügers Archiv. 2004;**447**:735-743

[70] Loffler M, Morote-Garcia JC, Eltzschig SA, Coe IR, Eltzschig HK. Physiological roles of vascular nucleoside transporters. Arteriosclerosis, Thrombosis, and Vascular Biology. 2007;**27**:1004-1013

[71] Sousa JB, Diniz C. The Adenosinergic system as a therapeutic target in the vasculature: New ligands and challenges. Molecules. 2017;**22**

[72] Wiklund NP, Cederqvist B, Gustafsson LE. Adenosine enhancement of adrenergic neuroeffector transmission in guinea-pig pulmonary artery. British Journal of Pharmacology. 1989;**96**:425-433

[73] Zhang GL, Miyahara H, Suzuki H. Inhibitory actions of adenosine differ between ear and mesenteric arteries in the rabbit. Pflügers Archiv. 1989;**415**:56-62

[74] Talaia C, Morato M, Quintas C, Goncalves J, Queiroz G. Functional crosstalk of prejunctional receptors on the modulation of noradrenaline release in mesenteric vessels: A differential study of artery and vein. European Journal of Pharmacology. 2011;**652**:33-39

[75] Rocha-Pereira C, Sousa JB, Vieira-Rocha MS, Fresco P, Goncalves J, Diniz C. Differential inhibition of noradrenaline release mediated by inhibitory a(1)-adenosine receptors in the mesenteric vein and artery from normotensive and hypertensive rats. Neurochemistry International. 2013;**62**:399-405

[76] Rocha-Pereira C, Arribas SM, Fresco P, Gonzalez MC, Goncalves J, Diniz C. Impaired inhibitory function of presynaptic A1-adenosine receptors in SHR mesenteric arteries. Journal of Pharmacological Sciences. 2013;**122**:59-70

[77] Sousa JB, Vieira-Rocha MS, Sa C, Ferreirinha F, Correia-de-Sa P, Fresco P, Diniz C. Lack of endogenous adenosine tonus on sympathetic neurotransmission in spontaneously hypertensive rat mesenteric artery. PLoS One. 2014;**9**:e105540

[78] Stoggall SM, Shaw JS. The coexistence of adenosine A1 and A2 receptors in guinea-pig aorta. European Journal of Pharmacology. 1990;**190**:329-335

[79] Goncalves J, Queiroz G. Purinoceptor modulation of noradrenaline release in rat tail artery: Tonic modulation mediated by inhibitory P2Y- and facilitatory A2A-purinoceptors. British Journal of Pharmacology. 1996;**117**:156-160

[80] Diniz C, Fresco P, Leal S, Goncalves J. Adenosine receptors involved in modulation of noradrenaline release in isolated rat tail artery. European Journal of Pharmacology. 2004;**504**:17-25

[81] Fresco P, Diniz C, Queiroz G, Goncalves J. Release inhibitory receptors activation favours the A2A-adenosine receptor-mediated facilitation of noradrenaline release in isolated rat tail artery. British Journal of Pharmacology. 2002;**136**:230-236

[82] Sangsiri S, Dong H, Swain GM, Galligan JJ, Xu H. Impaired function of prejunctional adenosine A1 receptors expressed by perivascular sympathetic nerves in DOCA-salt hypertensive rats. The Journal of Pharmacology and Experimental Therapeutics. 2013;**345**:32-40

[83] Jackson EK, Cheng D, Tofovic SP, Mi Z. Endogenous adenosine contributes to renal sympathetic neurotransmission via postjunctional A1 receptor-mediated coincident signaling. American Journal of Physiology. Renal Physiology. 2012;**302**:F466-F476

[84] Leal S, Sa C, Goncalves J, Fresco P, Diniz C. Immunohistochemical characterization of adenosine receptors in rat aorta and tail arteries. Microscopy Research and Technique. 2008;**71**:703-709

[85] Ansari HR, Nadeem A, Tilley SL, Mustafa SJ. Involvement of COX-1 in A3 adenosine receptor-mediated contraction through endothelium in mice aorta. American Journal of Physiology. Heart and Circulatory Physiology. 2007;**293**:H3448-H3455

[86] Balligand JL, Kelly RA, Marsden PA, Smith TW, Michel T. Control of cardiac muscle cell function by an endogenous nitric oxide signaling system. Proceedings of the National Academy of Sciences of the United States of America. 1993;**90**:347-351

[87] Conti V, Russomanno G, Corbi G, Izzo V, Vecchione C, Filippelli A. Adrenoreceptors and nitric oxide in the cardiovascular system. Frontiers in Physiology. 2013;**4**:321

Chapter 15

Endothelial Cell Dysfunction in HIV-1 Infection

Pietro Mazzuca, Arnaldo Caruso and
Francesca Caccuri

Additional information is available at the end of the chapter

http://dx.doi.org/10.5772/intechopen.73023

Abstract

Human immunodeficiency virus type 1 (HIV-1) promotes a generalized immune activation that alters the physiology of cells that are not sensitive to viral infection. Endothelial cells (ECs) display heavy dysfunctions in HIV-1-seropositive (HIV$^+$) patients that persist even in patients under successful combined antiretroviral therapy (cART). In vivo studies failed to demonstrate the presence of replicating virus in ECs suggesting that a direct role of the virus in vascular dysfunction is unlikely. This finding paves the way to the hypothesis of a key role of molecules released in the microenvironment by HIV-1-infected cells in sustaining aberrant EC function. Here we review the current understanding regarding the contribution of HIV-1 infection to vascular dysfunction. In particular, we argue that different HIV-1 proteins may play a key role in driving and sustaining inflammation and EC dysregulation, thus underlining the need to target them for therapeutic benefit.

Keywords: HIV-1, viral proteins, endothelial cells, vascular dysfunction, inflammation

1. Introduction

Human immunodeficiency virus type 1 (HIV-1) infection is highly pathogenic since it stimulates a generalized immune activation involving not only the main targets of HIV-1 infection, such as CD4$^+$ T cells and monocytes/macrophages, but also cells that are not sensitive to viral infection.

Endothelial cells (ECs) are not fully permissive to HIV-1 infection, and there are no in vivo evidences that demonstrate the presence of replicating virus in ECs. Nowadays, the number of HIV-1-seropositive (HIV$^+$) patients that exhibit EC dysfunction is increasing vertiginously. In this chapter, the actual knowledges of how HIV-1 can directly and/or indirectly contribute to vascular dysfunction are reviewed. In particular, we underline the emerging role played by some structural and regulatory HIV-1 proteins released in the microenvironment by infected cells in driving inflammation and EC dysregulation. This finding highlights the need to target these viral proteins for therapeutic benefit.

2. Endothelial dysfunction during HIV-1 infection

Chronic inflammation contributes to many leading causes of death, and in particular cardiovascular events have emerged as a clinically significant issue and have become the matter of several studies. HIV-1 infection is characterized by altered immune responses leading to a generalized chronic inflammation and, in particular, to a pro-inflammatory status in the vascular endothelium fostering the development of cardiovascular diseases [1]. A strong correlation between high plasma HIV-1 RNA levels and signs of endothelial dysfunction is known [2], and subclinical signs of atherosclerosis have been found in asymptomatic HIV^+ young men with long-standing HIV-1 disease [3]. As the efficacy of combined antiretroviral therapy (cART) improves and patients live longer, the prevalence of cardiovascular diseases is increasing in HIV^+ individuals [4, 5]. Moreover, many antiretroviral drugs, particularly HIV-1 protease inhibitors, can cause dyslipidemia, thus contributing to the increased risk for endothelial dysfunction. The high risk of endothelial dysfunction persists even in new-generation antiretroviral drugs era, despite the fact that several adverse metabolic effects (e.g., insulin resistance, dyslipidemia, and hypertension) are abolished [6]. In light of these considerations, the following paragraphs consider three essential factors in the development and pathogenesis of endothelial dysfunction during the natural course of HIV-1 infection: (a) the ability of HIV-1 to promote inflammation, (b) the HIV-mediated damage of endothelium, and (c) the capability of HIV-1 structural and regulatory proteins of affecting EC function.

2.1. HIV-1 and inflammatory microenvironment

Chronic activation of the immune system is a peculiar feature of HIV-1 infection. Persistent activation of immune cells is known to gain an elevated pro-inflammatory cytokine/chemokine release contributing to the development of a chronically inflamed microenvironment. HIV-1 virus cycle is dominated by a local replication at the transmission site and in local lymphoid tissues and then dissemination. Virus expansion is associated with a dramatic depletion of memory $CD4^+$ T cells, particularly from gut-associated lymphoid tissues and with increased plasma levels of pro-inflammatory cytokines and chemokines. During the early phase of infection, a pro-inflammatory cytokine storm contributes to the control of viral replication but also to the early immunopathology of the infection and to the associated long-term consequences. Many cell types contribute to the release of different pro-inflammatory cytokines and chemokines during HIV-1 infection [7] such as interferon (IFN)-α, tumor necrosis factor (TNF)-α, INF-γ, interleukin (IL)-1β, IL-10, interferon gamma-induced protein (IP)-10, IL-15, IL-8, IL-6, IL-18, and monocyte chemoattractant protein (MCP)-1 [8, 9]. Antiretroviral therapy usually controls and even abolishes HIV-1 replication, but does not completely recover immune dysfunction. Therefore, immune alteration and inflammation are common features of HIV^+ patients even under successful cART.

2.2. Role of inflammatory cytokines and chemokines in the HIV-1-triggered endothelial dysfunction

Endothelial dysfunction and vascular diseases such as atherosclerosis and arterial damage are predominantly enhanced during a systemic chronic inflammatory status. Elevated levels of IL-6 have been associated with carotid atherosclerosis and progressive stenosis of the carotid artery, thereby upregulating the lipid uptake in macrophages and inhibiting the activity of lipoprotein lipase [10]. Increased carotid intima-media thickness (IMT) and hypertension are common features of patients with increased plasma levels of IL-18 [11], whereas TNF-α has a key role in promoting atherosclerosis, myocardial ischemia/reperfusion, and heart failure via several mechanisms: increased cholesterol uptake and foam cell formation in macrophages, augmented leukocyte transmigration in subendothelial structures, and increased proliferation and migration of vascular smooth muscle cells [12].

HIV-1 infection generates a systemic chronic inflammatory disorder as a result of continuous alteration of the immune response, contributing to dyslipidemia, EC dysfunction, vascular smooth muscle cell proliferation and migration, and, ultimately, the atherosclerotic plaque formation. The virus itself promotes the release of IL-6, IL-18, and TNF-α, together with IFN-γ, IL-1β, IL-10, tumor necrosis factor-related apoptosis-inducing ligand (TRAIL), and macrophage colony-stimulating factor (M-CSF) by T cells and monocytes [13].

Liver-synthesized C-reactive protein (CRP) is a member of the pentraxin family factors and is considered a marker for coronary vascular disease and endothelial damage. CRP plasma levels are significantly upregulated in HIV^+ patients and inversely correlated with $CD4^+$ T lymphocyte count [14], and elevated CRP levels have been associated with an increased risk of myocardial infarction in HIV^+ patients [15]. It is noteworthy that increased levels of IL-6, IL-1, and TNF- α induce CRP, which in turn is able to activate pro-inflammatory cytokines such as IL-6 and M-CSF via a positive feedback loop.

The levels of cell adhesion molecules such as vascular cell adhesion protein 1 (VCAM-1) and intercellular adhesion molecule 1 (ICAM-1) are raised during HIV-1 infection, thus contributing to trans-endothelial migration of immune cells [16].

HIV-1 causes a continuous recruitment of monocytes that migrate across the endothelial barrier in blood vessels, differentiate into macrophages, and produce pro-inflammatory cytokines, thus determining the progressive damage of vessel structures. Furthermore, HIV-1 replicates in macrophages and induces activation and synthesis of several pro-inflammatory cytokines that in turn induce endothelial activation and leukocyte adhesion generating a positive feedback [17].

An important alteration in lipid metabolism is evident in more than 50% of HIV^+ patients. It likely relies on the upregulation of hepatic fatty acid synthesis and very low-density lipoprotein (VLDL) production, usually triggered by inflammatory cytokines as IFN-γ, TNF-α, and IL-1β [18]. At the same time, the continuous trans-endothelial migration of immune cells and their inhibited reverse transport determines the localization of monocytes inside the vessel wall and promotes the formation of foam cells, the fat-laden macrophages that are implicated in the buildup of an atheromatous plaque [17].

Monocytes, depending on the cytokine/chemokine stimulation, may differentiate into M1 macrophages, which promote inflammation or into M2 macrophages, which are inflammatory resolving cells [19]. In particular, IFN-γ and IL-1β drive monocytes to acquire an M1 profile, whereas IL-4 and IL-13 generate M2 macrophages. HIV-1, by infecting macrophages, polarizes these cells toward the M1 phenotype [20]. This leads to the imbalance of the M1/M2 ratio, a condition necessary for sustaining endothelial dysfunction [21].

Endothelin-1 (ET-1) is a potent vasoconstrictor that promotes migration and proliferation of smooth muscle cells. HIV-1-triggered secretion of ET-1 promotes a reduction of vascular nitric oxide (NO) production by ECs with the consequent proliferation and migration of smooth muscle cells leading to arterial vasoconstriction.

Altogether, these findings suggest that HIV-1 produces a general inflammatory microenvironment that contributes to dyslipidemia, EC dysfunction, chemotaxis, and vascular smooth muscle cell proliferation and migration. All these conditions are likely to foster endothelial degeneration and atherosclerotic plaque formation (**Figure 1**).

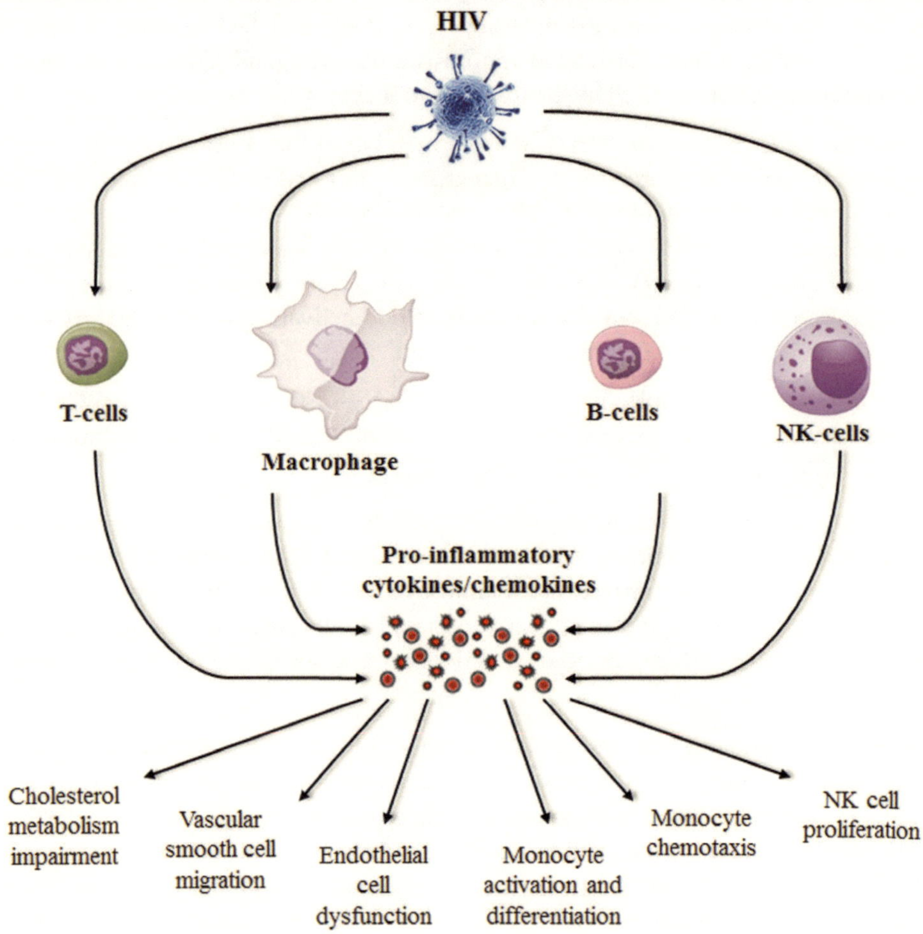

Figure 1. HIV-1 capability to promote inflammation, dyslipidemia, and endothelial dysfunction through the activation of different immune cells such as T and B cells, macrophages, and natural killer cells (NK cells).

2.3. HIV-1-triggered damage of ECs

HIV-1 is not an endothelium-tropic virus. It displays a narrow tropism predominantly determined by the cell surface receptors required for HIV-1 infection. CD4 and co-receptors are usually essential for HIV-1 to infect cells efficiently. The chemokine (C-C motif) receptor type 5 (CCR5) is the main co-receptor used in vivo, but variants that use another co-receptor, namely, chemokine (C-X-C motif) receptor type 4 (CXCR4), evolve during disease. In vitro, more than a dozen different co-receptors have been identified that support infection of cell lines by different HIV-1 strains. Moreover, HIV-1 particles interact with a range of cell surface receptors via interactions of its envelope glycoprotein gp120 with glycolipid galactocerebroside (gal)-C and its sulfated derivative.

HIV-1 capability to infect ECs in vitro depends on the tissue source of ECs and on their functional status. Microvascular ECs from the brain, kidney glomeruli, hepatic sinusoid, and bone marrow may be infected by HIV-1 in the absence of cytolysis [22, 23]. HIV-1 infection of brain ECs has been largely studied for its relevance in neurological diseases. T cell tropic but not brain-derived macrophage tropic HIV-1 strains selectively infect the brain endothelium in vitro, suggesting that T cell tropism may be important for HIV-1 entry through the blood-brain barrier [22] and spreading in the central nervous system [24]. However, it is important to underline that in vivo studies do not support the presence of replicating virus in ECs. Even if HIV-1 infection of ECs cannot be completely ruled out, this may suggest an indirect action of molecules released in the microenvironment by HIV-1-infected cells at the base of the mechanism for vascular dysfunction.

In the pathophysiology of cardiovascular disease, the damage of ECs assessed by responses to altered blood flow (e.g., flow-mediated dilatation) and differences in the levels of EC specific molecules released in the blood (e.g., von Willebrand factor) represent a hallmark. The equilibrium between the mechanisms of vascular damage and repair plays a crucial role during homeostasis of vascular integrity. Following a blood vessel injury, high levels of circulating ECs (cECs) and microvesicles are released from endothelium, and the reinstatement of the vascular integrity mainly implies activity of endothelial progenitor cells (EPCs), plaque neovascularization, and reverse cholesterol transport [25]. EPCs are key determinants of endothelial dysfunction and show a high predictive value of early vascular disease. Interestingly, all vascular repair mechanisms are impaired in HIV^+ individuals who have lower EPC levels than HIV-1-seronegative subjects [26]. Decrease in the number of EPCs is attributed to HIV-1, which seems to be able to infect these cells because of their chemokine receptor CCR5 and CXCR4 expressions.

Along with reduced EPC levels, HIV^+ individuals show high plasma levels of EC-derived microvesicles also known as microparticles that are small membranous structures released from ECs during apoptosis, which impair the restoration of physiological conditions and sustain endothelial dysfunction [27]. HIV^+ patients also exhibit high plasma concentrations of high sensitivity C-reactive protein (hsCRP), IL-6, TNF-α, D-dimer, fibrinogen, soluble ICAM, and VCAM, suggesting endothelial activation and damage. These molecules are also responsible for an increased interaction of infected monocytes with ECs, thereby disrupting the integrity of the EC monolayer and promoting extravasation of HIV-1-infected cells into peripheral tissues and viral dissemination [28].

2.4. Role of HIV-1 proteins in the pathogenesis of endothelial dysfunction

The HIV-1 genome encodes a total of three structural proteins, two envelope proteins, three enzymes, and six accessory proteins. HIV-1 has designed its structural and regulatory/accessory proteins to better adapt to the human host and to promote virus replication and transmission. Among the many functions in the virus life cycle, a major role played by different HIV-1 proteins in directly driving inflammation and EC dysregulation is strengthening (**Figure 2**), thus highlighting the need to target them for therapeutic benefit.

2.5. HIV-1 structural proteins

The HIV-1 gp120 is the key protein for viral entry by binding to the CD4 receptor and to the co-receptor CCR5 or CXCR4. The HIV-1 matrix protein p17 (p17) is a myristoylated protein that exerts many important and crucial functions during the virus cell cycle. It contributes to nuclear localization of the pre-integration complex after HIV-1 entry and promotes virus maturation and assembly [29]. In addition to its key role in the virus life cycle, p17 exerts a chemokine-like activity by binding to the chemokine receptor CXCR1 and CXCR2 and mimics some of the biological activities of IL-8, the CXCR1 and CXCR2 natural ligand.

Binding of gp120 and p17 to their receptors and/or co-receptors alters the biological activity of different cells. Extracellularly, p17 alters immune responses by activating different immune cells such as $CD4^+$ T cells, $CD8^+$ T cells, NK cells, plasmacytoid dendritic cells, monocytes, and B cells and contributing to the production and release of pro-inflammatory molecules and to the development of an inflammatory microenvironment [30–32]. Furthermore, p17 stimulates the rapid adhesion and chemotaxis of monocytes and B cells through activation of the Rho/

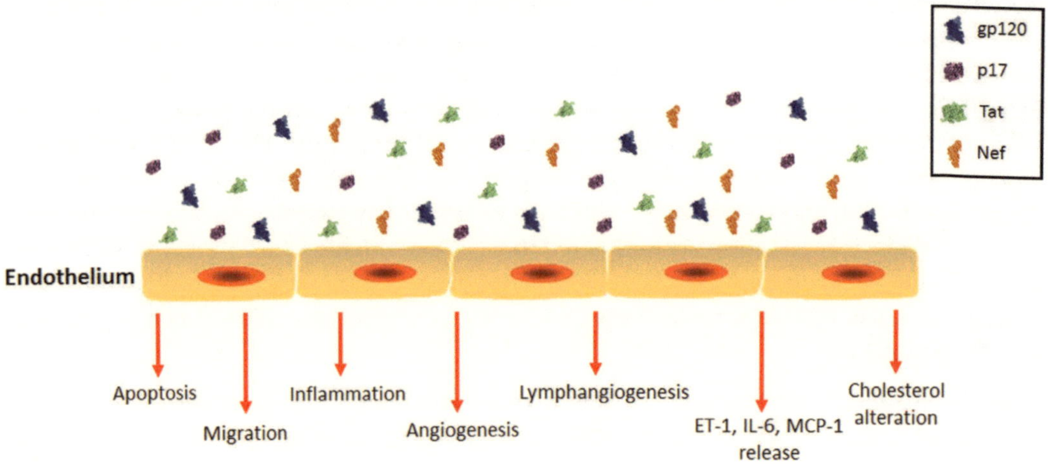

Figure 2. Role of HIV-1 structural and regulatory proteins in the pathogenesis of inflammation and endothelial cell (EC) dysfunction: endothelin-1 (ET-1), interleukin-6 (IL-6), monocyte chemoattractant protein-1 (MCP-1), HIV-1 glycoprotein-120 (gp120), HIV-1 matrix protein (p17), HIV-1 transactivator of transcription (Tat), and HIV-1 negative regulatory factor (Nef).

ROCK signaling pathway [33], suggesting that p17 may recruit activated monocytes and B cells in different tissues and organs to participate and/or sustain inflammatory processes.

On the other hand, gp120 is known to induce dysfunction of T cells, macrophages, cardiomyocytes, ECs, and central nervous system cells, when expressed on the viral particle, on the surface of infected cells, or as a viral-free soluble protein [34].

Endothelial dysfunction mediated by these two HIV-1 structural proteins results to occur through different mechanisms: gp120 is considered a direct and indirect proapoptotic factor favoring EC death, whereas p17 is a potent angiogenic and lymphangiogenic factor.

EC death by gp120 is mediated by its interaction with CXCR4 expressed on the endothelial cell surface that triggers different downstream effects, as activation of the CXCR4-dependent caspase and the mitogen-activated protein kinase (MAPK), or through protein kinase C (PKC) activation [35]. The indirect mechanism of gp120 apoptosis is based on the increased secretion of ET-1 [36, 37], inhibition of NO synthase [38], and a higher surface expression of endothelial monocyte-activating polypeptide II (EMAPII) [39]. In particular, EMAPII acts as proapoptotic factor following different types of stress including hypoxia and mechanical stress. It is worth noting that after its interaction with CXCR4, gp120 promotes p38 MAPK signaling pathway activation and a rapid surface expression and release of EMAPII, thus favoring apoptosis through a paracrine mechanism. In the context of an inflammatory microenvironment, gp120 may also contribute to reduce the EC-derived NO synthesized by the NO synthase that is a major mediator of endothelium-dependent vasorelaxation and endothelial dysfunction.

P17 is a potent angiogenic and lymphangiogenic molecule both in vitro and in vivo. Activity of p17 is dependent on its interaction with the chemokine receptors CXCR1 and CXCR2, expressed on ECs [40–42]. Angiogenesis and lymphangiogenesis promoted by p17 after its interaction with CXCR1 and/or CXCR2 involve activation of both MAPK/ERK and PI3K/Akt signaling pathways [40–42]. Lymphangiogenesis induced by p17 was found to be partly mediated by the selective release of the pro-angiogenic/lymphangiogenic factor ET-1 [42], which binds to its B receptor (ETBR) expressed on lymph node-derived ECs (LECs) and activates the downstream PI3K/Akt and MAPK/ERK signaling pathways.

Interestingly, many studies demonstrated a long-term persistence of these two structural HIV-1 proteins in lymph node germinal centers and lymphoid tissue of HIV^+ patients, even during successful cART and in the absence of any detectable viral replication [43, 44].

Interestingly, p17 is continuously released in the extracellular space even in the absence of viral replication and viral protease activity [45] and is detected at nanomolar concentrations in the blood of HIV^+ patients even in the presence of anti-p17 antibodies [46].

Altogether, these findings suggest that gp120 and p17 are released by infected cells even during cART, bind to ECs, and drive cell activation, angiogenesis, and/or apoptosis, leading to vascular disease. In addition, the capability of p17 to stimulate the immune system and promote a pro-inflammatory status highlights the key role played by this protein in driving endothelial dysfunction.

2.6. HIV-1 regulatory proteins

HIV-1 Tat protein is a trans-activating regulatory protein, which is essential for efficient transcription of the viral genome. Tat is a proto-cytokine promoting several disease conditions by modulating the function of immune cells, mesenchymal cells, and ECs [47, 48].

The HIV-1 viral protein Nef is a 27-kD myristoylated protein. It is not secreted by infected cells, but its interaction with membrane and host cell proteins is crucial to sustain its biological activity. Nef protein is involved in different intracellular functions including alteration of protein trafficking, cell signaling cascades, and inhibition of antibody maturation in B cells [49]. Nef is able to enhance HIV-1 infectivity by promoting the formation of nanotubes connecting HIV-1-infected cells to bystander cells [50]. In particular, transfer of Nef from a HIV-1-infected target cell to ECs through nanotubes supports EC activation, dysfunction, and death [51].

Similarly to many potent angiogenic growth factors such as vascular endothelial growth factor (VEGF) A, Tat has a basic domain rich in arginine and lysine residues that endows the viral protein of a potent and direct angiogenic activity [52, 53]. On the contrary, Nef contains multiple domains capable of interacting with the endocytic cellular machinery [54]. Tat and Nef are both capable of inducing apoptosis in ECs. Many studies demonstrate that Nef is able to induce and activate NADPH oxidase that drives ECs to go for apoptosis. Indeed, by significantly decreasing NO production and increasing superoxide anion production, Nef contributes to reactive oxygen species (ROS) production, cell oxidative stress, and cell death [55, 56]. Moreover, Nef was also found to potently induce EC apoptosis by activation of caspases [57]. Tat causes apoptotic death of ECs via either TNF-α secretion or through activation of the Fas-dependent pathway. Additionally, Tat is able to promote apoptosis in ECs by activating the MAPK/ERK signaling pathway and caspase-3 [58].

In contrast to its proapoptotic effect, Tat may also exert an angiogenic activity through a multi-signaling-dependent pathway. Angiogenic activity promoted by Tat depends on binding and activation of the Flk-1/kinase insert domain receptor (Flk-1/KDR), a VEGF-A tyrosine kinase receptor, and on binding to integrin $\alpha v\beta 5$ receptor and heparan sulfate proteoglycans. Tat interaction with cellular receptors leads to the activation of signaling pathways associated with EC growth, migration, and angiogenesis [59, 60].

Similarly to the HIV-1 structural protein p17, both Tat and Nef proteins trigger immune cells activation and inflammation. In fact, Tat promotes transmigration of monocytes through the endothelial barrier and inflammation by inducing ECs to express adhesion molecules as E-selectin, ICAM-1, VCAM-1, and ELAM-1 and to release IL-6 [61, 62]. Tat-induced EC activation is likely aimed to facilitate interaction of inflammatory cells with ECs and promote MCP-1 secretion by activation of PKC signaling pathway [63]. At the same time, Nef protein contributes to inflammation increasing the endothelial MCP-1 production through activation of the NF-kB signaling pathway [50]. It is worth noting that this activity is also promoted by the HIV-1 structural protein p17, following activation of the AP-1 signaling pathway [32] highlighting a remarkable redundancy in the biological activity of structural and regulatory proteins. Interestingly, it has been recently shown that Nef is also involved in the alteration of

EC cholesterol homeostasis by phosphorylation of Caveolin-1 (Cav-1) at Tyr14 that promotes Cav-1 redistribution and impairment of HDL-mediated cholesterol efflux in ECs [64].

Secretion of Tat in the microenvironment, even during antiretroviral therapy [65]; its direct involvement in endothelial homeostasis, acting as proapoptotic factors or as a pro-angiogenic factor; and its ability to generate an inflammatory status suggest that in the absence of HIV-1 detectable viremia, persistence of endothelial dysfunction in HIV^{+} patients may be, at least in part, ascribed to this (and *bona fide* to Nef) HIV-1 regulatory protein.

2.7. Animal models in HIV-1 endothelial dysfunction

Although many improvements have been made in the development of animal models to study HIV-1-associated endothelial dysfunction, these models do not completely reproduce the pathophysiological features of endothelial dysfunction in humans.

A model of transgenic mice partially reproduces, but below expectations, the features of endothelial dysfunction observed during HIV-1 infection in humans [66]. Indeed, HIV-1-infected mice develop an adventitial mixed inflammatory cell migration, medial hypocellularity, and intimal hyperplasia following smooth muscle infiltration with sparing of the ECs. Furthermore, viral components are observed in smooth muscle cells, which in some instances proliferate in the absence of inflammation, remarking the conceptual principles of viral invasion [66]. The model of macaque species infected with the simian immunodeficiency virus (SIV) shares many more similarities than the transgenic mouse model, in term of disease, with HIV-1 infection and vascular diseases in humans. In an animal model based on macaques infected with a chimeric viral construct containing the HIV-1 Nef gene in a SIV backbone (SHIV-1-nef), the presence of complex vascular lesions has been demonstrated that are not evident in SIV-infected animals [67]. These findings seem to highlight a possible role of HIV-1 Nef in endothelial dysfunction leading to severe arterial disease. Interestingly, vascular alterations, subendothelial infiltration of immune cells, and significantly reduced levels of NO have been found in a model of Rhesus macaques infected by SIV and SHIV-1 [68].

Vasculogenic activity of p17 has been recently demonstrated using ex vivo and in vivo model [40–42]. The ex vivo rat aortic ring assay showed that p17 was able to promote vasculogenesis as potent as that observed using VEGF-A [40]. Similar results were obtained in the in vivo chick chorioallantoic membrane (CAM) assay, which highlighted the capability of p17 to generate allantoic neovessels as compared to control CAMs [40]. Matrigel plug assay has been used to test the lymphangiogenic activity of p17 in mice. Matrigel plugs containing the viral matrix protein were implanted into the dorsal subcutaneous tissue of C57BL/6 mice and after 10 days from the injection; matrigel plugs were immunostained with polyclonal antibody to lymphatic vessel endothelial receptor-1 (LYVE-1) identifying pronounced lymphatic vessel formation in p17-treated mice, compared to controls [42]. Interestingly, matrigel plugs containing a p17 variant derived from an Ugandan clade A1, named S75X and endowed with B cell growth-promoting activity, showed the presence of adipocyte infiltration observed at the histological level, thus suggesting that at least some p17 variants may trigger a possible interplay between angiogenesis, lymphangiogenesis, and adipogenesis [41].

3. Conclusions

As described in the present chapter, endothelial dysfunction occurring in HIV+ patients may be considered as a multifactorial pathology in which the HIV-1 virus itself and, most of all, its structural and regulatory proteins are able to induce strong changes in the physiology and morphology of ECs by altering their homeostasis and function.

Interestingly, HIV+ patients have a high risk of endothelial dysfunction in the absence and in the presence of suppressive cART [69, 70], although low-level transcription of HIV-1 genes continues even after years of cART [71, 72]. Many studies demonstrated the persistence of HIV-1-encoded proteins in different tissues and organs also during pharmacological control of infection. Since these proteins are able to induce a direct endothelial damage and to develop an inflammatory microenvironment, it is possible to hypothesize that viral proteins are among the most important factors involved in endothelial dysfunction development. Although animal models have limitations and can never completely mimic HIV-1 infection of humans or the physiological relevance of a single protein product in the human microenvironment, they start to provide proof of concept for a general vascular dysregulation operated by HIV-1 and its products. Altogether, these data show that a microenvironment disposed to endothelial dysfunction is a common feature in HIV+ individuals (**Figure 3**). Recognizing the interaction of some HIV-1 protein products with their receptors as the key events in sustaining endothelial aberrant functioning could help us to identify new therapeutic strategies in combating and/or preventing HIV-1-related vascular disease.

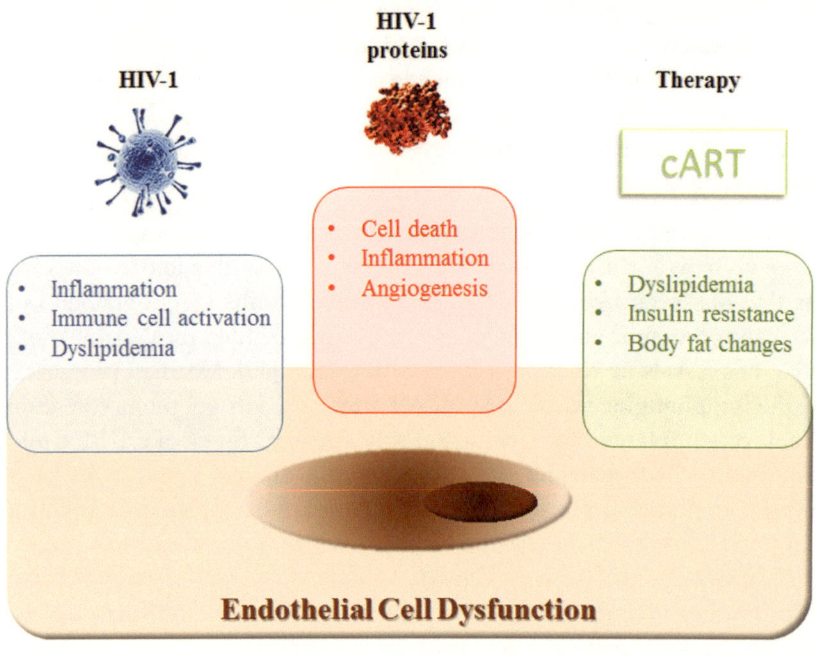

Figure 3. Endothelial dysfunction in HIV+ patients under combination antiretroviral therapy (cART) occurs following multiple trigger factors.

Author details

Pietro Mazzuca, Arnaldo Caruso and Francesca Caccuri*

*Address all correspondence to: francesca.caccuri@unibs.it

Department of Molecular and Translational Medicine, University of Brescia Medical School, Brescia, Italy

References

[1] Hsue PY, Hunt PW, Wu Y, Schnell A, Ho JE, Hatano H, Xie Y, Martin JN, Ganz P, Deeks SG. Role of viral replication, antiretroviral therapy, and immunodeficiency in HIV-1-associated atherosclerosis. World Journal of AIDS. 2009;**23**:1059-1067. DOI: 10.1097/QAD.0b013e32832b514b

[2] Funderburg NT, Mayne E, Sieg SF, Asaad R, Jiang W, Kalinowska M, Luciano AA, Stevens W, Rodriguez B, Brenchley JM, Douek DC, Lederman MM. Increased tissue factor expression on circulating monocytes in chronic HIV-1 infection: Relationship to in vivo coagulation and immune activation. Blood. 2010;**115**:161-167. DOI: 10.1182/blood-2009-03-210179

[3] Lo J, Abbara S, Shturman L, Soni A, Wei J, Rocha-Filho JA, Nasir K, Grinspoon SK. Increased prevalence of subclinical coronary atherosclerosis detected by coronary computed tomography angiography in HIV-1-infected men. World Journal of AIDS. 2010;**24**:243-253. DOI: 10.1097/QAD.0b013e328333ea9e

[4] d'Arminio A, Sabin CA, Phillips AN, Reiss P, Weber R, Kirk O, El-Sadr W, De Wit S, Mateu S, Petoumenos K, Dabis F, Pradier C, Morfeldt L, Lundgren JD, Friis-Møller N. Writing committee of the D:A:D: Study Group. Cardio- and cerebrovascular events in HIV-infected persons. World Journal of AIDS. 2004;**18**:1811-1817

[5] Rose H, Hoy J, Woolley I. HIV-1 infection and high density lipoprotein metabolism. Atherosclerosis. 2008;**199**:79-86. DOI: 10.1016/j.atherosclerosis.2007.10.018

[6] Cao R, Hu Y, Wang Y, Gurley EC, Studer EJ, Wang X, Hylemon PB, Pandak WM, Sanyal AJ, Zhang L, Zhou H. Prevention of HIV-1 protease inhibitor-induced dysregulation of hepatic lipid metabolism by raltegravir via endoplasmic reticulum stress signaling pathways. The Journal of Pharmacology and Experimental Therapeutics. 2010;**334**:530-539. DOI: 10.1124/jpet.110.168484

[7] McMichael AJ, Borrow P, Tomaras GD, Goonetilleke N, Haynes BF. The immune response during acute HIV-1 infection: Clues for vaccine development. Nature Reviews. Immunology. 2010;**10**:11-23. DOI: 10.1371/journal.ppat.1001273

[8] Gaines H, von Sydow MA, von Stedingk LV, Biberfeld G, Böttiger B, Hansson LO, Lundbergh P, Sönnerborg AB, Wasserman J, Strannegåard OO. Immunological changes in primary HIV-1-1 infection. World Journal of AIDS. 1990;**4**:995-999. PMID: 2261128

[9] Graziosi C, Gantt KR, Vaccarezza M, Demarest JF, Daucher M, Saag MS, Shaw GM, Quinn TC, Cohen OJ, Welbon CC, Pantaleo G, Fauci AS. Kinetics of cytokine expression during primary human immunodeficiency virus type 1 infection. Proceedings of the National Academy of Sciences of the United States of America. 1996;**93**:4386-4391. PMID: 8633076

[10] Thakore AH, Guo CY, Larson MG, Corey D, Wang TJ, Vasan RS, D'Agostino RB Sr, Lipinska I, Keaney JF Jr, Benjamin EJ, O'Donnell CJ. Association of multiple inflammatory markers with carotid intimal medial thickness and stenosis (from the Framingham Heart Study). The American Journal of Cardiology. 2007;**99**:1598-1602. DOI: 10.1016/j.amjcard.2007.01.036

[11] Rabkin SW. The role of interleukin 18 in the pathogenesis of hypertension-induced vascular disease. Nature Clinical Practice. Cardiovascular Medicine. 2009;**6**(3):192-199. DOI: 10.1038/ncpcardio1453

[12] Kleinbongard P, Heusch G, Schulz R. TNFa in atherosclerosis, myocardial ischemia/reperfusion and heart failure. Pharmacology & Therapeutics. 2010;**127**:295-314. DOI: 10.1016/j.pharmthera.2010.05.002

[13] Ford ES, Puronen CE, Sereti I. Immunopathogenesis of asymptomatic chronic HIV infection: The calm before the storm. Current Opinion in HIV and AIDS. 2009;**4**:206-214. DOI: 10.1097/COH.0b013e328329c68c

[14] De Lorenzo F, Boffito M, Collot-Teixeira S, Gazzard B, McGregor JL, Shotliff K, Xiao H. Prevention of atherosclerosis in patients living with HIV. Vascular Health and Risk Management. 2009;**5**(1):287-300. PMID: 19436663

[15] Triant VA, Meigs JB, Grinspoon SK. Association of C-reactive protein and HIV infection with acute myocardial infarction. Journal of Acquired Immune Deficiency Syndromes. 2009;**51**:268-273. DOI: 10.1097/QAI.0b013e3181a9992c

[16] Nordoy I, Aukrust P, Muller F, Frøland SS. Abnormal levels of circulating adhesion molecules in HIV-1 infection with characteristic alterations in opportunistic infections. Clinical Immunology and Immunopathology. 1996;**81**:16-21. PMID: 8808636

[17] Westhorpe CL, Zhou J, Webster NL, Kalionis B, Lewin SR, Jaworowski A, Muller WA, Crowe SM. Effects of HIV-1 infection in vitro on transendothelial migration by monocytes and monocyte derived macrophages. Journal of Leukocyte Biology. 2009;**85**:1027-1035

[18] Khovidhunkit W, Memon RA, Feingold KR, Grunfeld C. Infection and inflammation-induced proatherogenic changes of lipoproteins. The Journal of Infectious Diseases. 2000;**181**:462-472. DOI: 10.1086/315611

[19] Mantovani A, Sica A, Sozzani S, Allavena P, Vecchi A, Locati M. The chemokine system in diverse forms of macrophage activation and polarization. Trends in Immunology. 2004;**25**:677-686. DOI: 10.1016/j.it.2004.09.015

[20] Cassol E, Cassetta L, Alfano M, Poli G. Macrophage polarization and HIV-1 infection. Journal of Leukocyte Biology. 2010;**87**:599-608. DOI: 10.1189/jlb.1009673

[21] Tabas I. Macrophage death and defective inflammation resolution in atherosclerosis. Nature Reviews. Immunology. 2010;**10**:36-46. DOI: 10.1038/nri2675

[22] Moses AV, Bloom FE, Pauza CD, Nelson JA. Human immunodeficiency virus infection of human brain capillary endothelial cells occurs via a CD4/galactosylceramide-independent mechanism. Proceedings of the National Academy of Sciences of the United States of America. 1993;**90**:10474-10478. PMID: 7504264

[23] Lafon ME, Gendrault JL, Royer C, Jaeck D, Kirn A, Steffan AM. Human endothelial cells isolated from the hepatic sinusoids and the umbilical vein display a different permissiveness for HIV-1. Research in Virology. 1993;**144**:99-104. PMID: 8446785

[24] Bagasra O, Lavi E, Bobroski L, Khalili K, Pestaner JP, Tawadros R, Pomerantz RJ. Cellular reservoirs of HIV-1 in the central nervous system of infected individuals: Identification by the combination of in situ polymerase chain reaction and immunohistochemistry. World Journal of AIDS. 1996;**10**:573-385. PMID: 8780811

[25] Moreno PR, Sanz J, Fuster V. Promoting mechanisms of vascular health: circulating progenitor cells, angiogenesis, and reverse cholesterol transport. Journal of the American College of Cardiology. 2009;**53**:2315-2323. DOI: 10.1016/j.jacc.2009.02.057

[26] da Silva EF, Fonseca FA, França CN, Ferreira PR, Izar MC, Salomão R, Camargo LM, Tenore SB, Lewi DS. Imbalance between endothelial progenitors cells and microparticles in HIV-1-infected patients naive for antiretroviral therapy. World Journal of AIDS. 2011;**25**:1595-1601. DOI: 10.1097/QAD.0b013e32834980f4

[27] Kuller LH, Tracy R, Belloso W, De Wit S, Drummond F, Lane HC, Ledergerber B, Lundgren J, Neuhaus J, Nixon D, Paton NI, Neaton JD. Insight Smart Study Group: Inflammatory and coagulation biomarkers and mortality in patients with HIV-1 infection. PLoS Medicine. 2008;**5**:e203. DOI: 10.1371/journal.pmed.0050203

[28] Dhawan S, Weeks BS, Soderland C, Schnaper HW, Toro LA, Asthana SP, Hewlett IK, Stetler-Stevenson WG, Yamada SS, Yamada KM. HIV-1 infection alters monocyte interactions with human microvascular endothelial cells. Journal of Immunology. 1995;**154**:422-432. PMID: 7527819

[29] Fiorentini S, Marini E, Caracciolo S, Caruso A. Functions of the HIV-1 matrix protein p17. The New Microbiologica. 2006;**29**:1-10. PMID: 16608119

[30] De Francesco MA, Baronio M, Fiorentini S, Signorini C, Bonfanti C, Poiesi C, Popovic M, Grassi M, Garrafa E, Bozzo L, Lewis GK, Licenziati S, Gallo RC, Caruso A. HIV-1 matrix protein p17 increases the production of proinflammatory cytokines and counteracts IL-4 activity by binding to a cellular receptor. Proceedings of the National Academy of Sciences of the United States of America. 2002;**99**:9972-9977. DOI: 10.1073/pnas.142274699

[31] Vitale M, Caruso A, De Francesco MA, Rodella L, Bozzo L, Garrafa E, Grassi M, Gobbi G, Cacchioli A, Fiorentini S. HIV-1 matrix protein p17 enhances the proliferative activity of natural killer cells and increases their ability to secrete proinflammatory cytokines. British Journal of Haematology. 2003;**120**:337-343. PMID: 12542496

[32] Marini E, Tiberio L, Caracciolo S, Tosti G, Guzman CA, Schiaffonati L, Fiorentini S, Caruso A. HIV-1 matrix protein p17 binds to monocytes and selectively stimulates MCP-1 secretion: Role of transcriptional factor AP-1. Cellular Microbiology. 2008;**10**:655-666. DOI: 10.1111/j.1462-5822.2007.01073.x

[33] Giagulli C, Magiera AK, Bugatti A, Caccuri F, Marsico S, Rusnati M, Vermi W, Fiorentini S, Caruso A. HIV-1 matrix protein p17 binds to the IL-8 receptor CXCR1 and shows IL-8-like chemokine activity on monocytes through Rho/ROCK activation. Blood. 2012;**119**:2274-2283. DOI: 10.1182/blood-2011-06-364083

[34] Jiang J, Fu W, Wang X, Lin PH, Yao Q, Chen C. HIV-1 gp120 induces endothelial dysfunction in tumour necrosis factor-alpha-activated porcine and human endothelial cells. Cardiovascular Research. 2010;**87**:366-374. DOI: 10.1093/cvr/cvq013

[35] Huang MB, Bond VC. Involvement of protein kinase C in HIV-1 gp120-induced apoptosis in primary endothelium. Journal of Acquired Immune Deficiency Syndromes. 2000;**25**:375-389. PMID: 11141237

[36] Didier N, Banks WA, Créminon C, Dereuddre-Bosquet N, Mabondzo A. HIV-1-induced production of endothelin-1 in an in vitro model of the human blood-brain barrier. Neuroreport. 2002;**13**:1179-1183. PMID: 12151765

[37] Ehrenreich H, Rieckmann P, Sinowatz F, Weih KA, Arthur LO, Goebel FD, Burd PR, Coligan JE, Clouse KA. Potent stimulation of monocytic endothelin-1 production by HIV-1 glycoprotein 120. Journal of Immunology. 1993;**150**:4601-4609. PMID: 8482849

[38] Ahr B, Robert-Hebmann V, Devaux C, Biard-Piechaczyk M. Apoptosis of uninfected cells induced by HIV-1 envelope glycoproteins. Retrovirology. 2004;**1**:1-12. DOI: 10.1186/1742-4690-1-12

[39] Green LA, Yi R, Petrusca D, Wang T, Elghouche A, Gupta SK, Petrache I, Clauss M. HIV-1 envelope protein gp120-induced apoptosis in lung microvascular endothelial cells by 31 concerted upregulation of EMAP II and its receptor, CXCR3. American Journal of Physiology. Lung Cellular and Molecular Physiology. 2014;**306**:372-382. DOI: 10.1152/ajplung.00193.2013

[40] Caccuri F, Giagulli C, Bugatti A, Benetti A, Alessandri G, Ribatti D, Marsico S, Apostoli P, Slevin MA, Rusnati M, Guzman CA, Fiorentini S, Caruso A. HIV-1 matrix protein p17 promotes angiogenesis via chemokine receptors CXCR1 and CXCR2. Proceedings of the National Academy of Sciences of the United States of America. 2012;**109**:14580-14585. DOI: 10.1073/pnas.1206605109

[41] Basta D, Latinovic O, Lafferty MK, Sun L, Bryant J, Lu W, Caccuri F, Caruso A, Gallo R, Garzino-Demo A. Angiogenic, lymphangiogenic and adipogenic effects of HIV-1 matrix protein p17. Pathogens and Disease. 2015;**73**:ftv062. DOI: 10.1093/femspd/ftv062

[42] Caccuri F, Rueckert C, Giagulli C, Schulze K, Basta D, Zicari S, Marsico S, Cervi E, Fiorentini S, Slevin M, Guzman CA, Caruso A. HIV-1 matrix protein p17 promotes lymphangiogenesis

and activates the endothelin-1/endothelin B receptor axis. Arteriosclerosis, Thrombosis, and Vascular Biology. 2014;**34**:846-856. DOI: 10.1161/ATVBAHA.113.302478

[43] Popovic M, Tenner-Racz K, Pelser C, Stellbrink HJ, van Lunzen J, Lewis G, Kalyanaraman VS, Gallo RC, Racz P. Persistence of HIV-1 structural proteins and glycoproteins in lymph nodes of patients under highly active antiretroviral therapy. Proceedings of the National Academy of Sciences of the United States of America. 2005;**102**:14807-14812. DOI: 10.1073/pnas.0506857102

[44] Dolcetti R, Gloghini A, Caruso A, Carbone A. A lymphomagenic role for HIV beyond immune suppression? Blood. 2016;**127**(11):1403-1409. DOI: 10.1182/blood-2015-11-681411

[45] Caccuri F, Iaria ML, Campilongo F, Varney K, Rossi A, Mitola S, Schiarea S, Bugatti A, Mazzuca P, Giagulli C, Fiorentini S, Lu W, Salmona M, Caruso A. Cellular aspartyl proteases promote the unconventional secretion of biologically active HIV-1 matrix protein p17. Scientific Reports. 2016;**6**:38027. DOI: 10.1038/srep38027

[46] Fiorentini S, Riboldi E, Facchetti F, Avolio M, Fabbri M, Tosti G, Becker PD, Guzman CA, Sozzani S, Caruso A. HIV-1 matrix protein p17 induces human plasmacytoid dendritic cells to acquire a migratory immature cell phenotype. Proceedings of the National Academy of Sciences of the United States of America. 2008;**105**:3867-3872. DOI: 10.1073/pnas.0800370105

[47] Barillari G, Ensoli B. Angiogenic effects of extracellular human immunodeficiency virus type 1 Tat protein and its role in the pathogenesis of AIDS-associated Kaposi's sarcoma. Clinical Microbiology Reviews. 2002;**15**:310-326

[48] Liou LY, Herrmann CH, Rice AP. HIV-1 infection and regulation of Tat function in macrophages. The International Journal of Biochemistry & Cell Biology. 2004;**36**:1767-1775

[49] Qiao X, He B, Chiu A, Knowles DM, Chadburn A, Cerutti A. Human immunodeficiency virus 1 Nef suppresses CD40-dependent immunoglobulin class switching in bystander B cells. Nature Immunology. 2006;**7**:302-310. DOI: 10.1038/ni1302

[50] Qi M, Aiken C. Nef enhances HIV-1 infectivity via association with the virus assembly complex. Virology. 2008;**373**:287-297. DOI: 10.1016/j.virol.2007.12.001

[51] Wang T, Green LA, Gupta SK, Kim C, Wang L, Almodovar S, Flores SC, Prudovsky IA, Jolicoeur P, Liu Z, Clauss M. Transfer of intracellular HIV-1 Nef to endothelium causes endothelial dysfunction. PLoS One. 2014;**9**:e91063. DOI: 10.1371/journal.pone.0091063

[52] Albini A, Soldi R, Giunciuglio D, Giraudo E, Benelli R, Primo L, Noonan D, Salio M, Camussi G, Rockl W, Bussolino F. The angiogenesis induced by HIV-1 tat protein is mediated by the Flk-1/KDR receptor on vascular endothelial cells. Nature Medicine. 1996;**2**:1371-1375. PMID: 8946838

[53] Albini A, Benelli R, Presta M, Rusnati M, Ziche M, Rubartelli A, Paglialunga G, Bussolino F, Noonan D. HIV-1-tat protein is a heparin-binding angiogenic growth factor. Oncogene. 1996;**12**:2892-2897. PMID: 8570206

[54] Stoddart CA, Geleziunas R, Ferrell S, Linquist-Stepps V, Moreno ME, Bare C, Xu W, Yonemoto W, Bresnahan PA, McCune JM, Greene WC. Human immunodeficiency virus type 1 Nef-mediated downregulation of CD4 correlates with Nef enhancement of viral pathogenesis. Journal of Virology. 2003;**77**:2124-2133. PMID: 12525647

[55] Vilhardt F, Plastre O, Sawada M, Suzuki K, Wiznerowicz M, Kiyokawa E, Trono D, Krause KH. The HIV-1 Nef protein and phagocyte NADPH oxidase activation. The Journal of Biological Chemistry. 2002;**277**:42136-42143. DOI: 10.1074/jbc.M200862200

[56] Duffy P, Wang X, Lin PH, Yao Q, Chen C. HIV-1 Nef protein causes endothelial dysfunction in porcine pulmonary arteries and human pulmonary artery endothelial cells. The Journal of Surgical Research. 2009;**156**:257-264. DOI: 10.1016/j.jss.2009.02.005

[57] Acheampong EA, Parveen Z, Muthoga LW, Kalayeh M, Mukhtar M, Pomerantz RJ. Human immunodeficiency virus type 1 Nef potently induces apoptosis in primary human brain microvascular endothelial cells via the activation of caspases. Journal of Virology. 2005;**79**:4257-4269. DOI: 10.1128/JVI.79.7.4257-4269.2005

[58] Park IW, Ullrich CK, Schoenberger E, Ganju RK, Groopman JE. HIV-1 Tat induces microvascular endothelial apoptosis through caspase activation. Journal of Immunology. 2001;**167**:2766-2771. PMID: 11509621

[59] Herrmann CH, Rice AP. Specific interaction of the human immunodeficiency virus Tat proteins with a cellular protein kinase. Virology. 1993;**197**:601-608. DOI: 10.1006/viro.1993.1634

[60] Zidovetzki R, Wang JL, Chen P, Jeyaseelan R, Hofman F. Human immunodeficiency virus Tat protein induces interleukin 6 mRNA expression in human brain endothelial cells via protein kinase C- and cAMP-dependent protein kinase pathways. AIDS Research and Human Retroviruses. 1998;**14**:825-833. DOI: 10.1089/aid.1998.14.825

[61] Hofman FM, Wright AD, Dohadwala MM, Wong-Staal F, Walker SM. Exogenous tat protein activates human endothelial cells. Blood. 1993;**82**:2774-2780. PMID: 7693046

[62] Dhawan S, Puri RK, Kumar A, Duplan H, Masson JM, Aggarwal BB. Human immunodeficiency virus-1-tat protein induces the cell surface expression of endothelial leukocyte adhesion molecule-1, vascular cell adhesion molecule-1, and intercellular adhesion molecule-1 in human endothelial cells. Blood. 1997;**90**:1535-1544. PMID: 9269771

[63] Park IW, Wang JF, Groopman JE. HIV-1 Tat promotes monocyte chemoattractant protein-1 secretion followed by transmigration of monocytes. Blood. 2001;**97**:352-358. PMID: 11154208

[64] Lin S, Nadeau PE, Mergia A. HIV-1 inhibits endothelial reverse cholesterol transport through impacting subcellular Caveolin-1 trafficking. Retrovirology. 2015;**12**:62. DOI: 10.1186/s12977-015-0188-y

[65] Mediouni S, Darque A, Baillat G, Ravaux I, Dhiver C, Tissot-Dupont H, Mokhtari M, Moreau H, Tamalet C, Brunet C, Paul P, Dignat-George F, Stein A, Brouqui P, Spector SA,

Campbell GR, Loret EP. Antiretroviral therapy does not block the secretion of the human immunodeficiency virus tat protein. Infectious Disorders Drug Targets. 2012;**1**:81-86. DOI: 10.2174/187152612798994939

[66] Tinkle BT, Ngo L, Luciw PA, Maciag T, Jay G. Human immunodeficiency virus-associated vasculopathy in transgenic mice. Journal of Virology. 1997;**71**:4809-4814. PMID: 9151876

[67] Marecki JC, Cool CD, Parr JE, Beckey VE, Luciw PA, Tarantal AF, Carville A, Shannon RP, Cota-Gomez A, Tuder RM, Voelkel NF, Flores SC. HIV-1 Nef is associated with complex pulmonary vascular lesions in SHIV-1-nef-infected macaques. American Journal of Respiratory and Critical Care Medicine. 2006;**174**:437-445. DOI: 10.1164/rccm.200601-005OC

[68] Panigrahi S, Freeman ML, Funderburg NT, Mudd JC, Younes SA, Sieg SF, Zidar DA, Paiardini M, Villinger F, Calabrese LH, Ransohoff RM, Jain MK, Lederman MM. SIV/SHIV-1 infection triggers vascular inflammation, diminished expression of Krüppel-like factor 2 and endothelial dysfunction. The Journal of Infectious Diseases. 2016;**213**:1419-1427. DOI: 10.1093/infdis/jiv749

[69] Currier JS, Lundgren JD, Carr A, Klein D, Sabin CA, Sax PE, Schouten JT, Smieja M. Working Group 2: Epidemiological evidence for cardiovascular disease in HIV-1-infected patients and relationship to highly active antiretroviral therapy. Circulation. 2008;**118**:29-35. DOI: 10.1161/CIRCULATIONAHA.107.189624

[70] Obel N, Thomsen HF, Kronborg G, Larsen CS, Hildebrandt PR, Sørensen HT, Gerstoft J. Ischemic heart disease in HIV-1-infected and HIV-1-uninfected individuals: A population-based cohort study. Clinical Infectious Diseases. 2007;**44**:1625-1631. DOI: 10.1086/518285

[71] Furtado MR, Callaway DS, Phair JP, Kunstman KJ, Stanton JL, Macken CA, Perelson AS, Wolinsky SM. Persistence of HIV-1-1 transcription in peripheral-blood mononuclear cells in patients receiving potent antiretroviral therapy. The New England Journal of Medicine. 1999;**340**:1614-1622. DOI: 10.1056/NEJM199905273402102

[72] Fischer M, Günthard HF, Opravil M, Joos B, Huber W, Bisset LR, Ott P, Böni J, Weber R, Cone RW. Residual HIV-1-RNA levels persist for up to 2.5 years in peripheral blood mononuclear cells of patients on potent antiretroviral therapy. AIDS Research and Human Retroviruses. 2000;**16**:1135-1140. DOI: 10.1089/088922200414974

Chapter 16

Selected Endothelial Responses after Ionizing Radiation Exposure

Bjorn Baselet, Raghda Ramadan,
Abderrafi Mohammed Benotmane,
Pierre Sonveaux, Sarah Baatout and An Aerts

Additional information is available at the end of the chapter

http://dx.doi.org/10.5772/intechopen.72386

Abstract

Along with the development of novel chemotherapeutic agents, radiation therapy has revolutionized the prognosis of patients with various cancers. However, with a longer life expectancy, radiation treatment-related comorbidity, like cardiovascular diseases (CVDs), becomes an issue for cancer survivors. In addition, exposure to X-rays for medical diagnostics is dramatically increasing at the present times. A pressing question is whether or not exposure to these very low doses can cause health damage. Below 0.5 gray (Gy), an increased risk cannot be evidenced by epidemiology alone, and in vitro and in vivo mechanistic studies focused on the elucidation of molecular signaling pathways are needed. Given the critical role of the endothelium in normal vascular functions, a complete understanding of radiation-induced endothelial dysfunction is crucial. In this way, the current radiation protection system could be refined if needed, making it possible to more accurately assess the cardiovascular risk in the low-dose region. Finally, radiation-induced CVD, like CVD in general, is a progressive disorder that may take years to decades to manifest. Therefore, experimental studies are warranted to fulfill the urgent need to identify noninvasive biomarkers for an early detection and potential interventions—together with a healthy lifestyle—that may prevent or mitigate these adverse effects.

Keywords: ionizing radiation, radiation therapy, X-ray diagnostics, cardiovascular disease, atherosclerosis, endothelial dysfunction, inflammation, DNA damage, apoptosis, cell cycle, oxidative stress, mitochondrial dysfunction and metabolic changes, premature senescence, intercellular communication

1. Introduction

Cardiovascular disease (CVD) is the leading cause of morbidity and mortality in the Western world. It accounts for nearly one-third of all deaths worldwide. There are multiple contributory risk factors for heart disease. Some are of a controllable nature, such as lifestyle, dietary factors, and metabolic disorders, such as high cholesterol levels and hypertension. Others are noncontrollable risk factors, such as gender, age, and genetic predisposition [1, 2]. In addition, there are environmental factors affecting the risk of CVD, ionizing radiation being one such factor.

It has been known for a long time that high doses of radiation, such as those delivered during radiotherapy, cause damage to the heart and vasculature and thus increase the risk of CVD. Data from animal experiments have strongly supported this observation [3–6]. However, for doses <0.5 gray (Gy), epidemiological data are suggestive rather than persuasive. Therefore, the magnitude of CVD risk in the low-dose region where issues of radiation protection usually operate is not clear [3–6].

Various issues, such as occupational radiation exposure, future of nuclear power, manned space flights, and threat of radiological terrorism, call for a thorough understanding of low-dose health risks [7]. The main concern is, however, an increasing use of ionizing radiation for diagnostic medical purposes (**Figure 1**) [8]. For instance, since 1993, the number of computed tomography (CT) scans has increased four times in the United States, and a similar trend is observed in Europe [9]. Medical radiation is the largest source of radiation exposure in Western countries, accounting for a mean effective dose of 3.0 millisievert (mSv) on average per capita per year from diagnostic procedures only, corresponding to a radiological risk of 30 chest X-rays [10]. Of note, doses from therapeutic procedures are not taken into account in this number. Although the health benefits of these improved diagnostic procedures are huge, concerns are raised regarding "overuse" and potential associated health risks [11].

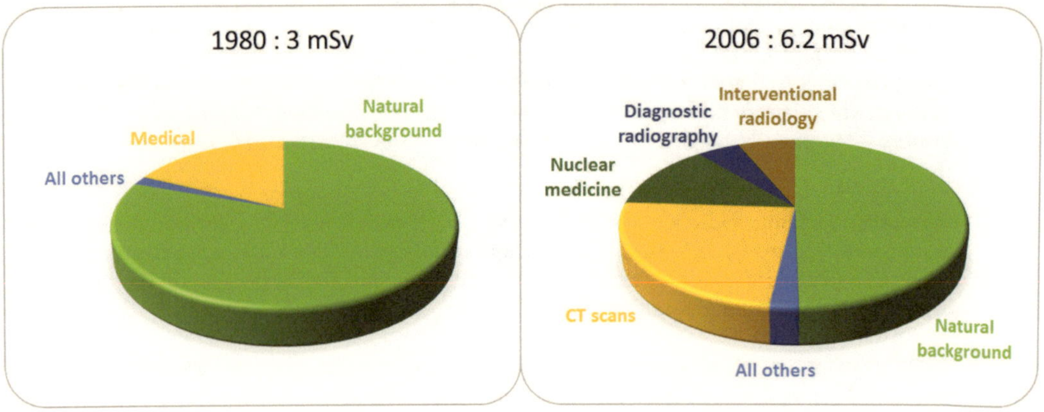

Figure 1. Average annual effective dose per person received in 1980 (left panel) and in 2006 (right panel) in the United States. The large increase in the use of ionizing radiation for medical purposes, in the period 1980–2006, contributed to a total increase from 3.0 mSv in 1980 to 6.2 mSv in 2006. Similar trends are observed in other industrialized countries [1].

1.1. What is ionizing radiation?

From natural to manufactured sources, life on earth is exposed on a daily basis to ionizing radiation. Defined as a type of energy released by atoms that travel in the form of electromagnetic or particles, this energy can eject tightly bound electrons from the orbit of an atom, causing the atom to become ionized [12]. In nature, one can distinguish three main types of ionizing radiation: alpha (α), beta (β) particles, and gamma (γ) rays. They are all produced by naturally occurring substances with unstable nuclei (e.g., cobalt-60 and cesium-137) that spontaneously undergo radioactive decay. During the decay process, energy is lost via emission of ionizing radiation in the form of electromagnetic γ-rays and/or charged particles (e.g., α- and β-particles) [13]. One of the most common manufactured forms of ionizing radiation is X-ray radiation. X-rays are in most aspects similar to γ-rays but differ in origin. While γ-rays are derived from the natural decay of radioactive elements, X-rays are artificially produced in X-ray generators by directing a stream of high-speed electrons at a target material, such as gold or tungsten [14]. When electrons interact with atomic particles of the target, X-radiation is produced [12]. In addition to the most common forms listed above, there are many other forms of ionizing radiation of human or natural origin. Examples are neutrons, accelerated ions and fission fragments [15, 16]. These less common forms can have different biological effects, which can be exploited, for example, in hadron therapy for cancer treatment [17].

1.2. Radiation metrics

Biological effects of ionizing radiation are related to energy deposition in matter. To assess the impact of ionizing radiation on human health and to set guidelines in radioprotection, units to measure a dose and its biological effects are required.

The absorbed dose is defined as the amount of energy, originating from any type of ionizing radiation and any irradiation geometry that is absorbed per unit mass of material. The international SI unit for absorbed dose is gray (Gy). One Gy represents the absorption of 1 joule of energy in 1 kilogram of mass (1 J/kg). This definition is pure physical, as it does not consider the quality of the ionizing radiation type and the extent of biological damage it inflicts to certain tissues and/or organs. As a result, the terms equivalent dose and effective dose have been introduced [18].

The equivalent dose takes into account the ability of a particular kind of ionizing radiation to cause damage. It is obtained by multiplying the absorbed dose (Gy) with a radiation-weighting factor (wR) attributed to each different radiation type (e.g., the wR of photons and electrons is 1, the wR of protons and charged ions is 2, and the wR of α particles and fission fragments is 20). The international SI unit for equivalent dose is the sievert (Sv) [18].

The effective dose is defined as the weighted sum of all tissue and organ equivalent doses multiplied by their respective tissue-weighting factor (wT). It expresses the biological effect that a certain type of ionizing radiation has on the human body. wT values have been defined to represent the contributions of individual organs and tissues to overall radiation effects on the human body. Similar to the equivalent dose, the effective dose has sievert (Sv) as international SI unit. Care should be taken with wT values because they constitute an average over both genders and adult ages to reflect the radiation burden to an average human adult [18, 19]. Examples of effective doses associated with different sources of ionizing radiation are presented in **Table 1**.

1.3. Protection against radiation exposure

Short after the discovery of ionizing radiation by Röntgen in 1895, its detrimental effects became apparent, and people tried to protect themselves [24]. Nowadays, the International Committee on Radiological Protection (ICRP) and the US National Council on Radiation Protection and Measurements (NCRP) aim to protect people by advising means for achieving this, e.g., regulatory and guidance limits [18, 25].

The major question that keeps radiation protection bodies busy and that became the foundation of radiation protection guidelines worldwide is "How much is harmful?" This question is particularly relevant for low-dose exposures for which health impact is not yet fully elucidated. Although a large number of epidemiological and radiobiological studies have been performed to date in order to investigate the effects of low doses of ionizing radiation [26–47], accurate risk assessment is not yet available [18]. Current guidelines for protection against low-dose radiation are based on cancer risk estimates from epidemiological studies. As discussed further, cohorts include atomic bomb survivors, occupationally exposed people, patients (diagnostics or therapeutics), and environmentally exposed people [48]. In general, an excess cancer

Source	Effective dose (mSv)*
Dental X-ray	0.005
Radiography of the chest	0.1
One return flight (New York-London)	0.1
Radiography of the abdomen	1.2
CT of the head	2
Natural background (per year)	2.4
Mammography	3
CT of the chest	7
CT of the abdomen	6–10
CT of the pelvis	8–10
Coronary CT angiography	12
Myocardial perfusion study	10–29
Myocardial viability study	14–41
Annual occupational dose limit	20
Radiotherapy (delivered in fractions)	40,000–70,000

*Doses are whole-body doses, except those of medical exposure, which are delivered to a specific organ. CT, computed tomography; Sv sievert [7, 19–23]

Table 1. Representative effective doses associated with different sources of ionizing radiation.

risk can be statistically evidenced for doses above 100 mGy. Nevertheless, doses below 100 mGy are inconclusive due to two practical limits of epidemiological studies: low statistical power that generates random errors and demography that gives rise to systematic errors. Due to a high natural incidence of cancer, a lifetime follow-up of larger cohorts would be needed to quantify excess cancer risks due to a low dose of ionizing radiation. This is practically infeasible. Furthermore, confounding factors, such as lifestyle risk factors for CVD, can hamper accuracy to confidently detect a small increase in cancer mortality (discussed in Section 2.4). Any inadequacy in matching between control and study groups may give rise to a bias that cannot be merely reduced by expanding the size of the groups [49]. As a consequence, risk assessment in the low-dose region (<100 mGy) is based on extrapolations made from high-dose risk estimates [50]. For cancer, it is widely accepted that the tumorigenic risk increases with radiation dose without the presence of a threshold (the stochastic linear non-threshold [LNT] model). This assumption implies that no dose is absolutely safe, resulting in implementation of the "as low as reasonably achievable" principle [51, 52].

In contrast to cancer, non-cancer diseases have for long not been considered as health risks following exposure to low doses of ionizing radiation. Consequently, they were believed to have a threshold dose below which no significant adverse risks are induced (deterministic linear threshold model) [18, 53]. This idea has been challenged by epidemiological findings showing an excess risk of non-cancer diseases following exposure to doses lower than previously thought [34, 54]. Epidemiological evidence suggests an excess risk of CVD mortality above 0.5 Gy [34, 54]. For doses below 0.5 Gy, the dose-risk relationship is still unclear. However, if the relationship proves to be without a threshold, this may have a considerable impact on the current radiation protection system, since the overall excess mortality risk following low-dose exposure could double [55].

2. Radiation-induced cardiovascular disease

2.1. Epidemiology of radiation-induced CVD

Current predictions indicate that in Western countries almost one of three people will develop cancer during their lifetime [56]. About 50–60% of all cancer patients will undergo radiotherapy with radiation doses averaging 1.8–2 Gy per fraction [57]. During the radiotherapeutic treatment of tumors located in the mediastinal region of the human body (breast, lung, and esophageal cancers), the heart and its blood vessels incidentally receive a part of the radiation dose [46]. Exposure of the cardiovascular system to these therapeutic doses is known to be associated with CVDs. The first epidemiological evidence of this association came from radiation-treated Hodgkin's lymphoma survivors in the 1960s. In a study of 258 Hodgkin's disease patients followed for a median of 14.2 years (range 0.7–26.2) after radiotherapy, cumulative risk for ischemic event increased from 6.4% (95% confidence interval (CI), 3.8 ± 10.7) at 10 years to 21.2% (95% CI, 15 ± 30) at 20–25 years after radiotherapy treatment. Risk for myocardial infarction was 3.4% (95% CI, 1.6 ± 7.0) at 10 years and 14.2% (95% CI, 9 ± 22) at 20–25 years, and risk for ischemic cardiac mortality was 2.6% (95% CI, 1.1 ± 6.1) at 10 years and 10.2% (95% CI, 5.3 ± 19) at 25 years (**Figure 2A**) [58]. Cardiac fibrosis, which causes cardiac dysfunction, arrhythmias, and heart failure, is also seen in Hodgkin's lymphoma survivors but is rather the result of the use of anthracyclines [59]. Radiation-induced cardiovascular disorders are based rather on the damage to the blood vessels. Later, in the study of Darby et al., 2168 breast cancer patients were followed between 5 and more than 20 years after radiotherapy. It was found that women irradiated for left breast cancer (estimated mean heart dose 6.6 Gy) had higher rates of major coronary events than women irradiated for right breast cancer (estimated mean heart dose 2.9 Gy; P = 0.002). Excess relative risk (ERR), a measure that quantifies how much the level of risk among persons with a given level of exposure exceeds the risk of nonexposed persons [60] for major coronary events was 7.4% per Gy (95% CI, 2.9–14.5) when all follow-up times and all breast cancer patients were included (**Figure 2B**) [54].

Additional proofs of increased risk of CVDs after high-dose exposure were provided during the follow-up of Japanese atomic bomb survivors. During a 53-year follow-up of 86,611 members of the Life Span Study cohort, excess relative risk of death from heart disease per Gy was 0.14 (95% CI 0.06–0.23) (**Figure 2C**) [34]. Although there is a large number of epidemiological studies showing a clear excess of CVD risk above 0.5 Gy, they are of limited use for quantitative risk assessment, because individual dosimetry has yet to be performed [35]. In addition, even if an adverse effect can be evidenced at relatively high doses of ionizing radiation, mechanisms by which therapeutic doses affect the cardiovascular system are still not completely understood [28].

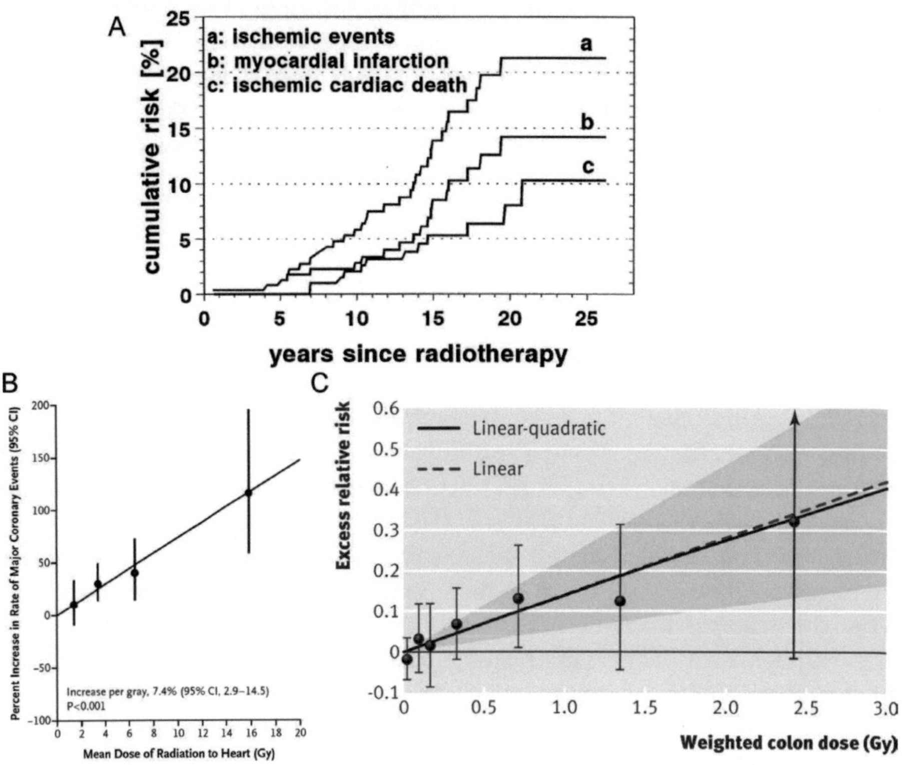

Figure 2. Epidemiological evidence for an increased risk of CVDs after exposure to ionizing radiation. (A) Cumulative risk curves for the occurrence of cardiac events in Hodgkin's lymphoma survivors [58]. (B) Rate of major coronary events according to mean radiation dose to the heart given during breast cancer radiotherapy, as compared with the estimated rate with no radiation exposure to the heart [54]. (C) Excess relative risk for death from heart disease in Japanese atomic bomb survivors. Shaded area is the 95% confidence region for the fitted lines [34].

When the heart receives a radiation dose lower than 0.5 Gy, epidemiological evidence is less strong than that for higher doses. The most informative cohort in this respect is composed of Japanese atomic bomb survivors. It is of high value for low-dose epidemiology as a source for risk estimation due to its large size, the presence of both sexes and all ages, and because irradiated people have well-characterized individual dose estimates [36]. Studies in occupationally exposed individuals are also of interest as they generally involve relatively low doses received during repeated exposures. Examples of such cohorts are nuclear industry workers from 15 countries (the 15-country study) [37], the UK National Registry for Radiation Workers [38], the National Dose Registry of Canada [39], the Chernobyl liquidator cohort [40], and the Mayak cohort [41–43]. The last cohort is composed of workers from Mayak PA, the first and largest Russian nuclear factory for plutonium production where the majority of workers were exposed to ionizing radiation during the first period of operation [61]. In addition, data can also be acquired from environmentally exposed groups, such as settlements located at the vicinity of the Techa River [44] and the Semipalatinsk nuclear test area [45].

When taking into account all epidemiological data on CVD effects of ionizing radiation, a small but highly statistically significant ERR of 0.09 per Gy (95% CI, 0.07–0.12) was observed at doses higher than 0.5 Gy [35]. In addition, ERR of CVD mortality was estimated at 0.08 (95% CI, 0.04–0.12). In other words, receiving 1 Gy of ionizing radiation to the heart and its blood vessels increases the risk of CVD mortality with 8% in comparison to nonexposed people. This assumed risk is rather large and may therefore have serious implications for public health. Indeed, considering the high background rate of CVD, the absolute number of excess cases could be substantial [62]. In order to find an association between low-level radiation exposure and CVD risk in a general unselected population, this meta-analysis was extended by Little et al. [55]. When taking into account 717,660 individuals from the Japanese atomic bomb survivor and occupational and environmental exposure studies listed above, a statistically significant ERR coefficient of 0.10 (95% CI, 0.05–0.15) for coronary artery disease was observed as a result of exposure to low-level radiation more than 5 years prior to death [55]. A linear association between ERR and radiation dose was assumed even in the low-dose range, because there was little evidence of nonlinearity in the dose-response curves for CVD in Japanese atomic bomb survivors [34, 63] and in Mayak workers [41]. Authors further argued that the consistency of ERR/Gy between Japanese atomic bomb survivors with moderate radiation doses [34, 63] and occupational cohorts with low doses could be used to support the notion of a linear relationship between ERR of CVD mortality and low doses of ionizing radiation [55]. In a recent third analysis of the Life Span Study cohort of atomic bomb survivors with 105,444 subjects, the shape of the dose-response curve for solid cancer incidence was found significantly different among males and females ($P = 0.02$). For females, dose-response was consistent with linearity, but for males dose-response best fitted a linear-quadratic model [64]. If this were to be confirmed, the overall excess risk of CVD-associated mortality after exposure to low doses of radiation would be about twice that associated to radiation-induced cancers, which ranges from 4.2% to 5.6% per Sv for the cohort populations discussed above [55, 65] and would even be different between both sexes.

2.2. Pathophysiology of radiation-induced CVD

Following radiotherapy of the thoracic part of the human body for mediastinal lymphoma, breast, lung, and esophageal cancers, the heart incidentally receives a part of the therapeutic dose [46].

As indicated in the epidemiology section, high-dose radiation exposure of the heart and its vessels is associated with a risk of radiation-induced CVD [34, 54, 55]. In this context, coronary artery disease is considered to be the major cardiovascular complication [28, 30, 54]. Two studies provide molecular and cellular mechanisms accounting for increased morbidity and mortality of coronary artery disease following radiation exposure. First, radiation can influence the pathogenesis of age-related atherosclerosis, thereby accelerating the development of atherosclerosis in coronary arteries [28]. Growing atherosclerotic plaques narrow the blood vessel and hamper the blood stream (**Figure 3**). Second, damage to the heart microvasculature can reduce blood flow to the myocardium, causing myocardial ischemia, which promotes acute infarction [30]. Because endothelial activation and dysfunction are major causes of atherosclerosis, much of the current radiobiological research is exploring the molecular and phenotypic effects of ionizing radiation in endothelial cells in the context of radiation-induced CVD [66, 67]. It should be noted, however, that there are also other clinical manifestations of radiation-related CVD, such as pericarditis, congestive heart failure, and heart fibrosis [30, 68, 69]. Radiation-induced pericarditis is caused by damage to the cardiac microvascular network in combination with fibrosis of cardiac venous and lymphatic channels. This ultimately leads to accumulation of a fibrin-rich exudate in the pericardium, causing pericardial tamponade. Congestive heart failure is attributed to radiation-induced fibrosis of the myocardium, which ultimately leads to decreased elasticity and extensibility of cardiac walls, thereby reducing the ejection fraction [70]. To learn more about putative mechanisms, the interested reader is referred to some excellent recent reviews [69, 71].

2.3. Gaps in the current knowledge of radiation-induced CVD

Available epidemiological studies have limited statistical power to detect a possible excess risk of CVD following exposure to radiation doses lower than 0.5 Gy. Limited power is due both to the high background level of CVD in studied populations and to the existence of many

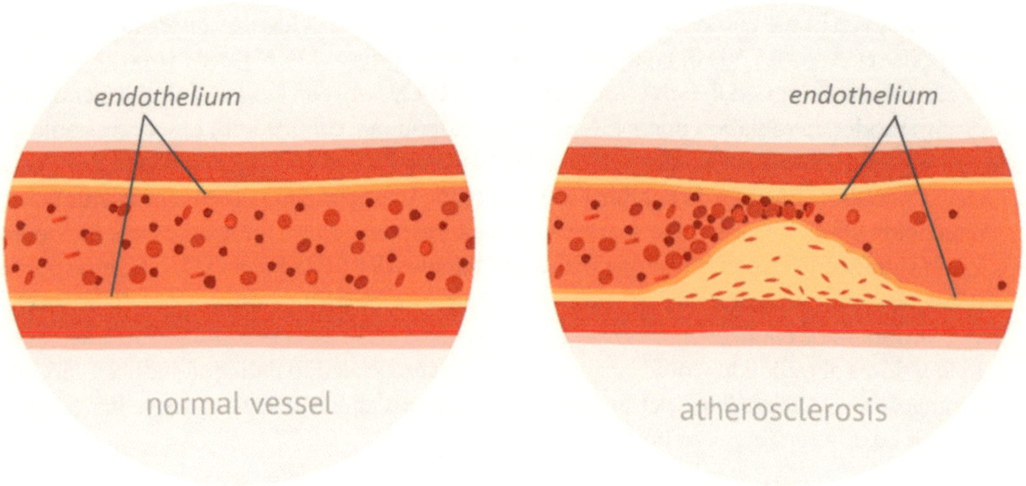

Figure 3. Longitudinal cut of a normal, healthy blood vessel (left) and of a blood vessel with an atherosclerotic plaque hampering the blood stream (right). Damage to the endothelium is an important trigger of atherosclerosis, itself a main cause of CVD.

potentially confounding risk factors. For example, occupational studies have to deal with the "healthy worker" effect, and the study of A-bomb survivors has to deal with the "healthy survivor" effect. Both selection effects occur when healthy individuals with lower mortality and morbidity rates are selectively retained at a specific site (work and living area, respectively) where they accumulate higher doses and therefore confound the dose-risk relationship [37]. Other potential confounders in epidemiological studies are lifestyle risk factors for CVD (e.g., smoking, alcohol consumption, obesity, diabetes, hypertension) [35, 55] prognosis of cancer treatment regimens [30], distribution of the dose range, accuracy of dosimetry, duration of follow-up after exposure, and correct assignment of the cause of mortality [62]. For these reasons, the number of people needed to quantify the excess risk of a dose <0.5 Gy is unfeasibly high. In the context of radiation-related cancer, for example, a cohort of 5 million people would be needed to quantify the excess risk of a 10 mGy dose, assuming that the excess risk is in proportion to the dose [7]. Moreover, CVD may occur a long time after exposure to doses below 30 Gy (approx. 10–30 year lag) [30, 72, 73]. As a result, a long follow-up period of time is needed to determine the nature and magnitude of risks following individual exposure to lower doses.

Despite the fact that epidemiological studies have led to significant insights in radiation-related CVD risk, there are still many uncertainties that need to be addressed. Does CVD risk occur only above a specific radiation dose? Is the latency of CVD development dependent on the dose? Which are the sensitive targets in the heart and vasculature (e.g., fibroblasts, vascular smooth muscle cells, and endothelial cells)? Does radiation exposure affect CVD incidence or progression or both? Is there a difference between single dose and fractionated and chronic exposure? How does the time interval between two consecutive dose fractionations play a role in the induction of damage? These questions need to be answered to provide a more accurate dose risk assessment in order to improve the current radiation protection system.

Classical epidemiological studies are not adapted to provide answers to these questions. There is, therefore, a clear need for more detailed epidemiological studies that would be capable of addressing potential confounding factors and selection biases that could influence results. Furthermore, there is a particular need for a better understanding of the biological and molecular mechanisms responsible for the association between ionizing radiation and CVD [6]. Hence, a more directed approach is required, such as molecular epidemiology that integrates epidemiology and biology [55]. Radiobiological research is thus essential for understanding the radiation-related CVD risks, both at high and low doses. In other words, accurate risk estimation will be possible only based on comprehensive biological and molecular understanding of what ionizing radiation does to the cardiovascular system. To date, the induction of radiation-related CVD risks is believed to be the result of endothelial dysfunction, which will be discussed in the next section [30].

3. Endothelial cell responses after ionizing radiation exposure

The endothelium could be a critical target in ionizing radiation-related CVD [74]. The endothelium is a single layer of cells that lines the interior of the vascular system and of the heart and has thus a strategic position between the blood and the surrounding tissues. It is a highly active organ system that is constantly sensing and responding to changes of the extracellular environment to maintain a normal function of the vascular system [75].

Endothelial cells are involved in a wide range of physiological processes, such as regulation of vascular tone, vascular permeability, blood coagulation/fibrinolysis, and inflammation, which are needed to maintain proper vascular functioning (**Figure 4**) [76]. Endothelial dysfunction has been observed in patients with atherosclerosis and in patients that exhibit CVD risk factors such as smoking, dyslipidemia, obesity, and diabetes mellitus [77] and is considered to be one of the first predictive indicators of cardiovascular morbidity and mortality [78].

A dysfunctional endothelium is characterized by inflammation, DNA damage, oxidative stress, alterations of coagulation and platelet pathways, senescence, and cell death, all of which are observed after radiation doses above 1–2 Gy, as shown in many in vitro and in vivo studies [6, 28, 79–81]. Comparatively, both protective and detrimental effects have been reported for low-dose exposure, suggesting that multiple mechanisms may influence radiation-induced atherosclerosis [6, 62]. Increasing evidence also suggests a role of intercellular communication in the endothelial cell response to ionizing radiation [82]. All of these endpoints are briefly discussed in the following paragraphs. In addition, other pathological effects of ionizing radiation on the endothelium are observed like impaired endothelial regulation of vascular tone [83–87], loss of the endothelial monolayer integrity [88–92], and procoagulant and prothrombic conditions [28, 93–108].

3.1. Inflammation

Endothelial expression of adhesion molecules plays an important role in recruiting inflammatory cells from the bloodstream into the vessel intima where they transform into foam cells, elements

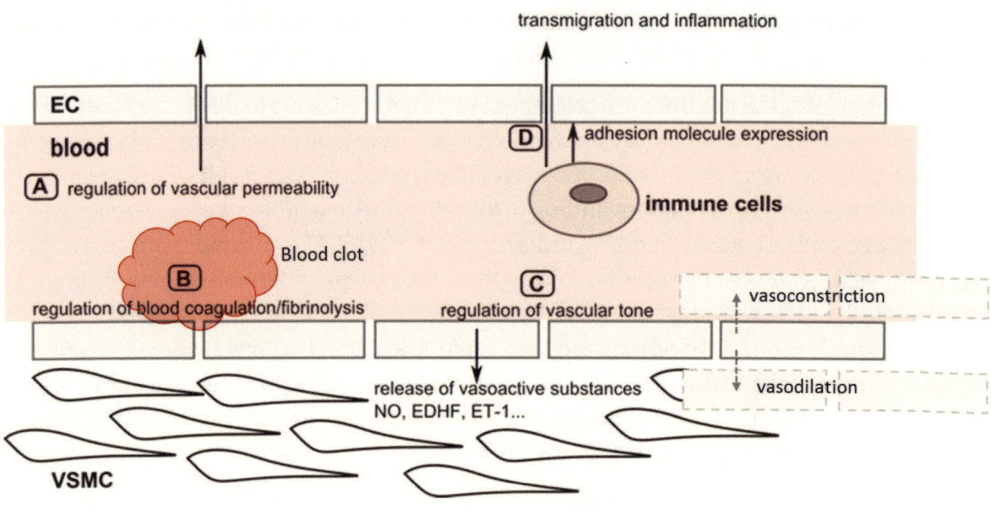

Figure 4. Overview of the major physiological functions of the arterial endothelium. (A) The endothelium (ECs, endothelial cells) forms a selective barrier regulating solute flux and fluid permeability between the blood and surrounding tissues [78]. (B) Formation of a thrombus or blood clot is referred to as intravascular coagulation, and the breakdown of a thrombus is referred to as fibrinolysis. Normal endothelium has antithrombotic and profibrinolytic properties and actively represses platelet adhesion and aggregation. Vessel damage or exposure to pro-inflammatory molecules shifts the balance toward more prothrombic/antifibrinolytic activities [75, 109]. (C) To regulate the vascular tone, the endothelium releases various vasodilatory agents, such as nitric oxide (NO) and endothelial-derived hyperpolarizing factor (EDHF), or vasoconstrictive agents, such as endothelin-1 (ET-1), which modify vascular smooth muscle cell (VSMC) contractility [110]. (D) In the case of inflammation, endothelial permeability is increased. Endothelial cells recruit immune cells via the expression of adhesion molecules and mediate their transmigration toward the inner vascular wall [75, 76] .

of the atherosclerotic plaque. Radiation has been shown to upregulate several of such adhesion molecules. For instance, exposure of endothelial cells to 5 Gy increases the expression of intercellular adhesion molecule-1 (ICAM-1) and E-selectin 6 h after irradiation [111]. Platelet endothelial cell adhesion molecule-1 (PECAM-1), ICAM-1 and ICAM-2, and vascular cellular adhesion molecule-1 (VCAM-1) were also observed to increase in mouse heart cells 10 weeks after local thorax irradiation with 8 Gy [112]. Interestingly, ICAM-1 and VCAM-1 remained upregulated 20 weeks after irradiation. Besides induction of adhesion molecules, the expression of cytokines, such as interleukin (IL)-6 and IL-8, and other inflammatory molecules such as transforming growth factor-β (TGF-β) was shown to increase after high and moderate irradiation doses in human endothelial cell cultures [113, 114]. In this context, the Japanese atomic bomb survivors' cohort also showed signs of a generally increased inflammation state, with increased levels of IL-6 and C-reactive protein (CRP) [115].

3.2. DNA damage and apoptosis

Ionizing radiation is known to induce a wide range of DNA lesions, of which double-strand breaks (DSBs) are most severe in a direct manner but also indirectly through the formation of reactive oxygen species (ROS) [116, 117]. Upon DNA damage, a response is initiated, and cells activate cell cycle checkpoints that slow down or stop cell cycle progression [118]. This gives them time to repair damaged DNA or to prevent division when chromosomes are damaged or incompletely replicated. If cells fail to repair their DNA, they undergo programmed cell death, apoptosis, or premature senescence (described below) [119]. Consequently, DSB leads to a high lethality of the affected cells.

Whereas high doses are known to induce apoptosis in endothelial cells [120], less is known about the effect of low radiation doses. A subtle but significant increase in DSBs was observed in human umbilical vein endothelial cells (HUVEC) and EA.hy926 endothelial cells 30 min after exposure to 0.05 Gy. In addition, irradiation with 0.05 Gy and 0.1 Gy induced relatively more DSB/Gy in comparison to 0.5 Gy and 2 Gy [121]. This observation could be caused either by an underestimation due to DNA damage spot merging [122] or by the induction of a global chromatin reorganization at low doses of ionizing radiation [123]. Furthermore, a dose-dependent increase in the number of apoptotic cells was observed, down to 0.5 Gy in HUVEC and 0.1 Gy in EA.hy926 cells [121]. Another study showed no increase in the number of apoptotic endothelial cells after exposure to 0.2 Gy, whereas apoptosis was observed after exposure to 5 Gy [124].

3.3. Oxidative stress, mitochondrial dysfunction, and metabolic changes

Mitochondria are often regarded as the powerhouse of the cell by generating the ultimate energy transfer molecule, adenosine triphosphate or ATP. Mitochondrial dysfunction is part of both normal and premature agings, but it can also contribute to inflammation, cell senescence, oxidative stress, and apoptosis. Increasing evidence indicates that mitochondrial damage and dysfunction occur in atherosclerosis and may contribute to the multiple pathological processes underlying the disease [125].

An increased accumulation of mitochondrial DNA damage was observed in several human fibroblast cell lines after exposure to doses as low as 0.1 Gy [126]. Furthermore, functional impairment of mitochondria (reduced mitochondrial respiration and electron transport chain activity) and alterations of the mitochondrial proteome were observed in isolated cardiac mouse mitochondria 4 and 40 weeks after a 2 Gy local heart irradiation. Only a few alterations of the mitochondrial proteome and no effect on mitochondrial function were observed with 0.2 Gy [127, 128]. Finally, alterations of energy and lipid metabolism and perturbations of the insulin/insulin growth factor—phosphatidylinositol-4,5-bisphosphate 3-kinase—RAC-alpha serine/threonine-protein kinase (IGP-PI3K-Akt) signaling pathway were suggested in proteomic studies using cell lines or cells isolated from mice after irradiation with doses ranging from 3 to 16 Gy [129–131].

Water radiolysis instantly causes the formation of ROS (e.g., $\bullet OH^-$, $\bullet O_2^-$, H_2O_2). However, cellular oxidative stress can also be observed long after irradiation, due to an increase in endogenous cellular ROS production [132]. Mitochondria are believed to be the major source of radiation-induced secondary ROS. For instance, Leach et al. have demonstrated that between 1 and 10 Gy, the amount of ROS-producing cells increased with the dose, which they suggested was dependent on radiation-induced propagation of mitochondrial permeability transition via a Ca^{2+}-dependent mechanism [133, 134]. It has further been suggested that ROS can be transferred from cell to cell by gap junctions and paracrine communication pathways in order to propagate radiation-induced biological effects at the intercellular level. This phenomenon is commonly referred to as the radiation-induced "bystander effect" [135]. Multiple molecular signaling mechanisms involving oxidative stress, various kinases, inflammatory molecules, and Ca^{2+} are postulated to contribute to this effect [136].

3.4. Premature senescence

The culprit of radiation-induced premature senescence is most likely severe irreparable DSB [137], even if accelerated telomere shortening has also been suggested [138]. Furthermore, oxidative stress is seen as a major player in radiation-induced senescence and is involved in both radiation-induced DNA damage and accelerated telomere attrition [138–140].

In several in vitro studies, it has been demonstrated that ionizing radiation induces endothelial cell senescence, mainly with exposure to higher radiation doses [141–144]. An interesting study was carried out to examine the effect of chronic low-dose rate irradiation (1.4, 2.4, and 4.1 mGy/h) during 10 weeks [145, 146]. Exposure to 1.4 mGy/h did not accelerate the onset of senescence, whereas exposure to 2.4 mGy/h and 4.1 mGy/h did. Remarkably, a senescent profile was observed when the accumulated doses received by the cells reached 4 Gy. Proteomic analysis revealed a role for radiation-induced oxidative stress and DNA damage, resulting in induction of the p53/p21 pathway. Also, a role for the PI3K/Akt/mechanistic target of rapamycin (mTOR) pathway was suggested. In a related transcriptomic study, authors suggested that premature senescence resulted from an early stress response with p53 signaling, cell cycle changes, DNA repair, and apoptosis observed after 1 week of exposure and an inflammation-related profile observed after 3 weeks. In addition, a possible role of insulin-like growth factor-binding protein 5 (IGFBP-5) signaling, known to be involved in the regulation of cellular senescence, was suggested for the induction of premature senescence after chronic low-dose rate irradiation [147].

Oxidative stress, inflammation, and cellular senescence are all consequences of a normal aging process but are observed early in irradiated tissues, including the heart, suggesting an intensification and acceleration of these molecular processes [71].

http://dx.doi.org/10.5772/intechopen.72386

3.5. Intercellular communication

Traditionally, it was accepted that exposure to ionizing radiation only directly affects irradiated cells. However, in 1992, it was found that irradiation of 1% cells with α-particles leads to genetic damage in more than 30% of cells [148]. Exposure of cells to ionizing radiation results in significant biological effects occurring in both irradiated and non-irradiated cells through the radiation-induced bystander effect [149, 150]. Although the mechanisms of this effect are not fully elucidated yet, oxidative stress, different cytokines (e.g., TNF-α, IL-1, and IL-6), Ca^{2+}, and kinases play a role in the damage to non-irradiated cells.

Intercellular communication through gap junctions and paracrine signaling through hemichannels have been suggested to mediate bystander responses. Gap junctions and hemichannels are composed of multimeric transmembrane structures made of connexin (Cx) [150, 151]. In human, 21 Cx proteins have been identified, which are present in most organs, and display a tissue/cellular specificity [152, 153]. There are three different Cx isotypes expressed in endothelial cells of major arteries, namely, Cx37, Cx40, and Cx43 [154–156]. Cxs have important physiological roles (e.g., they support longitudinal and radial cell-cell communication in the vascular wall), and changes of their expression patterns have been observed during atherosclerosis. Although healthy endothelial cells mainly express Cx37 and Cx40, both Cxs are lost in the endothelium covering advanced atherosclerotic plaques. On the contrary, Cx43 is detectable at specific regions of advanced atherosclerotic plaques [157]. The mechanisms responsible for modification of the Cx expression pattern in atherosclerosis are not fully understood. However, it has been recently demonstrated that Cx37 is a regulator of endothelial NO synthase (eNOS) [158]. The altered Cx37 expression level could be responsible for decreased eNOS activity and decreased NO bioavailability, which may cause endothelial cell dysfunction and increased susceptibility to atherosclerosis. Therefore, Cx37 may play a protective role against atherosclerosis. In addition, Cx40 may play a similar role, as endothelial-specific deletion of Cx40 was reported to promote atherosclerosis by increasing CD73-dependent leukocyte adhesion to the endothelium [155]. In contrast to the atheroprotective effects of Cx37 and Cx40, Cx43 has been suggested to be pro-atherosclerotic. Indeed, downregulation of Cx43 expression inhibited monocyte-endothelial adhesion by decreasing the expression levels of cell adhesion proteins, whereas its upregulation enhanced the adhesion of monocytes to endothelial cells [159]. Besides their roles in atherosclerosis, Cxs were reported to be highly sensitive to ionizing radiation [156]. Indeed, it was observed that a low-dose irradiation exposure induced activation of Cx43 in a time- and dose-dependent manner in human neonatal foreskin fibroblasts [160]. Moreover, upregulation of Cx43 was noticed after 5 Gy of X-ray exposure in mouse primary endothelial cells [161].

4. Conclusion

Research regarding CVD risk related to ionizing radiation is an important way forward to complement epidemiological data with the underlying biological and molecular mechanisms. This is especially important for doses <0.5 Gy, for which epidemiological data are suggestive rather than persuasive. Indeed, due to limited statistical power, the dose-risk relationship is undetermined below 0.5 Gy, but if this relationship proves to be without a threshold, it may have a considerable impact on current low-dose health risk estimates. In this regard, a complete understanding of the pathological effects of ionizing radiation regarding endothelial dysfunction is needed. In addition, it will help in the identification of protective strategies as well as a set of predictive biomarkers for radiation-induced cardiovascular disorders.

Acknowledgements

This review is written in the context of a study that was funded by EU FP7 DoReMi (grant agreement 249689) on "low dose research towards multidisciplinary integration,", by EU FP7 ProCardio project (grant agreement 295823) and by the Federal Agency of Nuclear Control (FANC-AFCN, Belgium) (grant agreement: CO-90-13-3289-00). R. Ramadam and B. Baselet are recipients of a doctoral SCK•CEN/Ghent University grant and of a doctoral SCK•CEN/ Université catholique de Louvain grant, respectively. P. Sonveaux is a Senior Research Associate of the Belgian National Fonds de la Recherche Scientifique.

Author details

Bjorn Baselet[1,2], Raghda Ramadan[1,3], Abderrafi Mohammed Benotmane[1], Pierre Sonveaux[2], Sarah Baatout[1,4] and An Aerts[1]*

*Address all correspondence to: an.aerts@sckcen.be

1 Radiobiology Unit, Institute for Environment, Health and Safety, Belgian Nuclear Research Centre (SCK•CEN), Mol, Belgium

2 Pole of Pharmacology and Therapeutics, Institut de Recherche Expérimentale et Clinique (IREC), Université catholique de Louvain (UCL), Belgium

3 Department of Basic Medical Sciences, Physiology Group, Faculty of Medicine and Health Sciences, Ghent University, Ghent, Belgium

4 Department of Molecular Biotechnology, Ghent University, Ghent, Belgium

References

[1] UNSCEAR United Nations Scientific Committee on the Effects of Atomic Radiation. Annex B. Epidemiological evaluation of cardiovascular disease and other non-cancer diseases following radiation exposure. UNSCEAR Report Vol 1. 2006

[2] Montgomery JE, Brown JR. Metabolic biomarkers for predicting cardiovascular disease. Vascular Health and Risk Management. 2013;**9**:37-45

[3] AGIR–Advisory Group on Ionising Radiation. Circulatory Disease Risk. Report of the independent Advisory Group on Ionizing Radiation. London: Health Protection Agency; 2010

[4] Authors of behalf of ICRP SF, Akleyev AV, Hauer-Jensen M, Henddy JH, Kleiman NJ, Macvittie TJ, Aleman BM, Edgar AB, Mabuchi K, Muirhead CR, et al. ICRP publication 118. ICRP statement on tissue reactions and early and late effects of radiation in normal tissue and organ—Threshold doses for tissue reactions in a radiation protection context. Annals of the ICRP. 2012;**41**:322

[5] Little MP. Radiation and circulatory disease. Mutation Research. 2016;**770**(Pt B):299-318

[6] Baselet B, Rombouts C, Benotmane AM, Baatout S, Aerts A. Cardiovascular diseases related to ionizing radiation: The risk of low-dose exposure (review). International Journal of Molecular Medicine. 2016;**38**(6):1623-1641

[7] Brenner DJ, Doll R, Goodhead DT, Hall EJ, Land CE, Little JB, et al. Cancer risks attributable to low doses of ionizing radiation: Assessing what we really know. Proceedings of the National Academy of Sciences of the United States of America. 2003;**100**(24):13761-13766

[8] UNSCEAR. Sources and effects of ionizing radiation. Annex A: medical radiation exposures. Report to the General Assembly with annexes. New york, NY: United Nations. 2008

[9] Hall EJ, Brenner DJ. Cancer risks from diagnostic radiology. The British Journal of Radiology. 2008;**81**(965):362-378

[10] Picano E, Vano E, Rehani MM, Cuocolo A, Mont L, Bodi V, et al. The appropriate and justified use of medical radiation in cardiovascular imaging: A position document of the ESC associations of cardiovascular imaging, percutaneous cardiovascular interventions and electrophysiology. European Heart Journal. 2014;**35**(10):665-672

[11] Shapiro BP, Mergo PJ, Snipelisky DF, Kantor B, Gerber TC. Radiation dose in cardiac imaging: How should it affect clinical decisions? American Journal of Roentgenology. 2013;**200**(3):508-514

[12] Hall EJ, Giaccia AJ. Radiobiology for the Radiologist. 7th ed. Philadelphia: Lippincott, Williams & Wilkins; 2012

[13] Martin A, Harbison S, Beach K, Cole P. An Introduction to Radiation Protection. 6th ed. London: Hodder Arnold; 2012. 256 p

[14] Dendy PP, Heaton B. Physics for Diagnostic Radiology. 3rd ed. Taylor & Francis Inc: Bosa Roca, US; 2012. 695 p

[15] Kudriashov IB, Kudriashov YB. Radiation Biophysics (Ionizing Radiations). 1st ed. New York: Nova Science Publishers Inc; 2008. 327 p

[16] Maalouf M, Durante M, Foray N. Biological effects of space radiation on human cells: History, advances and outcomes. Journal of Radiation Research. 2011;**52**(2):126-146

[17] Durante M, Loeffler JS. Charged particles in radiation oncology. Nature Reviews. Clinical Oncology. 2010;**7**(1):37-43

[18] ICRP. The 2007 recommendations of the international commission on radiological protection. ICRP publication 103. Annals of the ICRP. 2007;**37**(2-4):1-332

[19] Einstein AJ. Effects of radiation exposure from cardiac imaging: How good are the data? Journal of the American College of Cardiology. 2012;**59**(6):553-565

[20] Lin EC. Radiation risk from medical imaging. Mayo Clinic Proceedings. 2010;**85**(12):1142-1146 quiz 6

[21] Mullenders L, Atkinson M, Paretzke H, Sabatier L, Bouffler S. Assessing cancer risks of low-dose radiation. Nature Reviews. Cancer. 2009;**9**(8):596-604

[22] Paterick TE, Jan MF, Paterick ZR, Tajik AJ, Gerber TC. Cardiac imaging modalities with ionizing radiation: The role of informed consent. JACC: Cardiovascular Imaging. 2012;**5**(6):634-640

[23] Fazel R, Krumholz HM, Wang Y, Ross JS, Chen J, Ting HH, et al. Exposure to low-dose ionizing radiation from medical imaging procedures. The New England Journal of Medicine. 2009;**361**(9):849-857

[24] Thariat J, Hannoun-Levi JM, Sun Myint A, Vuong T, Gerard JP. Past, present, and future of radiotherapy for the benefit of patients. Nature Reviews. Clinical Oncology. 2013;**10**(1):52-60

[25] Walker JS. Permissible dose : a history of radiation protection in the twentieth century. Berkeley: University of California Press; 2000. xii, 168 pp

[26] Stewart JR, Fajardo LF. Radiation-induced heart disease. Clinical and experimental aspects. Radiologic Clinics of North America. 1971;**9**(3):511-531

[27] Stewart FA. Mechanisms and dose-response relationships for radiation-induced cardiovascular disease. Annals of the ICRP. 2012;**41**(3-4):72-79

[28] Schultz-Hector S, Trott KR. Radiation-induced cardiovascular diseases: Is the epidemiologic evidence compatible with the radiobiologic data? International Journal of Radiation Oncology, Biology, Physics. 2007;**67**(1):10-18

[29] Clarke M, Collins R, Darby S, Davies C, Elphinstone P, Evans E, et al. Effects of radiotherapy and of differences in the extent of surgery for early breast cancer on local recurrence and 15-year survival: An overview of the randomised trials. Lancet. 2005;**366**(9503):2087-2106

[30] Darby SC, Cutter DJ, Boerma M, Constine LS, Fajardo LF, Kodama K, et al. Radiation-related heart disease: Current knowledge and future prospects. International Journal of Radiation Oncology, Biology, Physics. 2010;**76**(3):656-665

[31] Darby SC, McGale P, Taylor CW, Peto R. Long-term mortality from heart disease and lung cancer after radiotherapy for early breast cancer: Prospective cohort study of about 300,000 women in US SEER cancer registries. Lancet Oncology. 2005;**6**(8):557-565

[32] McGale P, Darby SC, Hall P, Adolfsson J, Bengtsson NO, Bennet AM, et al. Incidence of heart disease in 35,000 women treated with radiotherapy for breast cancer in Denmark and Sweden. Radiotherapy and Oncology. 2011;**100**(2):167-175

[33] Carr ZA, Land CE, Kleinerman RA, Weinstock RW, Stovall M, Griem ML, et al. Coronary heart disease after radiotherapy for peptic ulcer disease. International Journal of Radiation Oncology, Biology, Physics. 2005;**61**(3):842-850

[34] Shimizu Y, Kodama K, Nishi N, Kasagi F, Suyama A, Soda M, et al. Radiation exposure and circulatory disease risk: Hiroshima and Nagasaki atomic bomb survivor data, 1950-2003. BMJ. 2010;**340**:b5349

[35] Radiation AGoI, editor. Circulatory Disease Risk. Report of the Independent Advisory Group on Ionising Radiation. Health Protection Agency; 2010

[36] Takahashi I, Abbott RD, Ohshita T, Takahashi T, Ozasa K, Akahoshi M, et al. A prospective follow-up study of the association of radiation exposure with fatal and non-fatal stroke among atomic bomb survivors in Hiroshima and Nagasaki (1980-2003). BMJ Open. 2012;**2**(1):e000654

[37] Vrijheid M, Cardis E, Ashmore P, Auvinen A, Bae JM, Engels H, et al. Mortality from diseases other than cancer following low doses of ionizing radiation: Results from the 15-country study of nuclear industry workers. International Journal of Epidemiology. 2007;**36**(5):1126-1135

[38] Muirhead CR, O'Hagan JA, Haylock RG, Phillipson MA, Willcock T, Berridge GL, et al. Mortality and cancer incidence following occupational radiation exposure: Third analysis of the National Registry for Radiation Workers. British Journal of Cancer. 2009;**100**(1):206-212

[39] Ashmore JP, Krewski D, Zielinski JM, Jiang H, Semenciw R, Band PR. First analysis of mortality and occupational radiation exposure based on the National Dose Registry of Canada. American Journal of Epidemiology. 1998;**148**(6):564-574

[40] Ivanov VK, Maksioutov MA, Chekin SY, Petrov AV, Biryukov AP, Kruglova ZG, et al. The risk of radiation-induced cerebrovascular disease in Chernobyl emergency workers. Health Physics. 2006;**90**(3):199-207

[41] Azizova TV, Muirhead CR, Druzhinina MB, Grigoryeva ES, Vlasenko EV, Sumina MV, et al. Cardiovascular diseases in the cohort of workers first employed at Mayak PA in 1948-1958. Radiation Research. 2010;**174**(2):155-168

[42] Azizova TV, Day RD, Wald N, Muirhead CR, O'Hagan JA, Sumina MV, et al. The "clinic" medical-dosimetric database of Mayak production association workers: Structure, characteristics and prospects of utilization. Health Physics. 2008;**94**(5):449-458

[43] Azizova TV, Muirhead CR, Moseeva MB, Grigoryeva ES, Vlasenko EV, Hunter N, et al. Ischemic heart disease in nuclear workers first employed at the Mayak PA in 1948-1972. Health Physics. 2012;**103**(1):3-14

[44] Krestinina LY, Epifanova S, Silkin S, Mikryukova L, Degteva M, Shagina N, et al. Chronic low-dose exposure in the Techa River Cohort: Risk of mortality from circulatory diseases. Radiation and Environmental Biophysics. 2013;**52**(1):47-57

[45] Grosche B, Lackland DT, Land CE, Simon SL, Apsalikov KN, Pivina LM, et al. Mortality from cardiovascular diseases in the Semipalatinsk historical cohort, 1960-1999, and its relationship to radiation exposure. Radiation Research. 2011;**176**(5):660-669

[46] Chargari C, Riet F, Mazevet M, Morel E, Lepechoux C, Deutsch E. Complications of thoracic radiotherapy. Presse Médicale. 2013;**42**(9 Pt 2):e342-e351

[47] Mancuso M, Pasquali E, Braga-Tanaka I 3rd, Tanaka S, Pannicelli A, Giardullo P, et al. Acceleration of atherogenesis in ApoE−/− mice exposed to acute or low-dose-rate ionizing radiation. Oncotarget. 2015;**6**(31):31263-31271

[48] United Nations. Scientific Committee on the Effects of Atomic Radiation. Sources and Effects of Ionizing Radiation : United Nations Scientific Committee on the Effects of Atomic Radiation : UNSCEAR 2008 Report to the General Assembly, with Scientific Annexes. New York: United Nations; 2010

[49] United Nations. Scientific Committee on the Effects of Atomic Radiation. Sources and Effects of Ionizing Radiation : United Nations Committee on the Effects of Atomic Radiation : UNSCEAR 1993 Report to the General Assembly, with Scientific Annexes. New York: United Nations; 1993. 922 p

[50] Committee to assess Health Risks from Exposure to Low Levels of Ionizing Radiation Research NRC. Health risks from exposure to low levels of ionizing radiation: BEIR VII—Phase 2. 2006

[51] Martin CJ. The LNT model provides the best approach for practical implementation of radiation protection. The British Journal of Radiology. 2005;**78**:14-16

[52] Martin CJ, Sutton DG, West CM, Wright EG. The radiobiology/radiation protection interface in healthcare. Journal of Radiological Protection: Official Journal of the Society for Radiological Protection. 2009;**29**:A1-A20

[53] Hildebrandt G. Non-cancer diseases and non-targeted effects. Mutation Research. 2010; **687**(1-2):73-77

[54] Darby SC, Ewertz M, McGale P, Bennet AM, Blom-Goldman U, Bronnum D, et al. Risk of ischemic heart disease in women after radiotherapy for breast cancer. The New England Journal of Medicine. 2013;**368**(11):987-998

[55] Little MP, Azizova TV, Bazyka D, Bouffler SD, Cardis E, Chekin S, et al. Systematic review and meta-analysis of circulatory disease from exposure to low-level ionizing radiation and estimates of potential population mortality risks. Environmental Health Perspectives. 2012;**120**(11):1503-1511

[56] Dale RG, Jones B, Carabe-Fernandez A. Why more needs to be known about RBE effects in modern radiotherapy. Applied Radiation and Isotopes. 2009;**67**(3):387-392

[57] Gottfried K-LD, Penn G. U.S. Nuclear Regulatory Commission. Medical Use Program., Institute of Medicine (U.S.). Committee for Review and Evaluation of the Medical Use Program of the Nuclear Regulatory Commission. Radiation in Medicine : A Need for Regulatory Reform. Washington, D.C.: National Academy Press; 1996. 308 p

[58] Reinders JG, Heijmen BJ, Olofsen-van Acht MJ, van Putten WL, Levendag PC. Ischemic heart disease after mantlefield irradiation for Hodgkin's disease in long-term follow-up. Radiotherapy and Oncology. 1999;**51**(1):35-42

[59] Ng AK, van Leeuwen FE. Hodgkin lymphoma: Late effects of treatment and guidelines for surveillance. Seminars in Hematology. 2016;**53**(3):209-215

[60] Lee WC. Excess relative risk as an effect measure in case-control studies of rare diseases. PLoS One. 2014;**10**(4):e0121141

[61] Azizova TV, Grigorieva ES, Hunter N, Pikulina MV, Moseeva MB. Risk of mortality from circulatory diseases in Mayak workers cohort following occupational radiation exposure. Journal of Radiological Protection. 2015;**35**(3):517-538

[62] Borghini A, Gianicolo EA, Picano E, Andreassi MG. Ionizing radiation and atherosclerosis: Current knowledge and future challenges. Atherosclerosis. 2013;**230**(1):40-47

[63] Yamada M, Wong FL, Fujiwara S, Akahoshi M, Suzuki G. Noncancer disease incidence in atomic bomb survivors, 1958-1998. Radiation Research. 2004;**161**(6):622-632

[64] Grant EJ, Brenner A, Sugiyama H, Sakata R, Sadakane A, Utada M, et al. Solid cancer incidence among the life span study of atomic bomb survivors: 1958-2009. Radiation Research. 2017;**187**(5):513-537

[65] Preston DL, Shimizu Y, Pierce DA, Suyama A, Mabuchi K. Studies of mortality of atomic bomb survivors. Report 13: Solid cancer and noncancer disease mortality: 1950-1997. Radiation Research. 2003;**160**(4):381-407

[66] Libby P, Ridker PM, Hansson GK. Progress and challenges in translating the biology of atherosclerosis. Nature. 2011;**473**(7347):317-325

[67] Bentzon JF, Otsuka F, Virmani R, Falk E. Mechanisms of plaque formation and rupture. Circulation Research. 2014;**114**(12):1852-1866

[68] Adams MJ, Lipshultz SE, Schwartz C, Fajardo LF, Coen V, Constine LS. Radiation-associated cardiovascular disease: Manifestations and management. Seminars in Radiation Oncology. 2003;**13**(3):346-356

[69] Taunk NK, Haffty BG, Kostis JB, Goyal S. Radiation-induced heart disease: Pathologic abnormalities and putative mechanisms. Frontiers in Oncology. 2015;**5**:39

[70] Adams MJ, Hardenbergh PH, Constine LS, Lipshultz SE. Radiation-associated cardiovascular disease. Critical Reviews in Oncology/Hematology. 2003;**45**(1):55-75

[71] Tapio S. Pathology and biology of radiation-induced cardiac disease. Journal of Radiation Research. 2016;**57**(5):439-448

[72] Little MP, Lipshultz SE. Low dose radiation and circulatory diseases: A brief narrative review. Cardio-Oncology. 2015;**1**(1):1-10

[73] Simonetto C, Azizova TV, Grigoryeva ES, Kaiser JC, Schollnberger H, Eidemuller M. Ischemic heart disease in workers at Mayak PA: Latency of incidence risk after radiation exposure. PLoS One. 2014;**9**(5):e96309

[74] Baselet B, Rombouts C, Benotmane AM, Baatout S, Aerts A. Cardiovascular diseases related to ionizing radiation: The risk of low-dose exposure (review). International Journal of Molecular Medicine. 2016

[75] Michiels C. Endothelial cell functions. Journal of Cellular Physiology. 2003;**196**(3):430-443

[76] Hirase T, Node K. Endothelial dysfunction as a cellular mechanism for vascular failure. American Journal of Physiology. Heart and Circulatory Physiology. 2012;**302**(3): H499-H505

[77] Flammer AJ, Luscher TF. Three decades of endothelium research: From the detection of nitric oxide to the everyday implementation of endothelial function measurements in cardiovascular diseases. Swiss Medical Weekly. 2010;**140**:w13122

[78] Triggle CR, Samuel SM, Ravishankar S, Marei I, Arunachalam G, Ding H. The endothelium: Influencing vascular smooth muscle in many ways. Canadian Journal of Physiology and Pharmacology. 2012;**90**(6):713-738

[79] Hendry JH, Akahoshi M, Wang LS, Lipshultz SE, Stewart FA, Trott KR. Radiation-induced cardiovascular injury. Radiation and Environmental Biophysics. 2008;**47**(2):189-193

[80] Little MP, Tawn EJ, Tzoulaki I, Wakeford R, Hildebrandt G, Paris F, et al. A systematic review of epidemiological associations between low and moderate doses of ionizing radiation and late cardiovascular effects, and their possible mechanisms. Radiation Research. 2008;**169**(1):99-109

[81] Bhatti P, Sigurdson AJ, Mabuchi K. Can low-dose radiation increase risk of cardiovascular disease? Lancet. 2008;**372**(9640):697-699

[82] Decrock E, Hoorelbeke D, Ramadan R, Delvaeye T, De Bock M, Wang N, et al. Calcium, oxidative stress and connexin channels, a harmonious orchestra directing the response to radiotherapy treatment? Biochimica et Biophysica Acta. 2017;**1864**(6):1099-1120

[83] Lerman A, Burnett JC Jr. Intact and altered endothelium in regulation of vasomotion. Circulation. 1992;**86**(6 Suppl):III12-III19

[84] Tousoulis D, Kampoli AM, Tentolouris C, Papageorgiou N, Stefanadis C. The role of nitric oxide on endothelial function. Current Vascular Pharmacology. 2012;**10**(1):4-18

[85] Bonetti PO, Lerman LO, Lerman A. Endothelial dysfunction: A marker of atherosclerotic risk. Arteriosclerosis, Thrombosis, and Vascular Biology. 2003;**23**(2):168-175

[86] Mombouli JV, Vanhoutte PM. Endothelial dysfunction: From physiology to therapy. Journal of Molecular and Cellular Cardiology. 1999;**31**(1):61-74

[87] Vanhoutte PM, Shimokawa H, Feletou M, Tang EH. Endothelial dysfunction and vascular disease—A 30th anniversary update. Acta Physiologica (Oxford, England). 2017; **219**(1):22-96

[88] Franken NA, Rodermond HM, Stap J, Haveman J, van Bree C. Clonogenic assay of cells in vitro. Nature Protocols 2006;**1**(5):2315-2319

[89] Park MT, ET O, Song MJ, Lee H, Park HJ. Radio-sensitivities and angiogenic signaling pathways of irradiated normal endothelial cells derived from diverse human organs. Journal of Radiation Research. 2012;**53**(4):570-580

[90] Riquier H, Wera AC, Heuskin AC, Feron O, Lucas S, Michiels C. Comparison of X-ray and alpha particle effects on a human cancer and endothelial cells: Survival curves and gene expression profiles. Radiotherapy and Oncology. 2013;**106**(3):397-403

[91] Haimovitz-Friedman A, Kan CC, Ehleiter D, Persaud RS, McLoughlin M, Fuks Z, et al. Ionizing radiation acts on cellular membranes to generate ceramide and initiate apoptosis. The Journal of Experimental Medicine. 1994;**180**(2):525-535

[92] Kolesnick R, Fuks Z. Radiation and ceramide-induced apoptosis. Oncogene. 2003; **22**(37):5897-5906

[93] Verheij M, Dewit LG, van Mourik JA. The effect of ionizing radiation on endothelial tissue factor activity and its cellular localization. Thrombosis and Haemostasis. 1995; **73**(5):894-895

[94] Wang J, Zheng H, Ou X, Albertson CM, Fink LM, Herbert JM, et al. Hirudin ameliorates intestinal radiation toxicity in the rat: Support for thrombin inhibition as strategy to minimize side-effects after radiation therapy and as countermeasure against radiation exposure. Journal of Thrombosis and Haemostasis. 2004;**2**(11):2027-2035

[95] van Kleef E, Verheij M, te Poele H, Oussoren Y, Dewit L, Stewart F. In vitro and in vivo expression of endothelial von Willebrand factor and leukocyte accumulation after fractionated irradiation. Radiation Research. 2000;**154**(4):375-381

[96] Boerma M, Kruse JJ, van Loenen M, Klein HR, Bart CI, Zurcher C, et al. Increased deposition of von Willebrand factor in the rat heart after local ionizing irradiation. Strahlentherapie und Onkologie. 2004;**180**(2):109-116

[97] Stewart FA, Te Poele JA, Van der Wal AF, Oussoren YG, Van Kleef EM, Kuin A, et al. Radiation nephropathy—The link between functional damage and vascular mediated inflammatory and thrombotic changes. Acta Oncologica. 2001;**40**(8):952-957

[98] Sporn LA, Rubin P, Marder VJ, Wagner DD. Irradiation induces release of von Willebrand protein from endothelial cells in culture. Blood. 1984;**64**(2):567-570

[99] Jahroudi N, Ardekani AM, Greenberger JS. Ionizing irradiation increases transcription of the von Willebrand factor gene in endothelial cells. Blood. 1996;**88**(10):3801-3814

[100] McManus LM, Ostrom KK, Lear C, Luce EB, Gander DL, Pinckard RN, et al. Radiation-induced increased platelet-activating factor activity in mixed saliva. Laboratory Investigation. 1993;**68**(1):118-124

[101] Wang J, Zheng H, Ou X, Fink LM, Hauer-Jensen M. Deficiency of microvascular thrombomodulin and up-regulation of protease-activated receptor-1 in irradiated rat intestine: Possible link between endothelial dysfunction and chronic radiation fibrosis. The American Journal of Pathology. 2002;**160**(6):2063-2072

[102] Zhou Q, Zhao Y, Li P, Bai X, Ruan C. Thrombomodulin as a marker of radiation-induced endothelial cell injury. Radiation Research. 1992;**131**(3):285-289

[103] Hosoi Y, Yamamoto M, Ono T, Sakamoto K. Prostacyclin production in cultured endothelial cells is highly sensitive to low doses of ionizing radiation. International Journal of Radiation Biology. 1993;**63**(5):631-638

[104] Leigh PJ, Cramp WA, MacDermot J. Identification of the prostacyclin receptor by radiation inactivation. The Journal of Biological Chemistry. 1984;**259**(20):12431-12436

[105] Eldor A, Vlodavsky I, Riklis E, Fuks Z. Recovery of prostacyclin capacity of irradiated endothelial cells and the protective effect of vitamin C. Prostaglandins. 1987; **34**(2):241-255

[106] Henderson BW, Bicher HI, Johnson RJ. Loss of vascular fibrinolytic activity following irradiation of the liver—An aspect of late radiation damage. Radiation Research. 1983;**95**(3):646-652

[107] Svanberg L, Astedt B, Kullander S. On radiation-decreased fibrinolytic activity of vessel walls. Acta Obstetricia et Gynecologica Scandinavica. 1976;**55**(1):49-51

[108] Ts'ao CH, Ward WF, Port CD. Radiation injury in rat lung. III. Plasminogen activator and fibrinolytic inhibitor activities. Radiation Research. 1983;**96**(2):301-308

[109] van Hinsbergh VW. Endothelium—Role in regulation of coagulation and inflammation. Seminars in Immunopathology. 2012;**34**(1):93-106

[110] Sandoo A, van Zanten JJ, Metsios GS, Carroll D, Kitas GD. The endothelium and its role in regulating vascular tone. Open Cardiovascular Medicine Journal. 2010;**4**:302-312

[111] Hildebrandt G, Maggiorella L, Rodel F, Rodel V, Willis D, Trott KR. Mononuclear cell adhesion and cell adhesion molecule liberation after X-irradiation of activated endothelial cells in vitro. International Journal of Radiation Biology. 2002;**78**(4):315-325

[112] Sievert W, Trott KR, Azimzadeh O, Tapio S, Zitzelsberger H, Multhoff G. Late proliferating and inflammatory effects on murine microvascular heart and lung endothelial cells after irradiation. Radiotherapy & Oncology. 2015;**117**(2):376-381

[113] Van Der Meeren A, Squiban C, Gourmelon P, Lafont H, Gaugler MH. Differential regulation by IL-4 and IL-10 of radiation-induced IL-6 and IL-8 production and ICAM-1 expression by human endothelial cells. Cytokine. 1999;**11**(11):831-838

[114] Milliat F, Francois A, Isoir M, Deutsch E, Tamarat R, Tarlet G, et al. Influence of endothelial cells on vascular smooth muscle cells phenotype after irradiation: Implication in radiation-induced vascular damages. The American Journal of Pathology. 2006; **169**(4):1484-1495

[115] Hayashi T, Morishita Y, Khattree R, Misumi M, Sasaki K, Hayashi I, et al. Evaluation of systemic markers of inflammation in atomic-bomb survivors with special reference to radiation and age effects. The FASEB Journal. 2012;**26**(11):4765-4773

[116] Jeggo P, Lobrich M. Radiation-induced DNA. damage responses. Radiation Protection Dosimetry. 2006;**122**(1-4):124-127

[117] Bolus NE. Basic review of radiation biology and terminology. Journal of Nuclear Medicine Technology. 2001;**29**(2):67-73 test 6-7

[118] Norbury CJ, Hickson ID. Cellular responses to DNA damage. Annual Review of Pharmacology and Toxicology. 2001;**41**:367-401

[119] Clarke PR, Allan LA. Cell-cycle control in the face of damage—A matter of life or death. Trends in Cell Biology. 2009;**19**(3):89-98

[120] Langley RE, Bump EA, Quartuccio SG, Medeiros D, Braunhut SJ. Radiation-induced apoptosis in microvascular endothelial cells. British Journal of Cancer. 1997;**75**(5):666-672

[121] Rombouts C, Aerts A, Beck M, De Vos WH, Van Oostveldt P, Benotmane MA, et al. Differential response to acute low dose radiation in primary and immortalized endothelial cells. International Journal of Radiation Biology. 2013;**89**(10):841-850

[122] Neumaier T, Swenson J, Pham C, Polyzos A, Lo AT, Yang P, et al. Evidence for formation of DNA repair centers and dose-response nonlinearity in human cells. Proceedings of the National Academy of Sciences of the United States of America. 2012;**109**(2):443-448

[123] Costes SV, Chiolo I, Pluth JM, Barcellos-Hoff MH, Jakob B. Spatiotemporal characterization of ionizing radiation induced DNA damage foci and their relation to chromatin organization. Mutation Research. 2010;**704**(1-3):78-87

[124] Pluder F, Barjaktarovic Z, Azimzadeh O, Mortl S, Kramer A, Steininger S, et al. Low-dose irradiation causes rapid alterations to the proteome of the human endothelial cell line EA.hy926. Radiation and Environmental Biophysics. 2011;**50**(1):155-166

[125] Yu E, Mercer J, Bennett M. Mitochondria in vascular disease. Cardiovascular Research. 2012;**95**(2):173-182

[126] Schilling-Toth B, Sandor N, Kis E, Kadhim M, Safrany G, Hegyesi H. Analysis of the common deletions in the mitochondrial DNA is a sensitive biomarker detecting direct and non-targeted cellular effects of low dose ionizing radiation. Mutation Research. 2011;**716**(1-2):33-39

[127] Barjaktarovic Z, Schmaltz D, Shyla A, Azimzadeh O, Schulz S, Haagen J, et al. Radiation-induced signaling results in mitochondrial impairment in mouse heart at 4 weeks after exposure to X-rays. PLoS One. 2011;**6**(12):e27811

[128] Barjaktarovic Z, Shyla A, Azimzadeh O, Schulz S, Haagen J, Dorr W, et al. Ionising radiation induces persistent alterations in the cardiac mitochondrial function of C57BL/6 mice 40 weeks after local heart exposure. Radiotherapy and Oncology: Journal of the European Society for Therapeutic Radiology and Oncology. 2013;**106**(3):404-410

[129] Azimzadeh O, Scherthan H, Sarioglu H, Barjaktarovic Z, Conrad M, Vogt A, et al. Rapid proteomic remodeling of cardiac tissue caused by total body ionizing radiation. Proteomics. 2011;**11**(16):3299-3311

[130] Azimzadeh O, Sievert W, Sarioglu H, Merl-Pham J, Yentrapalli R, Bakshi MV, et al. Integrative proteomics and targeted transcriptomics analyses in cardiac endothelial cells unravel mechanisms of long-term radiation-induced vascular dysfunction. Journal of Proteome Research. 2015;**14**(2):1203-1219

[131] Azimzadeh O, Sievert W, Sarioglu H, Yentrapalli R, Barjaktarovic Z, Sriharshan A, et al. PPAR alpha: A novel radiation target in locally exposed Mus musculus heart revealed by quantitative proteomics. Journal of Proteome Research. 2013;**12**(6):2700-2714

[132] Yamamori T, Yasui H, Yamazumi M, Wada Y, Nakamura Y, Nakamura H, et al. Ionizing radiation induces mitochondrial reactive oxygen species production accompanied by upregulation of mitochondrial electron transport chain function and mitochondrial content under control of the cell cycle checkpoint. Free Radical Biology & Medicine. 2012;**53**(2):260-270

[133] Bernardi P. The mitochondrial permeability transition pore: A mystery solved? Frontiers in Physiology. 2013;**4**:95

[134] Leach JK, Van Tuyle G, Lin PS, Schmidt-Ullrich R, Mikkelsen RB. Ionizing radiation-induced, mitochondria-dependent generation of reactive oxygen/nitrogen. Cancer Research. 2001;**61**(10):3894-3901

[135] Marin A, Martin M, Linan O, Alvarenga F, Lopez M, Fernandez L, et al. Bystander effects and radiotherapy. Reports of Practical Oncology and Radiotherapy. 2015;**20**(1):12-21

[136] Decrock E, Hoorelbeke D, Ramadan R, Delvaeye T, De Bock M, Wang N, et al. Calcium, oxidative stress and connexin channels, a harmonious orchestra directing the response to radiotherapy treatment? Biochimica et Biophysica Acta. 2017;**1864**(6):1099-1120

[137] Vavrova J, Rezacova M. The importance of senescence in ionizing radiation-induced tumour suppression. Folia Biologica. 2011;**57**(2):41-46

[138] Sabatino L, Picano E, Andreassi MG. Telomere shortening and ionizing radiation: A possible role in vascular dysfunction? International Journal of Radiation Biology. 2012;**88**(11):830-839

[139] Kurz DJ, Decary S, Hong Y, Trivier E, Akhmedov A, Erusalimsky JD. Chronic oxidative stress compromises telomere integrity and accelerates the onset of senescence in human endothelial cells. Journal of Cell Science. 2004;**117**(Pt 11):2417-2426

[140] Campisi J, d'Adda di Fagagna F. Cellular senescence: When bad things happen to good cells. Nature Reviews Molecular Cell Biology. 2007;**8**(9):729-740

[141] CW O, Bump EA, Kim JS, Janigro D, Mayberg MR. Induction of a senescence-like phenotype in bovine aortic endothelial cells by ionizing radiation. Radiation Research. 2001;**156**(3):232-240

[142] Panganiban RA, Mungunsukh O, Day RM. X-irradiation induces ER stress, apoptosis, and senescence in pulmonary artery endothelial cells. International Journal of Radiation Biology. 2013;**89**(8):656-667

[143] Igarashi K, Sakimoto I, Kataoka K, Ohta K, Miura M. Radiation-induced senescence-like phenotype in proliferating and plateau-phase vascular endothelial cells. Experimental Cell Research. 2007;**313**(15):3326-3336

[144] Kim KS, Kim JE, Choi KJ, Bae S, Kim DH. Characterization of DNA damage-induced cellular senescence by ionizing radiation in endothelial cells. International Journal of Radiation Biology. 2014;**90**(1):71-80

[145] Yentrapalli R, Azimzadeh O, Barjaktarovic Z, Sarioglu H, Wojcik A, Harms-Ringdahl M, et al. Quantitative proteomic analysis reveals induction of premature senescence in human umbilical vein endothelial cells exposed to chronic low-dose rate gamma-radiation. Proteomics. 2013;**13**(7):1096-1107

[146] Yentrapalli R, Azimzadeh O, Sriharshan A, Malinowsky K, Merl J, Wojcik A, et al. The PI3K/Akt/mTOR pathway is implicated in the premature senescence of primary human endothelial cells exposed to chronic radiation. PLoS One. 2013;**8**(8):e70024

[147] Rombouts C, Aerts A, Quintens R, Baselet B, El-Saghire H, Harms-Ringdahl M, et al. Transcriptomic profiling suggests a role for IGFBP5 in premature senescence of endothelial cells after chronic low dose rate irradiation. International Journal of Radiation Biology. 2014;**90**(7):560-574

[148] Nagasawa H, Little JB. Induction of sister chromatid exchanges by extremely low doses of alpha-particles. Cancer Research. 1992;**52**(22):6394-6396

[149] Mancuso M, Pasquali E, Leonardi S, Tanori M, Rebessi S, Di Majo V, et al. Oncogenic bystander radiation effects in patched heterozygous mouse cerebellum. Proceedings of the National Academy of Sciences of the United States of America. 2008;**105**(34):12445-12450

[150] Wang N, De Bock M, Decrock E, Bol M, Gadicherla A, Vinken M, et al. Paracrine signaling through plasma membrane hemichannels. Biochimica et Biophysica Acta. 2013;**1828**(1):35-50

[151] Herve JC, Derangeon M. Gap-junction-mediated cell-to-cell communication. Cell and Tissue Research. 2013;**352**(1):21-31

[152] Laird DW. Life cycle of connexins in health and disease. The Biochemical Journal. 2006;**394**(Pt 3):527-543

[153] Sohl G, Willecke K. An update on connexin genes and their nomenclature in mouse and man. Cell Communication & Adhesion. 2003;**10**(4-6):173-180

[154] Wong CW, Christen T, Roth I, Chadjichristos CE, Derouette JP, Foglia BF, et al. Connexin37 protects against atherosclerosis by regulating monocyte adhesion. Nature Medicine. 2006;**12**(8):950-954

[155] Chadjichristos CE, Scheckenbach KE, van Veen TA, Richani Sarieddine MZ, de Wit C, Yang Z, et al. Endothelial-specific deletion of connexin40 promotes atherosclerosis by increasing CD73-dependent leukocyte adhesion. Circulation. 2010;**121**(1):123-131

[156] Azzam EI, de Toledo SM, Little JB. Expression of CONNEXIN43 is highly sensitive to ionizing radiation and other environmental stresses. Cancer Research. 2003;**63**(21):7128-7135

[157] Kwak BR, Mulhaupt F, Veillard N, Gros DB, Mach F. Altered pattern of vascular connexin expression in atherosclerotic plaques. Arteriosclerosis, Thrombosis, and Vascular Biology. 2002;**22**(2):225-230

[158] Pfenniger A, Derouette JP, Verma V, Lin X, Foglia B, Coombs W, et al. Gap junction protein Cx37 interacts with endothelial nitric oxide synthase in endothelial cells. Arteriosclerosis, Thrombosis, and Vascular Biology. 2010;**30**(4):827-834

[159] Yuan D, Sun G, Zhang R, Luo C, Ge M, Luo G, et al. Connexin 43 expressed in endothelial cells modulates monocyteendothelial adhesion by regulating cell adhesion proteins. Molecular Medicine Reports. 2015;**12**(5):7146-7152

[160] Glover D, Little JB, Lavin MF, Gueven N. Low dose ionizing radiation-induced activation of connexin 43 expression. International Journal of Radiation Biology. 2003;**79**(12):955-964

[161] Banaz-Yasar F, Tischka R, Iliakis G, Winterhager E, Gellhaus A. Cell line specific modulation of connexin43 expression after exposure to ionizing radiation. Cell Communication & Adhesion. 2005;**12**(5-6):249-259

Chapter 17

The Markers of Endothelial Activation

Ines Drenjancevic, Ivana Jukic, Ana Stupin,
Anita Cosic, Marko Stupin and
Kristina Selthofer-Relatic

Additional information is available at the end of the chapter

http://dx.doi.org/10.5772/intechopen.74671

Abstract

Biomarkers are biological indicators of processes that are part of ethiopathogenesis of the diseases, and can, but do not have to be causal to diseases. One very important question is how specific and sensitive the marker is, since one molecule can appear in many conditions. Biomarkers of endothelial cell activation can be very diverse, from biochemical/metabolic to functional biomarkers. Activation of endothelial cells is part of physiological as well as pathophysiological response of cardiovascular system in conditions as physical activity, growth, pregnancy and in all cardiometabolic diseases (e.g., hypertension, diabetes mellitus, autoimmune inflammatory diseases, coronary artery disease, atherosclerosis, ischemia and reperfusion, etc.). During activation, there is a change in endothelial cell morphology and function, which could be a defensive response of endothelium to provoking factor or could lead to increased risk for the injury and end organ damage. This chapter aims to overview current knowledge on established biomarkers of normal and disease-related endothelial activation and to provide information on novel, potential biomarkers in common cardiometabolic diseases.

Keywords: endothelial activation, biomarkers, laser Doppler flowmetry, flow mediated dilation, pregnancy, exercise, cardiometabolic diseases, functional markers, nitric oxide, prostaglandins

1. Introduction

Vascular endothelium has a critical role in maintaining vascular tone, and changes in vascular flow are in complex interactions with endothelium. The importance of this particular function of the endothelium manifests in the fact that the term "endothelial function" is usually used to describe the ability of endothelium to release vasoactive substances and thereby regulate blood flow. The basic principle of vascular function is that healthy blood vessels dilate normally and the diseased blood vessels exhibit a dysfunctional vasodilation. Therefore, all methods for endothelial function assessment are based on the ability of endothelium to respond (vasodilation or vasoconstriction) to a specific stimulus (vascular occlusion, pharmacological vasodilators, heating, etc.).

Biomarkers are biological indicators of processes that are part of etiology of the diseases, and can, but do not have to be causal to diseases. One very important question is how specific and sensitive the marker is, since one molecule can appear in many conditions. Biomarkers of endothelial cell activation can be very diverse: biochemical/metabolic (such as plasma glucose, lipids, cytokines, asymmetric dimethylarginine (ADMA), high sensitive C-reactive protein (hsCRP), myeloperoxidase (MPO), cell adhesion molecules (CAMs), markers of coagulability, markers of oxidative stress, chemokines, microparticles, endothelial progenitor cells), functional biomarkers (such as flow-mediated dilation and other types of flowmetry, arteriographic measurements of vascular function) and structure (e.g., CIMT—carotid intima-media thickness, angiogenesis, or rarefaction).

2. Biochemical biomarkers of vascular (endothelial) function

Over the last three decades, a number of methodological approaches were developed in order to evaluate and measure (patho)physiological function of the endothelium in humans [1, 2]. Evidently, these new methods intensified research and brought novelties in the field of vascular physiology and pathophysiology, but still are not implemented as clinical tools in daily practice. The approaches for endothelial function assessment were designed to provide insight into vascular/endothelial function in different sites (vascular beds) and different blood vessel types (conductive, resistant, and microcirculation). Earlier methods were more invasive (e.g., intracoronary infusion of acetylcholine (ACh), and later developed techniques that were less invasive have focused on peripheral circulation (forearm circulation) as a surrogate for coronary arteries [3–5]. As expected, all of these methods have their advantages and accepted limitations, and neither of the developed methods does present the absolute standard for the evaluation of endothelial function, in both macro- and microcirculation.

There is an extensive body of evidence reporting that generalized endothelial dysfunction exhibited virtually in every arterial bed presents an early manifestation of a variety of cardiovascular diseases (CVDs) [6, 7]. Still, when investigating endothelial function in different CVDs, diverse (patho)physiological role of large conductance vessels and small microvasculature should be considered.

There are many various molecules which have been denoted as vascular or endothelial markers, e.g., lipids, cytokines, ADMA, hsCRP, MPO, CAMs, markers of coagulability, markers of oxidative stress, chemokines, microparticles, and endothelial progenitor cells. It has been demonstrated that reduced bioavailability of nitric oxide (NO) plays a central role in impaired vascular/endothelial response (endothelial dysfunction) in conduit arteries, while NO in the microcirculation primarily modulates tissue metabolism [8]. On the other hand, a number of

http://dx.doi.org/10.5772/intechopen.74671

studies indicate that endothelium-derived hyperpolarizing factor (EDHF) plays a major role in vasodilation in skin microcirculation [9], whereas the results are still conflicting concerning the implication of prostaglandins [10–12]. A study on coronary endothelial function in young smokers reported that they had epicardial coronary endothelial dysfunction but preserved microvascular endothelial function [13].

2.1. Biomarkers in pregnancy

The importance of maternal vascular adaptation to pregnancy is to increase blood flow and to assure the proper development of the fetus. Several possible biochemical biomarkers have been proposed to evaluate vascular/endothelial function in pregnancy. First among them is NO, one of most important endothelial vasodilators, which is produced by NO synthase (NOS). It is well accepted that NOS-3 expression levels are increased in uterine artery endothelium in pregnancy [14]. Prostacyclin (PGI2) also plays an important role in vasodilator response, and its concentration is elevated in pregnancy [15]. In order to estimate the real impact of prostacyclin on vascular tone, determination of thromboxane a2 (TXA2)/PGI2 ratio is needed. Since both TXA2 and PGI2 have very short half-life, only indirect measures can be made of stable metabolites in the blood (thromboxane b2 (TXB2) and 6-keto-prostaglandin F2a (6-ketoPGF2A)), and there is no technique which allows their monitoring in real time. It has been demonstrated that cyclooxygenase 1 (COX1) is upregulated in endothelial cells during pregnancy, and therefore induces a PGI2 increment [14]. EDHF is the third major player in endothelial vasodilation in pregnancy, causing smooth muscle relaxation. As it is not a single factor and there is still ongoing research to identify its specific components, it is described as spectrum of responses that are neither NO nor PGI2 mediated. Another limiting problem is that there is no appropriate method for its tracking. Although EDHF may seem as unnecessary pathway beside NO and PGI2, a number of studies showed an important role of EDHF in endothelium vasodilation in pregnancy, suggesting that without EDHF, there would not be sufficient blood flow to the fetus [16].

Endogenous eNOS inhibitor ADMA concentrations were found to be significantly lower in pregnant women. However, this did not explain the improved flow-mediated dilation (FMD) in the correlation analysis [17, 18]. Also, endothelial function in normal pregnancy was not attenuated despite the significant increase in hsCRP, and pregnancy-related changes in the concentrations of proinflammatory cytokines, e.g., tumor necrosis factor alpha (TNF-α) and interleukin 6 (IL-6), were nonsignificant [19].

2.2. Biomarkers in exercise

It has been reported that the regulation of the NO-dependent pathway presents a key mechanism mediating endothelial adaptations to shear stress, including increased NO synthesis, increased expression and activity of antioxidative enzymes (e.g., superoxide dismutase (SOD) and catalase), and decreased oxidative stress level (reactive oxygen species (ROS) production) which all increases NO bioavailability. However, recent studies demonstrated that COX-dependent pathway and increased PGI2 synthesis take part in endothelial adaptations to shear stress, as well. Furthermore, a growing body of evidence suggest that increased shear stress generated by increased blood flow during exercise, presents a prime signal for decreased level of vasoconstrictor endothelin 1 (ET1), and inflammatory markers such as vascular cell adhesion molecule 1 (VCAM-1) and monocyte chemotactic protein 1 (MCP-1) level [20]. Furthermore, increased endothelial NOS (eNOS) gene expression has been proposed to be a marker of anterograde shear stress-induced endothelial activation (result of repeated episodic increase in blood flow during exercise), and to have anti-atherogenic effect in endothelial cell cultures [21, 22].

On the other hand, rhythmic stretching (cyclic strain) provoked by systolic blood pressure changes during exercise affects endothelial cell growth and NO- and EDHF-dependent vasodilation pathway, and its effect depends on the blood pressure increment during exercise (e.g., >135 mmHg elicits inhibition of endothelial cell growth) [23]. Surprisingly, further studies on endothelial cell cultures have reported that rhythmic stretching can induce ROS production and increase the expression of cell adhesion molecules. On the other hand, ROS produced by cyclic strain may indirectly increase expression of eNOS [24]. It became evident that the time of exposure to high blood pressure/cyclic strain (continuous or pulsatile) is crucial for its final effect on endothelial function. Brief increases in blood pressure and ROS production associated with bouts of exercise may signal an increase in eNOS production and other beneficial effects resulting in improved endothelial function. Chronic increases in cyclic strain (e.g., hypertension) may elevate ROS chronically and finally provoke development of endothelial dysfunction. Thus, beside abovementioned endothelial biomarkers of inflammation and endothelial dysfunction, measurement of oxidative stress level and antioxidant capacity present suitable and commonly used markers of endothelial response to different exercise modes and patterns (shear stress) in both health and disease.

2.3. Biomarkers in cardiometabolic diseases

Oxidation of low density lipoproteins (oxLDL) and NO synthesis contribute to endothelial dysfunction, vascular aging, and disease. OxLDL and NO exert contradictory actions within the vascular endothelium such as: leukocyte adhesion, platelet aggregation, and vascular smooth muscle cell proliferation and migration [25, 26]. While oxLDL—an oxidative stress biomarker—has been identified as a pro-atherogenic risk factor for coronary artery disease (CAD), NO is a free radical signal-transducing molecule that maintains vasodilation, modulates *in vitro* lipid peroxidation reactions and alters pro-inflammatrory gene expression. Both are part of complex atherosclerotic process, from initiation to plaque destabilization and coronary artery disease [25, 26].

As already mentioned, ADMA is an endogenous inhibitor of NO synthase [27] and thus may cause endothelial dysfunction [28]. Increased plasma levels of ADMA are related with hyperlipidemia, hypertension, coronary artery disease, unstable angina, stroke and end-stage renal disease and diabetes [28]. Reduced plasma levels of ADMA after percutaneous coronary intervention could be indicative of a reduced risk of recurrent cardiovascular events. Although ADMA was significantly associated with all-cause mortality in patients with acute coronary syndrome and ischemic heart disease, there is no clear association between ADMA and cardiovascular disease incidence [29]. Type II diabetes has been associated with increased ADMA levels. ADMA and NO have been found to be significant determinants of insulin resistance [30]. A study performed in type 2 diabetes patients that used antidiabetic metformin for

3 months showed reduced serum ADMA levels for 30% [31]. Another study, from Stuhlinger et al. found that rosiglitazone reduced the level of ADMA by 30% in seven insulin-resistant non-diabetic hypertensive individuals [32].

Toll-like receptors (TLRs), such as toll-like receptors TLR2 and TLR4 have been found to have elevated expression in T2DM patients, which could be a possible underlying mechanism of inflammation in T2DM [33]. TLR-2 and TLR-4 activation has also been found in murine models of atherosclerosis [33, 34]. There are many unanswered questions: the consequences of activation/blockade of TLRs in atherosclerosis, relationship between innate and adaptive responses in atherosclerosis, and mechanistic insight on the intricate balance of direct and risk factor-mediated effects of TLRs in CVD [33, 34].

The over expression of TNF-alpha and its inflammatory and immunomodulatory effects have been implicated in the pathogenesis of CAD and myocardial dysfunction. Cardiovascular complications may be influenced by TNF-alpha gene polymorphisms. Certain studies failed to find a significant association between the TNF-alpha gene polymorphisms and CVD [35]. Further studies are required to resolve this controversy.

IL-6 is associated with the process of inflammation and coronary artery disease. Patients with high levels of IL-6 show worse in-hospital outcome following treatment in case of unstable angina. An association has been shown between the IL-6 promoter polymorphism −174G/C and hypertension, left ventricular hypertrophy and ischemic heart disease CAD [35].

Endothelial cells also express chemotactic factors: MCP-1, proinflammatory cytokines (macrophage colony-stimulating factor) and tumor necrosis factor-beta (TNF-β) [36]. Hyperglycemia promotes MCP-1 expression in vascular endothelial cells and has a pivotal role in the pathogenesis of diabetic vasculopathy [37]. Patients with diabetes mellitus or obesity have increased circulating levels of inflammatory markers, including C reactive protein (CRP), TNF-α, and IL-6 [38–40]. Blood level of CRP, as independent predictor of diabetes, is increased in both Type I and Type II diabetes [41, 42]. TNF-α can induce cytokines such as IL-6 which regulates the expression of CRP. They can impair endothelial function and contribute to atherothrombosis especially in patients with Type II diabetes, alone or in combination [43]. It was also found in male diabetic patients that increased levels of inflammatory markers predict cardiovascular risk in diabetic patients [44].

Microparticles, the membrane vesicles released by various cell types and circulating endothelial cells represent novel biomarkers of endothelial injury, associated with atherosclerosis and related complications (thrombosis, inflammation, and apoptosis). Microparticles are suggested to be biomarkers of vascular injury and inflammation [45]. Changes in circulating levels of microparticles might give an important clinical information in healthy subjects or patients with CVDs as a surrogate marker of vascular function, but it is still not clear whether it is a cause or effect of atherosclerosis [45].

Endocan or endothelial cell specific molecule-1 (ESM-1) is a novel endothelium-derived soluble proteoglycan [46]. It binds to a wide range of bioactive molecules associated with cellular signaling and adhesion. It is involved in regulation of proliferation, differentiation, migration, and adhesion of different types of cells in health and disease. The endocan concentration is related to endothelial activation and neovascularization [47]. Endocan levels are elevated in

Novel biomarkers	System/cells	Effect
Metabolic/biochemical		
ADMA	Inhibitor NOS	Endothelial dysfunction
MMP2, MMP9 TIMP2, TIMP9	Intercellular matrix	Intracellular matrix rearrangement
Myeloperoxidase (MPO)	Activated neutrophils and macrophages	Production of oxidative stress
ox-LDL, 8-hydroxy-2′-deoxygunosine. MDA (lipid peroxidation), protein carbonyl (PCO)	Lipids, activated proteins	Reactive oxygen species and products (with increased oxidative stress
IL-6, TNF-alfa	lymphocytes	Proinflammatory cytokines
Toll-like receptor 4	lymphocytes	Innate immunity
NO metabolites (nitrates, nitrites)	Endothelium (NO)	Vasodilation (NO) and nitrosylation
Functional/structural		
Flow-mediated dilation (FMD)	Blood vessels (endothelial function)	NO dependent, or COX, EDHF, EDCF dependent
Intima-media thickness (IMT)	Blood vessels (endothelial function + VSMC)	multifactorial

Table 1. Potential novel biomarkers of atherosclerosis.

conditions such as tumor progression, hypertension, chronic kidney disease, and renal transplant rejection [48]. Tadzic et al. [49] have described an increased expression of cell adhesion molecules, intracellular adhesion molecule's (ICAM) and vascular cell adhesion molecule's (VACM) ligands, together with decrease of sCAMs and endocan in hypertensive patients on amlodipine therapy with reduction in blood pressure, suggesting de-activation of endothelium. Systolic and diastolic blood pressure was positively correlated with ICAM-1 and VCAM-1, and systolic blood pressure was negatively correlated with CD11a/LFA-1. Endocan significantly positively correlated with ICAM-1 [49].

Diabetes is associated with increased circulating levels of endothelium-derived adhesion molecules and plasminogen activator inhibitor-1, which have pro-inflammatory and prothrombotic effects [50, 51]. In endothelial dysfunction, the endothelium can express adhesion molecules responsible for the withdrawal of leukocytes from vascular wall, such as VCAM-1 and ICAM-1 [36]. Also, E-selectin and platelet endothelial cell adhesion molecule have been expressed in atherosclerotic lesions and are involved in mononuclear cell adhesion to the vascular endothelium [52, 53]. The main difference in the activation of adhesion molecules is that the expression of ICAM-1 increases after cell activation, while E-selectin and VCAM-1 are only induced after cell activation. It is demonstrated that hyperglycemia results in the expression of adhesion molecules: endothelial-leukocyte adhesion molecule-1, VCAM-1, and ICAM-1 in human vascular endothelial cells [54]. In the rat mesenteric microcirculation, only intraperitoneal co-administration of IL-1β with D-glucose increased leukocyte rolling flux, adhesion, and migration, indicating that pro-inflammatory environment in diabetes is a critical factor in pro-atherosclerotic effects of hyperglycemia [54, 55].

Increased concentration of plasma glucose activates the endothelium [56–58]. Exposure of arterial tissue to increased glucose level induces superoxide production and impairs NO bioavailability in the vascular wall which leads to increased oxidative stress in these conditions [59]. In diabetes mellitus, the production of superoxide and NADPH oxidase activity are increased [60, 61] which promote activation of the pro-inflammatory transcription factor NFκB [56]. The transcription factor NFκB is one of key regulator of endothelial activation and is included in insulin resistance [62, 63]. This is supported by study in obese persons [64]. Salsalate (an anti-inflammatory drug) increased expression of the inhibitor of NF-κB and reduced NFκB activation in freshly isolated endothelial cells taken from obese persons. Salsalate increased brachial artery flow-mediated dilation and reduced nitrotyrosine and expression of NADPH oxidase p47(phox) in these endothelial cells [64]. **Table 1** presents some of the proposed novel biomarkers for atherosclerosis, which could also be related to other cardiometabolic diseases.

3. Functional biomarkers of vascular (endothelial) function

3.1. Assessment of microvascular endothelial function

3.1.1. Coronary microvascular function assessment

In the past, coronary angiography (of larger conductance arteries, i.e., coronary vessels) was considered a gold standard for evaluation of the severity and extent of CAD. However, in the last two decades, the attention was shifted to the coronary microcirculation as the possible site of anatomical and functional abnormalities crucial for the development and progression of final myocardial ischemia. Thus, functional assessment of coronary microcirculation and its endothelial function became a challenge. For a long time, measurement of changes in coronary blood flow (CBF) during coronary angiography (Doppler wires) has been used as a surrogate parameter for coronary microvascular function assessment [65]. The final result of this measurement is assessment of coronary flow reserve (CFR) which presents the ratio between the maximal CBF during maximal coronary hyperemia (provoked by adenosine infusion, pacing, or exercise) and the resting CBF. It has been demonstrated that CFR is both endothelium-dependent and endothelium-independent, and CFR below 2.0 is considered abnormal [66]. For coronary microvascular endothelium-dependent vasodilation assessment, instead of maximal CBF, CBF in response to endothelium-dependent vasodilator (commonly ACh) infused at increasing concentrations is calculated. Another method for the assessment of coronary microvascular function includes the measurement of the number of cineangiographic frames that it takes to fill a distal vessel with proximal injection of contrast. This method is named Thrombolysis in Myocardial Infarction (TIMI) and provides semi-quantitative assessment of epicardial coronary blood flow [67]. The main advantage of the abovementioned methods is to measure microvascular endothelial function directly in this clinically important vascular bed. However, main limitations are the cost, invasive nature, and therefore a limited population in which these measurements can be actually performed (symptomatic individuals requiring invasive coronary angiography) [68].

In recent years, a number of other methods have been developed among them: (a) blood oxygen level-dependent (BOLD) magnetic resonance imaging (MRI), a functional test that detects a dissociation of tissue hemoglobin from blood flow, is shown to be a useful tool for coronary endothelial function assessment [69]; (b) positron-emission tomography (PET) myocardial perfusion imaging that is based on the assessment of regional myocardial blood flow both at rest and during various forms of vasomotor stress [70] and presents a powerful tool to evaluate the effects of CV risk factors on the health of the microvasculature and its endothelium [71]; and (c) myocardial perfusion echocardiography, a bedside method with relatively low cost that is capable to detect myocardial perfusion abnormalities and quantify regional and global coronary blood flow [72]. Despite the fact that these new methods manage to provide noninvasive evaluation of coronary microvasculature directly at the site, they are still unacceptable for routine screening due to their limited availability, expensive equipment and associated costs, and lack of experienced/trained staff. Considering that endothelial function is a systemic disorder, peripheral vascular beds and their microcirculation present a good alternative that provides an easier access and need less elaborate equipment.

3.1.2. *Venous occlusion plethysmography*

Venous occlusion plethysmography presents a semi-invasive technique (arterial puncture) for assessment of forearm blood flow (and the corresponding microcirculation) changes before and after infusion of vasoactive substances into a cannulated brachial artery [3]. The method was introduced 90 years ago by Hewlett and van Zwaluwenburg [73], and the basic methodology has changed little since its first description. Basic principle of this method is to stop the return of venous blood from the forearm (inflating the cuff over the diastolic pressure value) with the preserved arterial blood inflow to the forearm, leading to a linear increase in blood flow at a given time, which is proportional to the arterial blood inflow. Another cuff excludes the blood flow through the hand to reduce the temperature fluctuations of the blood flow depending on the temperature. Changes in the flow are recorded by changing the electrical resistance of the plethysmograph located around the longest part of the forearm [74]. The main advantage of this method is that it provides assessment of endothelium-dependent and -independent vasodilation and mechanisms mediating it by intra-arterial infusion of vasoactive substances (e.g., ACh or sodium nitroprusside, and SNP), hormones, and drugs. However, its important limitation is that it could not strictly discern between macro- and microcirculation. Final results are expressed as ratio between blood flow changes in both arms and are well reproducible [75]. Regarding the mechanisms, some studies reported that ACh-induced dilation was inhibited by a NOS inhibitor, L-N^{G}-monomethyl Arginine citrate (L-NMMA) [76], suggesting that NO is the main vasodilator mediating endothelium-dependent vasodilation in this vascular bed. On the other hand, others reported that EDHF has a crucial role in mediating microvascular endothelial-dependent vasodilation, especially in population with multiple CV risk factors [77]. A large number of studies used venous occlusion plethysmography to assess the association between endothelial dysfunction and CV risk factors, and described it in hypercholesterolemia [78], diabetes mellitus [79], cigarette smoking [80], and aging [81], while the results in hypertensive patients were conflicting [3, 4, 82, 83]. Even though the method and pharmacologically induced vasodilation provide an insight into peripheral microvascular patho(physiology), venous occlusion plethysmography is characterized by several limitations and disadvantages, including its semi-invasive character, limited comparison between groups due to different initial blood pressure and forearm blood flow, different sizes of the forearm, etc., [68].

3.1.3. *Reactive hyperemia peripheral arterial tonometry (RH-PAT)*

RH-PAT is a noninvasive technique designed for assessment of peripheral microvascular function. This method reflects changes in finger pulse volume amplitude during reactive hyperemia (an equivalent to finger plethysmography). PAT device includes digital probes that are placed on the tip of each index finger and a blood pressure cuff (for provoking occlusion) that is placed around the upper arm of the study arm, while the other arm serves as a control [84, 85]. Vascular occlusion is provoked by inflation of the blood pressure cuff to a 50 mmHg above systolic blood pressure for 5 min. The PAT signal is recorded 10 min prior occlusion, and for 10 min after the cuff is deflated. The final result of this measurement is calculated as the ratio of average amplitude of the PAT signal over a period of 1 min, starting 1 min after cuff deflation to average amplitude of the PAT signal for 3 min at baseline (RH-PAT index) that is normalized to the control arm [84, 85]. Studies have shown that RH-PAT is at least partly NO dependent. Importantly, studies by Rubinshtein et al. and Akiyama et al. reported that RH-PAT may be a useful tool for prediction of future CV events in patients with CV risk [86, 87]. Advantages of this method are that it is noninvasive, it is very simple and reproducible, and that it is operator independent (RH-PAT index is measured automatically). Even though RH-PAT is very similar to FMD of the brachial artery, Framingham Heart Study has revealed that there was no significant correlation between RH-PAT and FMD [88]. Moreover, the same study reported that different CV risk factors contribute differently to changes in FMD and RH-PAT [89], suggesting that these two methods assess different vascular beds, and that macro- and microvascular endothelium is differently susceptible to various risk factors.

3.1.4. *Laser Doppler (LD) flowmetry*

Because of its easy accessibility, the skin presents an appropriate site to study peripheral microcirculation, which was proposed as a suitable marker of systemic microvascular function in various diseases [89]. Therefore, in recent years, a number of simple and noninvasive methods have been developed in order to assess peripheral microcirculation. Still, it is an open question whether skin microcirculation is actually a representative indicator of the microvascular function of other organs. Despite that skin microvascular function was extensively used over the past 30 years to investigate vascular mechanisms in various diseases including hypertension [90, 91], obesity [92], diabetes [93, 94], aging, kidney disease [95], etc.

The laser Doppler (LD) technique is based on the estimation of the flow rate in the skin microcirculation using the laser beam reflection from the erythrocyte in microcirculation and its wavelength change (Doppler's effect) [96]. Computer software determines the flow size, which is rather an index of skin perfusion (flux) than direct measure of skin blood flow. Results are commonly expressed in arbitrary units (perfusion units, PU) or as cutaneous vascular conductance (CVC; flux divided by arterial pressure in mV/mmHg) [96]. The first developed technique was the laser Doppler flowmetry (LDF) that measures blood flow in a single point and thus over a small volume but with a high sampling frequency. A major limitation of this technique is its spatial variability, due to regional heterogeneity of skin perfusion and blood flow measurement in a single point [97]. Later, laser Doppler imaging (LDI) was developed, which provides a 2D image of skin microvascular perfusion using the same principle as LDF. Since this method assess flow over larger surface than LDF, it managed to reduce spatial variability, but it appears to be much slower than LDF, making rapid changes in blood flow difficult to record [98]. Both techniques are commonly used for microvascular reactivity assessment in response to various stimuli, including iontophoresis of vasoactive drugs, post-occlusive reactive hyperemia (PORH), and thermal challenges [98].

Microdialysis is a technique based on intradermal insertion of small fibers for continuous delivery of drugs into a small area of tissue. This type of drug delivery provides avoiding its systemic effect [99] and it provides controlled drug application and absence of current-induced vasodilation, compared to iontophoresis. However, microdyalisis is invasive and painful, and justifies the use of local anesthesia which might also affect the blood flow and thus impact the results. It was commonly used to assess the role of NO in PORH and the thermal hyperemia response of skin microcirculation measured with LDF [98].

Iontophoresis is a method for noninvasive transdermal drug delivery (charged molecules) using low-density electric current. ACh and SNP iontophoresis are widely used for assessment of endothelium-dependent and endothelium-independent vasodilation of skin microcirculation [98, 100]. Regarding endothelium-dependent dilation, studies reported that ACh-induced dilation seems to be predominantly mediated by COX metabolites (although results are still conflicting) [101, 102], and NO does not extensively contribute to such dilation [103] in skin microcirculation. Beside endothelial-dependent vasodilation, ACh administration induces neural axon reflex-mediated dilation as well [104]. Iontophoresis is associated with several issues: (a) current itself may induce nonspecific vasodilation, which could interfere with the vasodilation potency of administrated drug, and it was suggested that it depends on the delivered electrical charge and the current delivery pattern [105]; (b) current-induced dilation also may depend on vehicles that have been used to dilute drugs (e.g., tap water, distilled water, deionized water, and saline), but this was not observed for ACh and SNP [106]; (c) skin resistance may influence drug delivery, and thus reduce skin resistance which was suggested as a part of good practice [100]; (d) spatial variability of ACh and SNP, suggesting that monitoring larger areas using LDI, rather than LDF provides better reproducibility [107, 108]; and (e) site of iontophoresis, since for example SNP-induced dilation could not be provoked on finger pulp, but it was provoked on the dorsum of the finger [109]. To summarize, ACh and SNP iontophoresis is widely used for endothelium-dependent and -independent microvascular vasodilation assessment in both healthy and various diseases. However, when interpreting results, complexity of mechanisms involved in these responses should be taken into account. Moreover, studies using iontophoresis should be carefully designed to reduce non-specific current-induced dilation by using low intensity current; saline should be rather

http://dx.doi.org/10.5772/intechopen.74671

used as vehicle than distilled water; pre-treatment with anesthetic should be considered; and, finally, skin resistance should be reduced as much as possible.

PORH refers to an increase in (micro)vascular blood flow due to transient short vascular occlusion, and represents a test that is commonly used for assessment of microvascular reactivity [98]. According to the literature, several mechanisms are involved in microvascular PORH response, including sensory nerves involvement via neural axon reflex [110], metabolic and myogenic component, and endothelial-dependent vasodilators production. Regarding endothelium, EDHF was suggested as an important mediator of PORH [9], while the role of prostaglandins is still not clarified [11, 12]. Studies have reported that eNOS inhibition does not alter PORH, suggesting that NO is not normally involved in forearm microvascular PORH [111]. It has been suggested that inhibition of COX inhibition may unmask the NO dependence of PORH in human cutaneous circulation [12]. Despite an evident role of endothelium-derived vasoactive mediators in skin microvascular PORH, it should be used as a tool for assessment of general microvascular reactivity, rather than a measure for microvascular endothelial function [89]. PORH can be used in conjunction with both LDF and LDI, but an advantage is given to the LDF, because LDI is considered too slow to track microvascular kinetics during PORH. Moreover, inter-day reproducibility of single-point LDF was excellent when the probe was placed on exactly the same site from one day to another [112]. While recording skin microvascular PORH homogenizing both skin and room temperature is important, since temperature plays a key role in regulation of baseline flux [97]. Another issue is related to the PORH measurement, and that is heterogeneity in study design, especially vascular occlusion duration (from 1 to 15 min) [113] and different cuff pressures used, ranging between 160 and 220 mmHg [114]. Although it is accepted as a good tool for microvascular reactivity assessment, this method still requires standardization.

Local thermal hyperemia (LTH) presents peripheral skin microvascular response to local heating mediated by joint effect of neural-dependent and NO-dependent vasodilator pathway [98]. LTH is characterized by initial peak (within the first 5 min) which depends on sensory nerves, and by sustained plateau which is mostly NO-dependent [115]. LTH has better reproducibility in conjunction with LDI, rather than a single-point LDF, and this reproducibility depends on the site of measurement too [97]. Similar to PORH, there is heterogeneity in the study design using LTH, including local warming temperature (42–43°C) [116], the time of heating, and the nature of the device used to heat the skin [89]. Another used thermal stimulus is local cooling that induces an initial vasoconstriction followed by transient vasodilation, and finally, prolonged vasoconstriction [116]. It has been demonstrated that initial vasoconstriction depends on norepinephrine, and prolonged vasoconstriction involved both norepinephrine and inhibition of NO system [116]. Results have shown that this method has the best reproducibility when the cooling protocol lasts for 30 min at 15°C [97].

Laser speckle contrast imaging is a novel technique that combines advantages of LDF and LDI, with very good inter-day reproducibility for both PORH and LTH measurements [117, 118]. This method is based on speckle contrast analysis that provides an index of blood blow. A potential limitation of this technique is its sensitivity to movements and potential challenging data analysis, but despite limitations, this method is expected to be a remarkable tool for microvascular function assessment, especially when coupled with PORH and/or LTH [89].

3.1.5. *Fingertip digital thermal monitoring (DTM)*

Fingertip digital thermal monitoring (DMT) of vascular reactivity represents a noninvasive, reproducible, operator-independent technique based on changes in fingertip temperature during cuff-occlusive reactive hyperemia [119]. This method relies on a premise that changes in fingertip temperature during and after vascular occlusion that reflects changes in blood flow and thus microvascular and endothelial function [120]. So far, studies have reported that vascular function measured by DTM correlate with Framingham Risk Score and coronary artery calcium score (a measurement of the amount of calcium in the walls of the coronary arteries using a special computed tomography (CT) scan of heart) independently of age, sex, and traditional cardiac risk factors [121]. Although clinical implications of DTM are promising, more studies on the mechanisms mediating this vascular response and large prospective trials are needed to establish the real research and clinical value of this method.

3.2. Assessment of macrovascular function

3.2.1. *Flow-mediated dilation*

FMD of the brachial artery is the most widely used noninvasive *in vivo* method for an indirect assessment of endothelial function of conduit vessels introduced by Celermajer and colleagues [5]. It provides decisive information about the ability of the endothelium to respond to particular stimulus (reactive hyperemia). In this method, an arterial occlusion cuff is placed to the forearm and inflated to stop the anterograde blood flow, thus generating ischemia. Consequently, distal from that the occlusion, in the resistance arteries, vasodilation occurs, and when the sphygmomanometer is deflated, reactive hyperemia occurs in the brachial artery. The method involves ultrasound arterial imaging in two conditions, at rest (baseline) and during reactive hyperemia after 5 min arterial occlusion, and FMD is expressed as the % difference between that two measured diameters [122]. The exact mechanism mediating FMD during reactive hyperemia has not been fully elucidated; it is considered that shear stress-induced NO is the main mediator [76, 85], but also other endothelium-derived vasodilator factors may also contribute [123]. Because reactive hyperemia flow, induces increased shear stress on endothelium challenges FMD, it might be a significant measure of peripheral microvascular function because reactive hyperemia is greatly dependent on maximal forearm resistance [124]. Furthermore, peripheral endothelial function as assessed by FMD correlates with vascular function of coronary artery [125]. In addition, impaired FMD is one of the early manifestations of vascular disease, and may be an important indicator of endothelium injury [126].

However, although the principle of this technique seems simple, its application is technically challenging and requires comprehensive practicing and standardization [127, 128]. Easy access of this noninvasive method is one of the main advantages of this method, while other advantages being a good correlation with invasive epicardial vascular function assessment, possibility to assess other important parameters (i.e., flow, baseline arterial diameters and flow-mediated constriction), and low costs [68].

To ensure that impaired FMD is not due to underlying vascular smooth muscle dysfunction or alterations in vascular structure but truly a consequence of endothelial dysfunction, response to nitroglycerine is used [127, 129, 130]. Nitroglycerine-induced vasodilation was significantly reduced in patients with cardiovascular disease [129]. Additionally, nitroglycerine-induced vasodilation was impaired in patients with atherosclerosis [131]. FMD should be interpreted as an index of vascular function reflecting both endothelium-dependent and -independent vasodilation in individuals with impaired nitroglycerine-induced vasodilation [129]. Furthermore, coronary artery dilation in response to nitroglycerine is impaired in patients with coronary heart disease which predicts long-term atherosclerotic disease progression and cardiovascular event rate [132]. These findings suggest that nitroglycerine-induced vasodilation *per se* may be a marker of the grade of atherosclerosis and predictor of cardiovascular events. However, the relationship between nitroglycerine-induced vasodilation and the risk for future cardiovascular events should still be established.

3.2.2. New method for assessment of endothelial function—measurement of ezFMD

Since FMD requires an expensive ultrasound system and high levels of technical skills, a novel method for measurement of endothelial function, namely, measurement of enclosed-zone flow-mediated dilatation (ezFMD) was developed [133]. ezFMD is a noninvasive method which assesses the level of vasodilatation from the oscillation signals transmitted to a sphygmomanometer cuff attached to the upper arm. In patients with cardiovascular diseases, ezFMD was significantly lower than in age- and gender-matched healthy individuals. In addition, cardiovascular risk factors were independent predictors of ezFMD. ezFMD was significantly correlated with conventional FMD [134]. Conventional measurement of FMD by ultrasound is measured by the change in vascular diameter, whereas ezFMD is based on the change in vascular volume. Both methods are equally valuable for assessing endothelial function, however, measurement of ezFMD is easier and less biased than measurement of FMD.

3.2.3. Coronary epicardial vasoreactivity

Quantitative coronary angiography (QCA) or intravascular ultrasound are methods for imaging vasomotor responses of epicardial coronary arteries, which enable tracing of changes in vessel diameters in response to endothelium-dependent interventions, e.g., intracoronary infusion of drugs or substances, such as acetylcholine [2]. Vessels with an intact endothelium vasodilate in response to ACh infusion, whereas segments with dysfunctional endothelial cells display abnormal vascular response [2]. Estimation of coronary endothelial function with intracoronary ACh provides diagnostic and prognostic data in patients with suspected coronary microvascular dysfunction.

Some of advantages of this method is direct assessment of the coronary vascular bed and represents gold standard for assessment of epicardial macrovasculature, while its disadvantage is invasiveness and limitation to those patients undergoing coronary angiography [68].

Physiologically, endothelium-dependent vasodilation occurs in response to exercise or tachycardia as a replacement for exercise, but also pacing induced tachycardia, and leads to increased flow-mediated endothelium-dependent vasomotion of the epicardial vessels that is impaired in atherosclerosis [68]. In healthy isolated intramyocardial porcine coronary resistance arteries, bradykinin, serotonin, and the alpha 2-adrenergic agonist clonidine evoked endothelium-dependent relaxations, which were fully (clonidine) or partially (serotonin) mediated by NO, while vasodilator response to bradykinin seems to be mediated by some other endothelium-derived mediator, different from NO [135]. Further, cold pressor test (CPT), in which the subject puts his hand into ice water, is another mode to assess epicardial vasoreactivity. In the study by Nabel et al., the response to CPT was assessed in patients with angiographically normal coronary arteries, in patients with mild coronary atherosclerosis and in patients with advanced coronary stenosis, using quantitative angiography and Doppler flow velocity measurements. Normal vessels exhibited vasodilation (partly related to beta-adrenergic receptor stimulation and partly due to flow-mediated dilation or alpha-2 adrenergic receptor activation) while atherosclerotic vessels exhibited vasoconstriction in response to CPT, possibly due to altered sensitivity to adrenergic stimulation and/or some other impairment of endothelium-dependent vasodilation [136].

3.2.4. Pulse wave velocity

Pulse wave velocity (PWV) is the velocity at which the pulse pressure wave spreads from the left ventricle (at the end of ventricular ejection) to the periphery. It results in an earlier return of the reflected wave which increases the pressure and subsequently the afterload of the left ventricle and reduces coronary artery perfusion pressure during diastole. One of the most frequently used noninvasive methods for the assessment of aortic stiffness is carotid-femoral (aortic) PWV [137]. It is a simple, noninvasive, and reproducible method which has been used as a gold standard and provides a predictive value of aortic stiffness for future cardiovascular events [138]. PWV has been used as significant marker of cardiovascular risk. Data indicate that increased arterial stiffness is being independently predictive of coronary artery disease, stroke, and cardiovascular events in general [139]. While PWV values are lower in healthy young individuals, the values of PWV increase with reduction of arterial elasticity [140].

Applanation tonometry is another method that is used for pulse wave analysis. Rather than directly assessing aortic pulse wave, it estimates aortic pulse wave from the common carotid artery or the radial artery pulse waves. As the measurement is easier, radial artery tonometry has been the most commonly recommended approach [137]. Since the method can detect changes that might be related to vascular health, even before the onset of signs and symptoms, yet, the PWV analysis occupies an important place in clinical practice [141]. This method has some limitations that are related to associated comorbidities, such as metabolic syndrome, obesity, and diabetes, because the femoral pressure waveform may be difficult to record accurately in these patients [137].

3.2.5. Intima-media thickness

Carotid intima-media thickness (CIMT) is a method that evaluates extra-cranial carotid arteries by high-resolution ultrasound, and represents an important marker of subclinical atherosclerosis [142]. CIMT is increased in atherosclerosis and also correlates with coronary artery disease [143] and cerebrovascular disease [144]. CIMT represents the combined width of the intima and media; in healthy individuals, it is composed almost entirely of media, with a progressive intimal thickening or hypertrophy of media, determined by age, gender, and hypertension [145]. The major advantage of CIMT is that it is noninvasive and reproducible, relatively inexpensive to perform, also widely available and well standardized [146].

3.2.6. *Functional endothelial biomarkers in cardiovascular diseases*

The baseline pathogenic process in cardiovascular diseases, such as atherosclerosis and coronary artery disease, is an endothelial dysfunction with complex underlying mechanisms: oxidative stress, diminished vasoreactivity, hemostatic disturbances, and inflammation leading to the disease progression by modulating the arterial wall, promoting lipoprotein retention, plaque formation and possibly its destabilization. Endothelial dysfunction is characterized by endothelial dysfunction, impaired vascular homeostasis and reduced "anti"-mechanisms (-oxidant, -inflammatory, -thrombotic) and activated "pro"-mechanisms. Diagnostic tools for detecting endothelial dysfunction in humans are limited. They should be safe, cost-effective, noninvasive, repeatable, reproducible, and standardized. Current diagnostic methods are FMD, forearm plethysmography, finger-pulse plethysmography, PWV analysis, and coronary angiography. However, there is a need for additional diagnostic tools, biomarkers. For everyday clinical use, more and larger human-based studies are necessary to validate clinical usefulness of biomarkers [147, 148].

4. Conclusion

To find a specific and sensitive biomarker for any disease sometimes looks like a search for the Holy Grail—something precious but impossible to find. The reason for that could be those cardiometabolic diseases, all having a common point—endothelial dysfunction and it is likely that they have common underlying mechanisms leading to endothelial dysfunction. These mechanisms may be redundant and not activated at the same time and the same order, but certainly end up with impaired endothelium, and inappropriate vascular response to physiological stimuli with inability to compensate for pathophysiological events, finally leading to manifested disease and organ damage. One can only take with "a grain of salt" as many different biomarkers as possible and build up a picture of their relationship to the disease's etiopathogenesis, development, and prognosis.

Acknowledgements

This work is supported by the European Structural and Investment Funds grant for the Croatian National Scientific Center of Excellence for Personalized Health Care, University of Josip Juraj Strossmayer Osijek (grant #KK.01.1.1.01.0010).

Author details

Ines Drenjancevic[1,4*], Ivana Jukic[1,2,4], Ana Stupin[1,2,4], Anita Cosic[1,4], Marko Stupin[1,3,4] and Kristina Selthofer-Relatic[1,3,4]

*Address all correspondence to: ines.drenjancevic@mefos.hr

1 Faculty of Medicine, University of Osijek, Osijek, Croatia

2 Faculty of Dental Medicine and Health Studies, University of Osijek, Osijek, Croatia

3 Internal Clinic, Clinical Hospital Center, Osijek, Croatia

4 Croatian National Scientific Center of Excellence for Personalized Health Care, University of Josip Juraj Strossmayer, Osijek, Croatia

References

[1] Flammer AJ, Luscher TF. Three decades of endothelium research: From the detection of nitric oxide to the everyday implementation of endothelial function measurements in cardiovascular diseases. Swiss Medical Weekly. 2010;**140**:w13122

[2] Ludmer PL, Selwyn AP, Shook TL, Wayne RR, Mudge GH, Alexander RW, Ganz P. Paradoxical vasoconstriction induced by acetylcholine in atherosclerotic coronary arteries. The New England Journal of Medicine. 1986 Oct 23;**315**(17):1046-1051

[3] Linder L, Kiowski W, Bühler FR, Lüscher TF. Indirect evidence for release of endothelium-derived relaxing factor in human forearm circulation in vivo: Blunted response in essential hypertension. Circulation. 1990;**81**:1762-1767

[4] Panza JA, Quyyumi AA, Brush JE Jr, Epstein SE. Abnormal endothelium-dependent vascular relaxation in patients with essential hypertension. The New England Journal of Medicine. 1990;**323**(1):22-27

[5] Celermajer DS, Sorensen KE, Gooch VM, Spiegelhalter DJ, Miller OI, Sullivan ID, Lloyd JK, Deanfield JE. Non-invasive detection of endothelial dysfunction in children and adults at risk of atherosclerosis. Lancet. 1992;**340**:1111-1115

[6] Anderson TJ, Gerhard MD, Meredith IT, Charbonneau F, Delagrange D, Creager MA, Selwyn AP, Ganz P. Systemic nature of endothelial dysfunction in atherosclerosis. The American Journal of Cardiology. 1995;**75**:71B-74B

[7] Brunner H, Cockcroft JR, Deanfield J, Donald A, Ferrannini E, Halcox J, Kiowski W, Luscher TF, Mancia G, Natali A, Oliver JJ, Pessina AC, Rizzoni D, Rossi GP, Salvetti A, Spieker LE, Taddei S, Webb DJ. Endothelial function and dysfunction, part II: Association with cardiovascular risk factors and diseases: A statement by the working group on Endothelins and endothelial factors of the European Society of Hypertension. Journal of Hypertension. 2005;**23**:233-246

[8] Trochu JN, Bouhour JB, Kaley G, Hintze TH. Role of endothelium-derived nitric oxide in the regulation of cardiac oxygen metabolism: Implications in health and disease. Circulation Research. 2000;**87**:1108-1117

[9] Lorenzo S, Minson CT. Human cutaneous reactive hyperaemia: Role of BKCa channels and sensory nerves. The Journal of Physiology. 2007;**585**:295-303

[10] Binggeli C, Spieker LE, Corti R, Sudano I, Stojanovic V, Hayoz D, Luscher TF, Noll G. Statins enhance postischemic hyperemia in the skin circulation of hypercholesterolemic patients: A monitoring test of endothelial dysfunction for clinical practice? Journal of the American College of Cardiology. 2003;**42**:71-77

[11] Dalle-Ave A, Kubli S, Golay S, Delachaux A, Liaudet L, Waeber B, Feihl F. Acetylcholine-induced vasodilation and reactive hyperemia are not affected by acute cyclo-oxygenase inhibition in human skin. Microcirculation. 2004;**11**:327-336

[12] Medow MS, Taneja SJM. Cyclooxygenase and nitric oxide synthase dependence of cutaneous reactive hyperemia in humans. American Journal of Physiology-Heart and Circulatory Physiology. 2007;**293**:H425-H432

[13] Lavi S, Prasad A, Yang EH, Mathew V, Simari RD, Rihal CS, Lerman LO, Lerman A. Smoking is associated with epicardial coronary endothelial dysfunction and elevated white blood cell count in patients with chest pain and early coronary artery disease. Circulation. 2007;**115**(20):2621-2627

[14] Magness RR, Shideman CR, Habermehl DA, Sullivan JA, Bird IM. Endothelial vasodilator production by uterine and systemic arteries. V. Effects of ovariectomy, the ovarian cycle, and pregnancy on prostacyclin synthase expression. Prostaglandins & Other Lipid Mediators. 2000;**60**(4-6):103-118

[15] Lewis PJ, Boylan P, Friedman LA, Hensby CN, Downing I. Prostacyclin in pregnancy. British Medical Journal. 1980;**280**:1581-1582

[16] Morton JS, Davidge ST. Arterial endothelium-derived hyperpolarization: Potential role in pregnancy adaptations and complications. Journal of Cardiovascular Pharmacology. 2013;**61**:197-203

[17] Juonala M, Viikari JSA, Alfthan G, Marniemi J, Kähönen M, Taittonen L, Laitinen T, Raitakari OT. Brachial artery flow-mediated dilation and asymmetrical Dimethylarginine in the cardiovascular risk in young Finns study. Circulation. 2007;**116**:1367-1373

[18] Rizos D, Eleftheriades M, Batakis E, Rizou M, Haliassos A, Hassioakos D, Botsis D. Levels of asymmetric dimethylarginine throughout normal pregnancy and in pregnancies complicated with preeclampsia or had small for gestational age baby. The Journal of Maternal-Fetal and Neonatal Medicine. 2012;**25**(8):1311-1315

[19] Coussons-Read ME, Lobel M, Carey JC, Kreither MO, D'Anna K, Argys L, Ross RG, Brandt C, Cole S. The occurrence of preterm delivery is linked to pregnancy-specific distress and elevated inflammatory markers across gestation. Brain, Behavior, and Immunity. 2012;**26**(4):650-659

[20] Himburg HA, Dowd SE, Friedman MH. Frequency-dependent response of the vascular endothelium to pulsatile shear stress. American Journal of Physiology. Heart and Circulatory Physiology. 2007;**293**:H645-H653

[21] Nishida K, Harrison DG, Navas JP, Fisher AA, Dockery SP, Uematsu M, Nerem RM, Alexander RW, Murphy TJ. Molecular cloning and characterization of the constitutive bovine aortic endothelial cell nitric oxide synthase. The Journal of Clinical Investigation. 1992;**90**:2092-2096

[22] Uematsu M, Ohara Y, Navas JP, Nishida K, Murphy TJ, Alexander RW, Nerem RM, Harrison DG. Regulation of endothelial cell nitric oxide synthase mRNA expression by shear stress. American Journal of Physiology. Cell Physiology. 1995;**269**:C1371-C1378

[23] Shin HY, Gerritsen ME, Bizios R. Regulation of endothelial cell proliferation and apoptosis by cyclic pressure. Annals of Biomedical Engineering. 2002;**30**:297-304

[24] Cheng JJ, Wung BS, Chao YJ, Wang DL. Cyclic strain-induced reactive oxygen species involved in ICAM-1 gene induction in endothelial cells. Hypertension. 1998;**31**:125-130

[25] Gradinaru D, Borsa C, Ionescu C, Prada GI. Oxidized LDL and NO synthesis-biomarkers of endothelial dysfunction and ageing. Mechanisms of Ageing and Development. 2015;**151**:101-113

[26] Mehta JL. The role of LOX-1, a novel lectin-like receptor for oxidized low density lipoprotein, in atherosclerosis. The Canadian Journal of Cardiology. 2004 Aug;**20** (Suppl B):32B-36B

[27] Vallance P, Leone A, Calver A, Collier J, Moncada S. Accumulation of an endogenous inhibitor of nitric oxide synthesis in chronic renal failure. Lancet. 1992 Mar 7; **339**(8793):572-575

[28] Stühlinger MC, Oka RK, Graf EE, Schmölzer I, Upson BM, Kapoor O, Szuba A, Malinow MR, Wascher TC, Pachinger O, Cooke JP. Endothelial dysfunction induced by hyperhomocyst(e)inemia: Role of asymmetric dimethylarginine. Circulation. 2003 Aug 26;**108**(8):933-938

[29] Boger RH, Sullivan LM, Schwedhelm E, Wang TJ, Maas R, Benjamin EJ, et al. Plasma asymmetric dimethylarginine and incidence of cardiovascular disease and death in the community. Circulation. 2009;**119**(12):1592-1600

[30] Cook S, Hugli O, Egli M, Ménard B, Thalmann S, Sartori C, Perrin C, Nicod P, Thorens B, Vollenweider P, Scherrer U, Burcelin R. Partial gene deletion of endothelial nitric oxide synthase predisposes to exaggerated high-fat diet-induced insulin resistance and arterial hypertension. Diabetes. 2004;**53**(8):2067-2072

[31] Asagami T, Abbasi F, Stuelinger M, Lamendola C, McLaughlin T, Cooke JP, Reaven GM, Tsao PS. Metformin treatment lowers asymmetric dimethylarginine concentrations in patients with type 2 diabetes. Metabolism. 2002;**51**(7):843-846

[32] Stühlinger MC, Abbasi F, Chu JW, Lamendola C, McLaughlin TL, Cooke JP, Reaven GM, Tsao PS. Relationship between insulin resistance and an endogenous nitric oxide synthase inhibitor. JAMA. 2002;**287**(11):1420-1426

[33] Falck-Hansen M, Kassiteridi C, Monaco C. Toll-like receptors in atherosclerosis. International Journal of Molecular Sciences. 2013;**14**(7):14008-14023

[34] Cole JE, Georgiou E, Monaco C. The expression and functions of toll-like receptors in atherosclerosis. Mediators of Inflammation. 2010;**2010**:393946

[35] Javed Q. Clinical implications of tumor necrosis factor-alpha, Interleukin-6 and resistin in coronary artery disease. World Journal of Cardiovascular Diseases. 2014;**4**:416-421

[36] Libby P, Ridker PM, Maseri A. Inflammation and atherosclerosis. Circulation. 2002;**105**:1135-1143

[37] Takaishi H, Taniguchi T, Takahashi A, et al. High glucose accelerates MCP-1 production via p38 MAPK in vascular endothelial cells. Biochemical and Biophysical Research Communications. 2003;**305**:122-130

[38] Festa A, D'Agostino R Jr, Howard G, Mykkanen L, Tracy RP, Haffner SM. Chronic subclinical inflammation as part of the insulin resistance syndrome: The insulin resistance atherosclerosis study (IRAS). Circulation. 2000;**102**:42-47

[39] Dandona P, Weinstock R, Thusu K, Abdel-Rahman E, Aljada A, Wadden T. Tumor necrosis factoralpha in sera of obese patients: Fall with weight loss. The Journal of Clinical Endocrinology and Metabolism. 1998;**83**:2907-2910

[40] Vozarova B, Weyer C, Hanson K, Tataranni PA, Bogardus C, Pratley RE. Circulating interleukin-6 in relation to adiposity, insulin action, and insulin secretion. Obesity Research. 2001;**9**:414-417

[41] Schalkwijk CG, Poland DC, van Dijk W et al. Plasma concentration of C-reactive protein is increased in type I diabetic patients without clinical macroangiopathy and correlates with markers of endothelial dysfunction: Evidence for chronic inflammation. Diabetologia 1999;**42**:351-357

[42] Ji SR, Wu Y, Potempa LA, Liang YH, Zhao J. Effect of modified C-reactive protein on complement activation: A possible complement regulatory role of modified or monomeric C-reactive protein in atherosclerotic lesions. Arteriosclerosis, Thrombosis, and Vascular Biology. 2006;**26**(4):935-941

[43] Pradhan AD, Manson JE, Rifai N, Buring JE, Ridker PM. C-reactive protein, interleukin 6, and risk of developing type 2 diabetes mellitus. Journal of the American Medical Association. 2001;**286**(3):327-334

[44] Schulze MB, Rimm EB, Li T, Rifai N, Stampfer MJ, Hu FB. C-reactive protein and incident cardiovascular events among men with diabetes. Diabetes Care. 2004;**27**:889-894

[45] Mahajan K. Microparticles in atherosclerosis: Biomarkers of disease. J Clin Exp Cardiolog. 2015;**6**:1 http://dx.doi.org/10.4172/2155-9880.1000356

[46] Sarrazin S, Adam E, Lyon M, Depontieu F, Motte V, Landolfi C, Lortat-Jacob H, Bechard D, Lassalle P, Delehedde M. Endocan or endothelial cell specific molecule-1 (ESM-1): A potential novel endothelial cell marker and a new target for cancer therapy. Biochimica et Biophysica Acta. 2006 Jan;**1765**(1):25-37

[47] Kali A, Shetty KS. Endocan: A novel circulating proteoglycan. Indian Journal of Pharmacology. 2014 Nov-Dec;**46**(6):579-583

[48] Balta S, Mikhailidis DP, Demirkol S, Ozturk C, Celik T, Iyisoy A. Endocan: A novel inflammatory indicator in cardiovascular disease? Atherosclerosis. 2015 Nov;**243**(1):339-343

[49] Tadzic R, Mihalj M, Vcev A, Ennen J, Tadzic A, Drenjancevic I. The effects of arterial blood pressure reduction on endocan and soluble endothelial cell adhesion molecules (CAMs) and CAMs ligands expression in hypertensive patients on Ca-channel blocker therapy. Kidney & Blood Pressure Research. 2013;**37**(2-3):103-115

[50] Keaney JF Jr, Massaro JM, Larson MG, et al. Heritability and correlates of intercellular adhesion molecule-1 in the Framingham offspring study. Journal of the American College of Cardiology 2004;**44**:168-173

[51] Meigs JB, Mittleman MA, Nathan DM, et al. Hyperinsulinemia, hyperglycemia, and impaired hemostasis: The Framingham offspring study. Journal of the American Medical Association. 2000;**283**:221-228

[52] Maugeri N, Rovere-Querini P, Baldini M, et al. Translational mini-review series on immunology of vascular disease: Mechanisim of vascular inflammation and remodeling in systemic vasculitis. Clinical and Experimental Immunology. 2009;**156**:395-404

[53] Chavakis T, Bierhaus A, Nawroth PP. RAGE (receptor for advanced glycation end products): A central player in the inflammatory response. Microbes and Infection. 2004:1219-1225

[54] Altannavch TS, Roubalová K, Kučera P, et al. Effect of high glucose concentrations on expression of ELAM-1, VCAM-1 and ICAM-1 in HUVEC with and without cytokine activation. Physiological Research. 2004;**53**:77-82

[55] Azcutia V, Abu-Taha M, Romacho T, et al. Inflammation determines the pro-adhesive properties of high extracellular D-glucose in human endothelial cells in vitro and rat microvessels in vivo. PLoS One. 2010;**5**:e1009

[56] Maloney E, Sweet IR, Hockenbery DM, et al. Activation of NF-kappaB by palmitate in endothelial cells: A key role for NADPH oxidase-derived superoxide in response to TLR4 activation. Arteriosclerosis, Thrombosis, and Vascular Biology. 2009;**29**:1370-1375

[57] Pieper GM, Riaz uH. Activation of nuclear factor-kappaB in cultured endothelial cells by increased glucose concentration: Prevention by calphostin C. Journal of Cardiovascular Pharmacology. 1997;**30**:528-532

[58] Piga R, Naito Y, Kokura S, Handa O, Yoshikawa T. Short-term high glucose exposure induces monocyte-endothelial cells adhesion and transmigration by increasing VCAM-1 and MCP-1 expression in human aortic endothelial cells. Atherosclerosis. 2007;**193**:328-334

[59] TS1 L, Pei YH, Peng YP, Chen J, Jiang SS, Gong JB. Oscillating high glucose enhances oxidative stress and apoptosis in human coronary artery endothelial cells. Journal of Endocrinological Investigation. 2014 Jul;**37**(7):645-651. DOI: 10.1007/s40618-014-0086-5

[60] San Martin A, Du P, Dikalova A, et al. Reactive oxygen species-selective regulation of aortic inflammatory gene expression in type 2 diabetes. American Journal of Physiology. Heart and Circulatory Physiology. 2007;**292**:H2073-H2082

[61] Gao L, Mann GE. Vascular NAD(P)H oxidase activation in diabetes: A double-edged sword in redox signalling. Cardiovascular Research. 2009;**82**:9-20

[62] Shoelson SE, Lee J, Goldfine AB. Inflammation and insulin resistance. The Journal of Clinical Investigation. 2006;**116**:1793-1801

[63] Read MA, Whitley MZ, Williams AJ, Collins T. NF-kappa B and I kappa B alpha: An inducible regulatory system in endothelial activation. The Journal of Experimental Medicine. 1994;**179**:503-512

[64] Pierce GL, Lesniewski LA, Lawson BR, Beske SD, Seals DR. Nuclear factor-{kappa}B activation contributes to vascular endothelial dysfunction via oxidative stress in overweight/obese middle aged and older humans. Circulation. 2009;**119**:1284-1292

[65] Beltrame JF, Crea F, Camici P. Advances in coronary microvascular dysfunction. Heart, Lung & Circulation. 2009;**18**:19-27

[66] Camici PG, Crea F. Coronary microvascular dysfunction. The New England Journal of Medicine. 2007;**356**:830-840

[67] Gibson CM, Cannon CP, Daley WL, Dodge JT, Jr, Alexander B, Jr, Marble SJ, McCabe CH, Raymond L, Fortin T, Poole WK, Braunwald E. TIMI frame count: A quantitative method of assessing coronary artery flow. Circulation 1996;**93**:879-888

[68] Flammer AJ, Anderson T, Celermajer DS, Creager MA, Deanfield J, Ganz P, Hamburg NM, Lüscher TF, Shechter M, Taddei S, Vita JA, Lerman A. The assessment of endothelial function: From research into clinical practice. Circulation. 2012;**126**(6):753-767

[69] Utz W, Jordan J, Niendorf T, Stoffels M, Luft FC, Dietz R, Friedrich MG. Blood oxygen level-dependent MRI of tissue oxygenation: Relation to endothelium-dependent and endothelium-independent blood flow changes. Arteriosclerosis, Thrombosis, and Vascular Biology. 2005;**25**:1408-1413

[70] Schindler TH, Schelbert HR, Quercioli A, Dilsizian V. Cardiac PET imaging for the detection and monitoring of coronary artery disease and microvascular health. JACC;**3**:623-640

[71] Al-Mallah MH, Sitek A, Moore SC, Di Carli M, Dorbala S. Assessment of myocardial perfusion and function with PET and PET/CT. Journal of Nuclear Cardiology. 2010;**17**(3):498-513

[72] Barletta G, Del Bene MR. Myocardial perfusion echocardiography and coronary microvascular dysfunction. World Journal of Cardiology. 2015;**7**(12):861-874

[73] Hewlett AW, van Zwaluwenburg JG. The rate of blood flow in the arm. Heart 1909;**1**:631-646

[74] Ian B. Wilkinson, David J Webb. Venous occlusion plethysmography in cardiovascular research: Methodology and clinical applications. British Journal of Clinical Pharmacology. 2001;**52**(6):631-646

[75] Petrie JR, Ueda S, Morris AD, Murray LS, Elliott HL, Connell JM. How reproducible is bilateral forearm plethysmography? British Journal of Clinical Pharmacology. 1998;**45**:131-139

[76] Joannides R, Haefeli WE, Linder L, Richard V, Bakkali EH, Thuillez C, Lüscher TF. Nitric oxide is responsible for flow-dependent dilatation of human peripheral conduit arteries in vivo. Circulation. 1995;**91**:1314-1319

[77] Ozkor MA, Murrow JR, Rahman AM, Kavtaradze N, Lin J, Manatunga A, Quyyumi AA. Endothelium-derived hyperpolarizing factor determines resting and stimulated forearm vasodilator tone in health and in disease. Circulation. 2011;**123**:2244-2253

[78] Chowienczyk PJ, Watts GF, Cockcroft JR, Ritter JM. Impaired endothelium-dependent vasodilation of forearm resistance vessels in hypercholesterolaemia. Lancet. 1992;**340**:1430-1432

[79] Makimattila S, Liu ML, Vakkilainen J, et al. Impaired endothelium-dependent vasodilation in type 2 diabetes. Relation to LDL size, oxidized LDL, and antioxidants. Diabetes Care. 1999;**22**:973-981

[80] Heitzer T, Yla-Herttuala S, Luoma J, et al. Cigarette smoking potentiates endothelial dysfunction of forearm resistance vessels in patients with hypercholesterolemia: Role of oxidized LDL. Circulation. 1996;**93**:1346-1353

[81] Taddei S, Virdis A, Mattei P, et al. Aging and endothelial function in normotensive subjects and patients with essential hypertension. Circulation. 1995;**91**:1981-1987

[82] Panza JA, Casino PR, Kilcoyne CM, Quyyumi AA. Impaired endothelium-dependent vasodilation in patients with essential hypertension: Evidence that the abnormality is not at the muscarinic receptor level. Journal of the American College of Cardiology. 1994;**23**:1610-1616

[83] Bruning TA, Chang PC, Hendriks MGC, Vermeij P, Pfaffendorf M, Van Zwieten PA. In vivo characterization of muscarinic receptor subtypes that mediate vasodilatation in patients with essential hypertension. Hypertension. 1995;**26**:70-77

[84] Bonetti PO, Pumper GM, Higano ST, Holmes DR Jr, Kuvin JT, Lerman A. Noninasive identification of patients with early coronary atherosclerosis by assessment of digital reactive hyperemia. Journal of the American College of Cardiology. 2004;**44**:2137-2141

[85] Higashi Y. Assessment of endothelial function. History, methodological aspects, and clinical perspectives. International Heart Journal. 2015;**56**(2):125-134

[86] Rubinshtein R, Kuvin JT, Soffler M, et al. Assessment of endothelial function by non-invasive peripheral arterial tonometry predicts late cardiovascular adverse events. European Heart Journal. 2010;**31**:1142-1148

[87] Akiyama E, Sugiyama S, Matsuzawa Y, et al. Incremental prognostic significance of peripheral endothelial dysfunction in patients with heart failure with normal left ventricular ejection fraction. Journal of the American College of Cardiology. 2012;**60**:1778-1786

[88] Hamburg NM, Palmisano J, Larson MG, et al. Relation of brachial and digital measures of vascular function in the community: The Framingham heart study. Hypertension. 2011;**57**:390-396

[89] Roustit M, Cracowski JL. Non-invasive assessment of skin microvascular function in humans: An insight into methods. Microcirculation. 2012;**19**(1):47-64

[90] Antonios TF, Singer DR, Markandu ND, Mortimer PS, MacGregor GA. Structural skin capillary rarefaction in essential hypertension. Hypertension. 1999;**33**:998-1001

[91] Feihl F, Liaudet L, Waeber B, Levy BI. Hypertension: A disease of the microcirculation? Hypertension. 2006;**48**:1012-1017

[92] Levy BI, Schiffrin EL, Mourad JJ, Agostini D, Vicaut E, Safar ME, Struijker-Boudier HA. Impaired tissue perfusion: A pathology common to hypertension, obesity, and diabetes mellitus. Circulation. 2008;**118**:968-976

[93] Chang CH, Tsai RK, Wu WC, Kuo SL, Yu HS. Use of dynamic capillaroscopy for studying cutaneous microcirculation in patients with diabetes mellitus. Microvascular Research. 1997;**53**:121-127

[94] Yamamoto-Suganuma R, Aso Y. Relationship between post-occlusive forearm skin reactive hyperaemia and vascular disease in patients with type 2 diabetes – A novel index for detecting micro- and macrovascular dysfunction using laser Doppler flowmetry. Diabetic Medicine. 2009;**26**:83-88

[95] Kruger A, Stewart J, Sahityani R, O'Riordan E, Thompson C, Adler S, Garrick R, Vallance P, Goligorsky MS. Laser Doppler flowmetry detection of endothelial dysfunction in end-stage renal disease patients: Correlation with cardiovascular risk. Kidney International. 2006;**70**:157-164

[96] Stern MD. In vivo evaluation of microcirculation by coherent light scattering. Nature. 1975;**254**:56-58

[97] Roustit M, Blaise S, Millet C, Cracowski JL. Reproducibility and methodological issues of skin post-occlusive and thermal hyperemia assessed by single-point laser Doppler flowmetry. Microvascular Research. 2010;**79**:102-108

[98] Cracowski JL, Minson CT, Salvat-Melis M, Halliwill JR. Methodological issues in the assessment of skin microvascular endothelial function in humans. Trends in Pharmacological Sciences. 2006;**27**:503-508

[99] Clough GF. Microdialysis of large molecules. The AAPS Journal. 2005;**7**:E686-E692

[100] Turner J, Belch JJ, Khan F. Current concepts in assessment of microvascular endothelial function using laser Doppler imaging and iontophoresis. Trends in Cardiovascular Medicine. 2008;**18**:109-116

[101] Durand S, Tartas M, Bouye P, Koitka A, Saumet JL, Abraham P. Prostaglandins participate in the late phase of the vascular response to acetylcholine iontophoresis in humans. The Journal of Physiology. 2004;**561**:811-819

[102] Holowatz LA, Thompson CS, Minson CT, Kenney WL. Mechanisms of acetylcholine-mediated vasodilatation in young and aged human skin. The Journal of Physiology. 2005;**563**:965-973

[103] Noon JP, Walker BR, Hand MF, Webb DJ. Studies with iontophoretic administration of drugs to human dermal vessels in vivo: Cholinergic vasodilatation is mediated by dilator prostanoids rather than nitric oxide. British Journal of Clinical Pharmacology. 1998;**45**:545-550

[104] Berghoff M, Kathpal M, Kilo S, Hilz MJ, Freeman R. Vascular and neural mechanisms of ACh-mediated vasodilation in the forearm cutaneous microcirculation. Journal of Applied Physiology. 2002;**92**:780-788

[105] Durand S, Fromy B, Bouye P, Saumet JL, Abraham P. Current-induced vasodilation during water iontophoresis (5 min, 0.10 mA) is delayed from current onset and involves aspirin sensitive mechanisms. Journal of Vascular Research. 2002;**39**:59-71

[106] Ferrell WR, Ramsay JE, Brooks N, Lockhart JC, Dickson S, McNeece GM, Greer IA, Sattar N. Elimination of electrically induced iontophoretic artefacts: Implications for non-invasive assessment of peripheral microvascular function. Journal of Vascular Research. 2002;**39**:447-455

[107] Agarwal SC, Allen J, Murray A, Purcell IF. Comparative reproducibility of dermal microvascular blood flow changes in response to acetylcholine iontophoresis, hyperthermia and reactive hyperaemia. Physiological Measurement. 2010;**31**:1-11

[108] Blaise S, Hellmann M, Roustit M, Isnard S, Cracowski JL. Oral sildenafil increases skin hyperaemia induced by iontophoresis of sodium nitroprusside in healthy volunteers. British Journal of Pharmacology. 2010;**160**:1128-1134

[109] Roustit M, Blaise S, Cracowski JL. Sodium nitroprusside iontophoresis on the finger pad does not consistently increase skin blood flow in healthy controls and patients with systemic sclerosis. Microvascular Research. 2009;**77**:260-264

[110] Larkin SW, Williams TJ. Evidence for sensory nerve involvement in cutaneous reactive hyperemia in humans. Circulation Research. 1993;**73**:147-154

[111] Wong BJ, Wilkins BW, Holowatz LA, Minson CT. Nitric oxide synthase inhibition does not alter the reactive hyperemic response in the cutaneous circulation. Journal of Applied Physiology. 2003;**95**:504-510

[112] Yvonne-Tee GB, Rasool AH, Halim AS, Rahman AR. Reproducibility of different laser Doppler fluximetry parameters of postocclusive reactive hyperemia in human forearm skin. Journal of Pharmacological and Toxicological Methods. 2005;**52**:286-292

[113] Yvonne-Tee GB, Rasool AH, Halim AS, Wong AR, Rahman AR. Method optimization on the use of postocclusive hyperemia model to assess microvascular function. Clinical Hemorheology and Microcirculation. 2008;**38**:119-133

[114] Keymel S, Sichwardt J, Balzer J, Stegemann E, Rassaf T, Kleinbongard P, Kelm M, Heiss C, Lauer T. Characterization of the non-invasive assessment of the cutaneous microcirculation by laser Doppler perfusion scanner. Microcirculation. 2010;**17**:358-366

[115] Minson CT, Berry LT, Joyner MJ. Nitric oxide and neurally mediated regulation of skin blood flow during local heating. Journal of Applied Physiology. 2001;**91**:1619-1626

[116] Johnson JM, Kellogg DL Jr. Local thermal control of the human cutaneous circulation. Journal of Applied Physiology 2010;**109**:1229-1238

[117] Briers JD. Laser Doppler, speckle and related techniques for blood perfusion mapping and imaging. Physiological Measurement. 2001;**22**:R35-R66

[118] Roustit M, Millet C, Blaise S, Dufournet B, Cracowski JL. Excellent reproducibility of laser speckle contrast imaging to assess skin microvascular reactivity. Microvascular Research. 2010;**80**:505-511

[119] Ahmadi N, McQuilkin GL, Akhtar MW, Hajsadeghi F, Kleis SJ, Hecht H, Naghavi M, Budoff M. Reproducibility and variability of digital thermal monitoring of vascular reactivity. Clinical Physiology and Functional Imaging. 2011;**31**(6):422-428

[120] Gul KM, Ahmadi N, Wang Z, Jamieson C, Nasir K, Metcalfe R. Digital thermal monitoring of vascular function: A novel tool to improve cardiovascular risk assessment. Vascular Medicine. 2009;**14**(2):143-148

[121] Ahmadi N, Hajsadeghi F, Gul K, Vane J, Usman N, Flores F, Nasir K, Hecht H, Naghavi M, Budoff M. Relations between digital thermal monitoring of vascular function, the Framingham risk score, and coronary artery calcium score. Journal of Cardiovascular Computed Tomography. 2008;**2**(6):382-388

[122] Alley H, Owens CD, Gasper WJ, Grenon SM. Ultrasound assessment of endothelial-dependent flow-mediated vasodilation of the brachial artery in clinical research. Journal of Visualized Experiments . 2014, 22;(92):e52070

[123] Parker BA, Tschakovsky ME, Augeri AL, Polk DM, Thompson PD, Kiernan FJ. Heterogenous vasodilator pathways underlie flow-mediated dilation in men and women. The American Journal of Physiology. 2011;**301**:H1118-H1126

[124] Bretón-Romero R, Wang N, Palmisano J, Larson MG, Vasan RS, Mitchell GF, Benjamin EJ, Vita JA, Hamburg NM. Cross-sectional associations of flow reversal, vascular function, and arterial stiffness in the Framingham heart study. Arteriosclerosis, Thrombosis, and Vascular Biology. 2016;**36**(12):2452-2459

[125] Takase B, Uehata A, Akima T, Nagai T, Nishioka T, Hamabe A, Satomura K, Ohsuzu F, Kurita A. Endothelium-dependent flow-mediated vasodilation in coronary and brachial arteries in suspected coronary artery disease. Am J Cardiol. 1998, 15;**82**(12):1535-9,A7-8

[126] Sorensen KE, Celermajer DS, Spiegelhalter DJ, Georgakopoulos D, Robinson J, Thomas O, Deanfield JE. Non-invasive measurement of human endothelium dependent arterial responses: Accuracy and reproducibility. British Heart Journal. 1995;**74**(3):247-253

[127] Corretti MC, Anderson TJ, Benjamin EJ, Celermajer D, Charbonneau F, Creager MA, Deanfield J, Drexler H, Gerhard-Herman M, Herrington D, Vallance P, Vita J, Vogel R. Guidelines for the ultrasound assessment of endothelial-dependent flow-mediated vasodilation of the brachial artery: A report of the international brachial artery reactivity task force. Journal of the American College of Cardiology. 2002;**39**:257-265

[128] Deanfield J, Donald A, Ferri C, Giannattasio C, Halcox J, Halligan S, Lerman A, Mancia G, Oliver JJ, Pessina AC, Rizzoni D, Rossi GP, Salvetti A, Schiffrin EL, Taddei S, Webb DJ. Endothelial function and dysfunction, part I: Methodological issues for assessment in the different vascular beds: A statement by the Working Group on Endothelin and Endothelial Factors of the European Society of Hypertension. Journal of Hypertension. 2005;**23**:7-17

[129] Maruhashi T, Soga J, Fujimura N, et al. Nitroglycerine-induced vasodilation for assessment of vascular function: A comparison with flow-mediated vasodilation. Arteriosclerosis, Thrombosis, and Vascular Biology. 2013;**33**:1401-1408

[130] Inoue T, Matsuoka H, Higashi Y, et al. Flow-mediated vasodilation as a diagnostic modality for vascular failure. Hypertension Research. 2008;**31**:2105-2113

[131] Raitakari OT, Seale JP, Celermajer DS. Impaired vascular responses to nitroglycerin in subjects with coronary atherosclerosis. The American Journal of Cardiology. 2001;**87**(2):217-219

[132] Schächinger V, Britten MB, Zeiher AM. Prognostic impact of coronary vasodilator dysfunction on adverse long-term outcome of coronary heart disease. Circulation. 2000;**101**:1899-1906

[133] Ukawa T, Takayanagi T, Morimoto H, Higashi Y, Idei N, Yoshizumi M, Tsuji T. Novel non-invasive method of measurement of endothelial function: Enclosed-zone flow-mediated dilatation (ezFMD). Medical & Biological Engineering & Computing. 2012;**50**(12):1239-1247

[134] Idei N, Ukawa T, Hata T, et al. A novel noninvasive and simple method for assessment of endothelial function: Enclosed zone flow-mediated vasodilation (ezFMD) using an oscillation amplitude measurement. Atherosclerosis. 2013;**229**:324-330

[135] Tschudi M, Richard V, Buhler FR, Luscher TF. Importance of endothelium-derived nitric oxide in porcine coronary resistance arteries. The American Journal of Physiology. 1991;**260**:H13-H20

[136] Nabel EG, Ganz P, Gordon JB, Alexander RW, Selwyn AP. Dilation of normal and constriction of atherosclerotic coronary arteries caused by the cold pressor test. Circulation. 1988;**77**:43-52

[137] Laurent S, Cockcroft J, Van BL, et al. Expert consensus document on arterial stiffness: Methodological issues and clinical applications. European Heart Journal. 2006;**27**(21):2588-2605

[138] Vlachopoulos C, Aznaouridis K, Stefanadis C. Prediction of cardiovascular events and all-cause mortality with arterial stiffness: A systematic review and meta-analysis. Journal of the American College of Cardiology. 2010;**55**(13):1318-1327

[139] Ben-Shlomo Y, Spears M, Boustred C, May M, Anderson SG, Benjamin EJ, Boutouyrie P, Cameron J, Chen CH, Cruickshank JK, Hwang SJ, Lakatta EG, Laurent S, Maldonado J, Mitchell GF, Najjar SS, Newman AB, Ohishi M, Pannier B, Pereira T, Vasan RS,

Shokawa T, Sutton-Tyrell K, Verbeke F, Wang K, Webb DJ, Willum Hansen T, Zoungas S, McEniery CM, Cockcroft JR, Wilkinson IB. Aortic pulse wave velocity improves cardiovascular event prediction: An individual participant meta-analysis of prospective observational data from 17,635 subjects. Journal of the American College of Cardiology. 2014;**63**(7):636-646

[140] Vlachopoulos C, O'Rourke M. Genesis of the normal and abnormal arterial pulse. Current Problems in Cardiology. 2000;**25**(5):303-367

[141] Husmann M, Jacomella V, Thalhammer C, Amann-Vesti BR. Markers of arterial stiffness in peripheral arterial disease. VASA. 2015;**44**:341-348

[142] Stein JH, Korcarz CE, Hurst RT, Lonn E, Kendall CB, Mohler ER, Najjar SS, Rembold CM, Post WS. Use of carotid ultrasound to identify subclinical vascular disease and evaluate cardiovascular disease risk: A consensus statement from the American Society of Echocardiography carotid intima-media thickness task force. Endorsed by the Society for Vascular Medicine. Journal of the American Society of Echocardiography. 2008;**21**(2):93-111

[143] Chambless LE, Heiss G, Folsom AR, Rosamond W, Szklo M, Sharrett AR, Clegg LX. Association of coronary heart disease incidence with carotid arterial wall thickness and major risk factors: The atherosclerosis risk in communities (ARIC) study, 1987-1993. American Journal of Epidemiology. 1997;**146**(6):483-494

[144] O'Leary DH, Polak JF, Kronmal RA, Manolio TA, Burke GL, Wolfson SK Jr. Carotid-artery intima and media thickness as a risk factor for myocardial infarction and stroke in older adults. Cardiovascular health study collaborative research group. The New England Journal of Medicine. 1999;**340**(1):14-22

[145] Finn AV, Kolodgie FD, Virmani R. Correlation between carotid intimal/ medial thickness and atherosclerosis: A point of view from pathology. Arteriosclerosis, Thrombosis, and Vascular Biology. 2010;**30**(2):177-181

[146] Onut R, Balanescu AP, Constantinescu D, Calmac L, Marinescu M, Dorobantu PM. Imaging atherosclerosis by carotid intima-media thickness in vivo: How to, where and in whom? Maedica (Buchar). 2012;**7**(2):153-162

[147] Mudau M, Genis A, Lochner A, Strijdom H. Endothelial dysfunction: The early predictor of atherosclerosis. CVJ Africa. 2012;**23**(4):222-229

[148] Deanfield JE, Halcox JP, Rabelink TJ. Endothelial function and dysfunction: Testing and clinical relevance. Circulation. 2007;**115**:1285-1295